COMPUTED TOMOGRAPHY

Physical Principles, Clinical Applications, and Quality Control

Third Edition

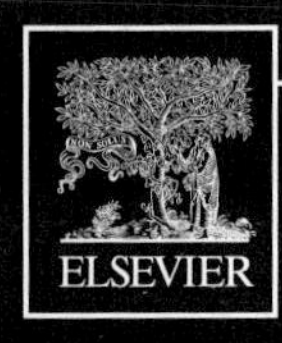

evolve

To access your Instructor Resources, visit:

http://evolve.elsevier.com/Seeram

Evolve Student Learning Resources for ***Seeram: Computed Tomography: Physical Principles, Clinical Applications, and Quality Control,* 3rd Edition,** offer the following features:

- **Practice Test**
  This 165-question practice test gives you the opportunity to reinforce what you have learned in the book, as well as to prepare you for the CT registry exam. The questions are organized by the ARRT CT exam categories, and the test can be sorted by category, enabling you to focus on specific area(s) as needed.
- **Weblinks**
  This exciting resource links you to websites that supplement the content of your book.
- **Image Collection**
  The figures from the book are posted electronically for convenient online access. Images can also be enlarged for enhanced viewing.

Third Edition

COMPUTED TOMOGRAPHY

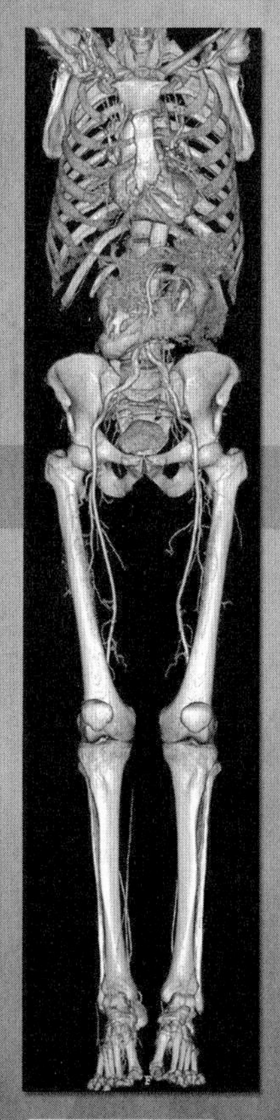

Physical Principles, Clinical Applications, and Quality Control

Euclid Seeram, RT (R), BSc, MSc, FCAMRT
Medical Imaging, Advanced Studies
British Columbia Institute of Technology
Burnaby, British Columbia, Canada

SAUNDERS

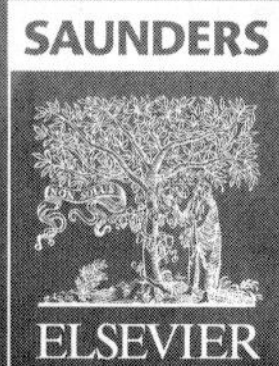

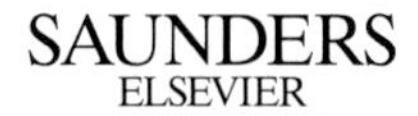

11830 Westline Industrial Drive
St. Louis, Missouri 63146

COMPUTED TOMOGRAPHY: PHYSICAL PRINCIPLES, CLINICAL APPLICATIONS, AND QUALITY CONTROL, THIRD EDITION ISBN: 978-1-4160-2895-6

Library of Congress Cataloging-in-Publication Data

Seeram, Euclid.
Computed tomography : physical principles, clinical applications, and quality control/ Euclid Seeram. – 3rd ed.
p. ; cm.
Includes bibliographical references and index.
ISBN 978-1-4160-2895-6 (pbk. : alk. paper) 1. Tomography. I. Title.
[DNLM: 1. Tomography, X-Ray Computed. WN 206 S453c 2009]
RC78.7.T6S36 2009
616.07′5722–dc22 2008036640

Acquisitions Editor: Jeanne Wilke
Developmental Editor: Luke Held
Publishing Services Manager: Patricia Tannian
Project Manager: Claire Kramer
Designer: Margaret Reid

Printed in United States of America
Last digit is the print number: 9 8 7 6 5 4 3 2 1

This book is dedicated with love and sincere appreciation to my mother, Betty Seeram, a caring, wise, and wonderful woman who graciously guided her six children toward achieving their life's goals, and to the memory of my father, the Rev. Samuel G. Seeram—the memories will last a lifetime, Dad.

Contributors

Frederic H. Fahey, DSc
Associate Professor of Radiology
Harvard Medical School
Director of Nuclear Medicine/PET Physics
Children's Hospital
Boston, Massachusetts

Borys Flak, MD, FRCP(C)
Associate Clinical Professor
Department of Radiology
University of British Columbia
Division Head
Department of Radiology
Vancouver Hospital
Vancouver, British Columbia, Canada

Jiang Hsieh, PhD
Chief Scientist
Applied Science Laboratory
General Electric Healthcare Technologies
Waukesha, Wisconsin

Jocelyne S. Lapointe, MD, FRCP(C)
Associate Professor
Radiology
University of British Columbia
Neuroradiologist
Vancouver General Hospital
Vancouver, British Columbia, Canada

Scott Lipson, MD
Associate Director of Imaging
Radiology
Long Beach Memorial Medical Center
Long Beach, California

Mahadevappa Mahesh, MS, PhD
Assistant Professor of Radiology
The Russell H. Morgan Department of Radiology and Radiological Science
Johns Hopkins University
Johns Hopkins Hospital
Baltimore, Maryland

Son Nguyen, MD
Staff Radiologist
Miller Children's Hospital
Long Beach Memorial Medical Center
Long Beach, California

Matthew R. Palmer, PhD
Instructor
Radiology
Harvard Medical School
Nuclear Medicine Physicist
Beth Israel Deaconess Medical Center
Boston, Massachusetts

Joey S. Battles, MAEd, RT(R)(CT)(QM)(MR)
Director
Medical Imaging
Clarkson College
Omaha, Nebraska

Joseph R. Bittengle, MEd, RT(R)(ARRT)
Division Director
Radiologic Imaging Sciences
University of Arkansas for Medical Sciences
Little Rock, Arkansas

Karen Bonsignore, MA, RT(R)(M)(QM)(MR)(CT)
Associate Professor
New York City College of Technology
Brooklyn, New York

Michael Eugene Dyches AS, AAS, BS, MEd, RT(R)(CT)(ARRT)
Assistant Professor of Medical Imaging Sciences
Computed Tomography Program Director
Greenville Technical College
Greenville, South Carolina

Kerry Greene-Donnelly MBA, RT (R)(M)(CT)(QM)
Instructor
Upstate Medical University
College of Health Professions
Syracuse, New York

Patty K. Hawley, MS, ED
Allied Health Instructor
Ferris State University, Mecosta-Osceola Career Center, and Spectrum Health
Big Rapids, Michigan

Patty Leary, MEd
Allied Health Technology Instructor
Mecosta-Osceola Career Center and Ferris State University
Big Rapids, Michigan

Cynthia L. Liotta, MS, RT(R)(T)
Assistant Professor and Program Director
Radiologic Sciences
Gannon University
Erie, Pennsylvania

Gary D. Morrison, MEd, RT(R)
Associate Professor
Radiologic Sciences
Midwestern State University
Wichita Falls, Texas

Bettye G. Wilson, MAEd, ARRT(R)(CT), RDMS
Associate Professor
University of Alabama
Birmingham, Alabama

Computed tomography (CT) is one of the most important diagnostic tools of the twenty-first century. Although it is not the most recent of devices found in imaging departments, recent technological developments in image acquisition in CT, which have extended the amount of anatomical, pathological, and functional data that is provided, will maintain its position in the forefront of radiological departments.

Such an effective tool requires competent and reflective operators. Initially, it would appear that the usability of radiological equipment becomes easier with subsequent technological generations, but this appearance is substantially undermined by the increased responsibilities generated by the advancement in CT techniques. The plethora of data generated, the expectation of useful image reconstructions by clinical staff, the move to automated segmentation and quantification procedures, the sophisticated quality assurance procedures, and the huge potential for excessive patient exposure require that technological staff be highly efficient and knowledgeable about the opportunities that this device offers.

The name Euclid Seeram has become synonymous with learning and teaching CT and other areas of medical imaging.

This third edition of his very well-known book, *Computed Tomography: Physical Principles, Clinical Applications, and Quality Control*, expands on previous editions. This book still covers the topics of earlier editions and now brings the reader up to date with the latest technologies. It also informs the reader of methods ensuring that these new technologies are implemented for the patient's greatest benefit. The focus of the previous editions had been on educating students; now, this edition will also be of benefit to current radiographers and clinicians so that they can update their CT knowledge.

Mr. Seeram is a distinguished and rigorous academic who has a proven track record in providing understandable and comprehensive radiological materials. A hallmark of his approach is the ability to convey complex topics in an easy-to-read and manageable way, and the current work is no exception. He presents his topics in an organized, progressive, and comprehensive manner so that at the end of each clearly defined chapter, the reader comes away with a solid and supported knowledge of specific topics. Euclid has decades of experience teaching CT and medical imaging and has gained international respect as an educator. Both clinicians and physicists in the field of medical imaging are in agreement as to the high level of influence that Euclid has on medical imaging education, and his contributions to the profession as a whole have been exceptional.

Euclid has the gift of being able to explain difficult concepts in a way that students can grasp. This ability has made the previous editions of this book highly desirable reading for learning CT. These earlier editions can be found on the syllabi of leading educational institutions throughout the world.

We are confident that this book will become essential reading for both undergraduate and graduate curricula and will be available in CT departments globally. We congratulate the author for adding another first-class tome to his already impressive collection. We highly recommend this book to students studying medical imaging; to those in allied fields where CT is becoming more important, such as nuclear medicine and radiation therapy; and to those already in the field who need an update or just want a great reference text.

A great book by a great educator.

Patrick Brennan, PhD
Professor
Head of Diagnostic Imaging/Biomedical Imaging Research
School of Medicine and Medical Science
University College Dublin
Dublin, Ireland

Stewart Carlyle Bushong, ScD, FAAPM, FACR
Professor of Radiologic Science
Baylor College of Medicine
Houston, Texas

Rob Davidson, PhD, MAppSc(MI), BBus, FIR
Associate Professor
Head, Discipline of Medical Radiations
RMIT University
Melbourne, Australia

The motivation for the third edition of *Computed Tomography: Physical Principles, Clinical Applications, and Quality Control* stems from the continued technical evolution of computed tomography (CT) to meet the needs of the clinical environment.

The continued evolution of CT is marked by the refinement of current physical principles, the introduction of new principles, and the development of engineering tools to make scanners consistently perform at a level that meets the needs of various clinical imaging requirements. One such notable technical evolution is the development of multislice CT scanners with more than four slices. Four-slice scanners were a key focus in the second edition. Of course, the third edition adds more scope to the content of the second edition by elaborating on new elements of the evolution of CT and deleting elements that some may now consider obsolete.

NEW TO THIS EDITION

Recent developments range across many aspects of CT, including the following:

- The design and implementation of multislice CT scanners capable of imaging 8, 16, 32, 40, 64, 256, and 320 slices per a 360-degree rotation
- The introduction of scanners especially dedicated to image the heart (cardiac CT) without motion artifacts
- The introduction of new dose reduction technology in an effort to address the concern that the dose in CT is high including one such notable technology, automated tube current modulation

Such new scanners include the dual-source CT (DSCT) scanner introduced by Siemens Medical Solutions and the 320-slice CT scanner developed by Toshiba Medical Systems. The clinical performance of 64- to 320-slice scanners requires several technical considerations such as the improvement of the detector technology from four-slice scanners, the goal of achieving the temporal resolution needed to image the heart without motion artifacts, isotropic data sets, and the development of new cone beam algorithms, as well as continued efforts to improve image quality and optimize the dose to the patient.

The use of CT in other imaging modalities receives increased attention in the third edition, including the following:

- Nuclear medicine (positron emission technology [PET]/CT)
- Radiation treatment planning (CT simulation)
- Flat-detector CT (FD-CT) in interventional radiology, breast imaging, and portable multislice CT scanning

Other recent improvements relate the continued development of image processing and visualization tools to enhance diagnostic interpretation of the increasing data sets that current multislice scanners generate. These include three-dimensional (3D) CT tools and virtual reality imaging tools that facilitate the following:

- Cardiac CT
- CT colonoscopy
- Computed tomography angiography (CTA)

The third edition keeps up with the latest advances in CT imaging with two new chapters on (1) other technical aspects of CT imaging and (2) PET/CT scanners.

In addition, each chapter from the previous edition has been expanded and updated to include state-of-the-art technology and the most current information on physical principles, instrumentation, clinical applications, and quality control. Numerous new images show the achievements of these technological advances. New line drawings provide a better representation of important concepts in the book. Last, but not least, a reasonable effort has been made to keep the cited literature current. These references are important because they serve two purposes:

1. To validate the statements made in the textbook regarding CT principles and applications
2. To guide students to the primary and secondary sources of information that serve as the

fundamental basis for pursuing their own research and presentations

Multislice CT has revolutionized CT scanning and has resulted in a wide range of new clinical applications that are examined in this book. This growth of CT technology and its clinical applications has resulted in a new, expanded edition of *Computed Tomography: Physical Principles, Clinical Applications, and Quality Control* that reflects the current state of CT technology.

Ancillaries

New ancillaries have also been added to this edition (available online on Evolve), including the following:

- A test bank of approximately 600 questions, available in both RTF (rich text format) and ExamView formats
- A practice test to help students reinforce what they have learned and prepare for the CT registry
- An image collection of the figures from the book

PURPOSE

The third edition has grown by including descriptions of new technology and the elaboration of some previous content to accommodate all the recent advances in CT. In this regard, the book remains dedicated to its original manifold purposes:

1. To provide comprehensive coverage of the physical principles of CT and its clinical applications for both adults and children
2. To lay the theoretical foundations necessary for the clinical practice of CT scanning
3. To enhance communication between the CT technologist and other related personnel, such as radiologists, medical physicists, and CT vendors
4. To promote an understanding of two-dimensional (2D) and 3D anatomical images as they relate to CT

CONTENT AND ORGANIZATION

Although much new and updated information is included in the third edition, the content and organization of the book have not been changed significantly. Nevertheless, certain chapters have been deleted, and some content has been reshaped and added to other chapters. For example, Chapters 9, 10, 14, 16, and 18 in the previous edition have been deleted; however, relevant content from all of them has been used and included in other chapters. Chapter 12, "Measuring Patient Dose from Computed Tomography Scanners," from the second edition has been totally reworked using some relevant content for the new dose chapter. The content and organization of the third edition are as follows.

Chapter 1 lays the foundations of CT by reviewing its history, including the introduction of the CT scanner as a diagnostic medical imaging tool. Because the digital computer is central to the CT scanner, Chapter 2 takes a closer look at the concepts of computer technology, including an overview of computer systems and computer applications in radiology, such as the picture archiving and communication system (PACS) and 3D imaging. Chapter 3 examines the topic of image processing and representation and explores the relevancy of CT to the technology of digital image processing.

Chapter 4 begins with a discussion of the limitations of radiography and conventional tomography followed by a more in-depth examination of the physical principles of CT, radiation attenuation, the meaning of CT numbers, and other technological considerations. It concludes with a list of the advantages and limitations of CT.

Chapter 5 addresses the concepts of data acquisition, the first step in image production, and also includes a description of CT detectors. Chapter 6 focuses on what the CT technologist needs to know to understand the process of image reconstruction and introduces the idea of cone-beam reconstruction. Chapter 7 is devoted to basic CT instrumentation and includes a description of the data acquisition; computer; and image display, storage, and communication systems. The discussion of image manipulation and visualization tools continues in Chapter 8, which includes an introduction to multiplanar reconstruction and 3D imaging. Chapter 9 describes the essentials on image quality and includes a discussion of image artifacts in CT. Chapter 10 deals with radiation dose in CT and is a completely rewritten chapter from the corresponding one in the second edition.

Chapters 11 through 15 are devoted to the physical concepts of volume CT scanning. Whereas Chapter 11 details the evolution and fundamentals of single-slice spiral/helical CT (also called *volume CT*), Chapter 12 outlines the major characteristics of multislice spiral/helical CT. This chapter is considered pivotal because most of the recent developments in multislice CT are described here. Chapter 13 continues the discussion by presenting other technical applications of multislice spiral/helical CT and includes a description of FD-CT, CT screening, breast CT imaging, and portable multislice CT scanning. Chapter 14 examines in depth 3D concepts in CT imaging because the advances in spiral/helical CT have resulted in an increased use of 3D display of sectional anatomy. Chapters 15 and 16 address virtual reality imaging and PET/CT, respectively.

The next three chapters include updated and expanded coverage of the clinical applications of CT: Chapter 17, "Computed Tomography of the Head, Cerebral Vessels, Neck, and Spine"; Chapter 18, "Computed Tomography of the Body"; and Chapter 19, "Pediatric Computed Tomography."

The final chapter in the book, Chapter 20, presents updated information on CT quality control.

Three appendixes include a discussion of the use of the terms *spiral* and *helical;* a summary of some of the historical and technical developments in CT; and finally, a detailed description of the physics of cardiac CT imaging.

USE AND SCOPE

This comprehensive book has been written to meet the wide and varied requirements of its users, including students, instructors, and practicing imaging professionals, and it is suitable for many different educational and program needs. *Computed Tomography: Physical Principles, Clinical Applications, and Quality Control* can be used as the primary text for introductory CT courses at the diploma, associate, and baccalaureate degree levels; it serves as a resource for continuing education programs; it functions as a reference for the CT technologist and other imaging personnel; and it provides the necessary overview of the physical and clinical aspects of CT, which is a prerequisite for graduate-level (master's degree) courses in CT.

The content is intended to meet the educational requirements of various radiological technology professional associations, including the American Society of Radiologic Technologists, the American Registry for Radiologic Technologists, the Canadian Association of Medical Radiation Technologists, the College of Radiographers in the United Kingdom, and those in Africa, Asia, Australia, and continental Europe.

CT has become an integral part of the education of radiologic technologists, who play a significant role in the care and management of patients undergoing sophisticated CT imaging procedures. Read on, learn, and enjoy. *Your patients will benefit from your wisdom.*

Euclid Seeram, RT (R), BSc, MSc, FCAMRT
British Columbia, Canada

Acknowledgments

The single most important and satisfying task in writing a book of this nature is to acknowledge the help and encouragement of those individuals who perceive the value of its contribution to the imaging sciences literature. It is indeed a pleasure to express sincere thanks to several individuals whose time and efforts have contributed tremendously to this third edition. First and foremost, I must thank all my contributing authors—three radiologists and four medical physicists—who gave their time and expertise to write selected chapters in this book. They are acknowledged individually elsewhere. In particular, I am indebted to Dr Jiang Hsieh, PhD, Chief Scientist with General Electric Healthcare Technologies, who took the time to answer several of my questions related to cone-beam reconstruction in CT and other related topics.

The content of this book is built around the works and expertise of several noted medical physicists, radiologists, computer scientists, and biomedical engineers who have done the original research. In reality, they are the tacit authors of this book, and I am truly grateful to all of them. In this regard, I owe a good deal of thanks to Dr. Godfrey Hounsfield and Dr. Allan Cormack, both of whom shared the Nobel Prize in medicine and physiology for their work in the invention and development of the CT scanner. I have been in personal communication with Dr. Hounsfield, and he has graciously provided me with details of his biography and his original experiments and signed his Nobel Lecture, which he sent to me. This signature is included in the book as an illustration. I am also grateful to several other physicists from whom I have learned much about CT physics through their writings. These include Professor Willi Kalender, PhD, of the Institute of Medical Physics in Germany; Mahadevappa Mahesh, PhD, Chief Physicist, John Hopkins Hospital in Baltimore; Michael McNitt-Gray, PhD, of the University of California; Cynthia McCollough, PhD, of the Mayo Clinic; Thomas Flohr, PhD, of Siemens Medical Solutions in Germany; and last, but not least, Shinichiro Mori, PhD, National Institutes of Radiologic Sciences, Japan. One more medical physicist to whom I owe thanks is John Aldrich, PhD, Vancouver General Hospital, University of British Columbia, whose seminars on radiation dose in CT and other topics have taught me quite a bit. Thanks, John.

In addition, I must acknowledge the efforts of all the individuals from CT vendors who have assisted me generously with technical details and photographs of their CT scanners for use in the book. In particular, I am grateful to Wes Henschel of Toshiba Medical Systems; Stephanie Row, Jason Plante, and Vickerie Williams of Philips Medical Systems; Kit Czarnecki of General Electric Healthcare; Nina Bastian of Siemens Medical Solutions in Germany; and Mark Morrison of NeuroLogica. Equally important are the individuals who provided me with several CT images for use in the second edition that are still being used in the third edition. Thanks so much for this assistance. These individuals are acknowledged in the respective figure legends.

In this book I have used several illustrations and quotes from original papers published in the professional literature, and I am indeed thankful to all the publishers and the authors who have done the original work and have provided me with permission to reproduce them in this book. I have purposely used several quotes so as not to detract from the authors' original meaning. I believe that these quotes and illustrations have added significantly to the clarity of the explanations. In this regard, I am appreciative of the Radiological Society of North America (RSNA) for use of materials from *Radiographics* and *Radiology*; Springer Science and Business Media, for materials from *European Radiology*; the American Association of Physicists in Medicine (AAPM), for materials from *Medical Physics*; Wiley-Blackwell Publishers Inc., for materials from *Australian Radiology*, ImPACT Scan from the United Kingdom, especially Sue Edyvean; and the American Thoracic Society. There are several radiologists who graciously gave their permission as well, and I would like to list some of their names here: Dr. Dalrymple, Dr. Silva, Dr. Kalra, and Dr. Van der Molen.

Additionally, I must acknowledge the work of the several reviewers of this book (listed separately) who offered constructive comments to help improve the quality of the chapters. Their efforts are very much appreciated.

The people at Elsevier deserve special thanks for their hard work, encouragement, and support of this project. They are Jeanne Wilke, Publisher, Health Professions; Christina Pryor, the original Developmental Editor for this edition who did significant work on the chapters as they were submitted; and Luke Held, current Developmental Editor who has provided the encouragement to keep me on track in meeting deadlines. Both Christina and Luke have offered sound and good advice. I must also thank the individuals in the production department at Elsevier for doing a wonderful job on the manuscript to bring it to its final form. In particular, I am grateful to Claire Kramer and the members of the production team who have worked exceptionally hard during the production of this book, especially in the page-proof stage.

Finally, my family deserves special mention for their love, support, and encouragement while I worked into the evenings on the manuscript. I appreciate the efforts of my lovely wife, Trish, a warm, caring, and overall special person in my life; our son David, a very smart and special young man; and our beautiful daughter-in-law, Priscilla, a remarkable and caring individual. Thanks for everything, especially for thinking that I am the greatest husband and dad. I would also like to acknowledge here the love, support, and encouragement of both my mother, Betty, and my father, Samuel, who passed away 5 years ago (thanks for having me and thanks for the memories, Dad); my father-in-law, Edward Penner; and my mother-in-law, Joan (who earned the title "the most well-read person I know" from me) and who passed away 5 years ago–I love all of you.

Furthermore, there are three additional individuals who deserve special recognition: Patrick Brennan, PhD, from Ireland, Rob Davidson, PhD, from Australia, and Stewart Bushong, ScD, from the United States. They have honored me by writing the foreword. Thanks, Patrick, for inviting me for the position of external examiner for the master's degree program in CT at the University College Dublin, Ireland. Rob was instrumental in getting me to be the keynote speaker at the Australian National Imaging and Therapy Conference in Perth, Australia, in March 2007. Thanks, Rob, for also inviting me to visit Melbourne and to present lectures on CT not only for your students at the Royal Melbourne Institute of Technology University, but also to the hospital imaging technologists. I appreciate your kind hospitality while in Melbourne. To my good friend and colleague Anthony Chan, PEng, CEng., MSc, a Canadian, award-winning biomedical engineer, I am grateful for the stimulating and useful discussions of various CT topics and for inviting me to present CT lectures to your biomedical engineering students.

Last but not least, I must thank the thousands of students who have diligently completed my CT physics course. Thanks for all of the challenging questions. Keep on learning and enjoy the pages that follow.

Euclid Seeram, RT (R), BSc, MSc, FCAMRT
British Columbia, Canada

SPECIAL ACKNOWLEDGMENT

A special thank you goes to Mahadevappa Mahesh, PhD, and Dianna Cody, PhD, whose paper "Physics of Cardiac Imaging with Multiple-Row Detector CT," published in *Radiographics*, has been reproduced in its entirety as an appendix in this book with their kind permission and the permission of the Radiological Society of North America.

COMPUTED TOMOGRAPHY

Physical Principles, Clinical Applications, and Quality Control

Third Edition

Computed Tomography: An Overview

Chapter Outline

Medical imaging has experienced significant changes in both the technologic and clinical arenas. Innovations have become commonplace in the radiology department, and today the introduction of new ideas, methods, and refinements in existing techniques is clearly apparent. The goal of these developments is to optimize the technical parameters of the examination to provide the acceptable image quality needed for diagnostic interpretation and, more importantly, to provide improved patient care services. One such development that is a revolutionary tool of medicine, particularly in medical imaging, is computed tomography (CT). This chapter explores the meaning of CT through a brief description of its fundamental principles and historical perspectives. In addition, it summarizes the growth of CT from its introduction in the 1970s to today's technology.

MEANING

The word *tomography* is not new. It can be traced back to the early 1920s, when a number of investigators were developing methods to image a specific layer or section of the body. At that time, terms such as "body section radiography" and "stratigraphy" (from *stratum*, meaning "layer") were used to describe the technique. In 1935 Grossman refined the technique and labeled it *tomography* (from the Greek *tomos*, meaning "section"). A conventional tomogram is an image of a section of the patient that is oriented parallel to the film.

In 1937, Watson developed another tomographic technique in which the sections were transverse sections (cross-sections); this technique was referred to as *transverse axial tomography*. However, these images lacked enough detail and clarity to be useful in diagnostic radiology, preventing the technique from being fully realized as a clinical tool.

Image Reconstruction from Projections

CT overcomes limitations in detail and clarity by using image reconstruction from projections to produce sharp, clear images of cross-sectional anatomy. Image reconstruction from projections had its theoretic roots in 1917 when the Austrian mathematician Radon proved it possible to reconstruct or build up an image of a two- or three-dimensional object from a large number of its projections from different directions. This procedure has been used in a number of fields, ranging from astronomy to electron microscopy. For example, in astronomy images of the sun have been reconstructed, and in microscopy images of the molecular structure of bacteria can be reconstructed.

Similarly, images of the human body can be reconstructed by using a large number of projections from different locations (Fig. 1-1). In simplified terms, radiation passes through each

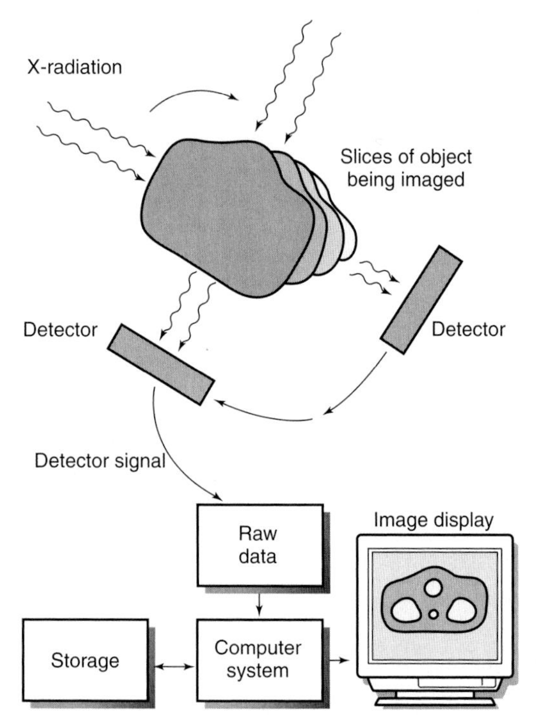

FIGURE 1-1 Image reconstruction from projections. From many different directions, radiation passes through each slice or cross-section of the object being imaged. This radiation is projected onto a detector that sends signals to a computer for processing into an image that reveals the internal structure of the object.

cross-section in a specific way and is projected onto a detector that sends signals to a computer for processing. The computer produces clear, sharp images of the internal structure of the object.

A more complete definition of this technique has been given by Herman (1980), who stated "Image reconstruction from projections is the process of producing an image of a two-dimensional distribution (usually some physical property) from estimates of its line integrals along a finite number of lines of known locations." The CT scanner uses this process to produce a variety of images ranging from cross-sectional two-dimensional images and three-dimensional (3D) images to virtual reality images of the anatomy or organ system under study.

Image reconstruction from projections finally found practical application in medicine in the 1960s through the work of investigators such as Oldendorf, Kuhl, and Edwards, who studied problems in nuclear medicine. In 1963, Cormack also applied reconstruction techniques to nuclear medicine. In 1967, Hounsfield finally applied reconstruction techniques to produce the world's first clinically useful CT scanner for imaging the brain (Fig. 1-2).

These studies resulted in two types of CT systems: emission CT, in which the radiation source is inside the patient (e.g., nuclear medicine), and transmission CT, in which the radiation source is outside the patient (e.g., x-ray imaging). Both involve image reconstruction. Image reconstruction has also been used in diagnostic medical sonography and magnetic resonance imaging (MRI). This book discusses only the fundamental principles and technology of x-ray transmission CT.

Evolution of Terms

Hounsfield's work produced a technique that revolutionized medicine and diagnostic radiology. He called the technique *computerized transverse axial scanning* (tomography) in his description of the system, which was first published in the *British Journal of Radiology* in 1973. Since then a number

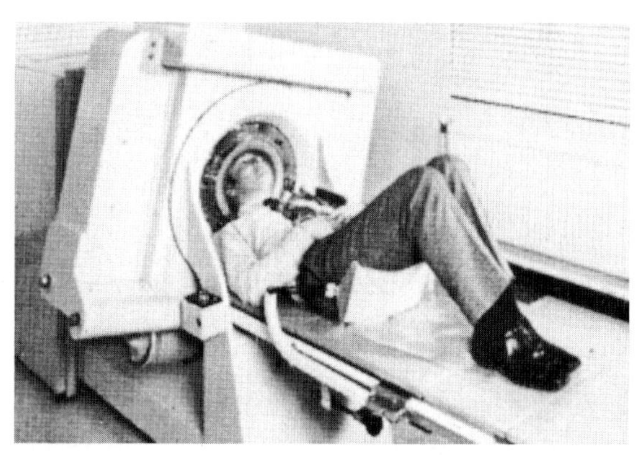

FIGURE 1-2 First-generation model of a CT head scanner. (Courtesy Thorn EMI, London, United Kingdom.)

of other terms have appeared in the literature. Terms such as "computerized transverse axial tomography," "computer-assisted tomography or computerized axial tomography," "computerized transaxial transmission reconstructive tomography," "computerized tomography," and "reconstructive tomography" were not uncommon. The term *computed tomography* was established by the Radiological Society of North America in its major journal *Radiology*. In addition, the *American Journal of Roentgenology* accepted this term, which has now gained widespread acceptance within the radiologic community. Throughout the remainder of this book the term *computed tomography* and its acronym, CT, are used.

PROCESS

The formation of CT images by a CT scanner involves three steps: data acquisition; image reconstruction; and image display, manipulation, storage, recording, and communication (Fig. 1-3).

Data Acquisition

The term *data acquisition* refers to the collection of x-ray transmission measurements from the patient. Once x-rays have passed through the

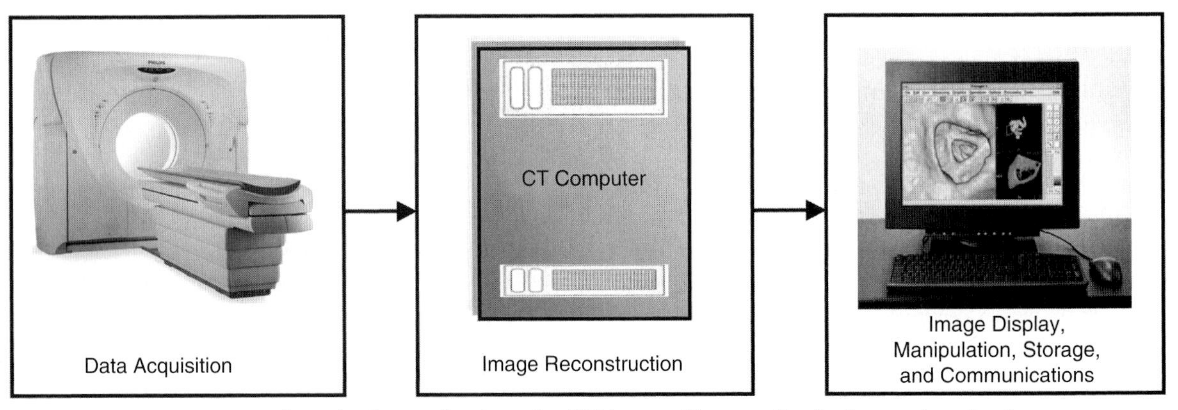

FIGURE 1-3 Steps in the production of a CT image. (See text for further explanation.)

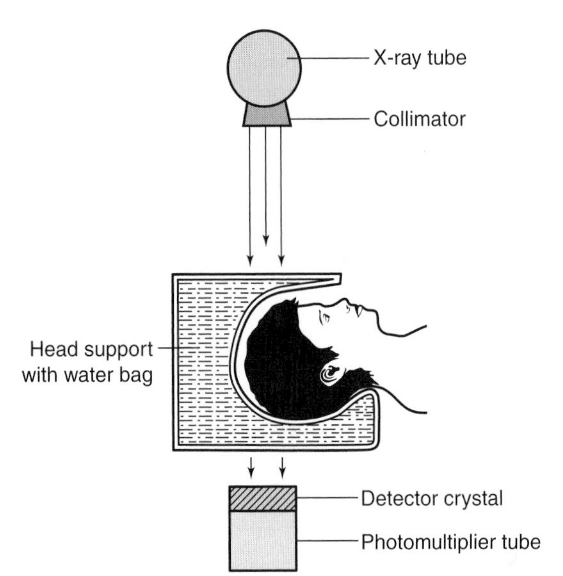

FIGURE 1-4 Data collection scheme in the first CT brain scanner.

patient, they fall onto special electronic detectors that measure the transmission values, or attenuation values. Enough transmission measurements or data must be recorded to meet the requirements of the reconstruction process. The first brain CT scanner used a data acquisition scheme where the x-ray tube and detectors moved in a straight line, or translated, across the patient's head, collecting a number of transmission measurements as they moved from left to right (Fig. 1-4). Then the x-ray tube and detector rotated 1 degree and started again to move across the patient's head, this time from right to left. This process of translate-rotate-stop-rotate, referred to as *scanning*, is repeated over 180 degrees.

The fundamental problem with this method of data collection was the length of time required to obtain enough data for image reconstruction. Later, more efficient schemes for scanning the patient were introduced (see Chapter 5). These schemes involve rotating the x-ray tube and detectors continuously as the patient moves through the scanner simultaneously. This process results in scanning a volume of tissue rather than a single slice of tissue characteristic of the early CT scanners. Acquiring a volume of tissue during the scanning is now referred to as *volume scanning*. The continuous rotation of the x-ray tube and detectors and the simultaneous movement of the patient result in a *spiral/helical* path traced by the x-ray beam. The goal of volume scanning is not only to improve the volume coverage speed but to provide new tools for clinical applications.

Data acquisition also involves the conversion of the electrical signals obtained from the electronic detectors to digital data that the computer can use to process the image.

Image Reconstruction

After enough transmission measurements have been collected by the detectors, they are sent to the computer for processing. The computer uses special mathematical techniques to reconstruct the CT image in a finite number of steps called *image reconstruction algorithms* (see Chapter 6). For example, the image reconstruction algorithm used by Hounsfield to develop the first CT scanner was called the *algebraic reconstruction technique*.

Today, a new set of image reconstruction algorithms have been developed for spiral/helical volume CT scanners. These include fan-beam filtered back projection algorithms, interpolation algorithms, and more recently, *cone-beam image reconstruction algorithms*.

A computer is central to the CT process. In general, this involves a minicomputer and associated microprocessors for performing a number of specific functions. In some CT scanners, array processors perform high-speed calculations, and specific microprocessors carry out image processing operations. Therefore, in this regard, computers are described briefly in Chapter 2.

Image Display, Manipulation, Storage, Recording, and Communications

After the computer has performed the image reconstruction process, the reconstructed image can be displayed and recorded for subsequent viewing and stored for later reanalysis. The image is usually displayed on a cathode ray tube, although other display technologies are now available; for example, touch screen technology is used for scan setup and control in some scanners. However, the cathode ray tube remains the best device for the display of gray-scale imagery, although LCDs are now being used. Display monitors are mounted onto control consoles that allow the technologist (operator's console) and radiologist (physician's console) to manipulate, store, and record images.

Image manipulation or digital image processing (see Chapter 3), as it is often referred to by some authors, has become popular in CT, and many computer software packages are now available. Images can be modified through image manipulation to make them more useful to the observer. For example, transverse axial images can be reformatted into coronal, sagittal, and paraxial sections. In addition, images can also be subjected to other image processing operations such as image smoothing, edge enhancement, gray-scale manipulation, and 3D processing.

Images can be recorded and subsequently stored in some form of archive. Images are usually recorded on x-ray film because of its wider gray scale compared with that of instant film. Such recording is accomplished by multiformat video cameras, although laser cameras have been developed and are now common in radiology departments. It is important to note, however, that film-based recording, as is described briefly below, has become obsolete.

CT images can be stored on magnetic tapes and magnetic disks. More recently, optical storage technology has added a new dimension to the storage of information from CT scanners. In optical storage the stored data are read by optical means such as a laser beam. In this case, storage is referred to as *laser storage*. Optical storage media include at least three formats: disk, tape, and card (see Chapter 7).

In CT, *communications* refers to the electronic transmission of text data and images from the CT scanner to other devices such as laser printers; diagnostic workstations; display monitors in the radiology department, intensive care unit, and operating and trauma rooms in the hospital; and computers outside the hospital. Electronic communications in CT require a standard protocol that facilitates connectivity (networking) among multimodalities (CT, magnetic resource imaging, digital radiography, and fluoroscopy) and multivendor equipment. The standard used for this purpose is the Digital Imaging and Communication in Medicine (DICOM) standard established by the

American College of Radiology (ACR) and the National Electrical Manufacturers Association. CT departments now operate in a Picture Archiving and Communications Systems (PACS) environment that allows the flow of CT data and images among devices and people not only in the radiology department but throughout the hospital as well. Additionally, the PACS is connected to a Radiology Information System, which in turn is connected to the Hospital Information System. (Networking and PACS are described in Chapter 2.)

HOW CT SCANNERS WORK

To enhance understanding of the early experiments and current technology, the technologist must be familiar with the way a CT scanner works (Fig. 1-5). The technologist first turns on the scanner's power and performs a quick test to ensure that the scanner is in good working order. The patient is in place in the scanner opening, with appropriate positioning for the particular examination. The technologist sets up the technical factors at the control console. Scanning can now begin.

When x rays pass through the patient, they are attenuated and subsequently measured by the detectors. The x-ray tube and detectors are inside the gantry of the scanner and rotate around the patient during scanning. The detectors convert the x-ray photons (attenuation data) into electrical signals, or analog signals, which in turn must be converted into digital (numerical) data for input into the computer. The computer then performs the image reconstruction process. The reconstructed image is in numerical form and must be converted into electrical signals for the technologist to view on a television monitor. The images and related data are then sent to the PACS, where a radiologist will be able to retrieve and

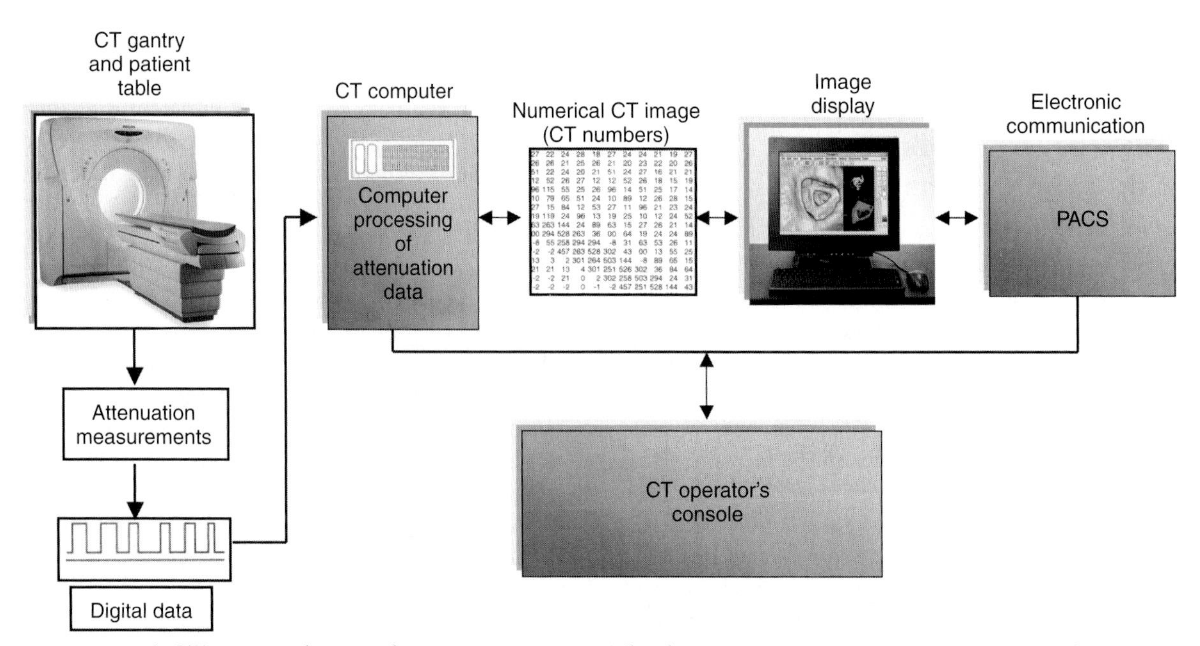

FIGURE 1-5 A CT scanner showing the main components. The data communications component is not shown.

interpret them. Finally, the image can be stored on magnetic tapes or optical disks.

HISTORICAL PERSPECTIVES

Early Experiments

The invention of the CT scanner has revolutionized the practice of radiology. CT is so remarkable that in many cases it generates a dramatic increase in diagnostic information compared with that obtained by conventional x-ray techniques. This extraordinary invention was made possible through the work of several individuals, most notably Godfrey Newbold Hounsfield and Allan MacLeod Cormack (Beckmann, 2006).

Godfrey Newbold Hounsfield

Godfrey Newbold Hounsfield (Fig. 1-6) was born in 1919 in Nottinghamshire, England. He studied electronics and electrical and mechanical engineering. In 1951, Hounsfield joined the staff at EMI Limited (Electric and Musical Industries [manufacturer of records and electronics, and recorded the Beatles under the EMI Label], now Thorn EMI) in Middlesex, where he began work on radar systems and later on computer technology. His research on computers led to the development of the EMIDEC 1100, the first solid-state business computer in Great Britain.

In 1967, Hounsfield was investigating pattern recognition and reconstruction techniques by using the computer. (In image processing, pattern recognition involves techniques for the observer to identify, describe, and classify various features represented in an image or a signal.) From this work, he deduced that, if an x-ray beam were passed through an object from all directions and measurements were made of all the x-ray transmission, information about the internal structures of that body could be obtained. This information would be presented to the radiologist in the form of pictures that would show 3D representations.

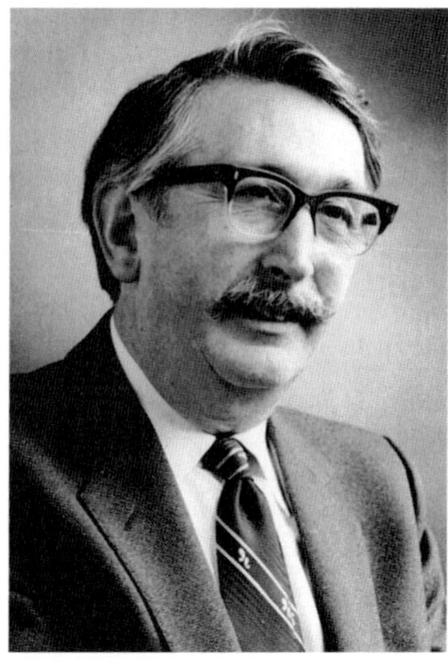

FIGURE 1-6 The inventor of clinical computed tomography, Dr. Godfrey Hounsfield. (Courtesy Thorn EMI, London, United Kingdom)

With encouragement from the British Department of Health and Social Security, an experimental apparatus was constructed to investigate the clinical feasibility of the technique (Fig. 1-7). The radiation used was from an americium gamma

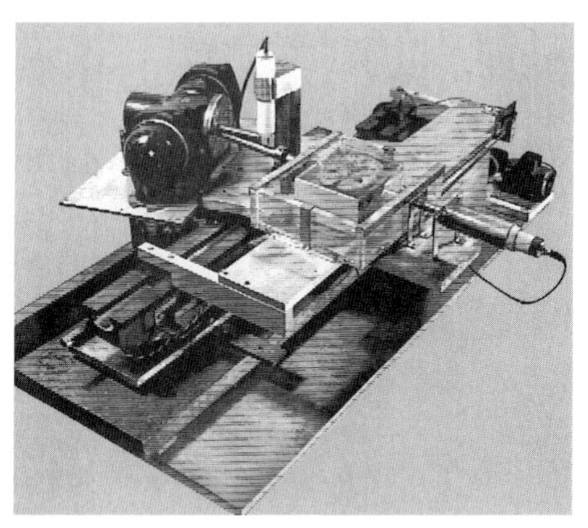

FIGURE 1-7 The original lathe bed scanner used in early CT experiments by Hounsfield. (Courtesy Thorn EMI, London, United Kingdom.)

source coupled with a crystal detector. Because of the low radiation output, the apparatus took about 9 days to scan the object. The computer needed 2.5 hours to process the 28,000 measurements collected by the detector. Because this procedure was too long, various modifications were made and the gamma radiation source was replaced by a powerful x-ray tube. The results of these experiments were more accurate, but it took 1 day to produce a picture (Hounsfield, 1980).

To evaluate the usefulness of this machine, Dr. James Ambrose, a consultant radiologist at Atkinson-Morley's Hospital, joined the study. Together, Hounsfield and Ambrose obtained readings from a specimen of human brain. The findings were encouraging in that tumor tissue was clearly differentiated from gray and white matter and controlled experiments with fresh brains from bullocks showed details such as the ventricles and pineal gland. Experiments were also done with kidney sections from pigs.

In 1971 the first clinical prototype CT brain scanner (EMI Mark 1) was installed at Atkinson-Morley's Hospital and clinical studies were conducted under the direction of Dr. Ambrose. The processing time for the picture was reduced to about 20 minutes. Later, with the introduction of minicomputers, the processing time was reduced further to 4.5 minutes.

In 1972 the first patient was scanned by this machine. This patient was a woman with a suspected brain lesion, and the picture showed clearly in detail a dark circular cyst in the brain. From this moment on, and as more patients were scanned, the machine's ability to distinguish the difference between normal and diseased tissue was evident (Hounsfield, 1980).

Dr. Hounsfield's research resulted in the development of a clinically useful CT scanner for imaging the brain. For this work, Hounsfield received the McRobert Award (akin to a Nobel Prize in engineering) in 1972. During the same year, he became a Fellow of the Royal Society and subsequently was awarded the Lasker Prize in the United States and, in 1977, Dr. Hounsfield was appointed Commander of the British Empire (CBE). In 1979, Hounsfield shared the Nobel Prize in medicine and physiology with Allan MacLeod Cormack, a physics professor at Tufts University in Medford, Massachusetts, for their contributions to the development of CT. Figure 1-8 shows a note sent to the author from Dr. Hounsfield in response to several questions. After receiving this prestigious prize, he was knighted by her majesty Queen Elizabeth and became an Honorary Fellow of the Royal Academy of Engineering. Dr. Hounsfield died on August 12, 2004, at the age of 84 years (Isherwood, 2004).

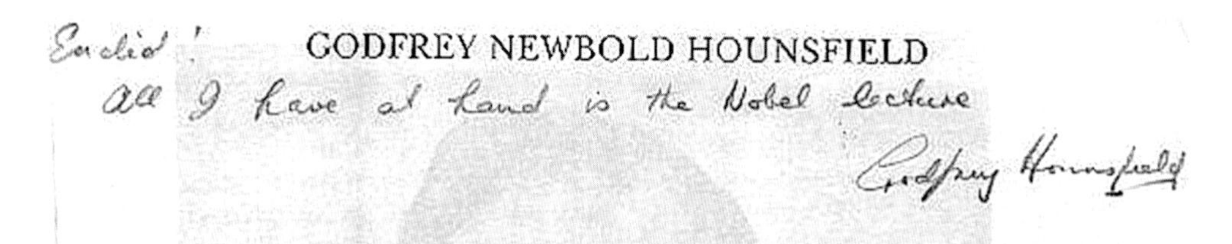

Euclid!

GODFREY NEWBOLD HOUNSFIELD

All I have at hand is the Nobel lecture

Godfrey Hounsfield

I was born and brought up near a village in Nottinghamshire and in my childhood enjoyed the freedom of the rather isolated country life. After the first world war, my father had bought a small farm, which became a marvellous playground for his five children. My two brothers and two sisters were all older than I and, as they naturally pursued their own more adult interests, this gave me the advantage of not being expected to join in, so I could go off and follow my own inclinations.

FIGURE 1-8 A personal note from Dr. Godfrey Hounsfield to the author, Euclid Seeram.

By developing the first practical CT scanner, Dr. Hounsfield opened up a new domain for technologists, radiologists, medical physicists, engineers, and other related scientists.

Allan MacLeod Cormack

Allan MacLeod Cormack (Fig. 1-9) was born in Johannesburg, South Africa, in 1924. He attended the University of Cape Town where he obtained a Bachelor of Science in Physics in 1944 and earned a Master of Science in Crystallography in 1945. He subsequently studied nuclear physics at Cambridge University before returning to the University of Cape Town as a physics lecturer. He later moved to the United States and was on sabbatical at Harvard University before joining the physics department at Tufts University in 1958.

Professor Cormack developed solutions to the mathematical problems in CT. Later, in 1963 and 1964, he published two papers in the *Journal of Applied Physics* on the subject, but they received little interest in the scientific community at that time. It was not until Hounsfield began work on the development of the first practical CT scanner that Dr. Cormack's work was viewed as the solution to the mathematical problem in CT (Cormack, 1980). Cormack died at age 74 years, in Massachusetts on May 7, 1998. Additionally, back in South Africa, Dr. Cormack was granted the Order of Mapungubwe, South Africa's highest honor, in December 2002, for his contribution to the invention of the CT scanner.

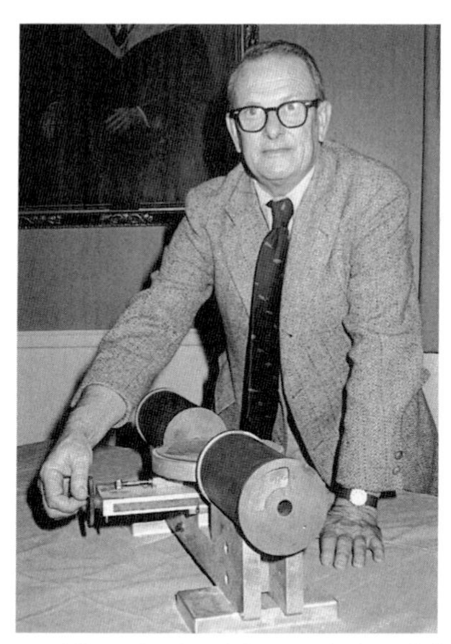

FIGURE 1-9 Allan MacLeod Cormack shared the Nobel Prize with Godfrey Hounsfield for his mathematical contributions to the problem in CT. (Courtesy Tufts University, Medford, Mass.)

Growth

First 10 Years

Between 1973 and 1983 the number of CT units installed worldwide increased dramatically. Perhaps the first significant technical development came in 1974 when Dr. Robert Ledley (Fig. 1-10), a professor of radiology, physiology, and biophysics at Georgetown University, developed the first whole-body CT scanner. (Hounsfield's EMI scanner scanned only the head.)

Dr. Ledley graduated with a doctorate in dental surgery from New York University in 1948, and in 1949 he earned a master's degree in theoretical physics from Columbia University. He holds

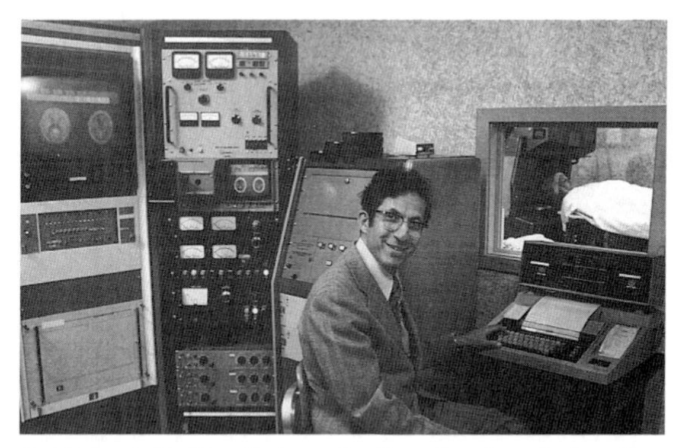

FIGURE 1-10 Dr. Robert Ledley developed the first whole-body CT scanner, the automatic computed transverse axial CT scanner. (Courtesy Robert Ledley, Washington, D.C.)

more than 60 patents on medical instrumentation and has written several books on the use of computers in biology and medicine.* In 1990 he was inducted into the National Inventors' Hall of Fame for the invention of the automatic computed transverse axial CT scanner. In 1997, Dr. Ledley won the National Medal of Technology, an honor awarded by the President of the United States for outstanding contributions to science and technology (Ledley, 1999). Currently, he is the president of the National Biomedical Research Foundation at Georgetown University Medical Center.

*One notable text by Dr. Ledley (coauthored by Dr. H. K. Huang) is *Cross-Sectional Anatomy: An Atlas for Computerized Tomography*, which provides radiologists and technologists with a tool to visualize sectional images. For detailed coverage of the pioneers of CT, the reader should refer to *Naked to the Bone* by Kelves (1999).

These pioneering works were followed by the introduction of three *generations* (a term used to refer to the method of scanning) of CT scanners. In 1974 a fourth-generation CT system was developed (Fig. 1-11).

A computer capable of performing multiple functions is central to the CT system. The CT computer has undergone several changes over time (see Chapter 7).

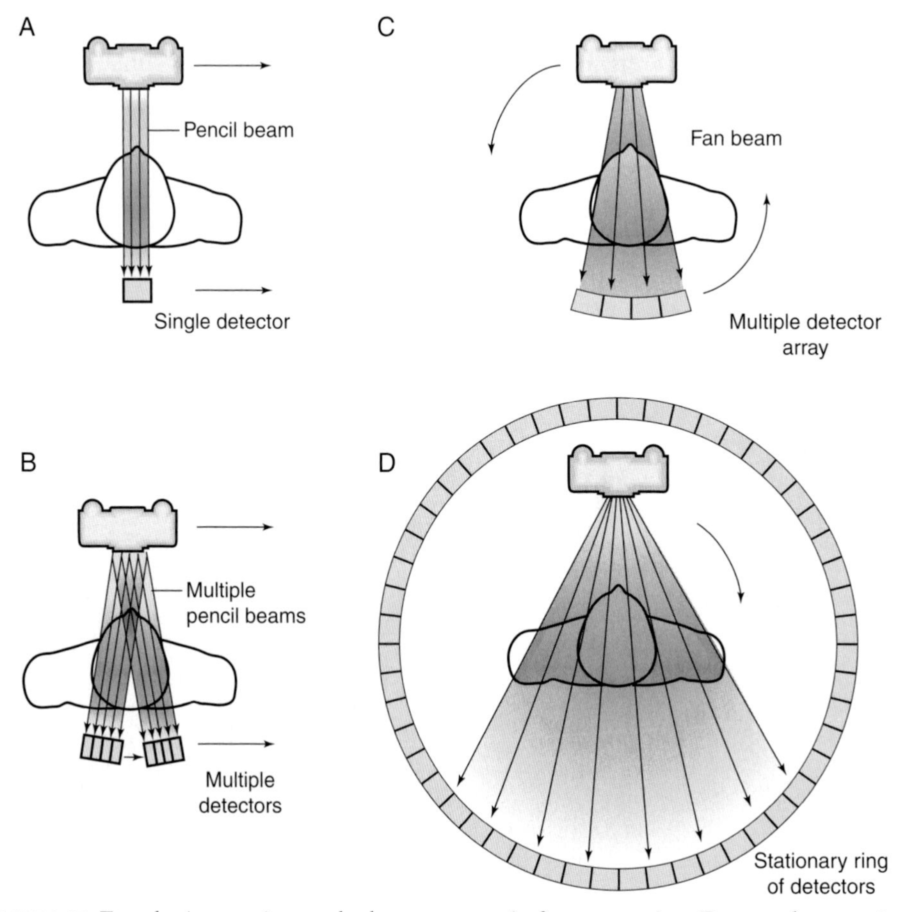

FIGURE 1-11 Four basic scanning methods or systems: **A,** first generation; **B,** second generation; **C,** third generation; **D,** fourth generation.

Image quality is another significant development as a result of technologic changes. Although earlier images appeared "blocky," images acquired later were remarkably improved (Fig. 1-12). Improvements in image quality included improved spatial resolution, decreased scan time, increased density resolution, and changes to the x-ray tube to facilitate the increased loadability required of whole-body scanners. For example, the matrix size in 1972 was 80 × 80; in 1993, it was 1024 × 1024. In addition, the spatial resolution and scan time in 1972 were reported to be three line pairs per centimeter (lp/cm) and 5 minutes, respectively, compared with 15 lp/cm and 1 second, respectively, in 1993 (Kalender, 1993). Increased loadability resulted in scanners capable of dynamic CT examinations that took a series of scans in rapid succession. Later-model CT scanners could operate in several modes such as the prescan localization mode, which produced a survey scan of the region of interest. Rapid reformatting of the axial scans into coronal, sagittal, and oblique sections also became possible.

High-Speed CT Scanners

In 1975 the dynamic spatial reconstructor (DSR) was installed in the biodynamics unit at the Mayo Clinic. The goal of the DSR was to carry out dynamic volume scanning to accommodate imaging of the dynamics of organ systems and the functional aspects of the cardiovascular and pulmonary systems with high temporal resolution as well as imaging anatomic details (Ritman et al, 1991; Robb and Morin, 1991). Research on this unit has since been discontinued.

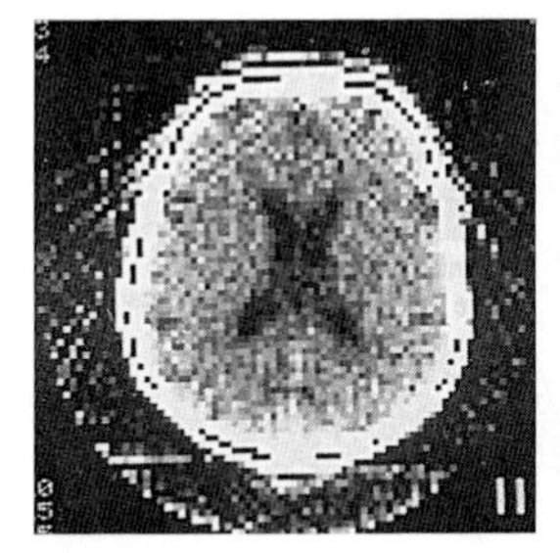
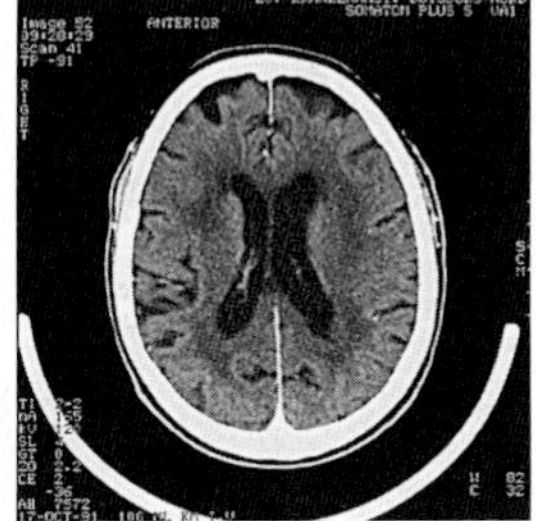

FIGURE 1-12 The appearance of early CT images *(left)* compared with those produced by a more recent CT scanner *(right)*. The difference in image quality is apparent. (From Schwierz G, Kirchgeorg M: The continuous evolution of medical x-ray imaging, I: the technically driven stage of development, *Electromedica* 63:2-7, 1995.)

In the mid 1980s, another high-speed CT scanner was introduced that used electron beam technology, a result of work by Dr. Douglas Boyd and colleagues during the late 1970s at the University of California at San Francisco. The scanner was invented to image the cardiovascular system without artifacts caused by motion. At that time the scanner was called the *cardiovascular CT scanner*. Later, this scanner was acquired and marketed by Siemens Medical Systems under the name *Evolution* and was subsequently referred to as the *electron beam CT (EBCT) scanner*. The most conspicuous difference between the EBCT scanner and conventional CT is the absence of moving parts. At that time, the EBCT scanner was capable of acquiring multislice images in as little as 50 and 100 milliseconds.

The U.S. Food and Drug Administration (FDA) cleared the EBCT scanner in 1983. As of 2007, the EBCT scanner is marketed by General Electric (GE) Healthcare under the name *e-Speed* and it now features proprietary technologies that play a significant role in imaging the heart. In October 2002, the e-Speed CT scanner received FDA clearance and it is now capable of 33-ms, 50-ms, and 100-ms True Temporal Resolution to produce images at up to 30 frames per second (GE Healthcare, 2007).

Because nearly 20 manufacturers made CT scanners between 1973 and 1983, a number of developments unique to particular manufacturers were also introduced (see Appendix B). The evolution of CT continued after 1983, with nearly 10 manufacturers competing for the CT market. (Box 1-1 highlights the developments from a major manufacturer actively involved in the research and development of the CT scanner).

BOX 1-1 *Milestones in Computed Tomography Development From Philips Medical Systems*

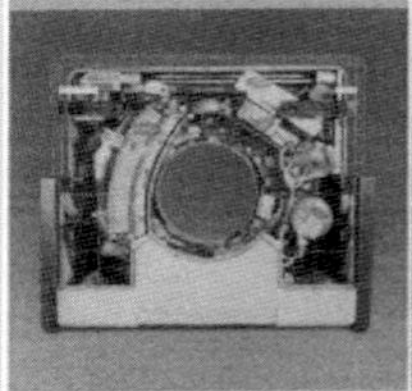

1988
R&D began on CT Twin™ multislice CT

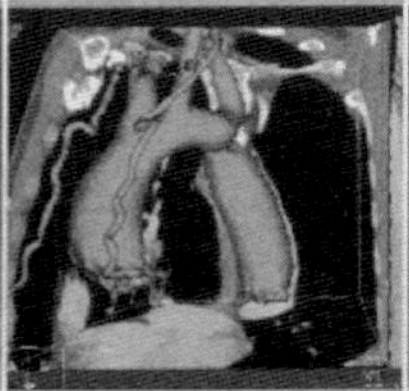

1991
Beta testing began for CT Twin

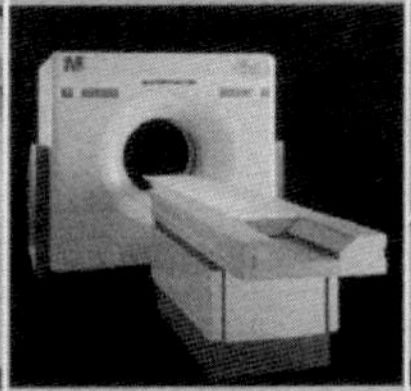

1992
CT Twin introduced to market and first units delivered

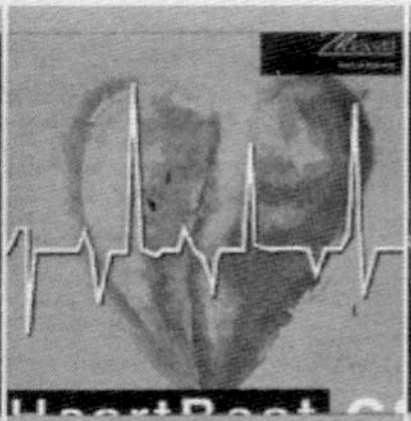

1993
HeartBeat-CS™ clinical trails started

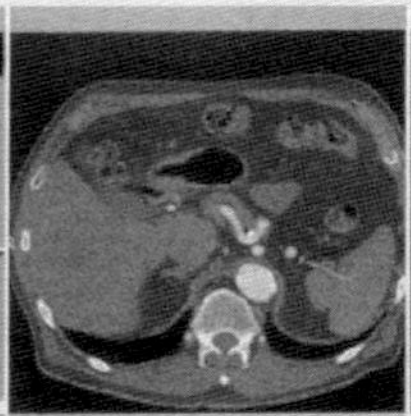

1994
Evolving Imaging™ real-time multislice introduced

1994
200th CT Twin multislice unit installed

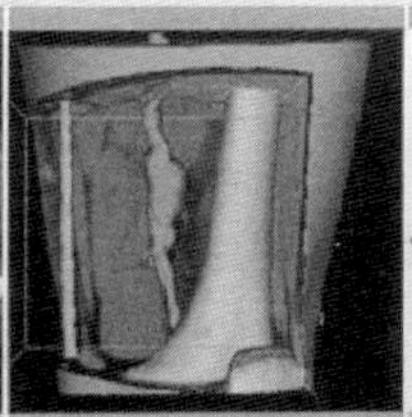

1995
First multislice clinical papers published using CT Twin

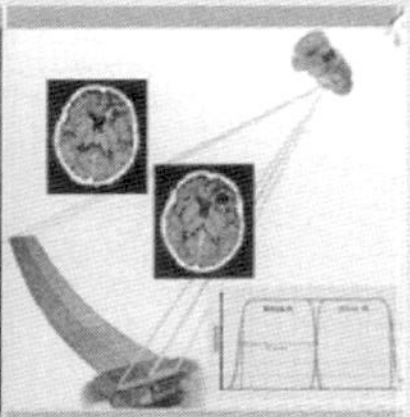

1998
Multislice Mx8000 introduced

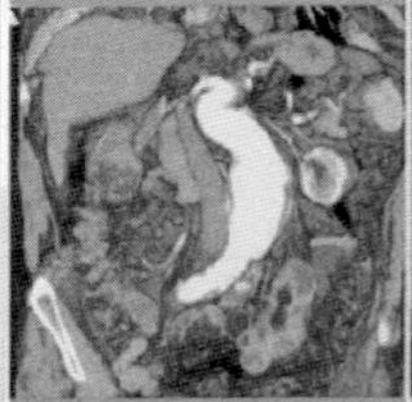

1999
Over 15.000.000 multislice exams completed using Philips multislice CT

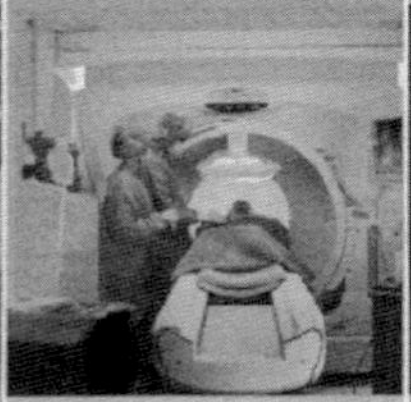

1999
LifeFlight™ trauma triage system

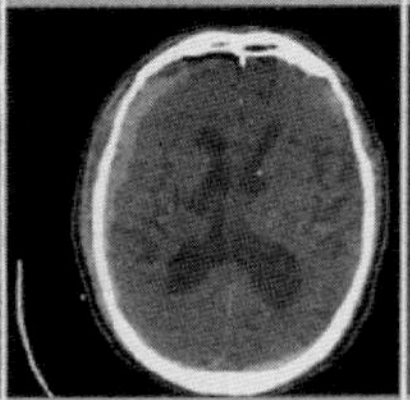

2000
Version 2.0 released with UltraImage™, perfusion, gated cardiac and other capabilities

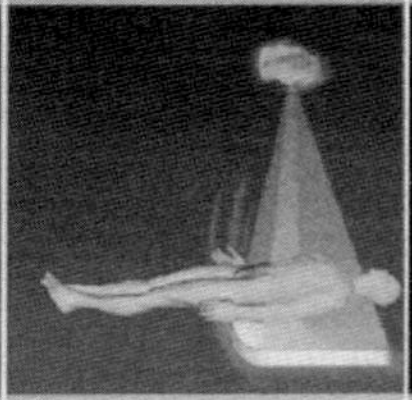

2000
Infinite Detector Technology introduced

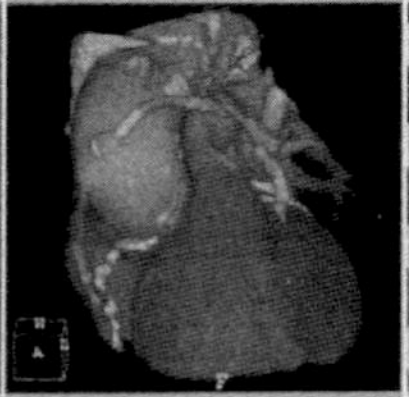

2000
Patented Heartbeat-RT cardiac gating algorithm

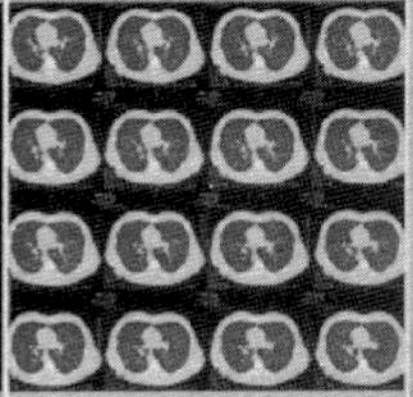

2001
World's first 16-slice CT images with IDT

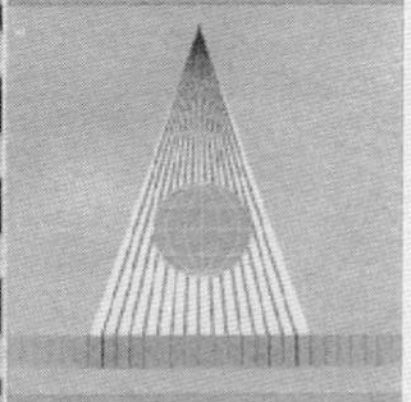

2001
Multi-patented 3-D Cone Beam Reconstruction Algorithm (COBRA)

Courtesy Philips Medical Systems.

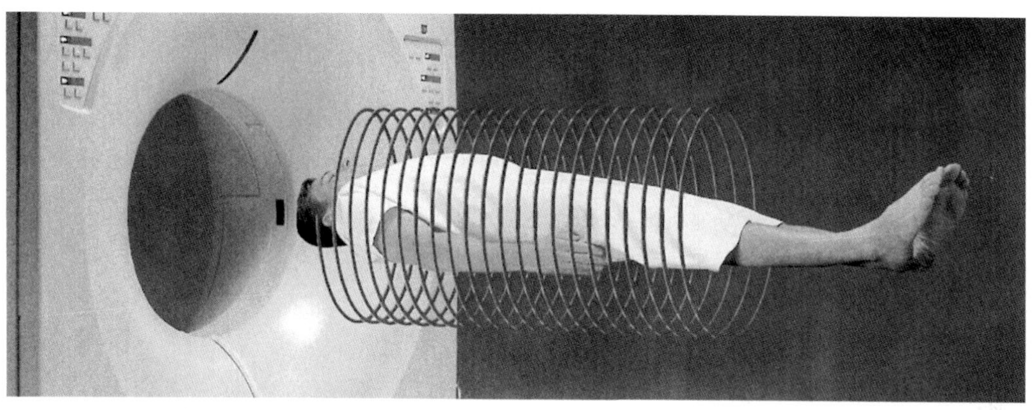

FIGURE 1-13 With volume CT scanners, the x-ray tube and detectors rotate continuously as the patient moves continuously through the gantry. As a result, the x-ray beam traces a path (beam geometry) around the patient. This method of scanning the patient is referred to as *helical* or *spiral CT*. (Courtesy Toshiba America Medical Systems, Tustin, Calif.)

Spiral/Helical CT Scanners: Volume Scanning

In conventional CT the patient is scanned one slice at a time. The x-ray tube and detectors rotate for 360 degrees or less to scan one slice while the table and patient remain stationary. This slice-by-slice scanning is time consuming, and therefore efforts were made to increase the scanning of larger volumes in less time. This notion led to the development of a technique in which a volume of tissue is scanned by moving the patient continuously through the gantry of the scanner while the x-ray tube and detectors rotate continuously for several rotations. As a result, the x-ray beam traces a path around the patient (Fig. 1-13). Although some manufacturers call this beam geometry *spiral CT* (the beam tracing a spiral path around the patient), others refer to it as *helical CT* (the beam tracing a helical path around the patient). This book uses both terms synonymously.

The idea of this approach to scanning can be traced to three sources (Kalender, 1995). In 1989, the first report of a practical spiral CT scanner was presented at the Radiological Society of North America (RSNA) meeting in Chicago by Dr. Willi Kalender (Fig. 1-14). Dr. Kalender has made significant contributions to the technical development and practical implementation of this approach to CT scanning. His main research interests are in the areas of diagnostic imaging, particularly the development and introduction of volumetric spiral CT.

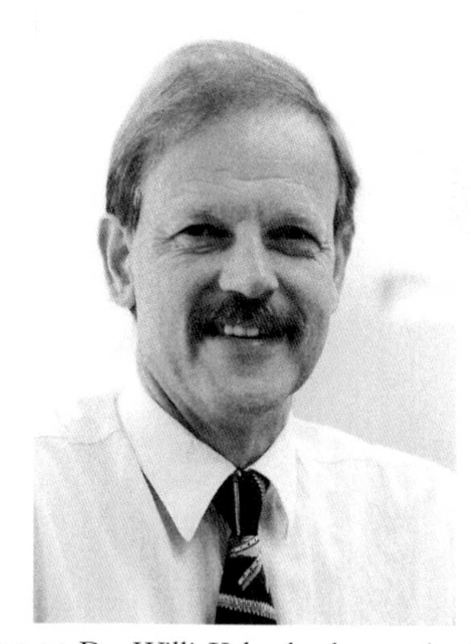

FIGURE 1-14 Dr. Willi Kalender has made significant contributions to the introduction and development of volume spiral CT scanning. (Courtesy Willi Kalender, Nürnberg, Germany.)

Dr. Kalender was born in 1949 and studied medical physics in Germany. Subsequently, he continued his studies at the University of Wisconsin in the United States. He later worked with Siemens Medical Solutions in the area of CT, and in 1995 he became professor and chairman of the Institute of Medical Physics, which is associated with the University of Erlanger, Nürnberg, Germany.

The spiral/helical CT scanners developed after 1989 were referred to as *single-slice spiral/helical* or *volume CT scanners*. In 1992 a dual-slice spiral/helical CT scanner (volume CT scanner) was introduced to scan two slices per 360-degree rotation, thus increasing the volume coverage speed compared with single-slice volume CT scanners.

In 1998 a new generation of CT scanners was introduced at the RSNA meeting in Chicago. These scanners are called *multislice CT (MSCT) scanners* because they are based on the use of multidetector technology to scan four or more slices per revolution of the x-ray tube and detectors, thus increasing the volume coverage speed of single-slice and dual-slice volume CT scanners. The number of slices per revolution has been increasing at a steady pace, as outlined in Figure 1-15. In 2004, a 256-slice prototype CT scanner was undergoing

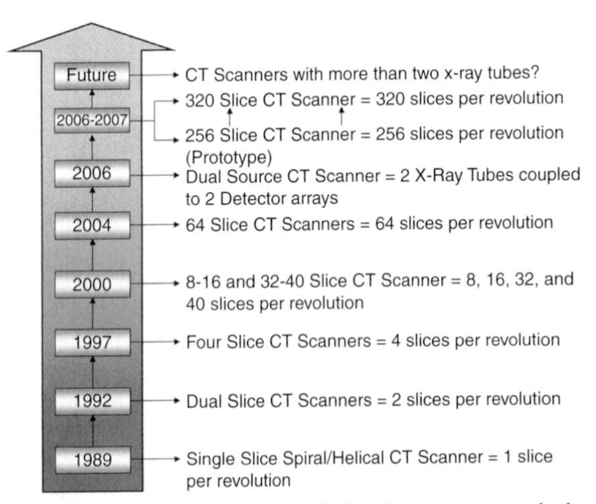

FIGURE 1-15 The evolution of MSCT scanners, including the DSCT scanner.

clinical tests and more recently, a comparison of the doses from the 256-slice CT scanner and a 16-slice CT scanner has been reported (Mori et al, 2006). The front view of the 256-slice CT scanner is shown in Figure 1-16, (*A*, the wide area 2D detector is shown in Figure 1-16, *B*.)

In addition to the improvements in the performance characteristics such as, for example, minimum scan time, data per 360° scan, image matrix, slice thickness, spatial and contrast resolution, from 1972 to 2004, MSCT scanners are now based on new technologies. These include new x-ray tube and detector technologies to accommodate high-speed imaging, large-bore gantry apertures to facilitate ease of patient positioning and patient access, improved z-axis resolution, radiation dose optimization with dose modulation techniques, integrated software featuring multiple software platforms, and intuitive interfacing and software for not only data management such as workflow optimization but also for image processing. Two notable new concepts for MSCT, particularly for scanners that have 16 or greater detector rows, are the reconstruction algorithm and the definition of an important parameter called the pitch. These scanners now use cone beam image reconstruction algorithms to address the cone beam geometry as the detector width increases to accommodate 16 to 64 detector rows. The pitch for volume scanners has now been defined by the International Electrotechnical Commission (IEC), after much debate in the literature as to what the exact definition should be. The IEC states that the pitch for MSCT scanners is the ratio of the table feed per revolution of the x-ray tube to the total width of the collimated beam. Pitch is described in a subsequent chapter.

One of the central goals in the development of the CT scanner is to achieve *isotropic resolution*, that is the voxel is a perfect cube (equal length, width, and height) as opposed to *nonisotropic resolution*, where the voxel is not a perfect cube, as is clearly illustrated in Figure 1-17. The impact of isotropic resolution on CT images is improved image quality in all three dimensions; hence, 3D images are sharp in appearance and do not exhibit

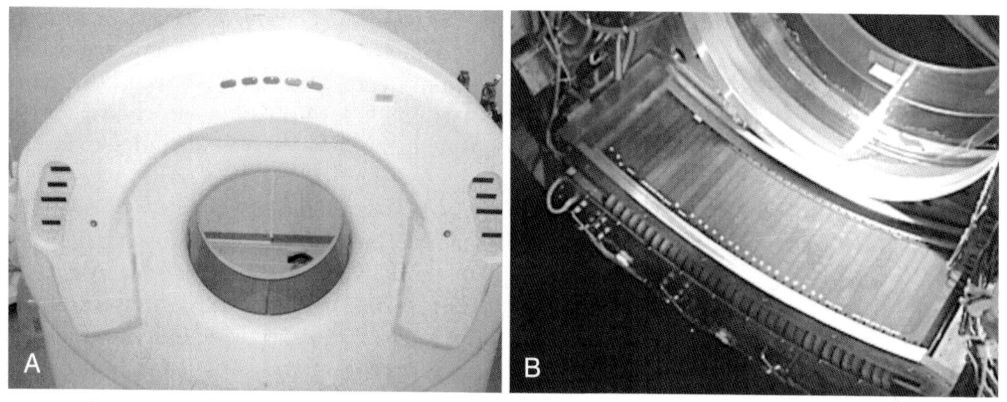

FIGURE 1-16 A front view of the 256-slice CT scanner gantry **(A)** and its wide area two-dimensional detector array **(B)**. (From Mori S et al: Comparison of patient doses in 256-slice CT and 16-slice CT scanners, *Br J Radiol* 79:56-61, 2006. Reproduced by permission.)

the stair-step artifacts seen in nonisotropic resolution 3D images. Scanners can now achieve isotropic resolution of less than 0.4 mm.

Dual Source CT Scanner

In 2005, Siemens Medical Solutions announced a new type of CT scanner at the RSNA, called the SOMATOM Definition. This is a *dual source CT* (DSCT) scanner that features two x-ray tubes and two detectors (Fig. 1-18) specifically intended for imaging cardiac patients in a very short time. As illustrated in Figure 1-19, the performance of the DSCT scanner compared with the single source CT (SSCT) scanner in imaging the beating heart at a low and stable heart rate (60 beats/min) is improved because of the higher temporal resolution of the DSCT scanner (Fig. 1-19, *A*). Furthermore, as the heart rate increases to 100 beats/min, the DSCT scanner offers much better image quality (sharpness) in both systolic and diastolic phases compared with the SSCT scanner, as illustrated in Figure 1-19, *B*.

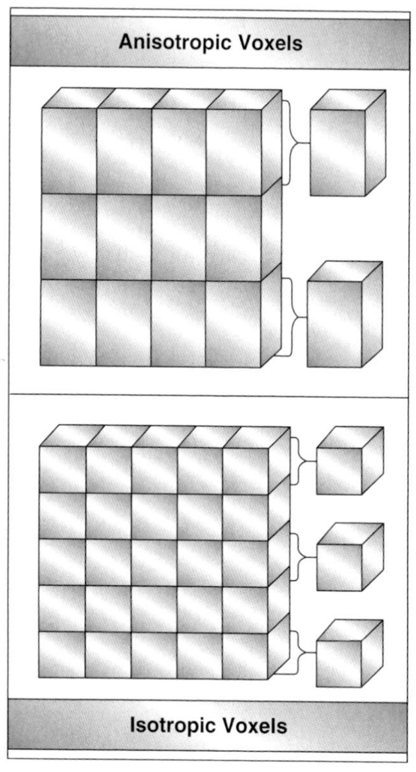

FIGURE 1-17 Isotropic resolution in CT implies that voxels are perfect cubes with all dimensions being equal, as opposed to anisotropic resolution where all dimensions are not equal.

Other Applications of Volume CT

Volume CT scanning has resulted in a wide range of applications such as CT fluoroscopy, CT angiography, 3D imaging, virtual reality imaging, and more recently improved cardiac CT imaging.

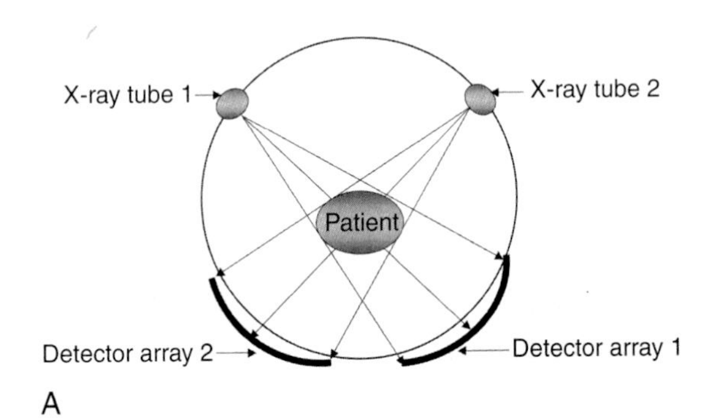

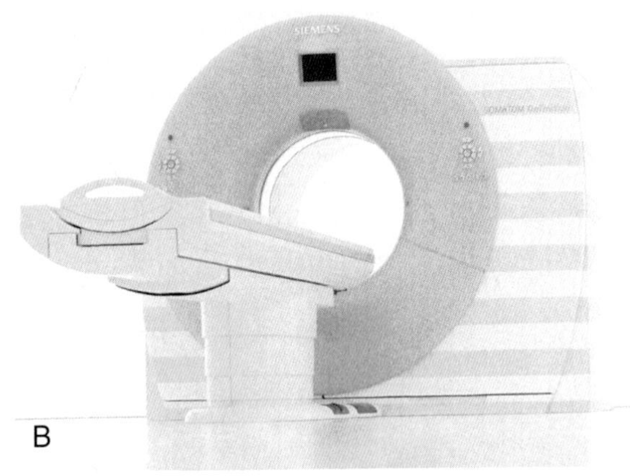

FIGURE 1-18 The basic concept of the DSCT scanner **(A)** and a full view of the scanner **(B)** introduced by Siemens Medical Solutions. (Courtesy of Siemens Medical Solutions.)

CT has found applications in radiation therapy and nuclear medicine technologies as well. In radiation therapy, for example, the CT scanner is now used in CT simulation process (Fig. 1-20). As noted, the *CT simulator* includes the CT scanner that is specially equipped with a *flat table top* and lasers that facilitate accurate positioning of the patient and is coupled to the radiation treatment planning virtual simulator. As noted by Mutic et al (2003), "the scanner is accompanied by specialized software which allows treatment planning on volumetric patient CT scans in a manner consistent with conventional radiation therapy simulators." This scanner can either be installed in the radiology department or in the radiation therapy department. In nuclear medicine, the CT scanner is combined with a positron emission tomography (PET) scanner (Ell, 2006) and single photon emission tomography (SPECT) to form single units referred to as a PET/CT scanner and a SPECT/CT scanner. PET/CT is described in detail in Chapter 16.

Mobile CT

A unique event in the evolution of CT technology was the development of a mobile CT scanner to image patients who are too ill or physically traumatized to be transported to a fixed CT scanner.

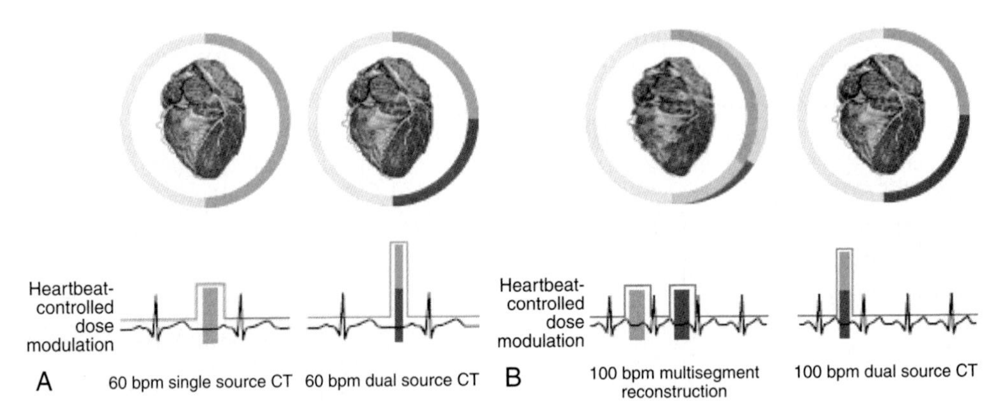

FIGURE 1-19 A visual comparison of the image quality of an SSCT scanner and the DSCT scanner in cardiac imaging. (Courtesy of Siemens Medical Solutions.)

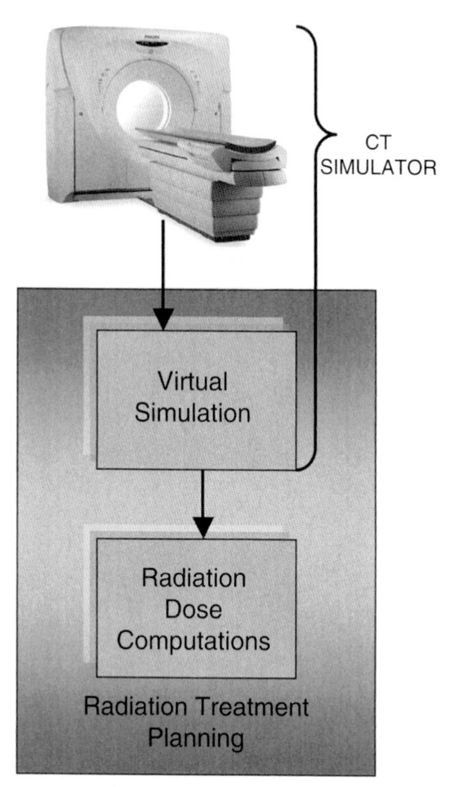

FIGURE 1-20 The CT simulation process in radiation therapy with a CT scanner.

Philips Medical Systems introduced one such scanner specifically for use in the operating room, intensive care unit, and emergency trauma unit. The portable CT scanner is compact and mounted on wheels to facilitate transportation of the unit to remote locations in the hospital by technologists.

Clinical Efficacy Studies

The term *efficacy* is synonymous with effectiveness, efficiency, and performance. A number of investigators designed efficacy studies to test the clinical usefulness of this new diagnostic technique. Studies reported the results of scanning the brain, spinal cord, neck, thorax, abdomen, retroperitoneum, pelvis, and extremities.

CT became well established in the diagnosis of diseases of the central nervous system, and in some cases, it eliminated the need for examinations such as pneumoencephalography and reduced the frequency of cerebral angiography. Disorders such as gliomas, metastases, intracranial lesions, aneurysms, infarctions, hemorrhage, and atrophy have been successfully detected by CT. Later, whole-body clinical applications (see Chapter 18) became effective. In addition, CT proved useful in radiation treatment planning to provide accurate isodose curves and in other areas, such as determination of the mineral salt content in bones, or quantitative CT. Studies using MSCT scanners clearly demonstrated their usefulness in a wide range of clinical applications, including playing a central role in cardiac imaging in applications such as coronary angiography, assessment of ventricular function and pulmonary veins, and calcium scoring (DeRoos, 2006).

Radiation Dose Studies

A fundamental goal of any new imaging technique is to provide maximum information content with the minimum radiation dose to the patient. Perry and Bridges (1973) measured both the cranial radiation dose and the gonadal radiation dose for a series of scans. Their results provided a foundation for future studies. Initially, the radiation dose to the patient was thought to be negligible because the beam in CT was tightly collimated, but the patient exposure for a series of CT scans usually exceeds that of film radiography of the same area (Seeram, 1982).

Radiation dose is an integral topic in CT technology because the CT beam geometry and method of acquiring images differ from those of conventional radiography. Several imaging parameters in CT affect dose, including slice thickness, noise, resolution detector efficiency, reconstruction algorithm, collimation, and filtration. Various dose studies have explored the ways in which these factors influence the dose.

These studies have also led to the development of special ways to measure and describe the dose (McNitt-Gray, 2002; Kalender, 2005; Seeram, 1999). Ionization chambers or thermoluminescent

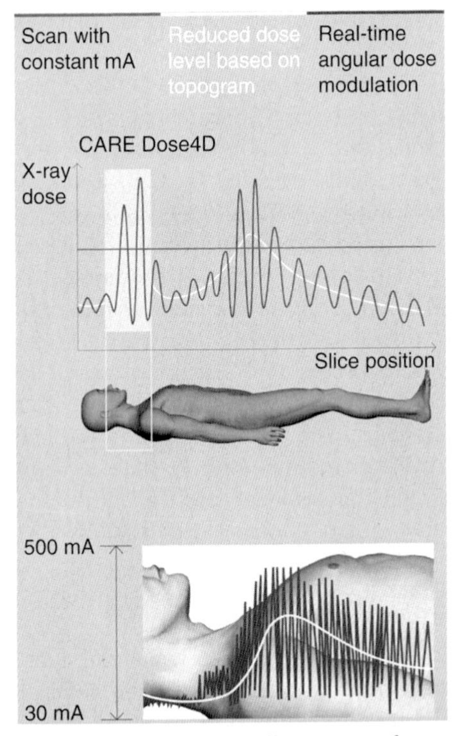

FIGURE 1-21 CAREDose4D illustration of automatic tube current modulation, a technique to reduce dose in CT. (Courtesy of Siemens Medical Solutions.)

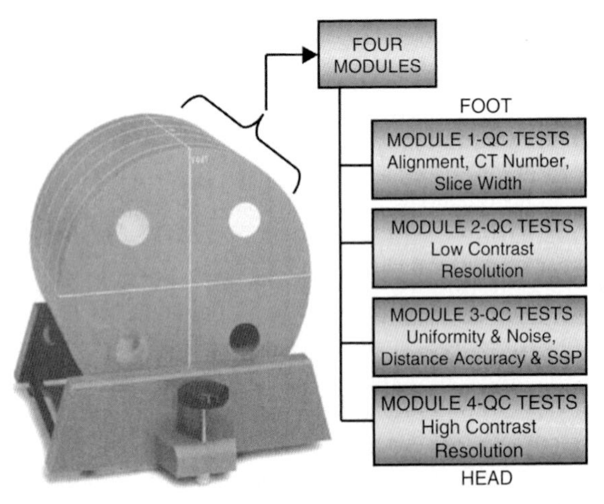

FIGURE 1-22 The ACR phantom used for CT quality control. The phantom consists of four sections (modules) for performing several quality control tests.

dosimeters are used to measure the dose. Dose descriptors include the single-scan dose profile, multiple-scan dose profile, CT dose index, multiple-scan average dose, and isodose curves.

Additionally, manufacturers have developed various schemes to reduce the dose in CT. One scheme uses three elements to keep the patient dose to a minimum during data acquisition: (1) combined applications to reduce exposure, a pre-patient filtering technique that reduces the dose by about 15% compared with conventional CT, (2) new ultrafast ceramic detectors that reduce the dose by another 25%, and (3) on-line dose modulation, whereby the milliamperage (mA) is optimized to the patient characteristics (diameter and absorption) to reduce the dose. This particular development in CT dose reduction is referred to as *automatic tube current modulation technique* (Iball et al, 2006; Rizzo et al, 2006). Different manufacturers have different methods to do *automatic exposure control* (AEC) in CT. For example, although Siemens Medical Solutions and GE Healthcare refer to their AEC packages as "CARE Dose 4D" and "SmartmA," respectively, Philips Medical Systems and Toshiba Medical Systems label their packages "DoseRight" and "SURE$_{\text{Exposure}}$," respectively. CARE Dose 4D is illustrated in Figure 1-21.

Quality Control

As with any medical imaging system, CT scanners are subject to quality control procedures and tests. Testing system performance is vital to maintain optimal image quality and minimize the production of image artifacts. Because the CT system consists of several mechanical and electronic components, many quality control tests are currently available. These range from simple tests, which the technologist can perform by using various phantoms provided by the manufacturers, to more complex tests that may require the expertise of the radiologic physicist or biomedical engineer. More recently, the ACR has introduced a CT phantom referred to as the ACR phantom, as illustrated in Figure 1-22, to be used for any

CT quality control program. The phantom basically consists of four sections which can be imaged simultaneously to generate several test results. Quality control for CT scanners will be described in detail in a later chapter.

Other Uses

CT is useful in areas other than medicine. For example, CT can be used to study internal log defects. Funt and Bryan (1987) investigated the use of CT technology in a sawmill. They developed and tested algorithms that automatically interpreted CT images of logs and stated, "The computer program uses the high density and elliptical shape of knots to distinguish them from good wood, and the low density and rough texture of rotten areas to separate rotten wood from sound wood." Habermehl and Ridder (1997) detailed the use of a portable CT scanner to take images of trees to determine wood rots; locate knots, hollows, and other defects; and determine water distribution inside the tree trunk (Fig. 1-23). These portable tree CT scanners use a cesium 137 gamma radiation source with a fan beam falling on an array of about 30 sodium iodide detectors.

CT has also been used in *paleoanthropology*. Zonneveld et al (1989) found that CT can visualize internal anatomy of completely preserved Egyptian mummies (Fig. 1-24) (Yasuda et al, 1992). Additionally, Hoffman et al (2002) report the use of CT in what they refer to as *paleoradiology*. Recently, a CT system for dedicated imaging of mummies has become available and will be used in a major research project planned by the Egyptian Supreme Council of Antiquities in conjunction with Siemens Medical Solutions (who donated an MSCT scanner) and the National Geographic Society.

Several cases report the use of CT in paleo-ornithology, oil exploration, fat stock breeding, and other animal investigations (Fig. 1-25). In fat stock breeding, pigs are scanned to determine the meat quality defined as the best combination of water, protein, and fat, thus eliminating the need to kill the pigs for this determination (Fig. 1-26).

Sirr and Waddle (1999) used CT to evaluate bowed stringed instruments such as violins. The scans demonstrated varying degrees of internal damage (e.g., wormholes, air gaps, and plastic deformities of wood) or those resulting from repair (e.g., glue lines, filler substances, and wooden cleats and

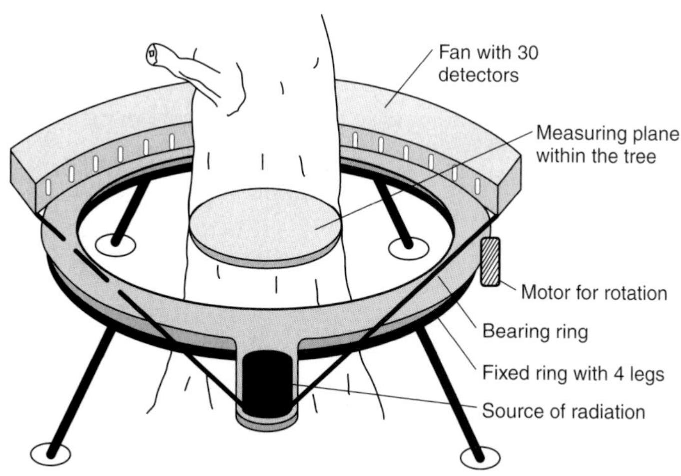

FIGURE 1-23 A portable CT scanner for imaging trees. (From Habermehl A, Ridder HW: γ-Ray tomography in forest and tree sciences. In Bonse U, editor: *Developments in x-ray tomography*. Proceedings of the International Society for Optical Engineering 3149:234-243, 1997.)

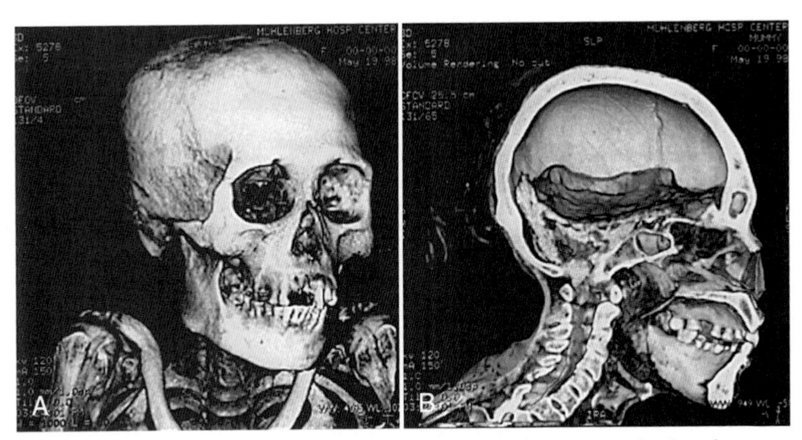

FIGURE 1-24 CT can be used to image mummies without destroying the bandages or plaster in which they are wrapped. **A,** 3D CT image of a 1000-year-old Peruvian mummy using volume rendering with a bone and detail filter. **B,** A lateral view of the same mummy shows residual brain in the posterior fossa. (Courtesy John Posh, Bethlehem, Pa.)

patches) not seen when the instruments are examined visually. The researchers also concluded that CT facilitated verification of authenticity and proof of ownership.

Another interesting and unique nonmedical use of CT is one by Meyer et al (2007). They used a 64-slice CT scanner to find out the combination of a bicycle lock belonging to the son of one of the authors who had forgotten the combination. Fortunately the lock was not on the bicycle. The lock was positioned on the scanner to show 0 on the right side of the lock. The lock was scanned with 350 mA, 120 kV, and a pitch of 0.33. The resulting images are shown in Fig. 1-27. As can be seen, the notches are clearly shown and reveal that the combination is 1789. This result must have made the little boy very happy.

More recently, CT scanners are now used at major airports for *automated explosives detection*. As baggage is scanned, the CT data (numbers) of the contents obtained as a result of the scanning are compared with CT numbers of known

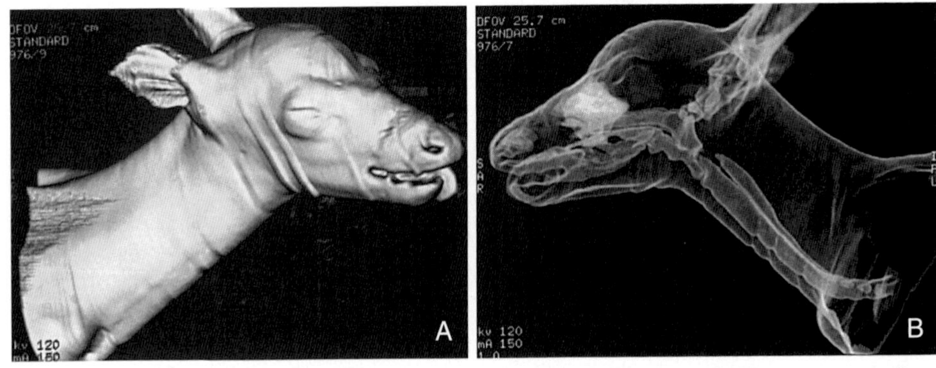

FIGURE 1-25 A, 3D surface rendering of a 2-month-old whitetail fawn mauled by a mountain lion. **B,** The same fawn examined by CT with a 3D transparency program to demonstrate the airways and other air-filled cavities. (Courtesy John Posh, Bethlehem, Pa.)

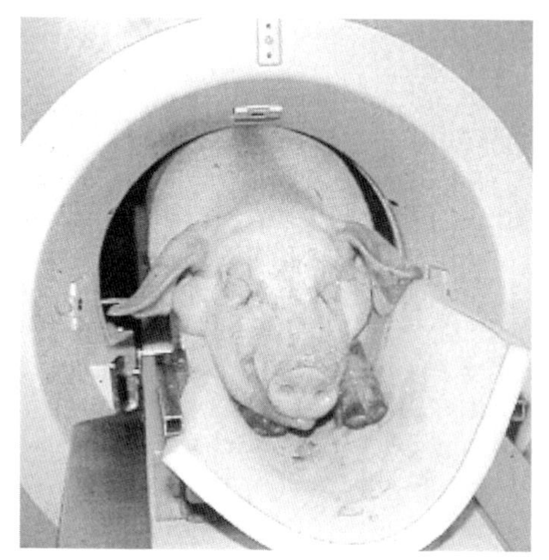

FIGURE 1-26 CT scanning of pigs in fat stock breeding to determine meat quality. (Courtesy Siemens Medical Systems, Iselin, N.J.)

explosives or contraband. If the two sets of CT numbers correspond, an alarm is sounded.

DIGITAL IMAGE PROCESSING

CT is an excellent example of digital image processing (Fig. 1-28). The x-ray beam passes through the patient and falls onto special detectors. These detectors convert the x-ray photons into electrical signals (analog signals) that must be converted into numerical data (digital data) for input into a digital computer.

Digital image processing involves the use of a digital computer to process and manipulate digital images. The computer receives an input of a digital image and performs specific operations on the data to produce an output image that is different from and more useful than the input image.

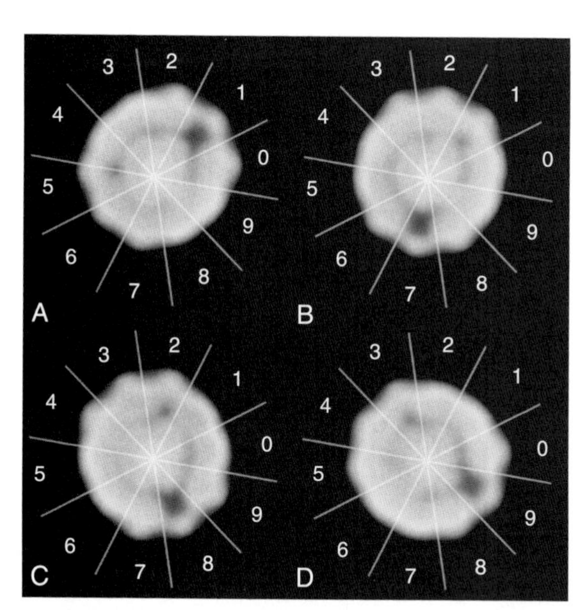

FIGURE 1-27 Images of a bicycle lock scanned by a 640-slice MSCT scanner to reveal the combination, 1789. (From Meyer H et al: How multidetector CT can help open bike locks, *Radiology* 245:921, 2007. Reproduced by permission of RSNA and the authors.)

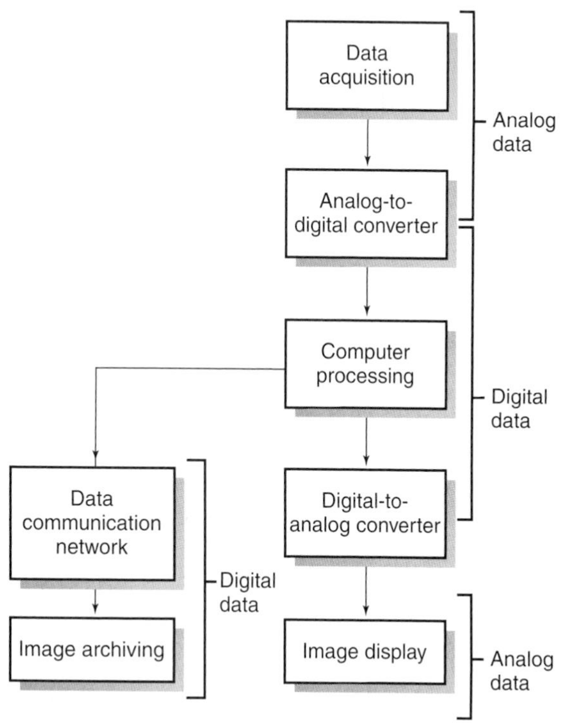

FIGURE 1-28 Major components of the digital imaging system on which CT is based.

The procedure had its origins at the National Aeronautics and Space Administration Jet Propulsion Laboratory at the California Institute of Technology, where it was used to enhance and restore images from space. Today, the space program generates and uses the largest amount of digital data.

The digital image processing of medical images dates back to the 1970s, about the time CT was introduced to the medical community. Today, digital radiography, digital fluoroscopy, digital subtraction angiography, and MRI use digital image processing techniques.

Digital image processing in radiology allows the observer to process images with use of a wide variety of algorithms to manipulate images to enhance diagnostic interpretation (Seeram, 2004; Seeram and Seeram, 2008). Such postprocessing can generate 3D images by use of the stack of sectional images or the volume data sets. Various 3D images such as surface-shaded display and volume-rendered images are now commonplace (Dalrymple et al, 2005). As noted by the expert CT researcher Dr. Kalender, "CT is fully 3D these days" (Kalender, 2005).

APPLICATIONS OF VOLUME SCANNING

Volume scanning from either single-slice spiral/helical or multislice spiral/helical CT generates vast amounts of data compared with slice-by-slice conventional CT scanning. Several new applications provide radiologists and other physicians with additional tools for taking images of patients with CT and enhancing their own diagnostic effectiveness. These new applications include continuous imaging or CT fluoroscopy, 3D imaging and visualization, CT angiography, and virtual reality imaging.

CT Fluoroscopy

CT fluoroscopy, or continuous imaging, depends on spiral/helical data acquisition methods, high-speed processing, and a fast image-processing algorithm for image reconstruction. In conventional CT, the time lag between data acquisition and image reconstruction makes real-time display of images impossible. CT fluoroscopy allows for the reconstruction and display of images in real-time with variable frame rates. In 1996 the U.S. FDA approved real-time CT fluoroscopy as a clinical tool for use in radiology (Katada et al, 1996).

CT fluoroscopy is based on three advances in CT technology: (1) fast, continuous scanning made possible by spiral/helical scanning principles, (2) fast image reconstruction made possible by special hardware performing quick calculations and a new image reconstruction algorithm, and (3) continuous image display by use of cine mode at frame rates of two to eight images per second (Daly and Templeton, 1999).

Other support tools were developed to facilitate interventional procedures in CT fluoroscopy. One such tool, the Fluoro Assisted Computed Tomography System, uses a unique flat-panel amorphous silicon digital detector coupled with an x-ray tube by a C-arm, which is a part of the CT gantry.

Three-Dimensional Imaging and Visualization

3D imaging is a popular technique in CT because of the availability of large amounts of digital data. 3D imaging is now possible on CT scanners and the results have been promising (Fishman et al, 1991). 3D CT is already used in radiation treatment planning, craniofacial imaging, surgical planning, and orthopedics.

3D images can be obtained by a hardware-based or a software-based approach. The hardware-based approach uses specialized equipment such as electronic computer display units to execute algorithms for 3D imaging, and the software-based approach uses computer programs or software-coded algorithms. These algorithms, or rendering techniques, transform the transaxial CT data into simulated 3D images. In general, two classes of techniques are available for the transformation: surface- and volume-based techniques. Each technique consists of three steps: volume formation, classification, and image projection. Although *volume formation* involves stacking images to form a volume with some preprocessing, *classification* refers to determining the tissue types in the slices. According to Fishman (1991), image projection consists of "projecting the classified volume data in such a manner that a two-dimensional (2D) representation or simulation of the 3D volume is formed." Additionally, Fishman (2004) reviews the essentials of 3D rendering describing the evolution and progress through the years.

Computer graphics has played a role in the evolution and refinement of 3D imaging (Rhodes, 1991). Computer graphics involves the creation, manipulation, and display of pictures or images with the computer. It allows the user to express ideas and information in a visual format and includes various ways to represent data to create and display images by use of graphics programming languages and image processing techniques.

3D CT has created a new area of interest for technologists (Seeram, 2004) who have the opportunity to participate in its development. Today, 3D articles are appearing more and more in the literature to support the increasing 3D applications that can make full use of the large data sets generated by the new MSCT scanners (Dalrymple et al, 2005).

Visualization is a term used in the discussion of the display of images in CT. It involves the use of computer programs, or visualization tools, that provide the observer-diagnostician with additional information from the image to facilitate diagnosis. These tools can be simple (e.g., image contrast and brightness [windowing] tools) or advanced (e.g., 3D imaging, interactive, and cine visualization tools). Examples of current state-of-the art CT images are shown in Figure 1-29.

CT Angiography

CT angiography is defined as CT imaging of blood vessels opacified by contrast media (Kalender, 1995). During contrast injection, the entire area of interest is scanned with spiral/helical CT and images are recorded when vessels are fully opacified to show arterial or venous phases of enhancement.

CT angiography uses 3D imaging principles to display images of the vasculature through intravenous injection of contrast media compared with those of intra-arterial angiograms. Four essential elements are patient preparation, selection of acquisition parameters (total spiral/helical scan time, slice thickness, table speed) to optimize the imaging process, contrast media injection, and postprocessing techniques and visualization tools such as algorithms to display 3D images in interactive cine modes, multiplanar reconstruction, maximum intensity projection, shaded surface display, and volume rendering, which are illustrated in Figure 1-30.

CT Endoscopy—Virtual Reality Imaging

Virtual reality is a branch of computer science that immerses users in a computer-generated environment and allows them to interact with 3D scenes. The application of virtual reality concepts to the creation of inner views of tubular structures is called *virtual endoscopy* (DeWever at al, 2005; Vining, 1999). Volume CT scanners produce large data sets (two-dimensional axial images) compared with their conventional slice-by-slice counterparts. Subsequently, volume CT scanners have allowed for improved 3D imaging, CT fluoroscopy, CT angiography, and CT virtual endoscopy (Fig. 1-31).

Cardiac CT Imaging

To image the beating heart with the goal of reducing motion artifacts and a loss of both spatial and contrast resolution, fast CT scanners such as the EBCT scanner were introduced to overcome these problems and produce good diagnostic images of the heart. Alternatively, the patient's electrocardiogram (ECG) is used to provide prospective imaging, after it is recorded at the same time with the scanning with stop and go scanners. Subsequently, retrospective imaging has been developed

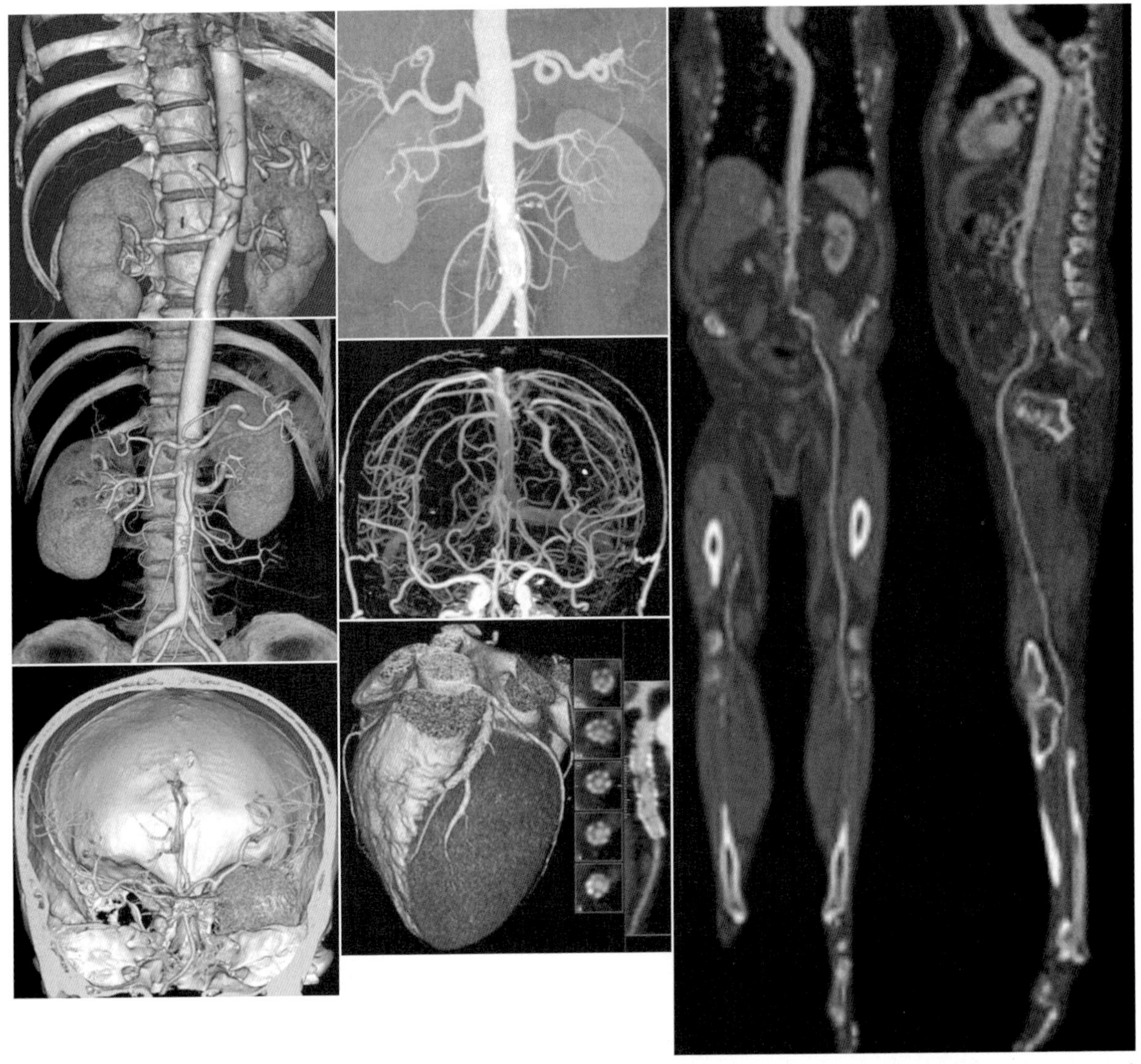

FIGURE 1-29 Examples of current state-of-the-art CT images. Note the 3D nature of these images. (Courtesy of Toshiba Medical Systems.)

where the ECG is correlated with image reconstruction in spiral/helical CT scanning.

The recent technical developments in MSCT scanners and the introduction of the DSCT scanner open up a whole new avenue for successful imaging the heart with excellent image quality that is based on meeting several technical requirements. These include low-contrast resolution to visualize small differences in tissue contrast, high-contrast resolution (spatial resolution) to visualize small structures in the anatomy scanned, and temporal resolution to image fast-moving objects to reduce motion artifacts. These have all been made possible by fast data acquisition and dedicated reconstruction algorithms, such as, for example, the segmented (multiple) algorithms that

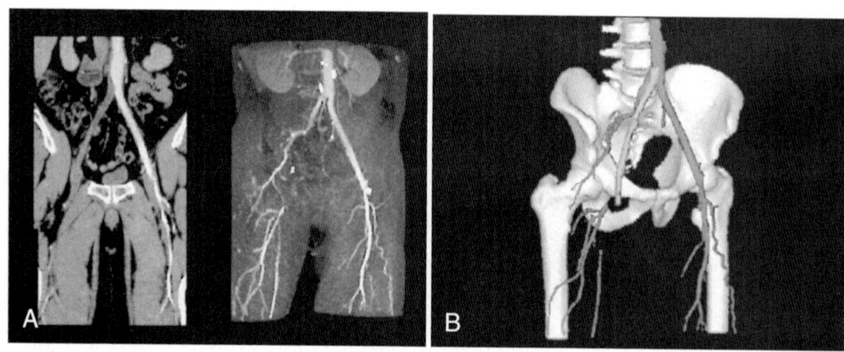

FIGURE 1-30 **A,** Multiplanar reconstruction *(left)* and maximum intensity projection *(right)* images. **B,** A 3D multitissue reconstruction image of an aortobifemoral bypass graft exhibiting a thrombosed right graft. (Courtesy Philips Medical Systems.)

"allow for merging synchronized transmission data from successive heart cycles. The more heart cycles that can be included in the reconstruction, the better the temporal resolution" (DeRoos et al, 2006). In addition, a low pitch factor (to be discussed later) is needed "to record at least two heart cycles and to achieve a temporal resolution in the order of magnitude of 100ms for typical heart rates between 60-80 beats per minute (BPM)" (DeRoos et al, 2006).

Finally, scan times in cardiac CT may vary from less than 30s "but preferably below 20s." Current 64-slice MSCT scanners are capable of shorter than 20-second scan times. For example, imaging for calcium scoring and coronary angiography use scan times of 2.5 and 10 seconds, respectively (DeRoos et al, 2006). Cardiac CT applications include quantitative assessment of coronary artery calcifications, ventricular function assessment, and coronary angiography assessment of pulmonary veins. Figure 1-32 illustrates a set of cardiac images from a current MSCT scanner.

The physics of cardiac CT imaging is described in the Appendix.

CT Screening

The excellent image quality and speed of current MSCT scanners has opened up yet another application of CT for imaging "healthy people as a

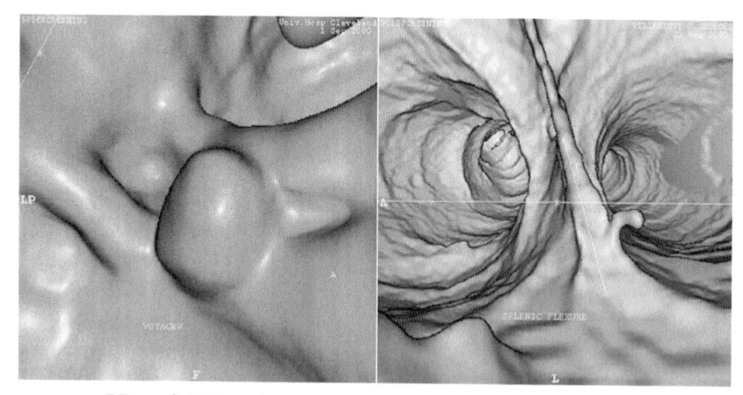

FIGURE 1-31 Virtual CT endoscopy images. (Courtesy Philips Medical Systems.)

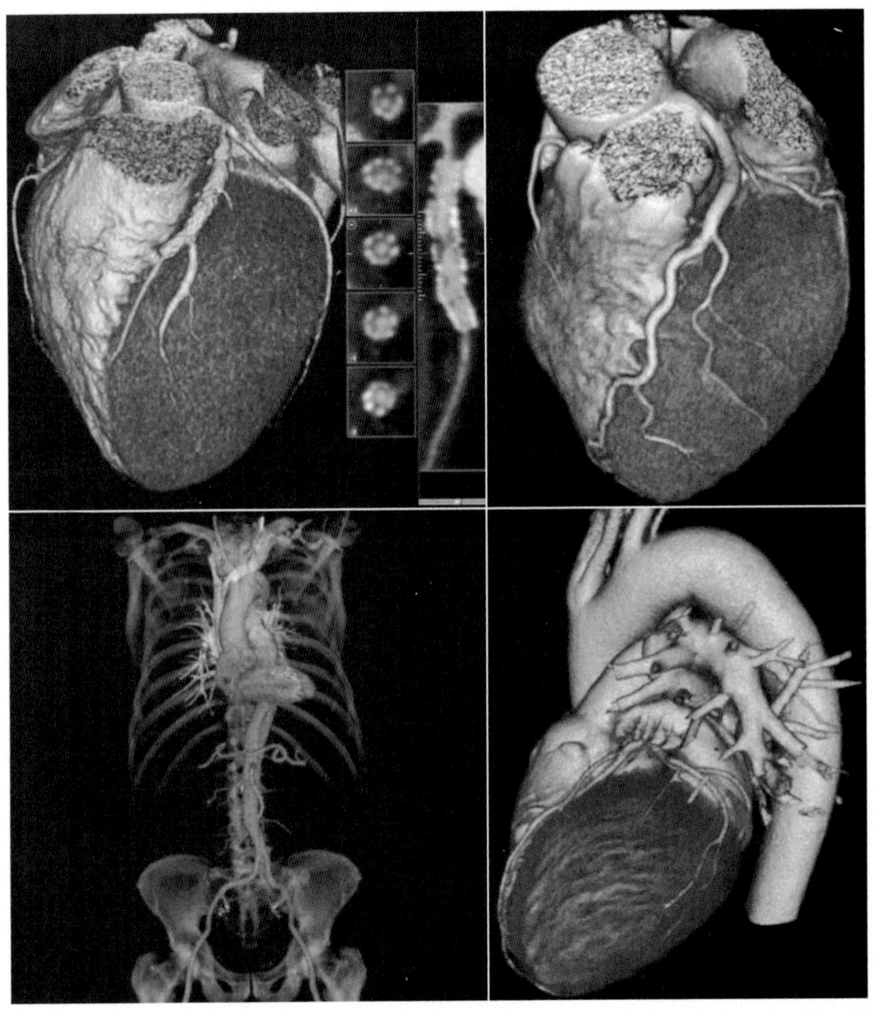

FIGURE 1-32 Examples of 3D images of the heart and great vessels. (Courtesy Toshiba Medical Systems.)

means to screen for early disease" (Horton et al, 2004). This concept is referred to as *CT screening*. CT screening is now being investigated as a potential tool for imaging asymptomatic individuals for the benefit related to cardiac screening, lung cancer screening, virtual colonoscopy, and whole body imaging (Furtado et al, 2005) for the primary purpose of the early detection of disease. However, CT screening has experienced significant controversy and debate to date, and therefore it will not be discussed further in this text.

REFERENCES

Beckmann EC: CT scanning in the early days, *Br J Radiol* 79: 5-8, 2006.

Cormack AM: Early two-dimensional reconstruction and recent topics stemming from it, Nobel Award address, *Med Phys* 7: 277-282, 1980.

Dalrymple NC et al: Introduction to the language of three-dimensional imaging with multidetector CT, *Radiographics* 25:1409-1428, 2005.

Daly B, Templeton PA: Real-time CT fluoroscopy: evaluation of an interventional tool, *Radiology* 211: 309-315, 1999.

DeRoos A et al: Cardiac applications of multislice computed tomography, *Br J Radiol* 79:9-16, 2006.

DeWever W et al: Virtual bronchoscopy: accuracy and usefulness—an overview, *Semin Ultrasound CT MRI* 26:364-373, 2005.

Ell PJ: The contribution of PET/CT to improved patient management, *Br J Radiol* 79:23-36, 2006.

Fishman EK: 3D rendering: principles and techniques, In Fishman EK, Jeffrey RB, editors: *Multidetector CT: principles, techniques, and clinical applications*, Philadelphia, 2004, Lippincott Williams & Wilkins.

Fishman EK et al: Three-dimensional imaging, *Radiology* 181:321-337, 1991.

Funt F, Bryant EC: Detection of internal log defects by automatic interpretation of computer tomography images, *Forest Prod J* 37:56-62, 1987.

Furtado CD et al: Whole-body CT screening: spectrum of findings and recommendations in 1192 patients, *Radiology* 237:385-394, 2005.

GE Healthcare: Personal communication, 2007.

Habermehl A, Ridder H-W: γ-Ray tomography in forest and tree sciences. In Bonse U, editor: *Developments in x-ray tomography: proceedings of the SPIE* 3149:234-243, 1997.

Herman GT: *Image reconstruction from projections: the fundamentals of computerized tomography*, New York, 1980, Academic Press.

Hounsfield GN: Computed medical imaging, Nobel Award address, *Med Phys* 7:283-290, 1980.

Hoffman H et al: Paleoradiology: advanced CT in the evaluation of nine Egyptian mummies, *Radiographics* 22:377-385, 2002.

Horton KM et al: CT screening: principles and controversies, In Fishman EK, Jeffrey RB, editors: *Multidetector CT: principles, techniques, and clinical applications*, Philadelphia, 2004, Lippincott Williams & Wilkins.

Iball GR et al: Assessment of tube current modulation in pelvic CT, *Br J Radiol* 79:62-70, 2006.

Isherwood I: Sir Godfrey Newbold Hounsfield—in memoriam, *Eur Radiol* 14:2152-2153, 2004.

Kalender W: Spiral CT angiography, In Goldman LW, Fowlkes JB, editors: *Medical CT and ultrasound: current technology and applications*, New London, Conn, 1995, American Association of Physicists in Medicine.

Kalender W: Personal communications, 1999 and 2006.

Kalender W: *Computed tomography—fundamentals, system technology, image quality, applications*, Erlangen, 2005, Publicis Corporate Publishing.

Katada K et al: Guidance with real-time CT fluoroscopy: early clinical experience, *Radiology* 200:851-856, 1996.

Kelves BH: *Naked to the bone*, New Brunswick, NJ, 1997, Rutgers University Press.

Ledley R: Personal communication, 1999.

McNitt-Gray MF: Radiation dose in CT, *Radiographics* 22:1541-1553, 2002.

Mori S et al: Comparison of patient doses in 256-slice CT and 16-slice CT scanners, *Br J Radiol* 79:56-61, 2006.

Mutic S et al: Quality assurance for computed tomography simulators and computed tomography simulation process: report of the AAPM Radiation Therapy Committee Task Group No 66, *Med Phys* 30: 2762-2792, 2004.

Perry BJ, Bridges C: Computerized transverse axial scanning (tomography), *part 3, Br J Radiol* 46: 1048-1051, 1973.

Posh J: Personal communication, 1999.

Rhodes ML: Computer graphics in medicine: the past decade, *IEEE Comput Graph Appl* 4:52-54, 1991.

Ritman et al: Synchronous volumetric imaging of noninvasive vivisection of cardiovascular and respiratory dynamics: evolution of current perspectives, In Giuliani ER, editor: *Cardiology: fundamentals and practice*, St Louis, 1991, Mosby.

Rizzo S et al: Comparison of angular and combined automatic tube current modulation techniques with constant tube current CT of the abdomen and pelvis, *AJR Am J Roentgenol* 186:673-679, 2006.

Robb RA, Morin RL: Principles and instrumentation for dynamic x-ray computed tomography. In Marcus ML, et al, editor: *Cardiac imaging: a comparison to Braunwald's heart disease*, Philadelphia, 1991, WB Saunders.

Seeram E: 3D Imaging: basic concepts for radiologic technologists, *Radiol Technol* 69:127-148, 1998.

Seeram E: Radiation dose in CT, *Radiol Technol* 70: 534-556, 1999.

Seeram E: Digital image processing, *Radiol Technol* 75: 435-452, 2004.

Seeram E, Seeram D: Image postprocessing in digital radiology: a primer for technologists, *Journal of Medical Imaging and Radiation Sciences* 39:23-41, 2008.

Siemens Medical Solutions: Archaeology—high tech meets history. SOMATOM Sessions No. 16: 33-34, 2005.

Sirr SA, Waddle JR: Use of CT in detection of internal damage and repair and determination of authenticity in high-quality bowed stringed instruments, *Radiographics* 19:639-646, 1999.

Vining DJ: Virtual colonoscopy, *Semin Ultrasound CT MRI* 20:56-60, 1999.

Yasuda T et al: 3D Visualization of an ancient Egyptian mummy, *IEEE Comput Graph Appl* 2:13-17, 1992.

Zonneveld FW et al: The use of the CT in the study of the internal morphology of hominid fossils, *Medicamundi* 34:117-127, 1989.

BIBLIOGRAPHY

Dümmling K: 10 years' computed tomography: a retrospective view, *Electromedica* 52:13-28, 1984.

Hounsfield GN: Computed medical imaging, Nobel Award address, *Med Phys* 7:283-290, 1980.

Klingenbeck-Regn K, Oppelt A: Dose in CT scanning-physical relationships and potentials for dose saving, *Electromedica* 66:26-30, 1998.

Schwierz G, Kirchgeorg M: The continuous evolution of medical x-ray imaging, I: the technically driven stage of development, *Electromedica* 63:2-7, 1995.

Chapter 2

Introduction to Computers

Chapter Outline

In Chapter 1, an overview of computed tomography (CT) was presented and a brief history reviewed, followed by an outline of the growth of CT technology from the time it was invented to its current clinical applications and its uses in nonclinical areas, such as scanning baggage at airports, for example. An important point made in Chapter 1 emphasized that computers play an important role in the production of a CT image, and they are a major component of the CT imaging system. With this in mind, it is mandatory for technologists to have a good understanding of what a computer is and how it works.

The purpose of this chapter is to outline the basic technical elements of computers and to highlight certain relevant characteristics that will serve to enhance the reader's understanding of CT principles.

COMPUTERS IN RADIOLOGY

Today, computers are used in all facets of human activity. They are successfully being used in government, education, energy, transportation, the military, robotics, the home, and health and medicine, to mention only a few. In 1955, computers were used to calculate radiation dose distributions in cancer patients (Seeram, 1989), which subsequently led to the use of computers in radiology. Radiology computer applications are now commonplace and currently fall into two categories: imaging and nonimaging applications. Therefore, technologists should have a certain degree of computer literacy that Capron (2005) defines as awareness (how they are used), knowledge (what they are and how they work), and interaction (being able to use the computer).

Imaging Applications

Imaging applications are those modalities in which the information acquired from the patient is subject to computer processing. Such processing involves digital image processing techniques to produce computer-generated or digital images. In medical imaging, computers are major components in digital imaging modalities such as CT, computed radiography, flat-panel digital radiography (DR), digital fluoroscopy, digital subtraction angiography, digital mammography, magnetic resonance imaging (MRI), nuclear medicine technologies such as single-photon emission tomography and positron emission tomography (PET), PET/CT, and diagnostic medical sonography. Computers also play an integral role in radiation therapy treatment planning.

The central role of the computer in digital imaging systems is to process and facilitate the display and to archive images and information. Additionally, computers are used as efficient vehicles for communicating images and information to remote areas in an effort to improve patient care by facilitating consultation and shared management of the patient's medical problem.

Nonimaging Applications

Two major nonimaging applications include a picture archiving and communication system (PACS) and a radiology information system (RIS). The central feature of the RIS is to address elements of patient admissions, scheduling, accounting, billing, film library functions, word processing, statistics, database management, and data communications. The RIS can connect to a hospital information system (HIS), which addresses the needs of all departments in the hospital including laboratory, pharmacy, finance, admissions, and hospital administration. On the other hand, a PACS is an electronic system for archiving, transmitting, viewing, and manipulating images acquired by the digital imaging modalities. PACS has now become commonplace in radiology and is an integral part of a CT imaging system and, of course, the other digital imaging modalities mentioned above. For this reason, it will be described in a little more detail later in the chapter.

COMPUTER SYSTEMS

Definition

A *computer* is a machine for solving problems. Specifically, the modern computer is a high-speed electronic computational machine that accepts information in the form of data and instructions through an input device and processes this information with arithmetic and logic operations from a program stored in its memory. The results of the processing can be displayed, stored, or recorded by use of suitable output devices or transmitted to another location.

Essentially, people can perform these same tasks; the word *computer* historically referred to a person. A *computer system*, on the other hand, consists of at least three elements: hardware, software, and computer users (Fig. 2-1). *Hardware* refers to the physical components of the machine, and *software* refers to the instructions that make the hardware work to solve problems. People are essential to computer systems because they design, develop, and operate hardware and software.

These elements result in three core characteristics that reflect the usefulness of computers: speed (solve problems very quickly), reliability (not prone to errors—computers are only as good as the people who program them), and storage capability (storage of a vast amount of data and information) (Capron, 2005).

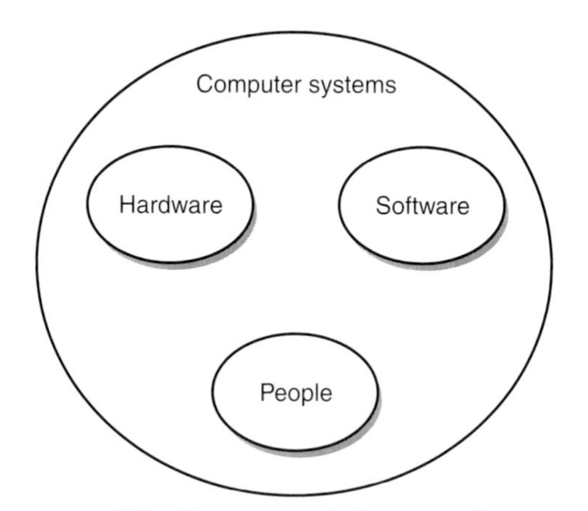

FIGURE 2-1 The three essential elements of a computer system.

Hardware Organization

A computer processes the data or information it receives from people or other computers and outputs the results in a form suitable to the needs of the user. This is a three-step process (Fig. 2-2).

The organization of a computer includes at least five hardware components: an input device, a central processing unit (CPU), internal memory, an output device, and external memory or storage (Fig. 2-3).

Input hardware refers to input devices such as a keyboard from which information can be sent to the processor. Processing hardware includes the CPU and internal memory. The CPU is the brain of the computer; it consists of a control unit that directs the activities of the machine and an arithmetic-logic unit (ALU) to perform mathematical calculations and data comparisons. In addition, the CPU includes an internal memory, or main memory, for the permanent storage of software instructions and data.

After data are processed, results are sent to an output device in the form of hard or soft copy. One popular hard copy output device is a printer. If the results are displayed on a monitor for direct viewing, then the term *soft copy* is used. Finally, processing results can be stored on external storage devices. These include magnetic storage devices, such as disks and tapes, and optical storage devices.

Software Concepts

The hardware receives its instructions from the software. The instructions are written in steps that specify ways to solve problems. These sets of instructions are called *programs*.

The three categories of software are (1) systems software, (2) applications software, and (3) software

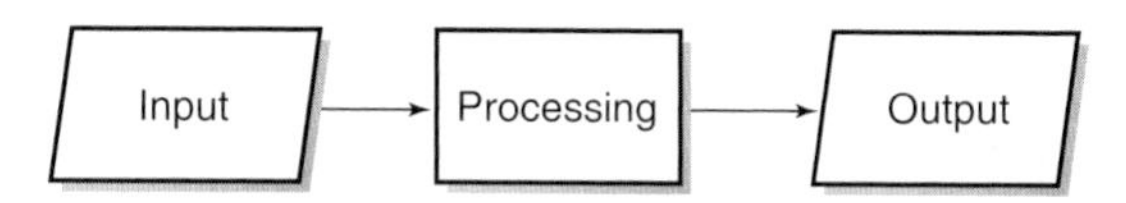

FIGURE 2-2 Computer processing involves input, processing, and output.

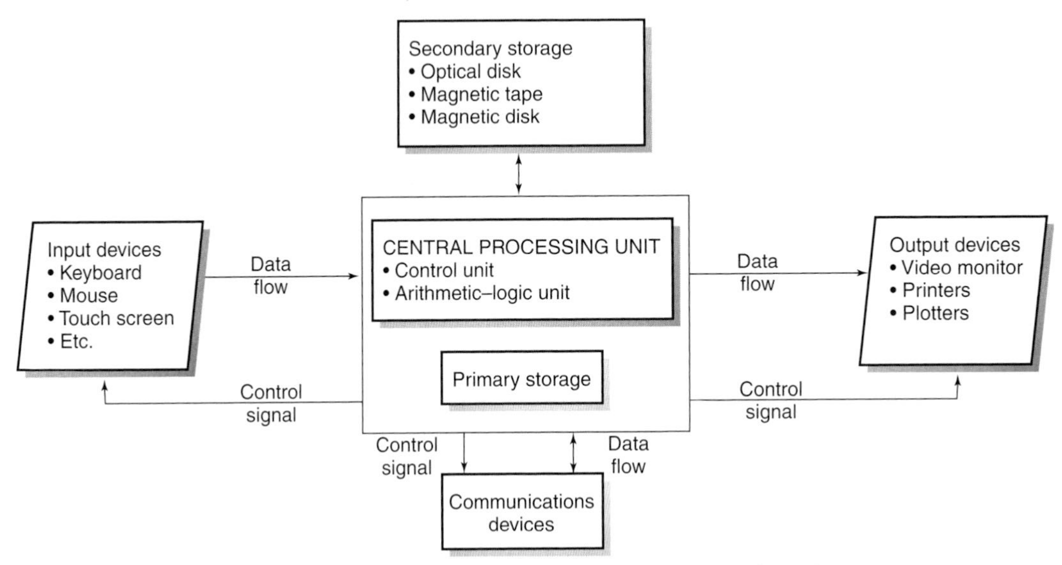

FIGURE 2-3 Organization of the hardware components of a computer.

development tools. *Systems software* refers to programs that start up the computer and coordinate the activities of all hardware components and applications software. *Applications software* refers to programs developed by computer systems users to solve specific problems. Software development tools include computer or programming languages such as BASIC, FORTRAN, COBOL, Pascal, DELPHI, C, and C++. Other tools are now available to simplify and expedite the software development process.

Historical Perspectives

The history of the computer dates back 2000 years to the abacus, a counting machine that is based on sliding beads on wires. In 1642, Blaise Pascal developed the arithmetic machine, and in 1694 Leibnitz developed a calculating machine to solve multiplication and division problems. In 1822, Charles Babbage invented the difference engine to calculate mathematical tables. He subsequently used punch card coding to develop the analytical engine, a machine that could solve mathematical problems automatically. During the United States census of 1890, Herman Hollerith introduced the first electronic tabulator based on punch card operation.

The development of computers progressed rapidly with Howard Aiken's MARK1, a large electromechanical calculator. Eckert and Mauchly's electronic numerical integrator and calculator and electronic variable automatic computer followed this. In 1951 the universal automatic computer became the first commercially available computer.

Today, computers are in their fifth generation. The term *generation* indicates a period of significant technical developments in hardware and software. These developments have been characterized by the following events:

- First-generation computers (1951-1958): The principal features were vacuum tubes used for memory. Punch cards and magnetic tape represented input-output media. These machines were large and slow and required an air-conditioned environment because of the amount of heat produced.
- Second-generation computers (1959-1963): These computers were characterized by solid-state devices such as transistors and magnetic cores used for internal memory. These machines were smaller and more reliable and

generated less heat than did first-generation computers. In addition, they required less power for operation.

- Third-generation computers (1963-1970): This period was marked by the introduction of the integrated circuit etched onto silicon chips. Magnetic disks were used for storage. These machines were smaller than second-generation computers and performed with greater speed and reliability. Major features included multiprocessing and the rapid evolution of systems and applications software.
- Fourth-generation computers (1971-1987): These computers were based on large-scale integration in which thousands of integrated circuits were set on a chip. The microprocessor was introduced in 1971.
- Fifth-generation computers: The Japanese labeled these computers as "intelligent" and subsequently applications were developed to have computers mimic human intelligence, something referred to as artificial intelligence (AI). AI includes a number of areas such as expert systems (the computer acts as an expert of a certain topic), natural language ("...the study of the person/computer interaction in unconstrained native language"), robotics ("computer-controlled machines with electronic capabilities for vision, speech, and touch"), and problem solving (Capron, 2005).

As noted by Capron (2005), "...the true focus of this ongoing fifth generation is connectivity, the massive industry effort to permit users to connect their computers to other computers. The concept of the information superhighway has captured the imaginations of both computer professionals and everyday computer users."

Classification

Computers are classified according to their processing capabilities, storage capacity, size, and cost. At present, computers are grouped in four main classes: supercomputers, mainframe computers, minicomputers, and microcomputers.

Supercomputers such as the CRAY-2 and the Blue Horizon supercomputer (IBM) are large, high-capacity computers that can process data at extremely high speeds. They are used in oil exploration studies, weather forecasts, research (especially in weapons), and scientific modeling.

Mainframe computers such as the IBM 3090/600 E are large, high-level computers capable of rigorous computations at high speeds. They have large primary memories and can support many pieces of peripheral equipment such as terminals, which enable multiple users to access the primary memory. Organizations such as banks, universities and colleges, large businesses, and governments use mainframe computers.

Midrange computers were once referred to as minicomputers, an old term that has been defined as "a mid-level computer built to perform complex computations while dealing efficiently with a high level of input and output from users connected via terminals (Microsoft, 2002). Midrange computers are also frequently connected to other midrange computers on a network and distribute processing among other computers such as personal computers (PCs). Midrange computers are used in CT and MRI.

Microcomputers, or PCs, are small digital computers available in a variety of sizes such as laptops or palmtops (notebooks). One category of microcomputers is the workstation, an upper-end PC. Workstations are now commonplace in radiology and are used in several digital imaging modalities including CT and MRI.

Microcomputers can be built with all circuitry on a single chip or on multiple circuit boards. A central feature is a microprocessor (Fig. 2-4). The microprocessor is a digital integrated circuit that processes data and controls the general workings of the microcomputer (Capron, 2005). Its processing capability is related to the number of bits, which are binary digits (0 and 1) used to represent data. A microprocessor can be either an eight-bit processor that represents 256 (2^8) numbers or a 16-bit processor that represents 65,536 (2^{16}) numbers. The 16-bit microprocessor therefore can process more data faster than an

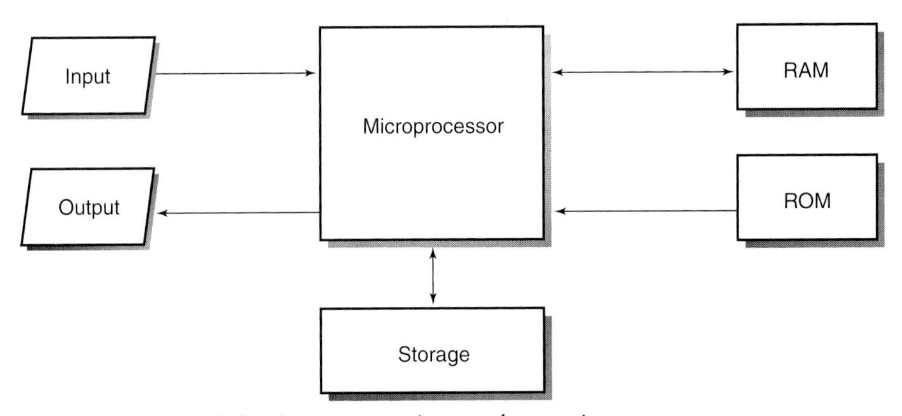

FIGURE 2-4 A microprocessor is central to a microcomputer system.

eight-bit microprocessor. Today, 32-bit microprocessors are available for specialized and dedicated applications. This information provides a rationale for why it is important for technologists to have a basic understanding of digital fundamentals, which will be covered later in this chapter.

COMPUTER ARCHITECTURES AND PROCESSING CAPABILITIES

Computer architecture refers to the general structure of a computer and includes both the elements of hardware and software. Specifically, it refers to computer systems, computer chips, circuitry, and systems software.

Types

Essentially, the two types of CPU architectures are complex instruction set computing (CISC) architecture and reduced instruction set computing (RISC) architecture. The CISC microprocessor design has more built-in operations compared with the RISC microprocessor design. Computers with CISC architecture include the IBM 3090 mainframe computer and nearly all microcomputers. Computers with RISC architecture are the IBM 6000, Sun Microsystems SPARC, and Motorola 88000. According to Covington (1991), "RISC is faster if memory is relatively fast so that no time is wasted fetching instructions. CISC is faster if memory is relatively slow because the same work can be done without fetching as many instruction codes."

These architectures are capable of processing operations such as serial or sequential processing, distributed processing, multiprocessing, multitasking, parallel processing, and pipelining. CT technologists should understand the meaning of these terms because they are used in the CT literature and manufacturers' brochures.

Terminology

Serial or sequential processing: Information (data and instructions) is processed in the order in which items are entered and stored in the computer. It is a simple form of processing data, one instruction at a time. The following definitions are taken from the most recent edition of the Microsoft Computer Dictionary, published by Microsoft Press.

Distributed processing: The information is processed by several computers connected by a network. True distributed processing "has separate computers that perform different tasks in such a way that their combined work can contribute to a larger goal....It requires a highly structured environment that allows hardware and software to communicate, share resources, and exchange information freely."

Multitasking: The computer works on more than one task at a time.

Multiprocessing: Multiprocessing uses two or more connected processing units. "In multiprocessing, each processing unit works on a different set of instructions (or on different parts of the same process). The objective is increased speed or computing power, the same as in parallel processing, and the use of special units called *co-processors.*"

Parallel Processing: This is a "method of processing that can run only on a type of computer containing two or more processors running simultaneously. Parallel processing differs from multiprocessing in the way a task is distributed over the available processors; in multiprocessing, a process might be divided up into sequential blocks, with one processor managing access to a database, another analyzing the data, and a third handling graphical output to the screen." A number of processes can be carried out at the same time.

Pipelining: A "method of fetching and decoding instructions in which, at any given time, several program instructions are in various stages of being fetched or decoded. Ideally, pipelining speeds execution time by ensuring that the microprocessor does not have to wait for instructions; when it completes execution of one instruction, the next is ready and waiting....In parallel processing, *pipelining* can also refer to a method in which instructions are passed from one processing unit to another, as on an assembly line, and each unit is specialized for performing a particular type of operation."

DIGITAL FUNDAMENTALS

The two main types of computers are digital and analog. Digital computers operate on digital data (discrete units), and analog computers operate on continuous physical quantities that are not digital but may have any value on a continuously variable scale (analog signals). Analog signals involve physical quantities such as electrical signals (voltage), speed, pressure, temperature, and displacement. An example of an analog computer is the slide rule, which compares the length on the rule and the logarithm of a number.

Digital computers are the most common type of computers; they operate on digital data through arithmetical and logical operations. Because the digital computer is used in all radiology applications, an understanding of the binary number system is important. This will provide a better insight on how computers work.

Binary Number System

An understanding of the decimal number system is necessary to then understand the binary number system. The decimal number system has a base 10, in which 10 values are represented as 0 through 9. Any decimal number can be written as a sum of these digits multiplied by a power of 10. For example, the number 321 can be written as follows:

$$(1 \times 10^0) + (2 \times 10^1) + (3 \times 10^2) = 321 =$$
$$(1 \times 1) + (2 \times 10) + (3 \times 100) = 321 =$$
$$1 + 20 + 300 = 321$$

The number 321 is thus formed from units (1), tens (20), and hundreds (300).

In the decimal system, any number can be expressed as units, tens, hundreds, thousands, tens of thousands, hundreds of thousands, millions, tens of millions, hundreds of millions, and so on. These are referred to as *powers of 10* and can be written as follows:

$$1 \times 10^0 = 1$$
$$1 \times 10^1 = 10$$
$$1 \times 10^2 = 100$$
$$1 \times 10^3 = 1000$$
$$1 \times 10^4 = 10{,}000$$
$$1 \times 10^5 = 100{,}000$$
$$1 \times 10^6 = 1{,}000{,}000$$

The binary number system, on the other hand, has a base 2, in which only two values, 0 and 1, are represented. A binary number can be 0, 1, a string of 0s, a string of 1s, or a string of 0s and 1s.

The conversion of the decimal numbers to binary numbers and binary numbers to decimal numbers is not within the scope of this chapter. The interested student should refer to any good computer textbook for an understanding of this process.

Other Number Systems

Binary numbers can become very long. For example, the binary number for 1025 is 1000000001. Because this can be time consuming with long numbers, other number systems have been developed, such as the octal and hexadecimal systems. In the octal system, groups of three binary digits are represented by one octal digit. The base of the octal system is 8, in which eight digits are represented by 0, 1, 2, 3, 4, 5, 6, and 7.

The hexadecimal system uses four binary digits (bits) to represent one hexadecimal digit, and the base is 16 in which the 16 digits are represented by 0, 1, 2, 3, 4, 5, 6, 7, 8, 9, 10, 11, 12, 13, 14, and 15. In this case the first 10 digits are represented by 0, 1, 2, 3, 4, 5, 6, 7, 8, and 9; and 10, 11, 12, 13, 14, and 15 are represented by the first six letters of the alphabet, A, B, C, D, E, and F, respectively.

Terminology

A binary digit, or a bit, is a single binary number. In computing, the grouping of bits is as follows:

4 binary bits (0.5 byte) = nibble
8 binary bits (1 byte) = byte
16 binary bits (2 bytes) = word
32 binary bits (4 bytes) = double word

Because binary numbers can be long, they are combined into groups of eight bits called *bytes*. A byte represents one addressable location in memory. Memory capacity is therefore measured in bytes, where

1 thousand bytes = 1 kilobyte (K or KB)
1 million bytes = 1 megabyte (MB)
1 billion bytes = 1 gigabyte (GB)
1 trillion bytes = 1 terabyte (TB)

Binary Coding Schemes

People enter information into a computer for processing in the form of characters (e.g., A, B, C), numbers (e.g., 1, 2, 3), or special characters (e.g., $, *, :, ;). These characters must be represented in binary code. Two popular binary coding schemes are extended binary coded decimal interchange code (EBCDIC) and American standard code for information interchange (ASCII) (Table 2-1). Although EBCDIC, developed by IBM, is the industry standard for minicomputers and mainframe computers, ASCII is widely used by microcomputers. When a character is entered into the computer, it is automatically converted into the ASCII or EBCDIC binary code, depending on the computer system.

Elements of a Digital Signal Processor

Information is entered into a computer in analog form. If the computer is an analog computer, then the results of processing are also analog. In this case, both the input and output are in analog form. However, if the computer is a digital computer and

TABLE 2-1 ASCII and EBCDIC Binary Coding Schemes for 12 Characters

	CODING SCHEME	
Character	**ASCII**	**EBCDIC**
A	0100 0001	1100 0001
B	0100 0010	1100 0010
C	0100 0011	1100 0011
D	0100 0100	1100 0100
E	0100 0101	1100 0101
F	0100 0110	1100 0110
1	0011 0000	1111 0000
2	0011 0001	1111 0001
3	0011 0010	1111 0010
4	0011 0011	1111 0100
5	0011 0100	1111 0101
6	0011 0101	1111 0110

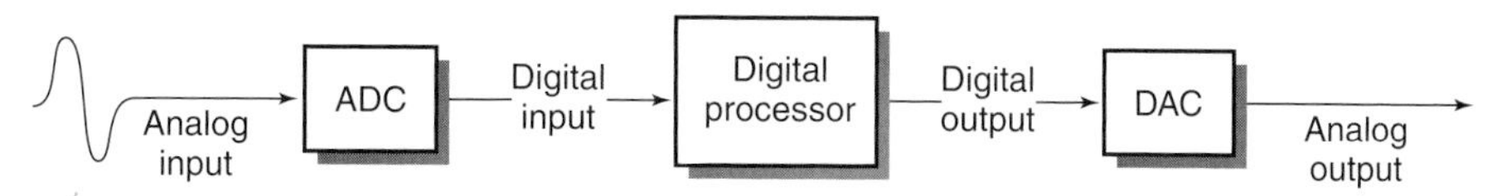

FIGURE 2-5 Elements of a digital signal processor.

the input is analog, an analog-to-digital converter (ADC) is needed to convert the analog input into digital data for processing. The results of digital processing are digital data that can be displayed as such but in most instances would have no meaning to an observer. Therefore an interface such as the digital-to-analog converter (DAC) is needed between the digital processor and the output display device. The ADC and DAC, coupled with a digital processor, constitute a *digital signal processor* (Fig. 2-5).

Analog-to-Digital Conversion

The ADC converts the analog signal into "a sequence of numbers having finite precision" (Proakis, 1992). This procedure is referred to as *analog-to-digital conversion*. The essential parts of an ADC include a sampler, a quantizer, and a coder (Fig. 2-6). These components perform the following three operations: sampling, quantization, and coding.

- *Sampling* is "the conversion of a continuous-time signal into a discrete signal obtained by taking 'samples' of the continuous-time signal at discrete time instants" (Proakis, 1992).
- *Quantization* is "the conversion of a discrete-time, discrete-valued (digital) signal. The value of each signal sample is represented by a value selected from a finite set of possible values" (Proakis, 1992).
- *Coding* is the assignment of a binary bit sequence to each discrete output from the quantizer.

Digital-to-Analog Conversion

The digital signal processor outputs digital data that are subsequently converted into the analog signals needed to operate analog display devices such as television monitors. This conversion requires a DAC, which is made of solid-state electronics that generate an output voltage proportional to the input digital number.

One important characteristic of the DAC is its resolution, that is, how finely an analog voltage may be represented, which is determined by the number of digital bits. For example, an 8-bit DAC outputs 256 (2^8) analog voltage as opposed to a 12-bit DAC, which outputs 4096 (2^{12}) analog voltages and indicates significantly better resolution.

COMPUTER HARDWARE

Input Hardware

In computing, *input* refers to information entered into the computer for processing. The information can be processed immediately or stored (usually on a magnetic medium such as a magnetic tape or disk) for later processing.

Input hardware can be placed in two categories: keyboard and nonkeyboard devices.

Keyboard Devices

A keyboard is a part of a terminal, which is an input-output device with a display screen. A keyboard

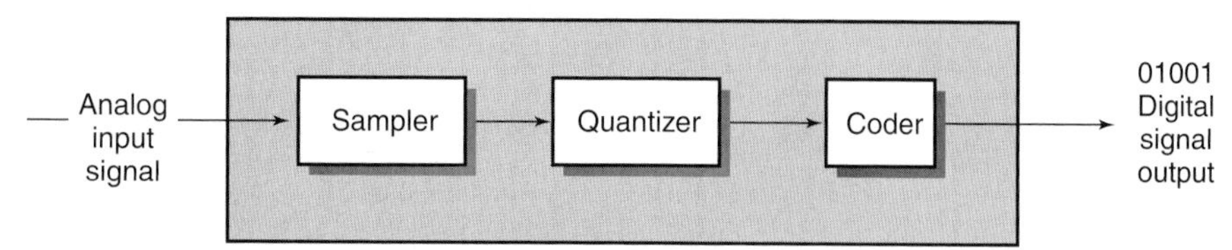

FIGURE 2-6 Essential parts of an ADC.

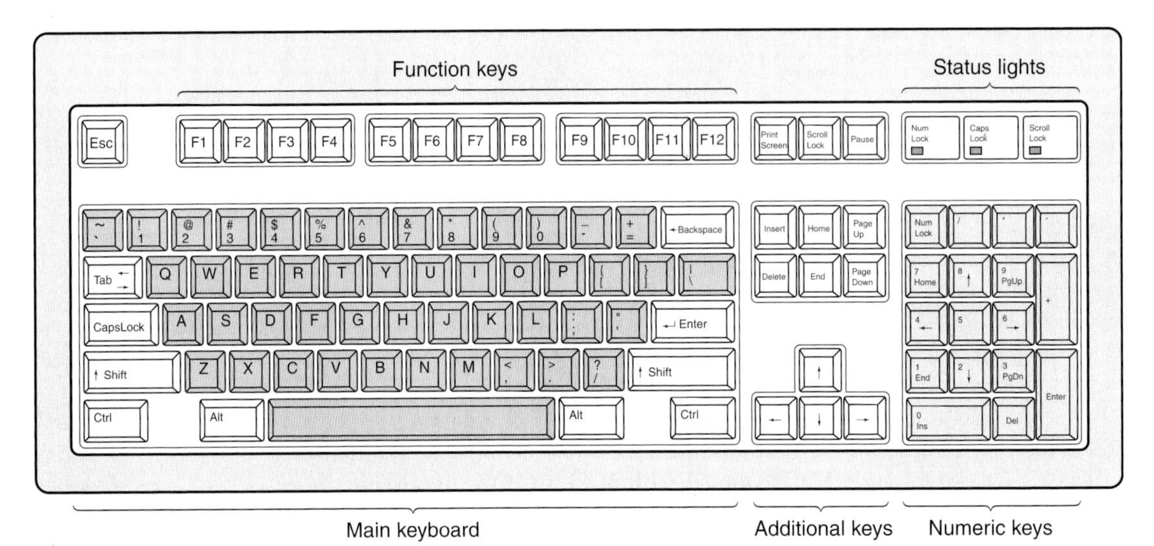

FIGURE 2-7 The main features of a computer keyboard. These include function keys, main keyboard, numerical keys, and additional keys.

is a special electromechanical device that resembles a typewriter keyboard with some additional features. Keyboards are available in different sizes and shapes, but all have at least four common features: (1) regular typewriter keys with alphabet characters, (2) numerical keys (numbers), (3) special function keys called *programmable keys*, and (4) cursor movement keys (Fig. 2-7). When characters are entered from the keyboard, they are converted into binary codes and are then sent to the CPU for processing.

There are three types of terminals, as follows:

1. *Dumb terminals* cannot process information and can only display the input received from the input hardware.
2. *Smart terminals* can process and store information but cannot perform any programming operations.
3. *Intelligent terminals* are microcomputers that can process data and store it internally and externally, and therefore they can carry out programming. Communication is also possible through a communications link (a modem).

Nonkeyboard Devices

Nonkeyboard input devices include pointing devices, scanning devices, and voice input devices. Pointing devices are commonly used because pointing appears to be a basic part of human behavior. These devices include light pens, digitizers, touch screens, and the mouse. Scanning devices include image scanners, fax machines, bar code readers (common in supermarkets), and character and mark recognition devices. Voice input devices change human speech into electrical signals, which can then be digitized for processing. These systems are also referred to as *voice recognition systems* and are an integral part of the digital radiology department (Fig. 2-8).

Input devices play an important role in computer systems, as noted by Stallings et al (1992): "The conversion of data into a computer-usable form is a vital part of a computer-based information system. Input control procedures are needed to safeguard the data's integrity and to ensure the production of complete and accurate information—inother words, to ensure no 'garbage in' to avoid getting 'garbage out.'"

Processing Hardware

Speed and power are two important characteristics of computers. *Speed* refers to how fast the computer processes data. *Power* includes speed and

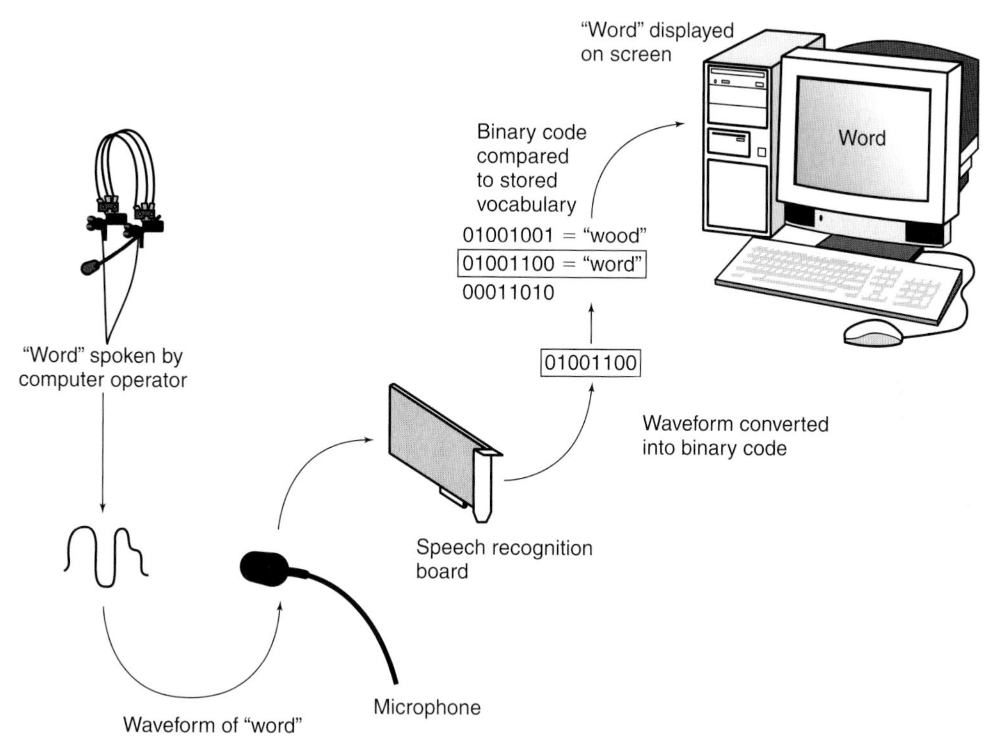

FIGURE 2-8 A voice input device works by translating the sound waves of spoken language into binary numbers that can be interpreted by the computer. If the binary code generated by the speech recognition board finds a match in the computer's stored vocabulary, that vocabulary word is displayed on the screen.

other characteristics such as storage capacity and memory size. Several factors affect the speed of a computer, including microprocessor speed, the bus line size, cache memory, flash memory, RISC architecture, and parallel processing of data.

Microprocessor speeds can range from 1 millisecond (ms = 10^{-3} seconds) to 1 microsecond (μs = 10^{-6} seconds) for early computers to 1 nanosecond (10^{-9} seconds) for modern computers. Research processing speeds continue to approach the picosecond (10^{-12} seconds) range. These speeds are expressed in cycles per second, megahertz (MHz), or gigahertz (GHz = 10^9 cycles per second). Additionally, computer speeds can be expressed in million instructions per second (MIPS) or megaflops (MFLOPs).

The processing hardware or CPU includes the control unit, ALU, registers, and memory (see Fig. 2-3).

The control unit directs the activities of the computer through programs stored in memory. For example, it indicates when information is to be moved from memory to the ALU and which operations the ALU should carry out. In addition, the control unit directs the flow of data from the CPU to the input-output hardware.

The ALU executes arithmetic and logic operations including addition, subtraction, multiplication, division, and comparisons such as "is equal to" (=), "is less than" (<), or "is greater than" (>).

Registers are temporary storage electronic devices. They hold the data for a short period and then send it to internal memory, where it is stored temporarily.

The movement of data among these components is accomplished by the bus or bus line, which provides a path for the flow of electrical signals between units. The amount of data transported at a single moment is called the *bus width*. As noted by Capron (2005), a computer with a larger bus size will be faster because it can transfer more data at one time, will have a larger memory, and can accommodate an increase in the number and variety of instructions.

A computer may have three types of buses: a data bus (data signals), an address bus that sends data from internal memory, and a control bus that sends signals from the control unit.

A major component of processing hardware is primary storage or internal memory, or simply *memory*. Its purpose is to store (1) the information entered into the computer for processing, (2) the program that provides the instructions for processing the input information, and (3) the results of the processing.

Internal memory is available in the form of chips, semiconductor chips, or integrated circuits. This type of memory is volatile, meaning that data are lost when the computer loses its electrical power. One semiconductor design, the complementary metal oxide semiconductor, requires very little power to operate.

There are two basic types of internal memory chips: read-only memory (ROM) and random-access memory (RAM). ROM chips contain data and programs to make the computer hardware work and cannot be changed, erased, or lost when the computer is turned off; RAM chips provide for temporary storage of data and programs that would be lost if the computer loses power. In addition, RAM can be static (SRAM) or dynamic (DRAM). Although SRAM is faster than DRAM, it does not require refreshing of its contents by the CPU, as does DRAM.

Three additional classes of ROM chips are available: programmable read-only memory (PROM), erasable programmable read-only memory (EPROM), and electrically erasable programmable read-only memory (EEPROM). PROM chips allow users to write their own data and programs but not to change or erase these instructions. With EPROM chips, data can be erased with an ultraviolet light after the EPROM chip is removed from the computer. Finally, EEPROM chips use special software that permit data and programs to be changed electronically without removal.

The storage capacity of RAM chips is expressed in megabytes (MB). Computer programs specify the RAM capacity needed for operation.

Two other types of memory are cache memory and flash memory. Cache memory is very fast memory for the storage of information and data that are used most of the time. It can be internal or external and available on separate chips. Flash memory is nonvolatile. Flash memory chips are being developed for computers and already are used in cellular telephones and flight recorders in airplanes.

Output Hardware

After the input data and instructions have been processed by the CPU, the results can be stored permanently or made available as soft copy or hard copy output. *Hard copy* refers to printed output on permanent media, such as paper and film, and *soft copy* refers to output "information that has been produced in a seemingly intangible form" (Stallings et al, 1992).

Hard copy output devices include printers, plotters, camera output microforms such as microfiche and microfilm, and voice output devices. Printers fall into two categories: impact and nonimpact. Impact printers make contact with the paper and include letter quality, dot matrix, and high-speed printers. Nonimpact printers include inkjet, thermal, and laser printers. Plotters produce graphics such as three-dimensional drawings, bar charts (graphs), and maps and are categorized as drum, flat bed, and electrostatic. Drum and flat-bed plotters use pens for drawings, and electrostatic plotters use electrostatic charges on a special paper to produce drawings. Voice output devices are based on prerecorded vocalized sounds, and the computer can output synthesized words in response to certain codes.

Soft copy output hardware is based on video display technology. Two common types of video display devices are the cathode ray tube (CRT) and flat-panel or flat-screen devices.

The CRT consists of an electron gun that directs a stream of electrons to strike a phosphor-coated screen located at the opposite end of the gun. Positioned in front of the screen is a shadow mask, which consists of numerous tiny holes that direct a small part of the beam to strike the screen. Each tiny spot that glows on the screen is called a *picture element*, or pixel. The displayed image on the screen is thus composed of pixels in both the horizontal and the vertical directions. The number of pixels determines the resolution, or sharpness, of the CRT image. In general, the greater the number of pixels (vertical and horizontal), the better the resolution.

Flat-screen output devices are based on flat-screen technologies and were developed primarily for portable computers. Flat-screen display technologies include the liquid crystal display (LCD), electroluminescent (EL) display, and gas plasma display. "LCDs use a clear liquid chemical trapped in tiny pockets between two pieces of glass. Each pocket of liquid is covered both front and back by very thin wires. When a small amount of current is applied to both wires, a chemical reaction turns the chemical a dark color—thereby blocking light. The point of blocked light is the pixel" (Stallings et al, 1992). An EL display panel consists of a phosphor layer that emits light when activated by a current. Two sets of electrodes are arranged with the phosphor layer to form columns and rows. A pixel glows when current flows to the electrodes that address that particular location. The gas plasma display screen is the best of the flat-screen displays. Usually a mixture of argon and neon gases is sandwiched between two glass plates with wire grids. A pixel is displayed when its address location has been charged.

Storage Hardware

Storage hardware devices include magnetic tapes and disks and optical disks. These devices constitute secondary storage (auxiliary storage), which is nonvolatile, as opposed to primary storage, which is volatile.

DATA STORAGE TECHNOLOGIES

Approaches to Secondary Storage

There are generally two approaches to secondary storage of information: the sequential access approach and the direct access method. The sequential or serial access method is analogous to finding a favorite song on an audiotape. In this method, information is stored in a specific sequence, such as alphabetically, and the information is therefore retrieved alphabetically. Tape storage is characteristic of this type of storage.

In the direct or random access method, the desired information is accessed directly, so therefore this method is much faster than sequential access. Disk storage is characteristic of this type of storage.

Magnetic Tape Storage

Magnetic tape storage requires a magnetic tape unit with a magnetic tape drive. Magnetic tape is made of Mylar polyester film (DuPont), a plastic-like material coated with particles that magnetize the tape to record information. The tape is threaded from a supply reel to pass by the read-write head and then moves onto a take-up reel.

The read-write head is a wire wrapped around an iron core with one or more small gaps. When information is recorded onto the tape, the electrical signal passing through the wire produces a varying magnetic field that magnetizes the particles on the tape. The direction of the magnetization on the tape represents binary code. When the tape is played back, the magnetization on the tape results in electrical signals that are sent to a display device or audio speakers. Magnetic tape used in conjunction with minicomputers and mainframes is about ½-inch wide and ½-mile long and can store a wide range of characters (O'Leary et al, 1992).

Magnetic tape streamers, also referred to as *back-up tape cartridge units*, are also available for use with microcomputers. Popular tape cartridges use 0.25-inch wide tape and are available in 1000-foot reels. The data recording method is based on the streaming tape method. According to Stallings et al (1992), "In this method, the data [are] written onto the tape in one continuous stream. There is no starting or stopping, no gaps between blocks (or records) of data being recorded." The amount of data that can be stored on the tape is its *density*, or the number of characters per inch (cpi) or bytes per inch (bpi). Today, digital audio tape drives are available to facilitate back-up storage. These tapes are high-capacity tapes and provide very fast access to the data stored on them.

Magnetic Disk Storage

Magnetic disks include floppy disks and hard disks. Floppy disks are made of flexible Mylar plastic, whereas hard disks are metal platters. Both are coated with magnetizable particles that allow data to be recorded and stored as binary code. Each disk consists of concentric tracks and preshaped sectors. A typical disk includes about 17 sectors per track and 512 bytes (4096 bits) of information per sector. Magnetic disks are random access devices, which means that any sector of the disk can be accessed quickly. The tracks on the disk contain dots, each of which represents a bit. The packing density of a track is about 4000 bits per inch.

Floppy disks or diskettes are available in two sizes: the 3½-inch microfloppy disk and the 5¼-inch minifloppy disk (Fig. 2-9). Both disks are made of Mylar plastic encased in plastic jacket covers. Data are stored and retrieved from these disks by means of the head window, where the read-write head of the disk drive makes contact with the disk. Microfloppy disks are commonly used in computing and can store much more data than minifloppy disks. Currently, two-inch microfloppy disks are available in some electronic cameras and personal computers. Iomega created the Zip drive, which can hold nearly 100-megabyte disks, a capacity about 70 times that of the 3½-inch diskettes.

When data files are too large to fit on these diskettes, compression programs are available to remove certain data without loss. Compression is also important when large data files are transmitted to remote locations.

Hard disks are high-capacity storage disks capable of storing more data than floppy disks. They are available as internal hard disks, hard disk cartridges, or hard disk packs. Internal hard disks consist of one or more metal platters positioned in a sealed container that also houses the read-write head. These common disk units are known as *Winchester disks*. Although internal hard disks have a fixed storage capacity, hard disk cartridges are self-contained and can be easily removed from their drives. In addition, they facilitate the storage of an unlimited amount of data. Hard disk packs have several stacked platters with read-write heads positioned so that as one head reads the underside of the disk above it, the other reads the surface of the disk below it. Hard disks are hermetically sealed to prevent smoke, dust, or other particles from entering the container. These particles may cause a head crash, in which case data are lost.

Redundant Array of Independent Disks

Safety is one problem of data and information storage on single disk systems. The redundant array of independent disks (RAID) system overcomes this problem through the use of hard disk technology.

There are several levels of RAID organization (Fig. 2-10). The first level uses disk mirroring in

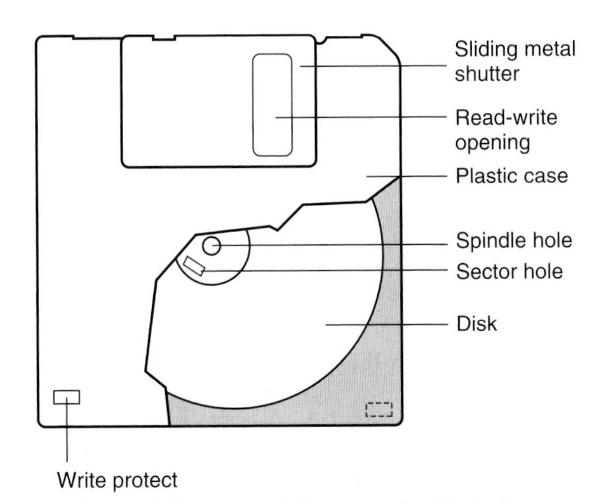

FIGURE 2-9 The external features of a 3½-inch microfloppy disk.

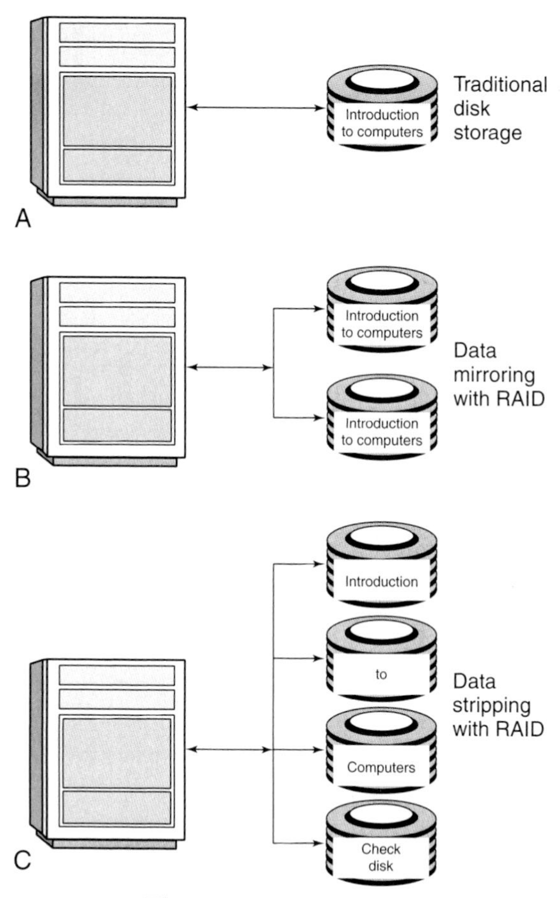

FIGURE 2-10 The concept of RAID storage compared with traditional storage. (From Capron HL: *Computers: tools for an information age*, Upper Saddle River, NJ, 2004, Prentice Hall.)

which data are copied onto another set of disks (Fig. 2-10, *B*). Should one disk fail in this situation, the data are not lost because they are stored on the other disk system. Another level uses data stripping (Fig. 2-10, *C*). The data are now distributed across several disks "with one disk used solely as a check disk, to keep track of what data is where. If a disk fails, the check disk can reconstitute the data" (Capron, 2005). RAID is now common in the digital imaging department, where vast amounts of data from several imaging modalities are stored in a safe and secure environment.

Optical Disk Storage

The most recent storage technology is optical storage, which is based on the use of optical rather than magnetic technology. It is a technology in which stored data are read by optical means.

Optical disk storage involves the use of a laser beam (e.g., from a helium-neon laser) to write the data on the surface of a metallic disk. The laser beam is tightly focused to form a spot of light, or the optical stylus, which burns tiny pits onto the concentric tracks (rings) on the disk to write data. The laser beam scans the pits, which reflect light from the disk to a photodetector to read data. The output electrical signal from the detector depends on the geometry and distribution of the pits.

Optical disks are available in diameters of 3½, 4¾, 5¼, 8, 12, and 14 inches. Three types of optical disks are available: compact disc; read-only memory (CD-ROM); write once, read many (WORM); and erasable optical disks. Information can only be read from a CD-ROM by optical means and cannot be recorded or erased. WORM optical disks can write data once to be read multiple times but not erased, which makes this disk suitable for information archives.

Erasable optical disks are made of magneto-optical materials (e.g., gadolinium, terbium, or iron). To write data on the disk, a focused laser beam heats a small region of magnetized ferromagnetic film and causes it to lose its magnetization. The region becomes magnetized in the opposite direction during cooling and in the presence of a magnetic field. In addition, the power of the laser used to write the data is much greater than that used to read the data, which ensures that stored data are not destroyed.

Storage Capacity

The storage capacity of the different storage devices is determined by the number of bytes that the device can hold. Storage capacities are expressed in kilobytes (K), MB, gigabytes (GB), and terabytes (TB). For example, secondary storage capacities for desktop microcomputers are now in the GB range.

COMPUTER SOFTWARE

Programming

The programmer follows a six-step developmental procedure for programming: (1) define the problem, (2) make or buy the decision, (3) design the program, (4) code the program, (5) debug the program, and (6) document (Fig. 2-11). Step 3 deserves a brief description. Programming techniques such as top-down program design, pseudocode, flow charting, and logic structures are used to arrive at a solution. Although the first two techniques concern major processing steps and a story or narrative of the program logic, respectively, flow charting involves the use of graphical symbols to indicate the sequence of operations needed to solve the problem. The program flow chart includes at least three logic structures: sequence (a program statement), decision, and a loop (the repetition of a process when the condition is true).

The program is coded or written in a programming language available to the computer system. Five generations of programming languages are now available, as follows (see following box):

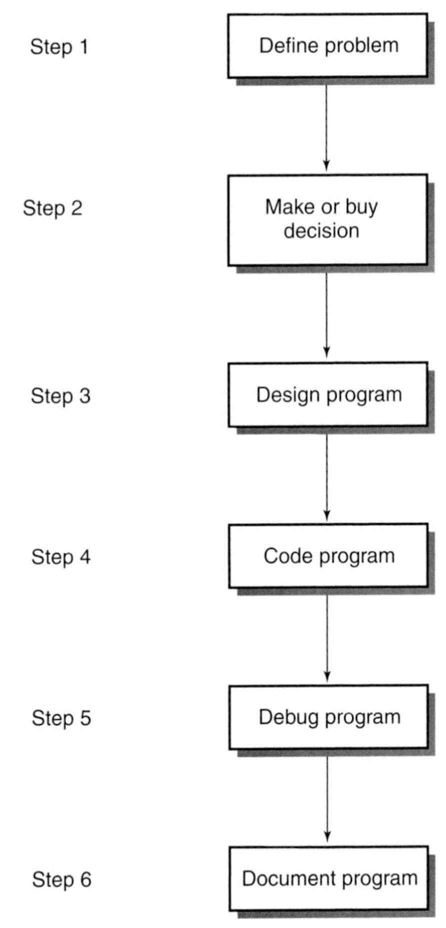

FIGURE 2-11 The programming procedure involves at least six steps.

Programming Languages

Machine—first generation (least advanced)
Assembly—second generation
Procedural—third generation
Problem oriented—fourth generation
Natural—fifth generation (most advanced)

Machine language, or machine code, is the only language that a computer can understand. It is a low-level language based on sequences of 0s and 1s, which can be represented by on (1) and off (0) switches.

Assembly language is another low-level language that uses abbreviations to develop the program. These must subsequently be converted into machine code with a special program called an *assembler*.

Procedural languages are considered high-level languages because they are similar to human languages (see following box). According to O'Leary (1992), procedural languages are so named because "they are designed to express the logic—the procedures—that can solve general problems." Procedural languages include BASIC, COBOL, and FORTRAN, which must be converted into machine code that the computer can process. This conversion is

Procedural Languages

BASIC (beginners' all-purpose symbolic instruction code)—developed in the mid 1960s at Dartmouth College; common in microcomputing
COBOL (common business-oriented language)—a language common to business applications
FORTRAN (formula translation)—developed 1954-1958; a compiled structured language; used specifically for scientific and engineering applications
Pascal—a popular language for use in microcomputing, developed by Niklaus Wirth (1967-1971); a compiled structured language
C—popular for microcomputers; a compiled language developed by Dennis Ritchie at Bell Laboratories in 1972

accomplished by either a compiler or an interpreter. A compiler converts the programmer's procedural language program, or source code, into a machine language code called the *object code*. This object code can then be saved and run later.

Problem-oriented languages were developed to simplify the programming process and are intended for use in specific applications. Examples are dBASE and Lotus 1-2-3.

Natural languages are the highest level of programmable languages. These are fifth-generation languages such as Clout and Intellect. The goal of these languages is to resemble human speech. Natural language is now applied to expert systems and artificial intelligence applications.

Applications Software

Applications software refers to programs developed to perform specific types of work such as the creation of text and images, manipulation of words and numbers, or communication of information. Five general-purpose applications programs are common. These are intended for word processing, spreadsheets, graphics, database management, and communications. If all these applications programs are available in one package, the package is referred to as *integrated software*. Examples include Microsoft Works, First Choice, Framework, and Symphony.

Systems Software

An operating system (OS) is a program that controls "the allocation and usage of computer hardware resources such as memory, central processing unit (CPU) time, disk space, and peripheral devices" (see box below) (Microsoft, 2002). *Systems software* are programs and data that comprise and relate to the OS. Systems software include at least four types of programs: (1) a bootstrap loader, (2) diagnostic routines, (3) input-output system programs, and (4) the OS.

The *bootstrap loader* is a program stored in ROM that starts up the computer and loads the OS into primary memory. Diagnostic routines ensure the CPU, primary memory, and other internal hardware are in proper working order. In addition, input-output system programs interpret and input characters and send these characters to output devices. The OS performs system initialization, memory and file management, and input-output control. It also facilitates multitasking and multiprocessing, depending on its capabilities.

Major Operating Systems

- Apple DOS—Apple Disk Operating System
- CP/M—Control Program/Microcomputers
- MS-DOS—Microsoft Disk Operating System
- Mac OS—operating system (for Macintosh computers only)
- OS/2—operating system for microcomputers and networking
- UNIX—a portable operating system that can be shared by several users simultaneously

Software Interfacing

As defined in the *Microsoft Press Computer Dictionary* (2002), an *interface* is the point at which a connection is made between two elements so that they can work together.

Software provides the connection between computer users. Essentially, there are three types of software interfaces: command driven, menu driven, and graphical interfaces. A command-driven interface is characteristic of command-driven programs, which require the user to type in commands from the computer console to initiate the operation of the system. The user must therefore learn and remember a set of commands for various programs. For example, the command *DIR*, or *dir*, enables the user of an IBM or IBM-compatible microcomputer to look at the system's directory.

Menu-driven programs use menu-driven interfaces that allow the user to select commands from a displayed list, menu list, displayed bar, or menu bar. This makes it easier for people to use the system because they do not have to remember numerous commands. In this respect, menu-driven programs are considered user friendly and easier to learn than are command-driven programs.

A graphical user interface enables the user to choose commands, start programs, and see lists of files and other options by pointing to pictorial representations (icons) and lists of menu items on the screen. The concept of a graphical interface was developed at Xerox (Palo Alto Research Center) and originally used by Apple to develop the Macintosh operating system (Arnold, 1991). It is also available for IBM microcomputers as Microsoft Windows or Windows.

Windows can be found on most personal computers. Two important characteristics of Windows are its (1) plug-and-play technology and (2) object-linking and embedding technology. Plug-and-play enables the computer to automatically configure itself when anything new is added; object linking and embedding allows the user to link or embed documents.

Windows NT is noted for its stability and is best suited to networked environments, making it a candidate for use in the digital radiology department. Windows NT is already used in several workstations for medical imaging.

DATA COMMUNICATIONS

Data Transmission Media

Data communications involves the transmission of data from one location to another through the use of pathways. These pathways are referred to as *transmission media* or *channels* and include telephone lines, coaxial cables, microwaves, satellites and radio waves, and optical fibers.

The choice of communication channel depends on several factors, of which data transmission speed is relatively important. Data transmission speed is influenced by the baud rate and the bandwidth of the communications channel (Arnold, 1991). The *baud rate* refers to the number of discrete signal elements (bauds) transmitted per second. The *bandwidth* refers to the frequency capacity of the channel and is expressed in bits per second (bps) (Arnold, 1991). There are essentially three types of bandwidths: voice band (e.g., a telephone line), which can transmit about 110 to 9600 bps; medium band, which can transmit 9600 to 256,000 bps; and broad band (e.g., coaxial cable, fiberoptics, and microwave), which can transmit 256,000 to 1,000,000 bps.

Data Communications Hardware

A typical data communications scheme sends data from computer A to computer B through the telephone line (Fig. 2-12). The modem modulates, or converts digital data to analog signals, and demodulates, or converts analog signals to digital data; both signals are to be transmitted and received.

Other hardware components include multiplexers, concentrators, controllers, and front-end

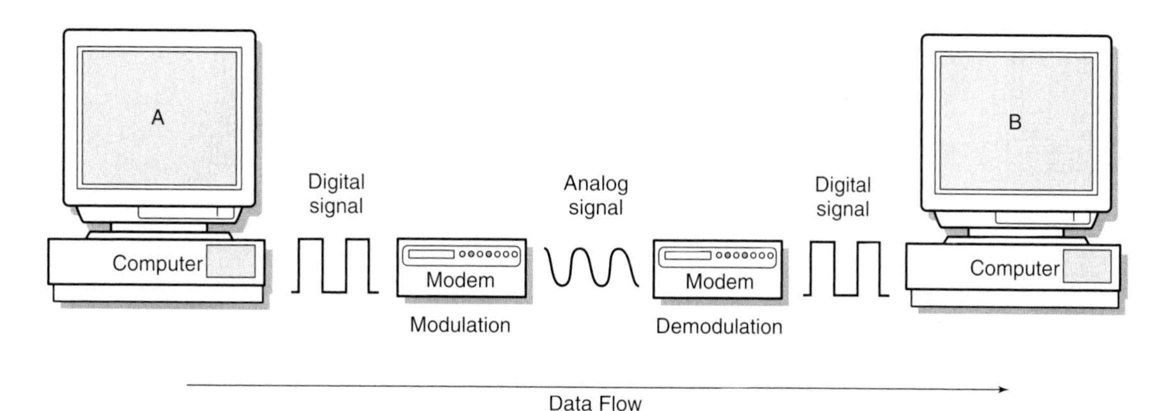

FIGURE 2-12 Typical scheme for data communication using computers.

processors. A multiplexer allows several computers to share a single communications line. A concentrator allows many devices to share a single communications line and is more "intelligent" than a multiplexer because it can store and forward transmissions (Capron, 2005). A controller supports a group of devices such as terminals and printers connected to a computer (Capron, 2005). A front-end processor is a small computer that performs several data management and communications functions, thus relieving the host or main computer of these processing tasks. Telephone companies are now replacing analog phone networks with integrated services digital networks (ISDN), which can handle data communications and also allow audio and video signals to be transmitted simultaneously over cable.

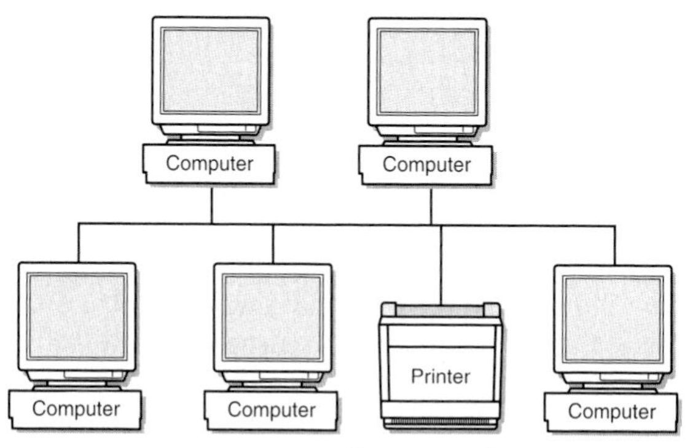

FIGURE 2-13 Bus network.

Network Topologies

There are four network topologies or configurations: bus, star, ring, and hierarchical. In a bus network (Fig. 2-13), devices such as computers and printers are connected so that each is responsible for its own communications control. The bus cable connects the devices, and there is no host computer or file server. The star network (Fig. 2-14) is characterized by a host computer or file server to which several computers are connected. In a ring network topology, the devices (mostly mainframes) are connected to form a ring without a host computer or file server (Fig. 2-15). The hierarchical network (Fig. 2-16) consists of a central host computer to which other computers are connected. These computers then serve as hosts to several smaller machines. In a typical system, a host computer represents a mainframe that plays host to two minicomputers, which in turn play host to several microcomputers (Capron, 2005; Davidson-Shivers and Rasmussen, 2006).

When computers and other hardware located in the same building are linked through a topology, they create a local area network (LAN) (Fig. 2-17). Figure 2-17 also includes a network gateway that allows the LAN to be connected to other LANs. If the LANs are connected across a region or city, a metropolitan area network (MAN) is created. Similarly, a wide area network (WAN) is created

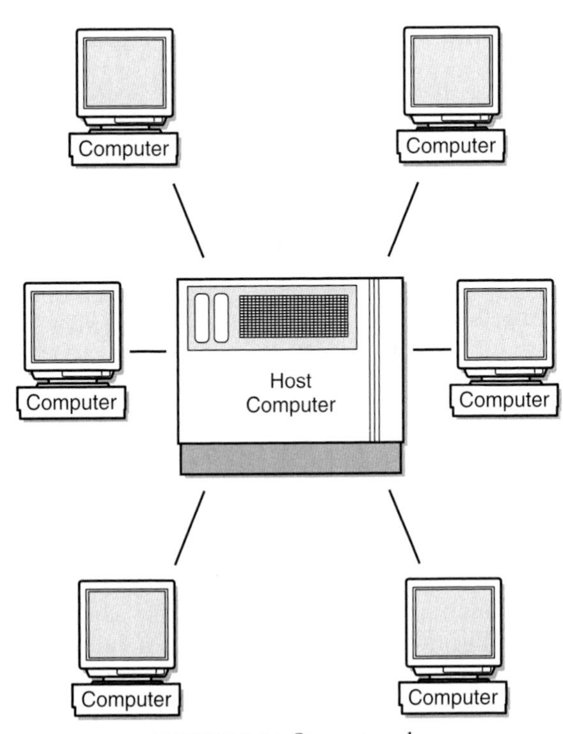

FIGURE 2-14 Star network.

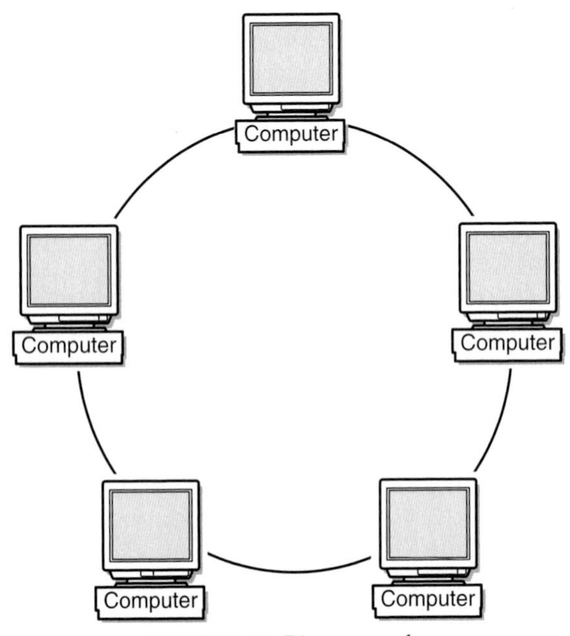

FIGURE 2-15 Ring network.

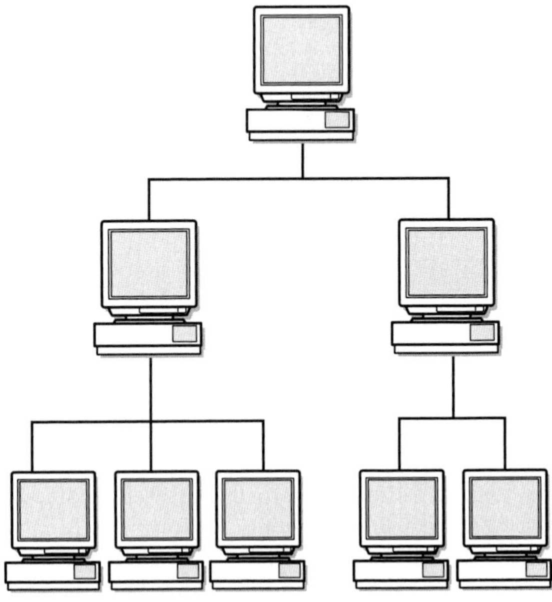

FIGURE 2-16 Hierarchical network.

when computers are connected across the country (Davidson-Shivers and Rasmussen, 2006).

LANs, MANs, and WANs require a technology that allows fast communication of the signals. One such technology common to LANs is Ethernet. Ethernet is based on a bus topology in which computers share the same cable to send data. Other technologies include Bitnet and Internet, which are characteristic of WANs.

THE INTERNET

History

The Internet is the largest computer network system in existence because it connects users all over the world (Davidson-Shivers and Rasmussen, 2006). Concern that a single bomb could destroy the computing facilities of the U.S. Department of Defense led to the creation and development of the Internet in 1959. Efforts were made to rely on one computer system at a single

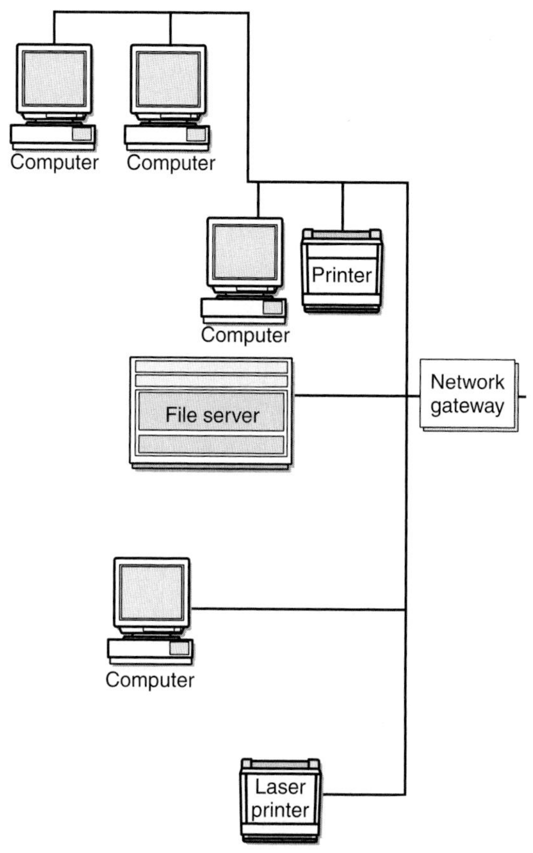

FIGURE 2-17 LAN with a bus topology. The network gateway allows the network to connect to other networks.

location and a large number of computers at remote locations. Communications between these computers breaks down messages into packets, each of which has a specific destination address and is subsequently reassembled when it arrives at its destination address. Software was then developed to facilitate the communication process. This software is referred to as *transmission control protocol/Internet protocol* (TCP/IP). TCP manages the packets and their reassembly, and the IP component ensures the packets arrive at their appropriate remote computers.

In 1990, Dr. Berners-Lee developed the worldwide web (www) to facilitate communications with remote computers through a set of links. (The name *web* refers to his vision of these links as a spider's web.) Dr. Berners-Lee's goal was to communicate more easily with his colleagues by linking with their computers.

Major Components

The Internet user must first access a server computer called the *Internet service provider* (ISP) by a phone line or a direct cable connection. The server computer relays the user's message to the Internet. Finally, the Internet returns electronic mail (e-mail) or requested information to the user through the ISP server (Fig. 2-18).

A web browser allows the user to use a mouse to point and click on text, drawings, and pictures to facilitate an Internet search. Two popular browsers are Netscape and Internet Explorer. Websites can be located with a uniform resource locator (URL) that must conform to a specific format to ensure successful communications (Davidson-Shivers and Rasmussen, 2006). The URL is the address of the site or file on the Internet. An example of a URL is as follows:

http://www.med.harvard.edu/AANLIB/
home.html

The parts of the URL that enable users to access a web page or file include the protocol for communicating links (http://[hypertext transfer protocol]), the ISP address or domain name (www.med.harvard.edu), and the final portion of the domain name, or top-level domain, which demonstrates the type and purpose of the organization. In the above URL, *edu* indicates an educational institution. The URL ends with path, directory, and file name (AANLIB/home.html). This site features "The Whole Brain Atlas."

The Internet also features search engines to help users find information in a systematic and organized manner. These are "software programs that assist users in connecting to databases of Web addresses (uniform resource locators, or URLs and that help users locate information on the

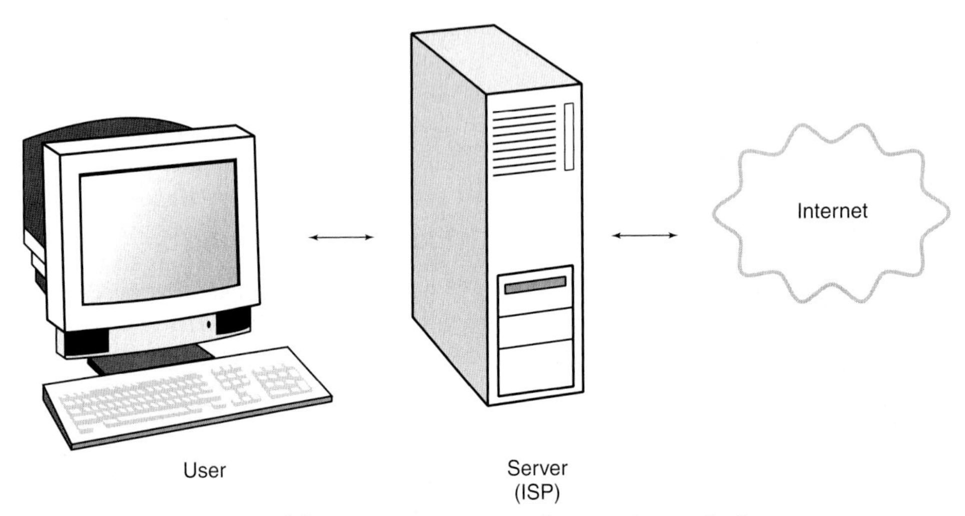

FIGURE 2-18 The major components of connecting to the Internet.

Web and Internet....Search engines, therefore, can in turn provide large numbers of pages (called *hits*) in response to a single search in both text and graphical formats" (Davidson-Shivers and Rasmussen, 2006). Examples of search engines include the popular Google, Alta Vista, Lycos, Yahoo!, Excite, Infoseek, HotBot, Northern Light, and WebCrawler (Davidson-Shivers and Rasmussen, 2006).

To access a search engine, computer users must have the capability of being able to connect to the worldwide web. This connection is facilitated via a browser, popularly referred to as a web browser, such as Netscape *Navigator*, Microsoft *Internet Explorer*, and Apple *Safari*, to mention the more popular ones.

CT AND PICTURE ARCHIVING AND COMMUNICATIONS SYSTEMS

The CT scanner is now connected to the PACS and for this reason a brief overview of PACS is worthwhile here.

Picture Archiving and Communications Systems: A Definition

What is PACS exactly? Some researchers believe that perhaps it should be called IMACS (image management and communication systems); however, the more popular acronym is PACS.

There are several comprehensive definitions of PACS. One such definition, for example, is "...PACS refer to a computer system that is used to capture, store, distribute, and then display medical images. For diagnostic imaging applications, PACS technology can be utilized to achieve near filmless operation" (Siegel, and Reiner, 2002).

A more detailed definition as provided by Arenson et al (2000) is that PACS "...are a collection of technologies used to carry out digital medical imaging. PACS are used to digitally acquire medical images from various modalities such as CT, MRI, Ultrasound (US), Nuclear Medicine (NM), and digital projection radiography. The image data and pertinent information are transmitted to other and possibly remote locations over network, where they can be displayed on computer workstations for soft-copy viewing in multiple locations simultaneously.

Data are secured and archived on digital media such as optical disks or tape and can be automatically retrieved as necessary."

Basically, the two definitions convey the same notion and meaning of PACS except that the second one offers a more detailed picture of PACS.

Picture Archiving and Communications Systems: Major Components

The major components of a PACS and their functional relationships are shown in Figure 2-19. These include digital image acquisition modalities, network switches, PACS controller (as it is often referred to) that includes a database/image server, archive server, short- and long-term archives, RIS/PACS broker, web server, primary and secondary image displays, printer, web-based clinical review, all connected by computer networks. To extend its functionality and usefulness, the PACS is integrated with the RIS and HIS again through computer communication networks. Note that the devices within the PACS communicate with each other, whereas the PACS is integrated with the RIS/HIS. This communication and integration requires the use of communication protocol standards. In this regard, two *communication protocol standards* are now commonplace in the digital radiology environment.

Communication Protocol Standards

Connectivity refers to a measure of the effectiveness and efficiency of computers and computer-based devices to communicate and share information

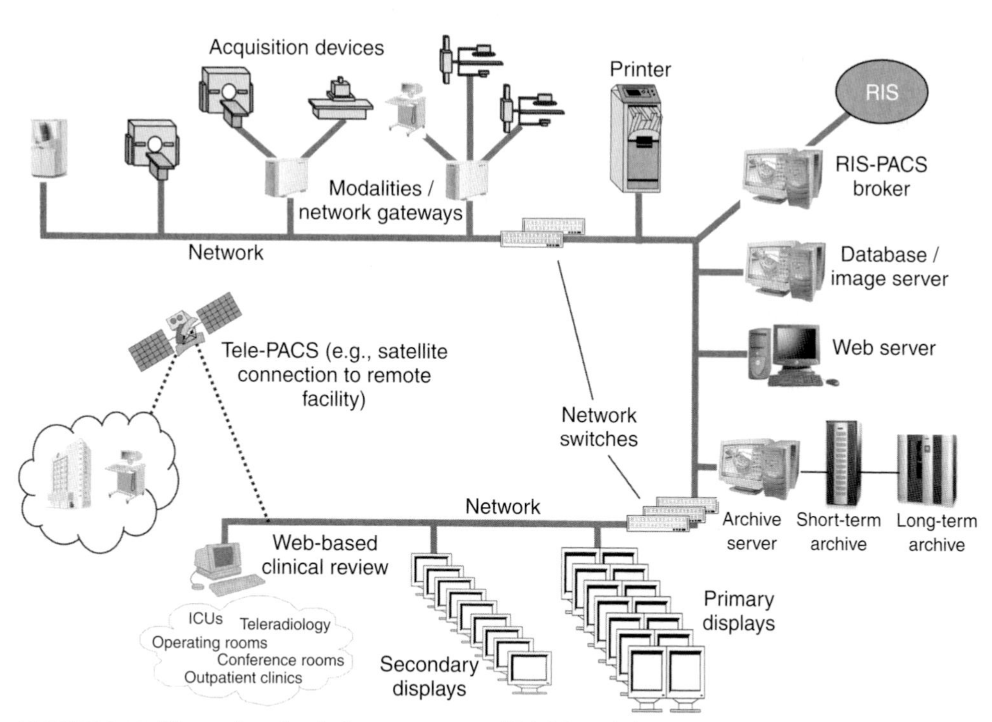

FIGURE 2-19 The major physical components of PACS and their functional relationships. (From Samei E et al: PACS equipment overview general guidelines for purchasing and acceptance testing of PACS equipment, *Radiographics* 24:313-334, 2004. Reproduced by permission.)

and messages without human intervention (Capron, 2005; Davidson-Shivers and Rasmussen, 2006; Laudon, 1994).

The use of communication protocol standards is integral to achieving connectivity. Although a *protocol* deals with the specifics of how a certain task will be done, a *standard* is an "approved reference model and protocol determined by standard-setting groups for building or developing products and services" (Laudon, 1994).

In health care, HIS, RIS, and PACS, integration is based on different communication protocol standards. Two such popular standards are health level 7 (HL-7) and digital imaging and communications in medicine (DICOM). HL-7 is the standard application protocol for use in most HIS and RIS; DICOM is the imaging communication protocol for PACS (Creighton, 1999). DICOM was developed by the American College of Radiology and the National Electrical Manufacturers Association. Of course in a PACS environment DICOM conformance is mandatory. In a CT-PACS environment, certain DICOM standards are applicable to CT. Some examples of these include storage service class, query and retrieve, print, HIS/RIS, and worklist.

Essential features of an image management and archiving system that is compliant with DICOM and compatible with HIS and RIS include examination acquisition (acquisition of patient demographics) and image acquisition; workflow management; diagnostic, clinical, and enterprise display; and hard copy output. The enterprise display component allows users to view, retrieve, and distribute image data and radiology reports on-line by using the DICOM web server. The nature of possible network systems in radiology is complex.

PACS can be classified according to the size and scope. If a PACS is dedicated to a single digital imaging modality such as CT or MRI scanner, for example, it is usually called a mini-PACS, in which case a single LAN is a central feature.

Networking consists of both hardware components and the necessary software to enable the hardware to function. Networking was described earlier in the chapter. In review, networks can be discussed in terms of LANs or WANs. The basis for this classification is the distance covered by the network. A LAN, for example, connects computers that are separated by short distances such as in a radiology department or in a building or two or more buildings. A WAN, on the other hand, connects computers that are separated by large distances, such as in another province or country. The Internet is a perfect example of a WAN. The network topology for LANs include bus, star, or ring as shown in Figures 2-14, 2-15, and 2-16, respectively.

Image Compression

Once images are acquired and sent through the computer network, they are generally displayed for viewing and stored temporarily or permanently for retrospective viewing and analysis.

The digital images acquired in a total DR department are large files with varying matrix sizes. For example, a typical CT image is usually 512 × 512 matrix by 2 bytes per pixel. These two characteristics alone (matrix size and bit depth) place huge demands not only on storage requirements but also on the speed of transmission over the network.

One effective way to manage the size of image files for transmission and storage is that of image compression. Image compression is a topic in itself that is quite complex and beyond the scope of this chapter; however, it is described in a little more detail in Chapter 3. In this chapter, the following basic facts are noteworthy for CT technologists:

- The purpose of compression is to speed up transmission of information (textual data and images) and to reduce storage requirements
- Several image compression methods are available, each providing advantages and
- disadvantages. Compression can be either:
  1. *lossless or reversible* compression, where no information is lost in the process
  2. *lossy or irreversible* compression, where some information is lost in the process (Seeram and Seeram, 2008)

Picture Archiving and Communications Systems and CT Interfacing

There are several issues related to interfacing a CT scanner to the PACS. These are related to the CT workstation, worklists, image distribution, information systems (RIS/HIS), RIS/HIS/PACS integration, and DICOM specifications. Each of these will be reviewed briefly.

Workstations will be used for primary diagnosis and other viewing tasks, and therefore an immediate concern is to orient radiologists and others such as other physicians and technologists to the nature of the workstation for soft-copy display of images. General hardware and software concerns must be addressed, especially software that allows sophisticated image processing such as three-dimensional imaging and virtual reality imaging.

Worklists are used to match cases from the CT scanner to various workstations, and therefore a PACS must be capable of creating and using worklists effectively (the worklist assignment algorithm is critical).

Image distribution is an important issue for CT PACS and it is the ability of the system to send images to referring physician and the radiation treatment planning department, for example. In this case, DICOM conformance is critical. Additionally, a PACS should be capable of teleradiology applications as well. Images from a CT scanner, for example, can be sent to a radiologist's home, where he can download them for interpretation. This would certainly save radiologists travel time late at night.

Picture Archiving and Communications Systems and Information Systems Integration

The integration of a CT scanner and PACS is quite critical. Equally important is the PACS integration with the HIS/RIS. Therefore connectivity is important. Several authors such as Bushberg et al (2004) and Dreyer et al (2006), have discussed the role of information systems integration in radiology. They have identified at least five separate information systems for DR, including PACS, RIS, HIS, a voice-recognition direction system, and the electronic teaching/research file system.

Integration of these systems is essential because it is intended to solve many problems in DR. It is not within the scope of this chapter to elaborate on these information systems; however, it is important to delineate between a HIS and a RIS. According to the experts (Van Bemmel and Musen, 1997), HIS is "an information system used to collect, store, process, retrieve, and communicate patient care and administrative information for all hospital-affiliated activities and to satisfy the functional requirements of all authorized users."

An RIS could be a stand-alone system or it may be integrated into a HIS. Some of the functions performed by the RIS are patient registration, examination scheduling, patient tracking, film archiving, report generation, administration and billing, and documentation, to mention only a few.

OTHER TOPICS

Many other topics in computer science are gaining attention in medical imaging. For example, computer graphics is the basis for three-dimensional rendering techniques such as shaded surface displays and volume rendering, which have become common in three-dimensional CT.

Artificial intelligence: AI is the branch of computer science that deals with enabling computers to emulate such aspects of intelligence as speech recognition, deduction, inference, creative response, the ability to learn from experience, and the ability to make reasonable inferences from incomplete information. AI is a complex arena that includes work in two related areas—one involved with understanding how living things think and the other with finding ways to impart similar capabilities to computer programs. Some tasks that used to be considered very difficult for a computer to perform, such as playing chess, have turned out to be relatively easy to program, and some tasks that were once thought easy to program, such as speech recognition and language translation, have turned out to be extremely difficult. Practical applications in this area include computer-based chess games and diagnostic aids, called *expert systems*, that are used by physicians and other professionals (Microsoft, 2002).

Computer graphics: Broadly, the term computer graphics refers to the display of "pictures" as opposed to only alphabetical and numerical characters on a computer screen. It encompasses different methods of generating, displaying, and storing information (Microsoft, 2002).

Expert system: An expert system is a type of application program that makes decisions or solves problems in a particular field, such as finance or medicine, by using knowledge and analytical rules defined by experts in the field. Human experts solve problems by using a combination of factual knowledge and reasoning ability. In an expert system, these two essentials are contained in two separate but related components, a knowledge base and an inference engine. The knowledge base provides specific facts and rules about the subject, and the inference engine provides the reasoning ability that enables the expert system to form conclusions (Microsoft, 2002).

Virus (computer): A computer virus is a set of illicit instructions that passes itself onto other programs with which it comes into contact (Capron, 2005).

Virtual reality: a system in which the user is immersed in a computer-created environment so that the user physically interacts with the computer-produced three-dimensional scene (Capron, 2005).

Computer-Aided Detection and Diagnosis: Computer-aided detection and diagnosis (CAD) is now being used in CT, especially in the area of lung nodule detection and in CT colonoscopy (Kalender, 2005; Yoshida and Dachman, 2004). In CAD, the computer (software) is used as a tool to provide additional information to the radiologist and other related individuals to make a diagnosis. In other words, the computer output is regarded as a "second opinion." The purpose of CAD is to improve diagnostic accuracy and to improve the consistency of image interpretation by using the computer results as a guide (Seeram, 2005).

CAD systems are essentially based on two approaches: those that use location of lesions by using the computer to search for abnormal patterns and those that quantify the image features of normal or abnormal patterns There are three major components of a CAD system: image processing, quantitation of image features, and data processing. The computer uses image processing algorithms such as filtering-based Fourier analysis, artificial neural networks, wavelet transform, and so forth, to enhance and extract lesions. Quantitation involves at least three steps to distinguish between lesions and normal anatomical structures. Finally, data processing uses techniques such as rule-based methods and other approaches such as discriminant analysis, artificial neural networks, and the decision tree method to distinguish between normal and abnormal patterns on the basis of features obtained in quantitation (Seeram, 2005).

REFERENCES

Arenson RL et al: Computers in imaging and health care: now and in the future. *J Digit Imaging* 13: 145-156, 2000.

Arnold DO: *Computers and society: impact*, New York, 1991, Mitchell McGraw-Hill.

Bushberg JT et al: *The essential physics of medical imaging*, ed 2, Philadelphia, 2004. Lippincott Williams & Wilkins.

Capron HL: *Computers: tools for an information age*, Upper Saddle River, NJ, 2005, Prentice Hall.

Covington MA: *Computer science—outline notes*, New York, 1991, Barron's.

Creighton C: A literature review on communications between picture archiving and communications systems and radiology information systems and/or hospital information systems. *J Dig Imaging* 12: 138-143, 1999.

Davidson-Shivers GV, Rasmussen KL: *Web-based learning: design, implementation, and evaluation*, Upper Saddle River, NJ, 2006, Pearson Education.

Dreyer KJ et al, editors: *PACS: a guide to the digital revolution*, ed 2, New York, 2006, Springer Science + Business Media.

Kalender W: *Computed tomography*, Munchen, 2005, Publicis MCD.

Laudon KC: *Management information systems: organization and technology*, Englewood Cliffs, NJ, 1994, Macmillan.

Microsoft: *Microsoft Press computer dictionary*, Redmond, Calif, 2002, Microsoft Press.

O'Leary TJ et al: *McGraw-Hill computing essentials, 1992-1993*, New York, 1992, Mitchell McGraw-Hill.

Proakis JG: *Digital signal processing: principles, algorithms, and applications*, New York, 1992, Macmillan.

Seeram E, editor: *Computers in diagnostic radiology—a book of selected readings*, Springfield, Ill, 1989, Charles C. Thomas.

Seeram E: Digital mammography—an overview. *Can J Med Radiat Technol* 36:15-23, 2005.

Seeram E, Seeram D: Image postprocessing in digital radiology: a primer for technologists, *Journal of Medical Imaging and Radiation Sciences* 39:23-41, 2008.

Van Bemmel JH, Musen MA, editors: *Handbook of medical informatics*, Heidelberg, 1997, Springer-Verlag.

Yoshida H, Dachman AH: Computer-aided diagnosis for CT colonoscopy. *Semin Ultrasound CT MRI* 25: 419-431, 2004.

Chapter 3

Digital Image Processing

Chapter Outline

LIMITATIONS OF FILM-BASED IMAGING

Film-based imaging has been the workhorse of radiology ever since the discovery of x rays in 1895. Applications of film-based imaging include conventional radiography and tomography, fluoroscopy, and special procedures imaging (angiography, for example). Additionally, nuclear medicine, ultrasound, computed tomography (CT), and magnetic resonance imaging (MRI) use film to record images from which a radiologist can make a diagnosis.

The steps in the production of a film-based radiographic image are very familiar to radiologic technologists. First, the patient is exposed to a predetermined amount of radiation that is needed to provide the required diagnostic image quality. A latent image is formed on the film that is subsequently processed by chemicals in a processor to render the image visible. The processed image is then ready for viewing by a radiologist, who makes a diagnosis of the patient's medical condition.

The imaging process can also result in poor image quality if the initial radiation exposure has not been accurately determined. For example, if the radiation exposure is too high, the film is overexposed and the processed image appears too dark; thus, the radiologist cannot make a diagnosis from such an image. Alternatively, if the radiation exposure is too low, the processed image appears too light and is not useful to the radiologist. In both these situations the images lack the proper image density and contrast and imaging would have to be repeated to provide an acceptable image quality needed to make a diagnosis. Additionally, the patient would be subjected to increased radiation exposure.

Despite the above problems, film-based imaging has been successful for the past 100 years and it is still being used today in many departments. There are other problems associated with film-based imaging. For example, film is not the ideal vehicle to perform the three basic functions of radiation detection, image display, and image archiving.

As a radiation detector, film-screen cannot show differences in tissue contrast that are less than 10%. This means that film-based imaging is limited in its contrast resolution. The spatial resolution of film-screen systems, however, is the highest of all imaging modalities, and this is the main reason that radiography has played a significant role in imaging patients through the years.

As a display medium, the optical range and contrast for film are fixed and limited. Film can only display once—the optical range and contrast determined by the exposure technique factors used to produce the image. To change the image display (optical range and contrast), another set of exposure technique factors would have to be used, thus increasing the dose to the patient by virtue of a repeat exposure.

As an archive medium, film is usually stored in envelopes and housed in a large room. It thus requires manual handling for archiving and retrieval by an individual.

A digital imaging system and digital image processing can overcome these problems.

GENERIC DIGITAL IMAGING SYSTEM

The major components of a generic digital imaging system for use in radiology are shown in Figure 3-1. These include data acquisition, image processing, image display/storage/archiving, and image communication. As noted in Chapter 1, CT consists of these major components (to be described in detail later in subsequent chapters) and can therefore be classified as a digital imaging system because it uses computers to process images. Each of these components will be described briefly.

Data Acquisition

The term data acquisition refers to a systematic method of collecting data from the patient. For projection digital radiography and CT, the data are the electron density of the tissues, which is

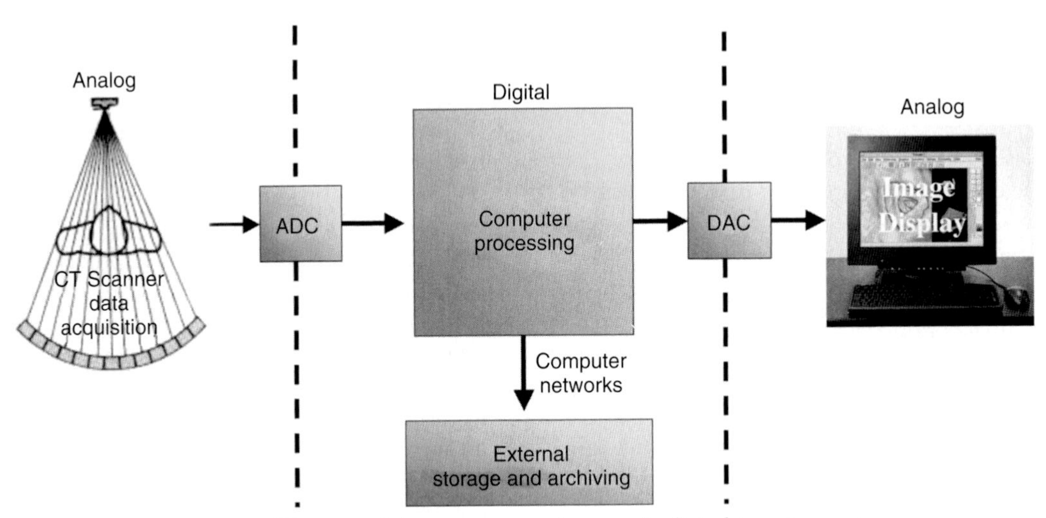

FIGURE 3-1 The essential components of a generic digital imaging system.

related to the linear attenuation coefficient (μ) of the various tissues. In other words, it is attenuation data that is collected for these imaging modalities. Data acquisition components for these modalities include the x-ray tube and the digital image detectors. The output signal from the detectors is an electrical signal (an analog signal that varies continuously in time). Because a digital computer is used in these imaging systems, the analog signal must be converted into a digital signal (discrete units) for processing by a digital computer. This conversion is performed by an analog-to-digital converter (ADC).

Image Processing

Image processing is performed by a digital computer that takes an input digital image and processes it to produce an output digital image by using the binary number system. Although we typically use the decimal number system (which operates with base 10, that is, 10 different numbers: 0,1,2,3,4,5,6,7,8,9), computers use the binary number system (which operates with base 2, that is, 0 or 1). These two digits are referred to as binary digits or bits. Bits are not continuous but rather they are discrete units. Computers operate with binary numbers, 0 and 1, discrete units that are processed and transformed into other discrete units. To process the word Euclid, it would have to be converted into digital data (binary representation). Thus the binary representation for the word Euclid is 01000101 01010101 01000011 01001100 01001001 01000100.

The ADC sends digital data for digital image processing by a digital computer. Such processing is accomplished by a set of operations and techniques to transform the input image into an output image that suits the needs of the observer (radiologist) to enhance diagnosis. For example, these operations can be used to reduce the noise in the input image, enhance the sharpness of the input image, or change the contrast of the input image. This chapter is concerned primarily with these digital image processing operations and techniques.

Image Display, Storage, and Communication

The output of computer processing, that is, the output digital image, must first be converted into an analog signal before it can be displayed on a monitor for viewing by the observer. Such conversion is the function of the digital-to-analog conversion (DAC). This image can be stored and archived on magnetic data carriers (magnetic tapes/disks) and laser optical disks for retrospective viewing and manipulation. Additionally, these images can be communicated electronically through computer networks to observers at remote sites. In this regard, picture archiving and communication systems (PACS) are becoming commonplace in the modern radiology department.

This chapter explores the fundamentals of digital image processing through a brief history and a description of related topics such as image representation, the digitizing process, image processing operations, and image processing hardware considerations.

HISTORICAL PERSPECTIVES

The history of digital image processing dates to the early 1960s, when the National Aeronautics and Space Administration (NASA) was developing its lunar and planetary exploration program. The Ranger spacecraft returned images of the lunar surface to Earth. These analog images taken by a television camera were converted into digital images and subsequently processed by the digital computer to obtain more information about the moon's surface.

The development of digital image processing techniques can be attributed to work at NASA's Jet Propulsion Laboratory at the California Institute of Technology. The technology of digital processing continues to expand rapidly and its applications extend into fields such as astronomy, geology, forestry, agriculture, cartography, military science, and medicine. (An overview of the history of digital image processing technology is shown in Fig. 3-2.) The technology has found widespread applications in medicine and particularly in diagnostic imaging, where it has been successfully applied to ultrasound, digital radiography, nuclear medicine, CT, and MRI (Huang, 2004). Digital image processing is a multidisciplinary subject that includes physics, mathematics, engineering, and computer science.

IMAGE FORMATION AND REPRESENTATION

An understanding of images is necessary to define digital image processing. Castleman (1996) has classified images on the basis of their form or method of generation. He used set theory to explain image types. According to this theory, images are a subset of all objects. Within the set of images, there are other subsets such as visible images (e.g., paintings, drawings, or photographs), optical images (e.g., holograms), nonvisible physical images (e.g., temperature, pressure, or elevation maps), and mathematical images (e.g., continuous functions and discrete functions). The sine wave is an example of a continuous function (analog signal), whereas a discrete function represents a digital image, as shown in Figure 3-3. Castleman noted that "only the digital images can be processed by computer."

Analog Images

Analog images are continuous images. For example, a black-and-white photograph of a chest x ray is an analog image because it represents a continuous distribution of light intensity as a function of position on the radiograph.

In photography, images are formed when light is focused on film. In radiography, x rays pass through the patient and are projected onto x-ray film. In both cases, films are processed in chemical solutions to render them visible and the images are formed by a photochemical process. Images can also be formed by photoelectronic means, in which the images may be represented as electrical signals (analog signals) that emerge from the photoelectronic device.

Digital Images

Digital images are numerical representations or images of objects. The formation of digital images requires a digital computer. Any information that enters the computer for processing must

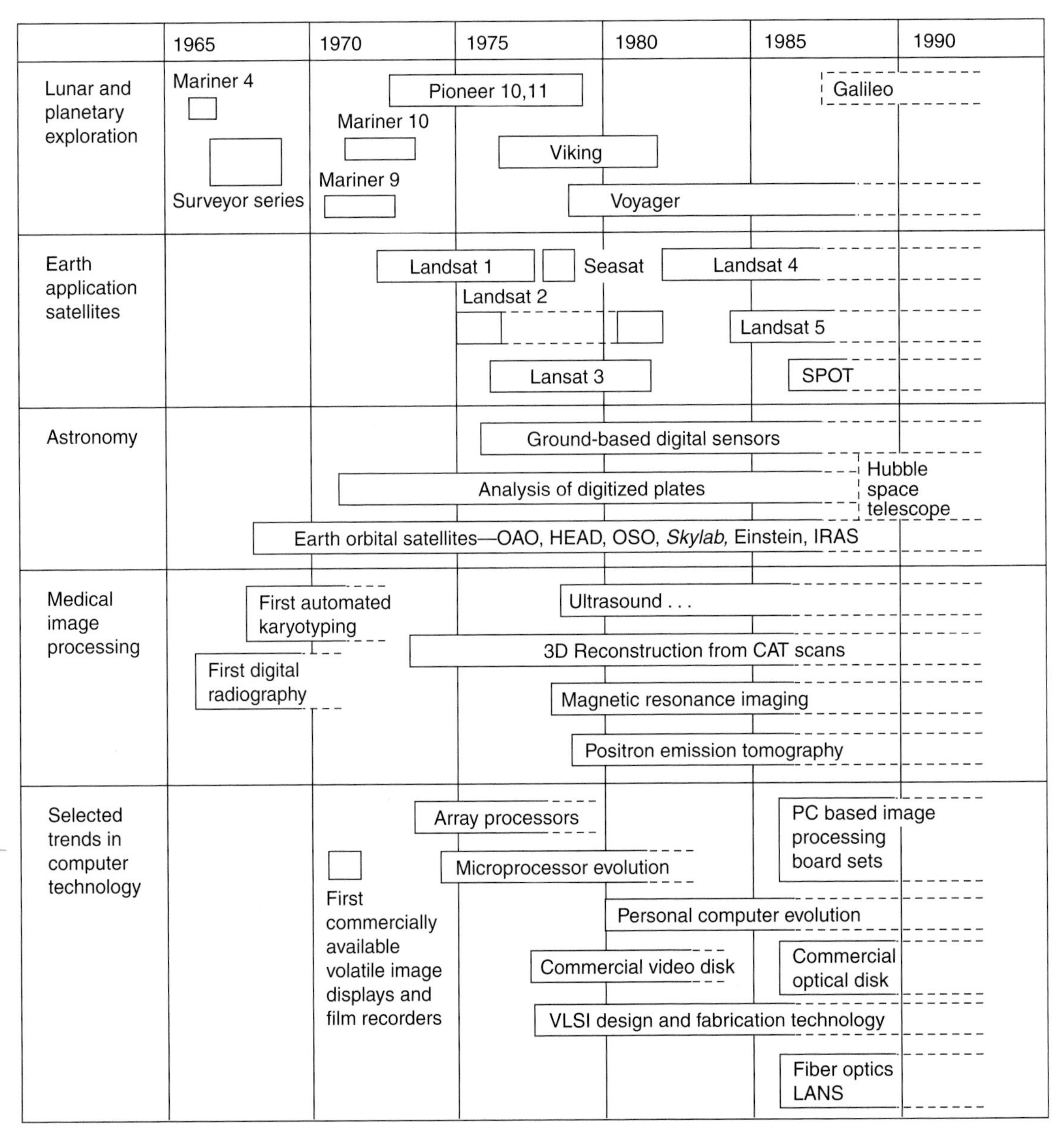

FIGURE 3-2 Overview of the first 20 years of important developments in digital image processing. (From Green WB: *Digital image processing: a systems approach*, ed 2, New York, 1989, Van Nostrand Reinhold.)

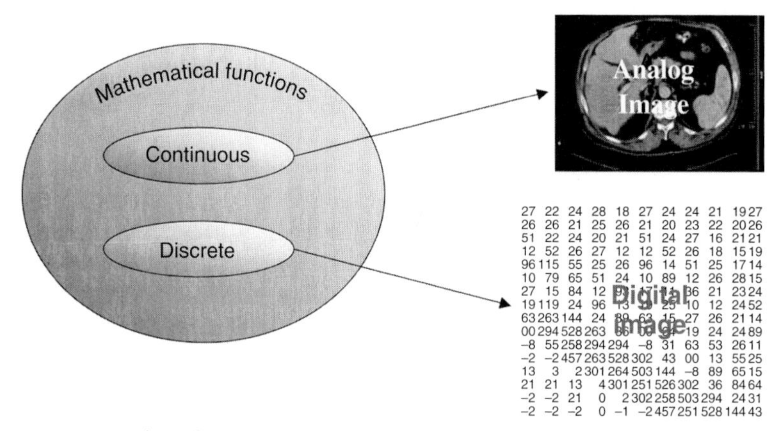

FIGURE 3-3 Two examples of continuous and discrete images. See text for further explanation.

first be converted into digital form, or numbers (Fig. 3-4). An important component is the ADC, which converts continuous signals to discrete signals, or digital data (Luiten, 1995).

The computer receives the digital data and performs the necessary processing. The results of this processing are always digital and can be displayed as a digital image (Fig. 3-5).

WHAT IS DIGITAL IMAGE PROCESSING?

Definitions

In image processing it is necessary to convert an input image into an output image. If both the input image and output image are analog, this is referred to as *analog processing*. If both the input image and output image are discrete, this is referred to as *digital processing*. In cases where an analog image must be converted into digital data for input to the computer, a digitization system is required. CT is based on a reconstruction process whereby a digital image is changed into a visible physical image (Fig. 3-6).

Castleman (1996) defined a *process* as "a series of actions or operations leading to a desired result; thus, a series of actions or operations are performed upon an object to alter its form in a desired manner." Castleman also defined *digital image processing* as "subjecting numerical representations of objects to a series of operations in order to obtain a desired result."

Given the variety of possible operations (Baxes, 1994), image processing has emerged as a discipline in itself (see box below).

Image Processing Operations

- Image generation
- Image modification
  - Image enhancement
  - Image combination
  - Image restoration
- Image analysis
  - Pattern recognition
  - Image interpretation
  - Feature extraction

Image Domains

Images can be represented in two domains on the basis of how they are acquired (Huang, 2004). These domains include the spatial location domain and the spatial frequency domain. All images displayed for viewing by humans are in the spatial location domain. Radiography and CT, for example, acquire images in the spatial location domain.

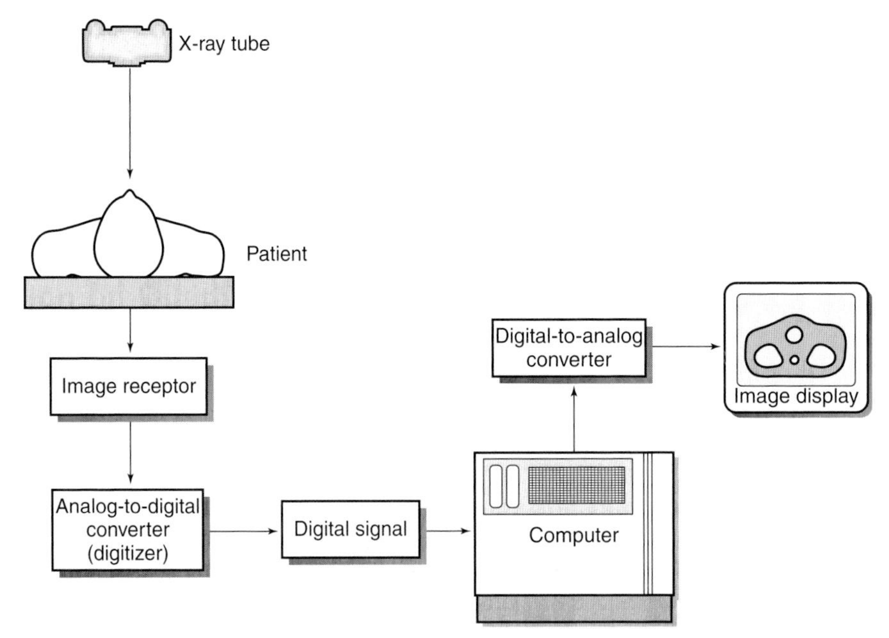

FIGURE 3-4 The conversion of analog data into digital data for input to a digital computer.

As mentioned earlier, the digital image is a numerical image arranged in such a manner that the location of each number in the image can be identified by using a right-handed x-y coordinate system, where the x-axis describes the rows or lines placed on the image and the y-axis describes the columns, as shown in Figure 3-7. For example, the first pixel in the upper left corner of the image is always identified as 0,0. The spatial location 9,4 will describe a pixel that is located nine pixels to the right of the left-hand side of the image and four lines down from the top of the image. Such an image is said to be in the spatial location domain.

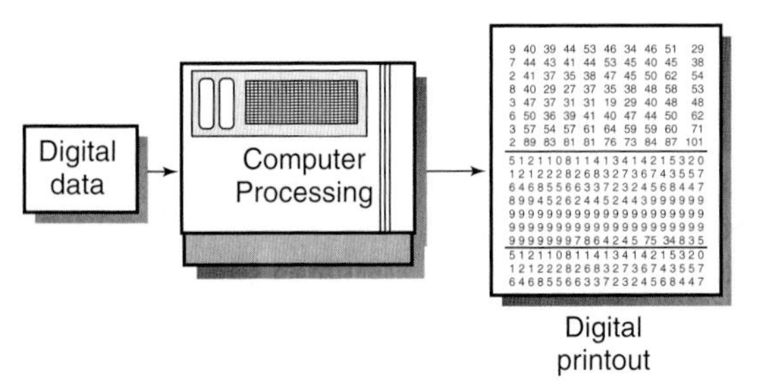

FIGURE 3-5 Input digital data can be displayed in digital form after computer processing.

Images can also be acquired in the spatial frequency domain, such as those acquired in MRI. The term frequency refers to the number of cycles per unit length, that is, the number of times a signal changes per unit length. Although small structures within an object (patient) produce high frequencies that represent the detail in the image, large structures produce low frequencies and represent contrast information in the image.

Digital image processing can transform one image domain into another image domain. For example, an image in the spatial location domain can be transformed into a spatial frequency domain image, as is illustrated in Figure 3-8. The Fourier transform (FT) is used to perform this task. The FT is mathematically rigorous and will not be covered in this article. The FT converts a function in the time domain, (say signal intensity versus time) to a function in frequency domain (say, signal intensity

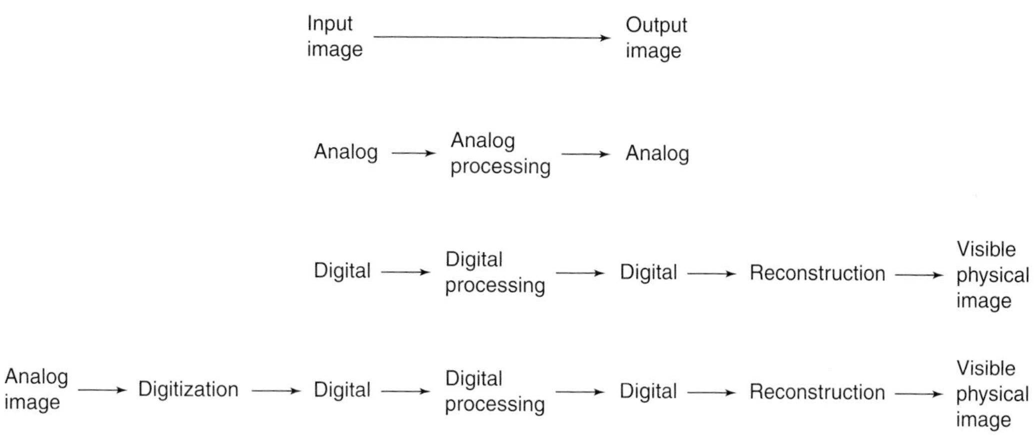

FIGURE 3-6 Digital image processing.

versus frequency). The inverse FT denoted by FT^{-1} is used to transform an image in the frequency domain back to the spatial location domain for viewing by radiologists and technologists. Physicists and engineers, on the other hand, would probably prefer to view images in the frequency domain.

The major reason for doing this is to facilitate image processing that can enhance or suppress certain features of the image. For example, Huang (2004) points out:

> One can use information appearing in the frequency domain, and not easily available in the spatial domain, to detect some inherent characteristics of each type of radiological image. If the image has many edges, there would be many high-frequency components. On the other hand, if the image has only uniform materials, like water or plastic, then it has low-frequency components. On the basis of this frequency in the image, we can selectively change the frequency components to enhance the image. To obtain a smoother appearing image we can increase the amplitude of the low-frequency components, whereas to enhance the edges of bones in the hand x-ray image, we can magnify the amplitude of the high-frequency components.

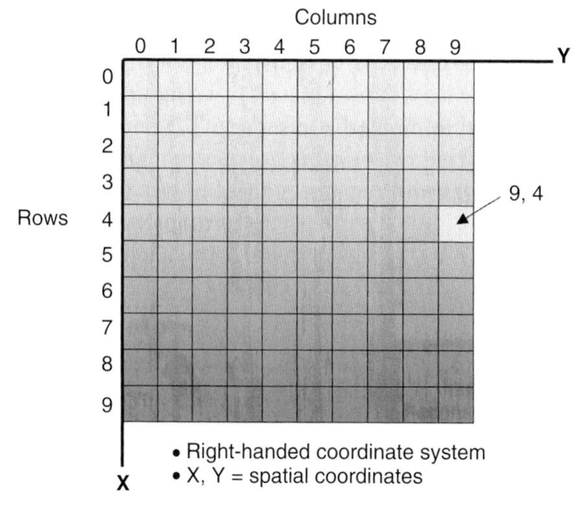

FIGURE 3-7 A right-handed coordinate system used to describe digital images in the spatial location domain. The exact location of a pixel can be found using columns and rows. See text for further explanation.

CHARACTERISTICS OF THE DIGITAL IMAGE

The structure of a digital image can be described with respect to several characteristics or fundamental parameters, including the matrix, pixels, voxels, and the bit depth (Castleman, 1996; Pooley et al, 2001; Seeram and Seeram, 2008; Seibert, 1995).

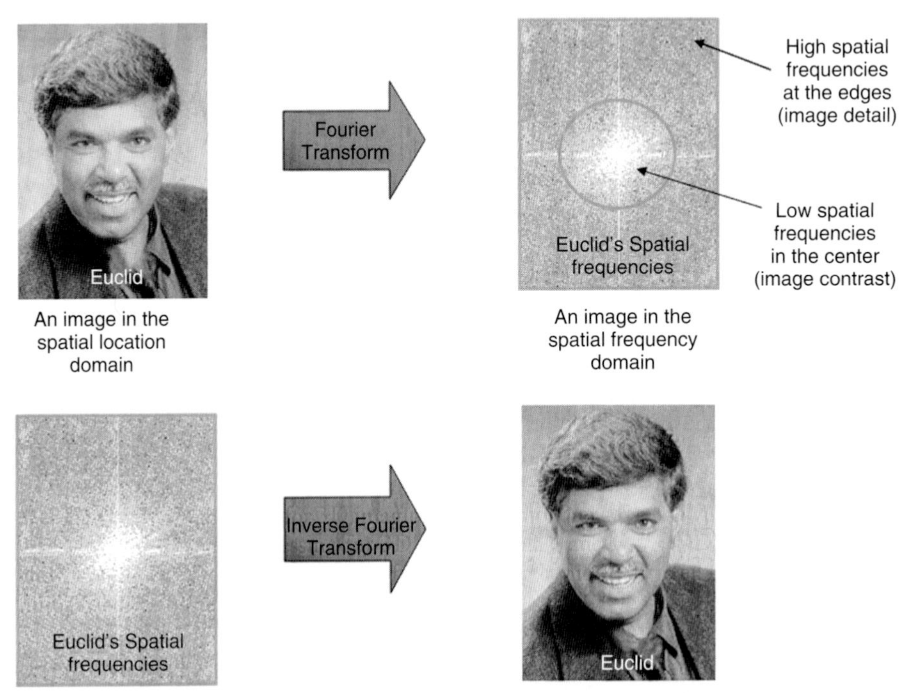

FIGURE 3-8 The Fourier transform is used to convert an image in the spatial location domain into an image in the spatial frequency domain for processing by a computer. The inverse Fourier transform (FT^{-1}) is used to convert the spatial frequency domain image back into a spatial location image for viewing by humans. (From Seeram E: Digital image processing, *Radiol Technol* 75:435-455, 2004. Reproduced by permission of the American Society of Radiologic Technologists.)

Matrix

Apart from being a numerical image, there are other elements of a digital image that are important to our understanding of digital image processing. A digital image is made up of a two-dimensional array of numbers, called a matrix. The matrix consists of columns (M) and rows (N) that define small square regions called picture elements, or pixels. The dimension of the image can be described by M, N, and the size of the image is given by the following relationship:

$$M \times N \times k \text{ bits}$$

When M = N, the image is square. Generally, diagnostic digital images are rectangular in shape. When imaging a patient with a digital imaging modality, the operator selects the matrix size, sometimes referred to as the field-of-view (FOV). Typical matrix sizes are shown in Table 3-1. It is important to note that as images become larger, they require more processing time and more storage space. Additionally, larger images will take more time to be transmitted to remote locations. In this regard, image compression is needed to facilitate storage and transmission requirements.

Pixels

The pixels that make up the matrix are generally square. Each pixel contains a number (discrete value) that represents a brightness level. The numbers represent tissue characteristics being imaged. For example, in radiography and CT, these numbers are related to the atomic number and mass density of the tissues, and in MRI they represent other

TABLE 3-1 Typical Matrix Sizes for Different Types of Digital Diagnostic Images

Digital Imaging Modality	Matrix Size	Typical Bit Depth
Nuclear medicine	128 × 128	12
MRI	256 × 256	12
CT	512 × 512	12
Digital subtraction angiography	1024 × 1024	10
Computed radiography	2048 × 2048	12
Digital radiography	2048 × 2048	12
Digital angiography	4096 × 4096	12

characteristics of tissues, such as proton density and relaxation times.

The pixel size can be calculated according to the following relationship:

$$\text{Pixel size} = \text{FOV}/\text{Matrix size}$$

For digital imaging modalities, the larger the matrix size, the smaller the pixel size (for the same FOV) and the better the spatial resolution. The effect of the matrix size on picture clarity can be seen in Figure 3-9.

Voxels

Pixels in a digital image represent the information contained in a volume of tissue in the patient. Such volume is referred to as a voxel (contraction for **vol**ume **el**ement). Voxel information is converted into numerical values contained in the pixels, and these numbers are assigned brightness levels, as illustrated in Figure 3-10.

Bit Depth

In the relationship $M \times N \times k\ bits$, the term "k bits" implies that every pixel in the digital image matrix $M \times N$ is represented by k binary digits. The number of bits per pixel is the bit depth. Because the binary number system uses the base 2, k bits = 2^k. Therefore each pixel will have 2^k gray levels. For example, in a digital image with a bit depth of 2, each pixel will have 2^2 (4) gray levels (density). Similarly, a bit depth of 8 implies that each pixel will have 2^8 (256) gray levels or shades of gray. The effect of bit depth is clearly seen in Figure 3-11. Table 3-1 also provides the typical bit depth for diagnostic digital images.

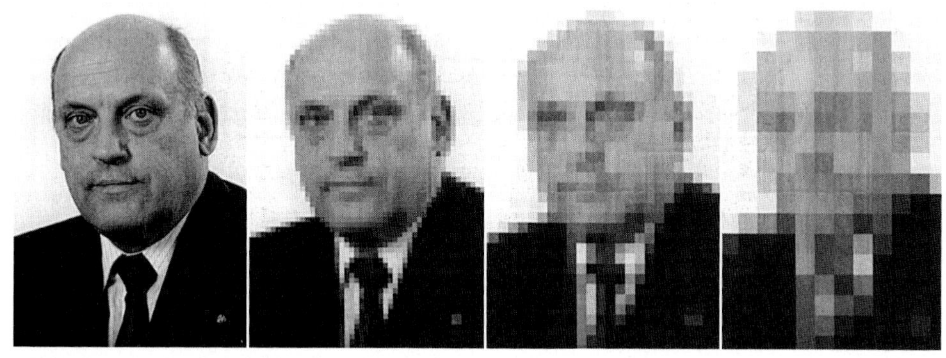

FIGURE 3-9 An increased number of pixels in the image matrix improves the picture quality and enhances the perception of details in the image. (From Luiten AL: Digital: discrete perfection, *Medicamundi* 40:95-100, 1995.)

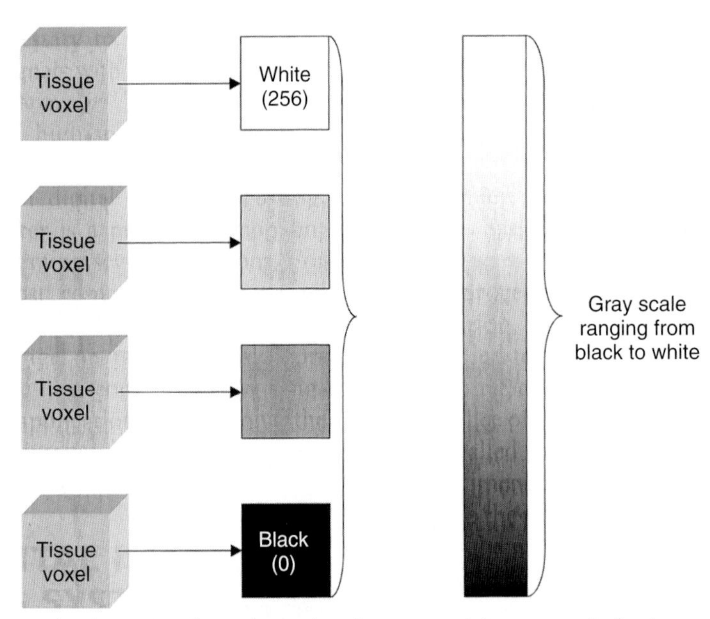

FIGURE 3-10 Voxel information from the patient is converted into numerical values contained in the pixels, and these numbers are assigned brightness levels. The higher numbers represent high signal intensity (from the detectors) and are shaded white (bright) while the low numbers represent low signal intensity, and are shaded dark (black).

Effect of Digital Image Parameters on the Appearance of Digital Images

The characteristics of a digital image, that is, the matrix size, the pixel size, and the bit depth, can affect the appearance of the digital image, particularly its spatial resolution and its density resolution.

The matrix size has an effect on the detail or spatial resolution of the image. The larger the matrix size (for the same FOV), the smaller pixel size, hence the better the appearance of detail. Additionally, as the FOV decreases without a change in matrix size, the size of the pixel decreases as well (recall the relationship pixel size = FOV/matrix size), thus improving detail. The operator selects a larger matrix size when imaging larger body parts, such as a chest, to show small details in the anatomy.

The bit depth has an effect on the number of shades of gray, hence the contrast resolution of the image. This is clearly apparent in Figure 3-11.

IMAGE DIGITIZATION

The primary objective during image digitization is to convert an analog image into numerical data for processing by the computer (Seibert, 1995). Digitization consists of three distinct steps: scanning, sampling, and quantization.

Scanning

Consider an image (Fig. 3-12). The first step in digitization is the division of the picture into small regions, or scanning. Each small region of the picture is a picture element, or pixel. Scanning results in a grid characterized by rows and columns.

The size of the grid usually depends on the number of pixels on each side of the grid. In Figure 3-12 the grid size is 9 × 9, which results in 81 pixels. The rows and columns identify a particular pixel by providing an address for that pixel. The rows and columns comprise a matrix; in this case, the matrix is 9 × 9. As the number of pixels in the image matrix increases, the image becomes more recognizable and facilitates better perception of image details.

Sampling

The second step in image digitization is sampling, which measures the brightness of each pixel in the entire image (see Fig. 3-12). A small spot of light is projected onto the transparency and the transmitted light is detected by a photomultiplier tube positioned behind the picture. The output of the photomultiplier tube is an electrical (analog) signal.

Quantization

Quantization is the final step, in which the brightness value of each sampled pixel is assigned an integer (0, or a positive or negative number) called a *gray level*. The result is a range of numbers or gray levels, each of which has a precise location on the rectangular grid of pixels. The total number of gray levels is called the *gray scale*, such as eight-level gray scale (see Fig. 3-12). The gray scale is based on the value of the gray levels; 0 represents black and 255 represents white. The numbers in between 0 and 255 represent shades of gray. In the case of two gray levels, the picture would show only black and white. An image can therefore be composed of any number of gray levels, depending on the bit depth.

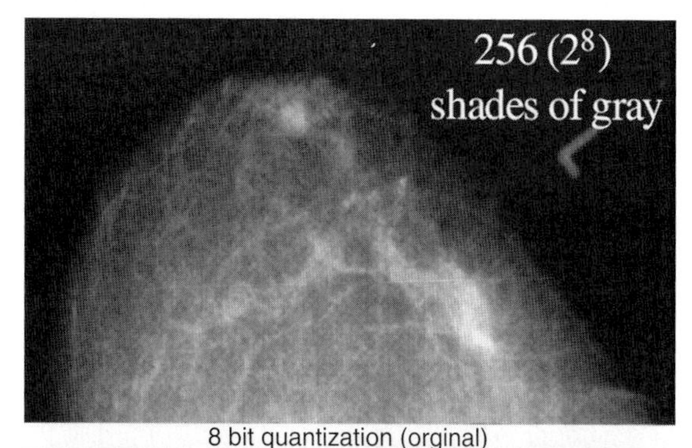

8 bit quantization (orginal)

64 (2^6)
shades of gray

6 bit quantization

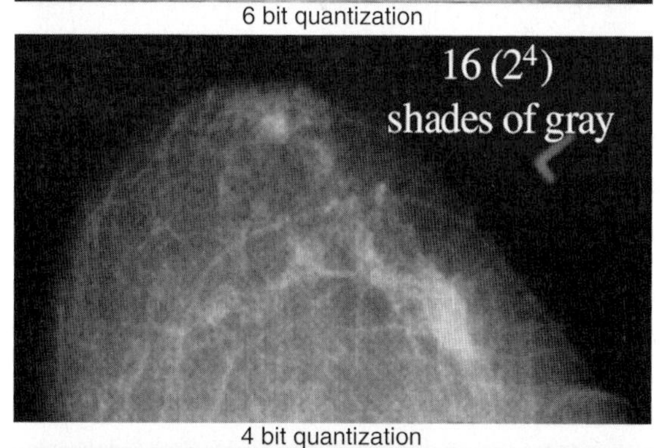

4 bit quantization

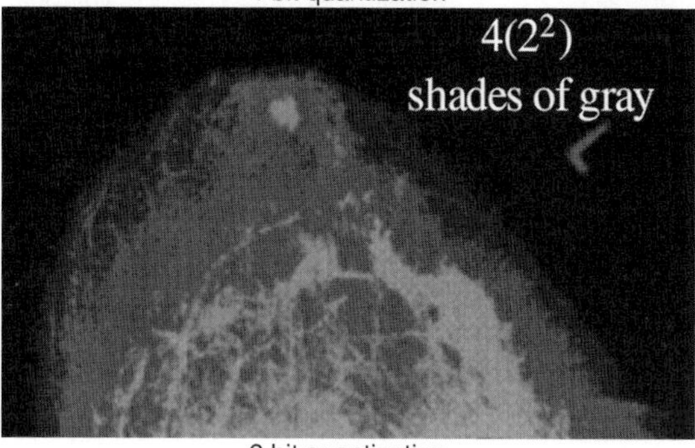

2 bit quantization

FIGURE 3-11 The effect of bit depth on the quality of the digital image. Higher bit depths result in better image quality. (Images courtesy of Bruno Jaagi, P.Eng-Biomedical Engineering Technology, British Columbia Institute of Technology.)

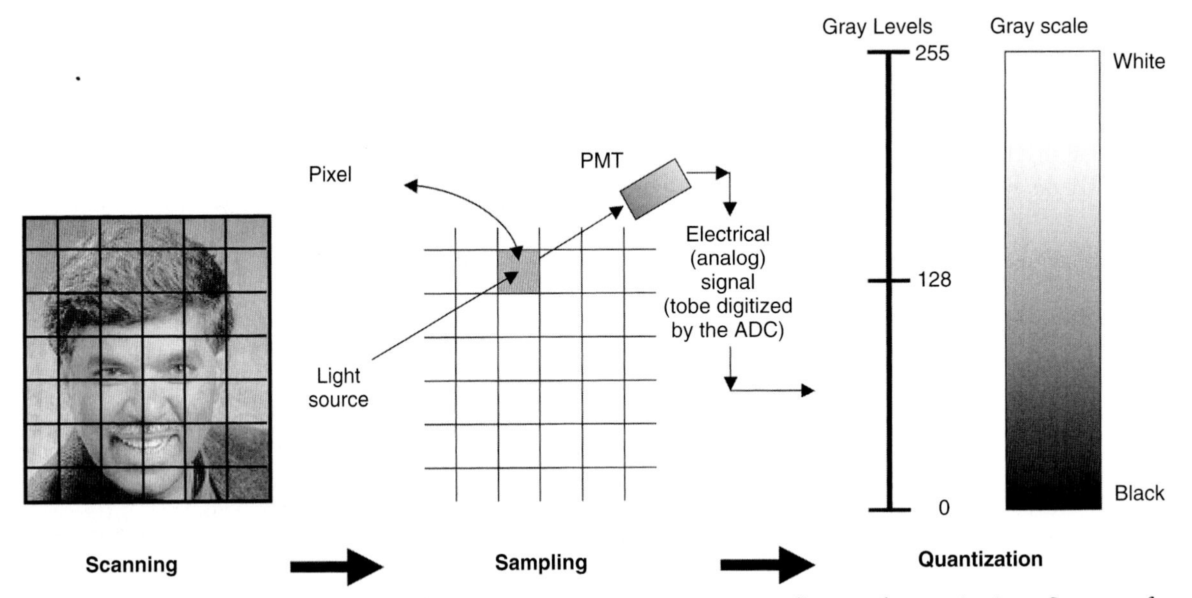

FIGURE 3-12 Three general steps in digitizing an image; scanning, sampling, and quantization. See text for further explanation. Similar steps apply to digital diagnostic techniques. (From Seeram E: Digital image processing, *Radiol Technol* 75: 435-455, 2004. Reproduced by permission of the American Society of Radiologic Technologists.)

In quantization, the electrical signal obtained from sampling is assigned an integer that is based on the strength of the signal. In general, the value of the integer is proportional to the signal strength (Seibert, 1995).

The result of the quantization process is a digital image, an array of numbers representing the analog image that was scanned, sampled, and quantized. This array of numbers is sent to the computer for further processing.

Analog-to-Digital Conversion

The conversion of analog signals to digital information is accomplished by the ADC. The ADC samples the analog signal at various times to measure its strength at different points. The more points sampled, the better the representation of the signal. This sampling process is followed by quantization.

Two important characteristics of the ADC are speed and accuracy. *Accuracy* refers to the sampling of the signal. The more samples taken, the more accurate the representation of the digital image (Fig. 3-13). If enough samples are not taken, the representation of the original signal will be inaccurate after computer processing (Fig. 3-14). This sampling error is referred to as *aliasing*, and it appears as an artifact on the image. Aliasing artifacts appear as Moiré patterns on the image (Baxes, 1994).

The sampling results in the division of the signal. The more parts to the signal, the greater the accuracy of the ADC. The measurement unit for these parts is the bit. Recall that a bit can be either 0 or 1. In a 1-bit ADC, the signal is divided in two parts ($2^1 = 2$). A 2-bit ADC generates four equal parts ($2^2 = 4$). An 8-bit ADC generates 256 equal parts ($2^8 = 256$). The higher the number of bits, the more accurate the ADC.

The ADC also determines the number of levels or shades of gray represented in the image. A 1-bit ADC results in two integers (0 and 1), which are represented as black and white. A 2-bit ADC results in four numbers, which produce a gray scale with four shades. An 8-bit ADC results in

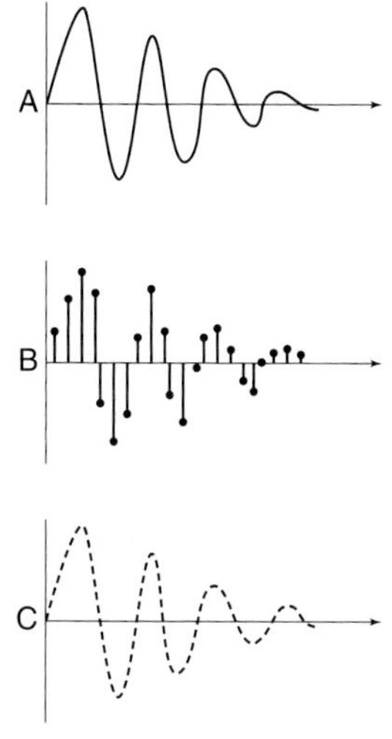

FIGURE 3-13 Good sampling (B) of original analog signal (A) produces an accurate representation of the original signal (C) after computer processing.

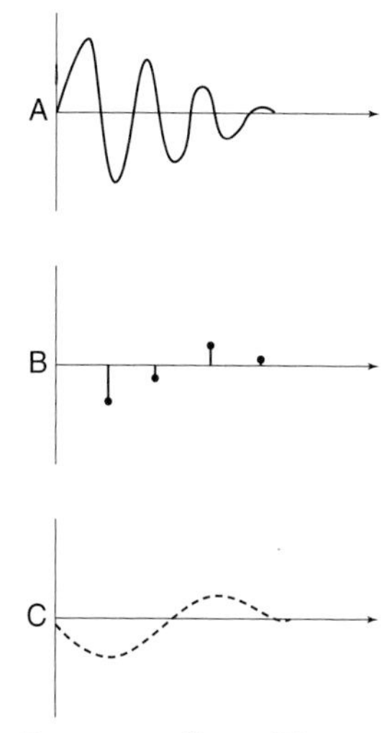

FIGURE 3-14 Poor sampling (B) misrepresents the shape of the original (A) after computer processing (C).

256 integers (2^8), ranging from 0 to 255, with 256 shades of gray (see Fig. 3-10).

The other characteristic of the ADC is *speed*, or the time taken to digitize the analog signal. In the ADC, speed and accuracy are inversely related—that is, the greater the accuracy, the longer it takes to digitize the signal.

Why Digitize Images?

The operations used in digital image processing to transform an input image into an output image to suit the needs of the human observer are several. Baxes (1994) identifies at least five fundamental classes of operations, including image enhancement, image restoration, image analysis, image compression, and image synthesis. Although it is not within the scope of this chapter to describe all of these in any great detail, it is noteworthy to mention the purpose of each of them and state their particular operations. For a more complete and thorough description of these, the interested reader should refer to the work of Baxes (1994).

1. *Image enhancement*: The purpose of this class of processing is to generate an image that is more pleasing to the observer. Certain characteristics such as contours and shapes can be enhanced to improve the overall quality of the image. The operations include contrast enhancement, edge enhancement, spatial and frequency filtering, image combining, and noise reduction.
2. *Image restoration*: The purpose of image restoration is to improve the quality of images that have distortions or degradations. Image restoration is commonplace in spacecraft imagery. Images sent to Earth from various camera systems on spacecrafts have distortions/degradations that must be corrected for proper viewing. Blurred images, for example, can be filtered to make them sharper.
3. *Image analysis*: This class of digital image processing allows measurements and statistics to be performed, as well as image segmentation, feature extraction, and classification of objects. Baxes (1994) indicates that "the process of analyzing objects in an image begins with image segmentation operations, such as image enhancement or restoration operations. These operations are used to isolate

and highlight the objects of interest. Then the features of the objects are extracted resulting in object outlines or other object measures. These measures describe and characterize the objects in the image. Finally, the object measures are used to classify the objects into specific categories." Segmentation operations are used in three-dimensional (3D) medical imaging (Seeram, 2001).

4. *Image compression*: The purpose of image compression of digital images is to reduce the size of the image to decrease transmission time and reduce storage space. In general, there are two forms of image compression, lossy and lossless compression (Fig. 3-15). In lossless compression there is no loss of any information in the image (detail is not compromised) when the image is decompressed. In lossy compression, there is some loss of image details when the image is decompressed. The latter has specific uses especially in situations when it is not necessary to have exact details of the original image. A more recent form of compression that has been receiving attention in digital diagnostic imaging is that of wavelet (special waveforms) compression. The main advantage of this form of compression is that there is no loss in both spatial and frequency information. Compression has received a good deal of attention in the digital radiology department, including the PACS environment, especially because image data sets are becoming increasingly larger. For this reason it will be described further later in this chapter.
5. *Image synthesis*: These processing operations "create images from other images or non-image data. These operations are used when a desired image is either physically impossible or impractical to acquire, or does not exist in a physical form at all" (Baxes, 1994). Examples of operations are image reconstruction techniques that are

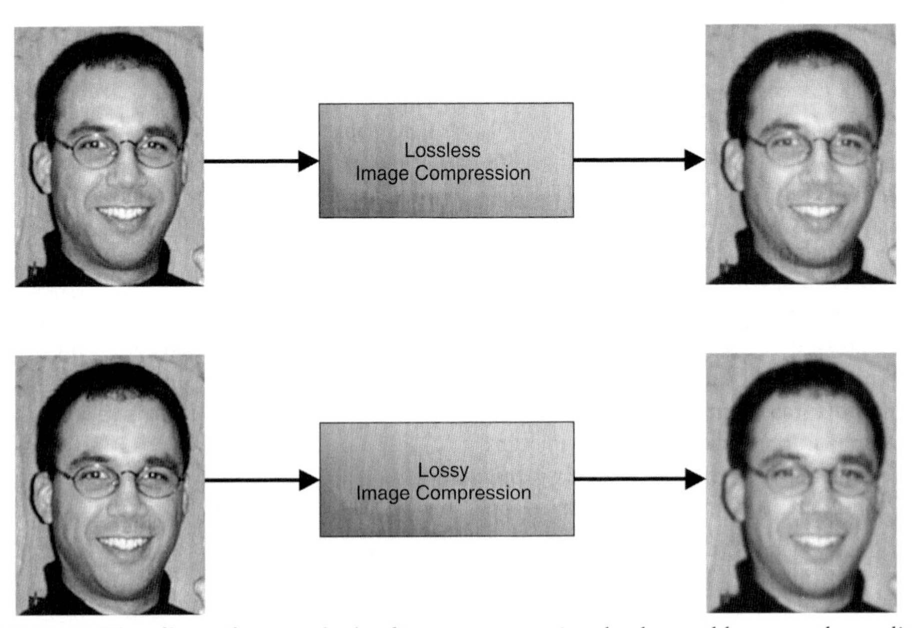

FIGURE 3-15 The effects of two methods of image compression, lossless and lossy, on the quality of the image (visual appearance of the image) of Euclid's son David, a brilliant, caring, and absolutely wonderful young man. (Images courtesy David Seeram.)

the basis for the production of CT and MRI images and 3D visualization techniques, which are based on computer graphics technology.

IMAGE PROCESSING TECHNIQUES

In general, image processing techniques are based on three types of operations: point operations (point processes), local operations (area processes), and global operations (frame processes). The image processing algorithms on which these operations are based alter the pixel intensity values (Baxes, 1994; Lindley, 1991; Marion, 1991). The exception is the geometric processing algorithm, which changes the position (spatial position or arrangement) of the pixel.

Point Operations

Point operations are perhaps the least complicated and most frequently used image processing technique. The value of the input image pixel is mapped on the corresponding output image pixel (Fig. 3-16). The algorithms for point operations enable the input image matrix to be scanned, pixel by pixel, until the entire image is transformed.

The most commonly used point processing technique is called *gray-level mapping*. This is also referred to as "contrast enhancement," "contrast stretching," "histogram modification," "histogram stretching," or "windowing." Gray-level mapping uses a look-up table (LUT), which plots the output and input gray levels against each other (Fig. 3-17).

LUTs can be implemented with hardware or software for gray-level transformation. Figure 3-18 illustrates the transformation process. Gray-level mapping changes the brightness of the image and results in the enhancement of the display image.

Gray-level mapping results in a modification of the histogram of the pixel values. A histogram is a graph of the pixels in all or part of the image, plotted as a function of the gray level. A histogram can be created as follows:

1. Observe the image matrix (Fig. 3-19) and create a table of the number of pixels with a specific intensity value, as shown.
2. Plot a graph of the number of pixels versus the gray levels (intensity or density values).

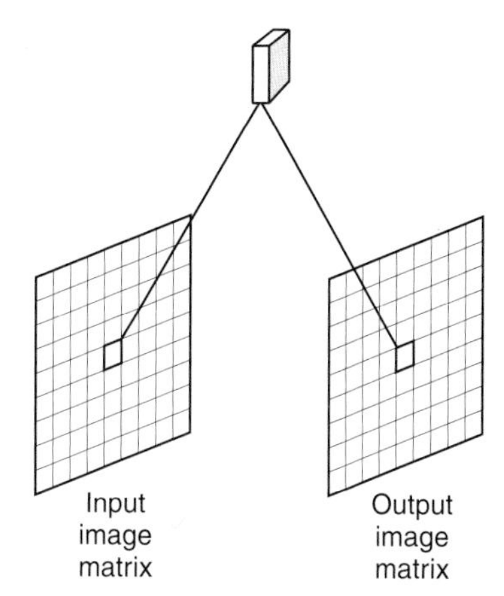

FIGURE 3-16 In a point operation, the value of the input image pixel is mapped onto the corresponding output image pixel.

Histograms indicate the overall brightness and contrast of an image. If the histogram is modified or changed, the brightness and contrast of the image can be altered, a technique referred to as *histogram modification*, or histogram stretching. This is also an example of a point operation in digital image processing. If the histogram is wide, the resulting image has high contrast. If the histogram is narrow, the resulting image has low contrast. On the other hand, if the histogram values are closer to the lower end of the range of values, the image appears dark, as opposed to a bright image, in which the values are weighted toward the higher end of the range of values.

Local Operations

A *local operation* is an image processing operation in which the output image pixel value

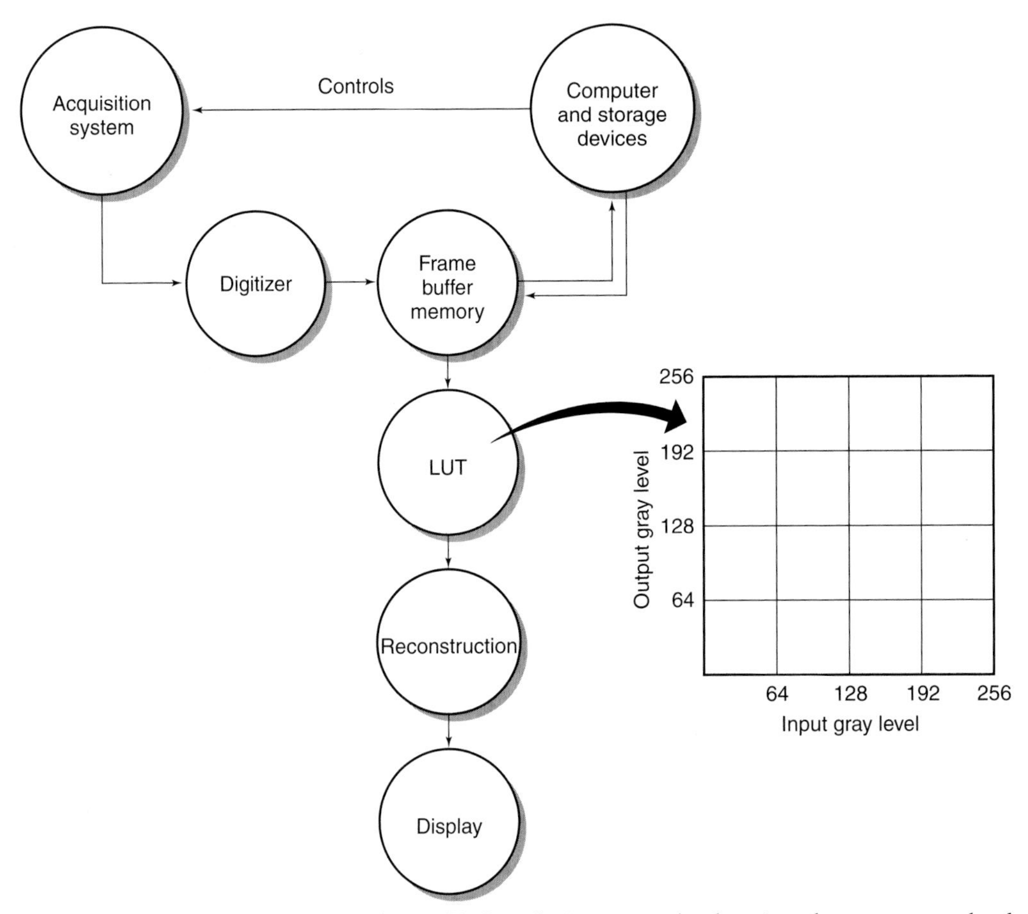

FIGURE 3-17 Gray-level mapping. The LUT plots the input gray level against the output gray level.

is determined from a small area of pixels around the corresponding input pixel (Fig. 3-20). These operations are also referred to as *area processes* or *group processes* because a group of pixels is used in the transformation calculation.

Spatial frequency filtering is an example of a local operation that concerns brightness information in an image. If the brightness of an image changes rapidly with distance in the horizontal or vertical direction, the image is said to have *high spatial frequency*. (An image with smaller pixels has higher frequency information than an image with larger pixels.) When the brightness changes slowly or at a constant rate, the image is said to have *low spatial frequency*. Spatial frequency filtering can alter images in several ways such as image sharpening, image smoothing, image blurring, noise reduction, and feature extraction (edge enhancement and detection).

There are two places to perform spatial frequency filtering: (1) in the frequency domain, which considers the FT, or (2) in the spatial domain, which uses the pixel values (gray levels) themselves.

Spatial Location Filtering: Convolution

Convolution, a general-purpose algorithm, is a technique of filtering in the space domain as illustrated in Figure 3-21.

The value of the output pixel depends on a group of pixels in the input image that surround

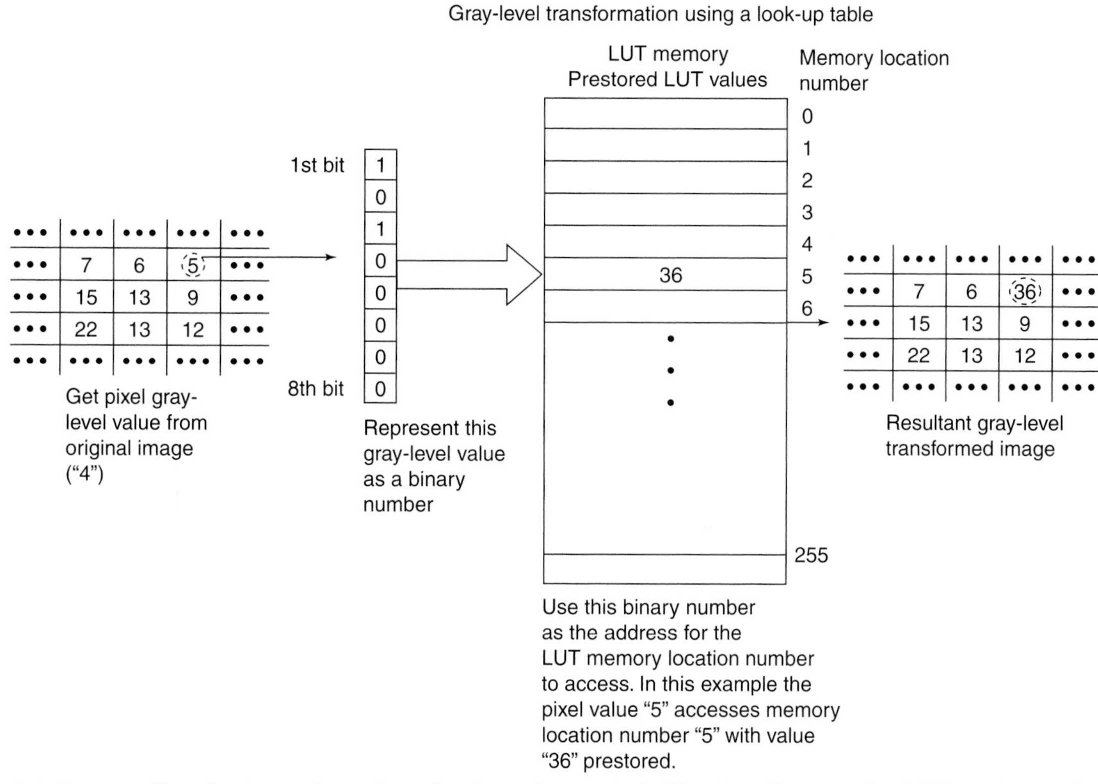

FIGURE 3-18 Gray-level transformation of an input image pixel. The algorithm uses the LUT to change the value of the input pixel (5) to 36, the new value of the output pixel. (From Huang HK: *PACS and imaging informatics: basic principles and applications*, Hoboken, NJ, 2004, John Wiley.)

the input pixel of interest: in this case, pixel P5. The new value for P5 in the output image is calculated by obtaining its weighted average and that of its surrounding pixels. The average is computed by using a group of pixels called a *convolution kernel*, in which each pixel in the kernel is a weighting factor, or convolution coefficient. In general, the size of the kernel is a 3×3 matrix. Depending on the type of processing, different types of convolution kernels can be used, in which case the weighting factors are different.

During convolution, the convolution kernel moves across the image, pixel by pixel. Each pixel in the input image, its surrounding neighbors, and the kernels are used to compute the value of the corresponding output pixel—that is, each pixel is multiplied by its respective weighting factor and then summed. The resulting number is the value of the center output pixel. This process is applied to all pixels in the input image; each calculation requires nine multiplications and nine additions. This can be time consuming, but special hardware can speed up this process.

Spatial Frequency Filtering: High Pass Filtering

The high pass filtering process, also known as edge enhancement or sharpness, is intended to sharpen an input image in the spatial domain that appears blurred. The algorithm is such that first the spatial location image is converted into spatial frequencies by using the FT, followed by the use of a high pass filter that suppresses the low

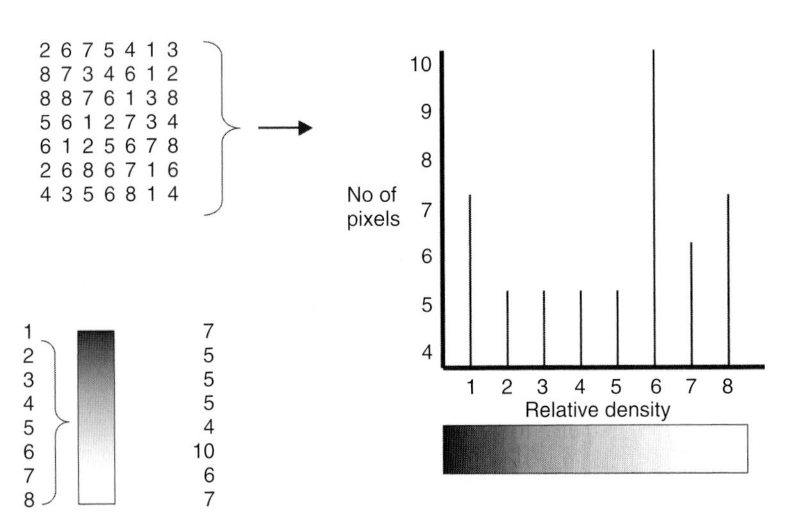

FIGURE 3-19 The creation of a histogram. A histogram is a graph of the number of pixels in the entire image or part of the image having the same gray levels (density values), plotted as a function of the gray levels. (From Seeram E: Digital image processing, *Radiol Technol* 75:435-455, 2004. Reproduced by permission of the American Society of Radiologic Technologists.)

spatial frequencies to produce a sharper output image. This process is shown in Figure 3-22. The high pass filter kernel is also shown.

Spatial Frequency Filtering: Low Pass Filtering

A low pass filtering process makes use of a low pass filter to operate on the input image with the goal of smoothing. The output image will appear blurred. Smoothing is intended to reduce noise and the displayed brightness levels of pixels; however, image detail is compromised. This is illustrated in Figure 3-23. The low pass filter kernel is also shown.

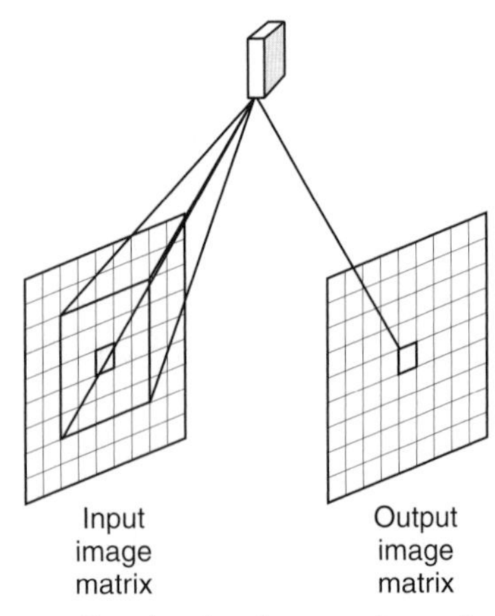

FIGURE 3-20 In the local operation, the value is determined from a small area of pixels surrounding the corresponding input pixel.

Spatial Frequency Processing: Unsharp (Blurred) Masking

The digital image processing technique of unsharp (blurred) masking uses the blurred image produced from the low pass filtering process and subtracts it from the original image to produce a sharp image, as illustrated in Figure 3-24. It can be see that the output image appears sharper.

Global Operations

In global operations, the entire input image is used to compute the value of the pixel in the output image (Fig. 3-25). A common global operation is Fourier domain processing, or the FT, which uses filtering in the frequency domain rather than the space domain (Baxes, 1994). Fourier domain image processing techniques can provide

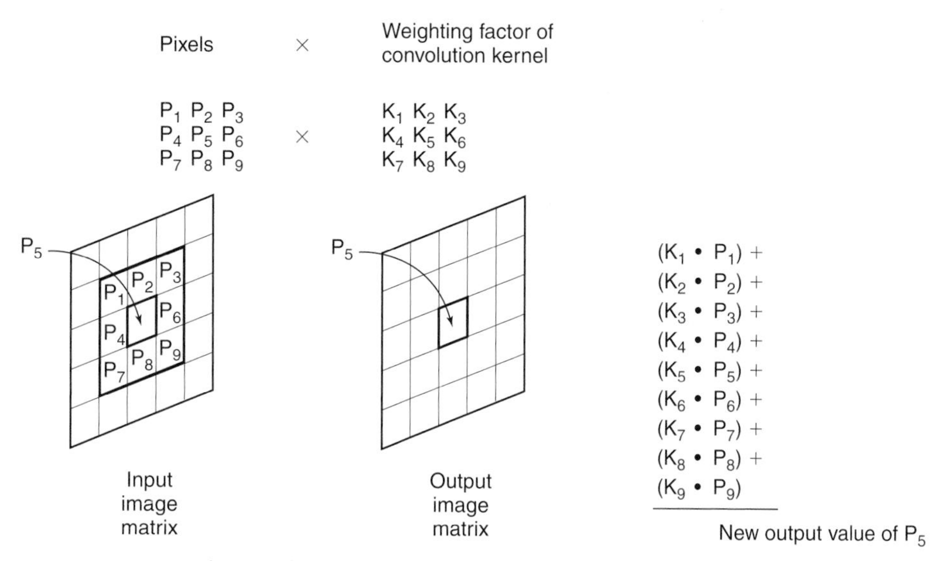

FIGURE 3-21 In convolution, the value of the output pixel is calculated by multiplying each input pixel by its corresponding weighting factor of the convolution kernel (usually a 3 × 3 matrix). These products are then summed.

edge enhancement, image sharpening, and image restoration.

Geometric Operations

Geometric operations are intended to modify the spatial position or orientation of the pixels in an image. These algorithms change the position rather than the intensity of the pixels, which is also a characteristic of point, local, and global operations. Geometric operations can result in the scaling and sizing of images and image rotation and translation (Castleman, 1996).

IMAGE COMPRESSION OVERVIEW

The evolving nature of digital image acquisition, processing, display, storage, and communications in diagnostic radiology has resulted in an exponential increase in digital image files. For example, the number of images generated in a multislice CT examination can range from 40 to 3000. If the image size is 512 × 512 × 12, then one examination can generate 20 megabytes (MB) of data, and up. A CT examination consisting of two images per

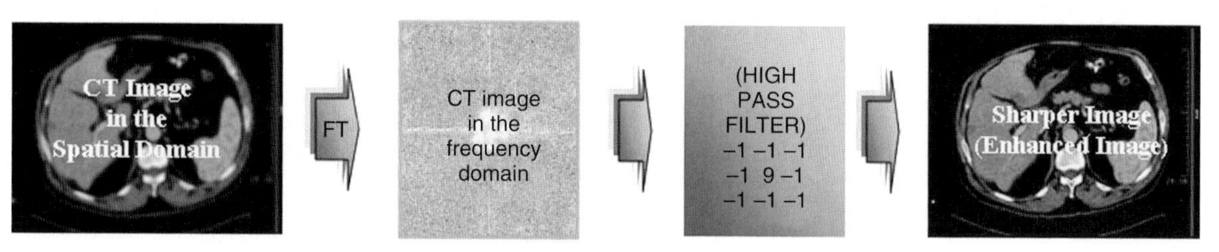

FIGURE 3-22 The use of a high pass filter to produce a sharper image. The filter is called a kernel and it suppresses the low spatial frequencies in the image.

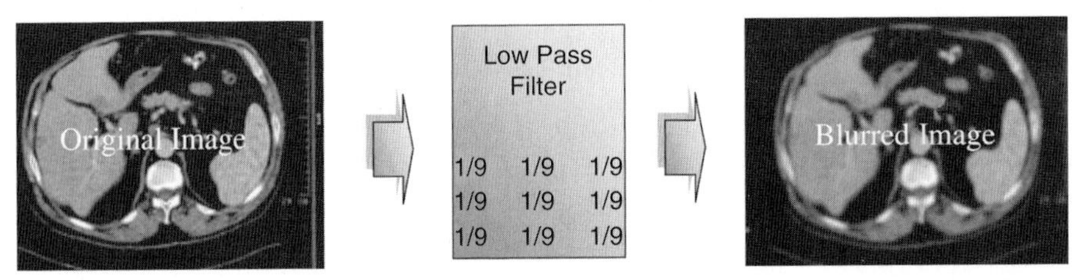

FIGURE 3-23 The effect of a low pass filter on picture quality. The low pass filter kernel suppresses the high spatial frequencies in the image.

examination with an image size of 2048 × 2048 × 12 will result in 16 MB of data. A digital mammography examination can now generate 160 MB of data. Additionally, Huang (2004) points out that "the number of digital medical images captured per year in the US alone is over pentabytes that is, 10^{15}, and is increasing rapidly every year." In this regard, it can safely be assumed that perhaps similar trends apply to Canada.

With the above in mind, image compression can solve the problems of image data storage and improve communication speed requirements for huge amounts of digital data (Seeram, 2004; Seeram and Seeram, 2008).

What Is Image Compression?

The literature is replete with definitions of image compression; however, one that stands out in terms of clarity is offered by Alan Rowberg, MD, of the Department of Radiology, University of Washington: "Digital compression refers to using one or more of many software and/or hardware techniques to reduce information by removing unnecessary data. The remaining information is then encoded and either transmitted or stored in an archive or storage media, such as tape or disk. In a process called decompression, the user's equipment later decodes the information and fills

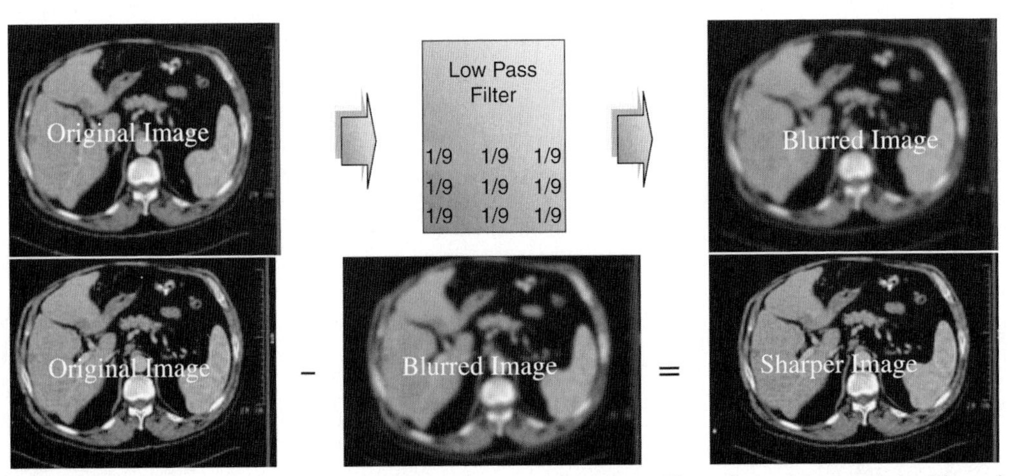

FIGURE 3-24 The digital image processing technique of unsharp (blurred) masking uses the blurred image produced from the low pass filtering process and subtracts it from the original image to produce a sharp image.

in a representation of the data that was removed during compression."

The above definition will serve as the basis for understanding what is meant by image compression.

Types of Image Compression

As mentioned earlier in this chapter, there are two types of image data compression; lossless or reversible compression, and lossy or irreversible compression. In the former, no information is lost when the image is decompressed or reconstructed; in the latter, there is some loss of information, when the image is decompressed (see Fig. 3-15).

Although it is not within the scope of this section to describe the technical details of the steps involved in image compression, the following points are noteworthy:

- In lossless or reversible compression, there is no loss of information in the compressed image data. Furthermore, lossless compression does not involve the process of quantization but makes use of image transformation and encoding to provide a compressed image.
- Lossy or irreversible compression involves at least three steps: image transformation, quantization, and encoding. As noted by Erickson (2002),

> Transformation is a lossless step in which the image is transformed from gray scale values in the spatial domain to coefficients in some other domain. One familiar transformation is the Fourier Transform used in reconstruction Magnetic Resonance Images (MRI). Other transforms such as the Discrete Cosine Transform (DCT) and the Discrete Wavelet Transform (DWT) are commonly used for image compression. No loss of information occurs in the transformation step. Quantization is the step in which the data integrity is lost. It attempts to minimize information loss by preferentially preserving the most important coefficients where less important coefficients are roughly approximated, often as zero. Quantization may be as simple as converting floating point values to integer values. Finally, these quantized coefficients are compactly represented for efficient storage or transmission of the image.

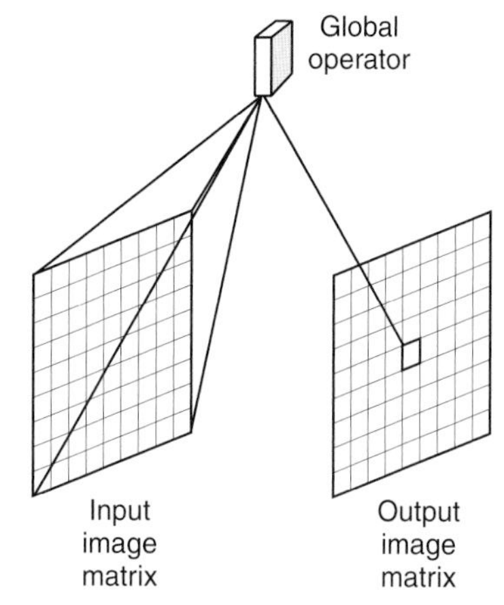

FIGURE 3-25 In a global operation, the entire input image is used to compute the value of the pixel in the output image.

There are a number of other issues relating to the use of irreversible compression in digital radiology, including the visual impact of compression (lossy compression) on diagnostic digital images and methods used to evaluate the effects of compression (Seeram, 2006). It is also well established that the quality of digital images plays an important role in helping the radiologist to provide an accurate diagnosis. At low compression ratios (8:1 or less), the loss of image quality is such that the image is still "visually acceptable" (Huang, 2004). The obvious concern that now comes to mind is related to what Erickson (2002) refers to as "compression tolerance," a term he defines as "the maximum compression in which the decompressed image is acceptable for interpretation and aesthetics."

Because lossy compression methods provide high to very high compression ratios compared with lossless methods, and keeping the term "compression tolerance" in mind, Huang (2004) points out that "currently lossy algorithms are not used by radiologists in primary diagnosis, because physicians and radiologists are concerned with the legal consequences of an incorrect diagnosis based on a lossy compressed image."

Visual Impact of Irreversible Compression on Digital Images

The goal of both lossless and lossy compression techniques is to reduce the size of the compressed image, to reduce storage requirements, and to increase image transmission speed.

The size of the compressed image is influenced by the compression ratio (see definition of terms), with lossless compression methods yielding ratios of 2:1 to 3:1 (Huang, 2004), and lossy or irreversible compression having ratios ranging from 10:1 to 50:1 or more (Huang, 2004). It is well known that as the compression ratio increases, less storage space is required and faster transmission speeds are possible but at the expense of image quality degradation.

A recent survey of the opinions of expert radiologists in the United States and Canada (Seeram, 2006), on the use of irreversible compression in clinical practice showed that the opinions are wide and varied. This indicates that there is no consensus of opinion on the use of irreversible compression in primary diagnosis. Opinions are generally positive on the notion of image storage and image transmission advantages of image compression. Finally, almost all radiologists are concerned with the litigation potential of an incorrect diagnosis that is based on irreversible compressed images.

In providing a rationale for examining the tradeoffs between image quality and compression ratio, an interesting experiment is suggested by Huang (2004) using five compressed CT images (512 × 512 × 12) with compression ratios of 4:1, 8:1, 17:1, 26:1, and 37:1 together with the original image. Next, determine the order of quality of the images, and finally, determine which compression ratio provides an image quality that can be used to provide a diagnosis. In the generalized results of this simple experiment, Huang states that "reconstructed images with compression ratios less than or equal to 8:1 do not exhibit visible deterioration in image quality. In other words, a compression ratio of 8:1 or less is visually acceptable. But visually unacceptable does not necessarily mean that the ratio is not suitable for diagnosis because this depends on what diseases are under consideration."

IMAGE SYNTHESIS OVERVIEW

One of the advantages of digital image processing is image synthesis, and examples of image synthesis are the image reconstruction methods used in CT and MRI, and 3D imaging operations. Although image reconstruction is based on mathematical procedures, 3D techniques are based on computer graphics technology. Both CT image reconstruction and 3D imaging will be described in detail in later chapters, and therefore only highlights will be mentioned here.

Magnetic Resonance Imaging

The major system processes of MRI signal acquisition to image display are shown in Figure 3-26. First, magnetic resonance signals are acquired from the patient, who is placed in the magnet during the imaging procedure. These signals are high and low frequencies collected from the patient. The signals are subsequently digitized and stored in what is referred to as "k" space, which is a frequency domain space. Once k space is filled, the FT algorithm uses the data in k space to reconstruct magnetic resonance images, which are displayed on the monitor for viewing by a radiologist or technologist.

Once displayed, images can be manipulated with special digital image processing software to perform such processing as windowing, and 3D image visualization, for example.

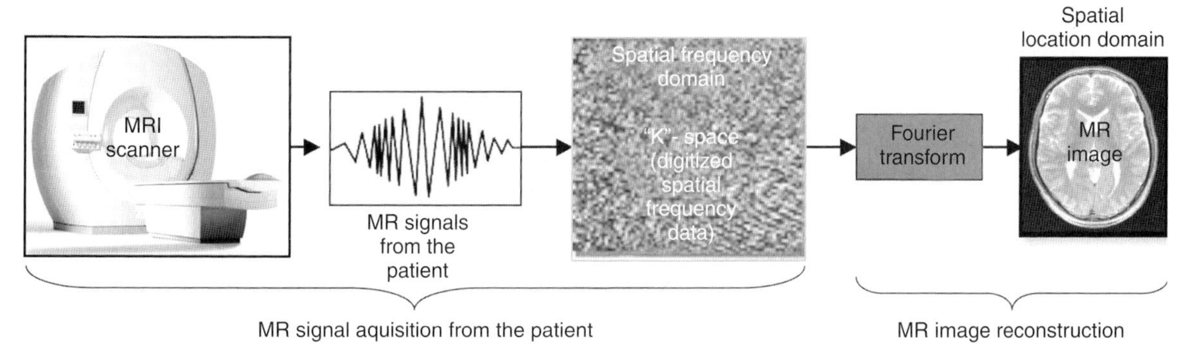

FIGURE 3-26 The major processes of MRI signal acquisition to image display. First, magnetic resonance (MR) signals are acquired from the patient, who is placed in the magnet during the imaging procedure. These signals are high and low frequencies collected from the patient. The signals are subsequently digitized and stored in what is referred to as "k" space, a frequency domain space. (Image courtesy Philips Medical Systems.)

CT Imaging

A conceptual overview of CT imaging is shown in Figure 3-27. Attenuation data are collected from the patient by the detectors that send their electronic signals to the computer, having been digitized by the ADC. The computer then uses a special image reconstruction algorithm, referred to as the filtered back projection algorithm, to build up a digital CT image. This image must be converted to a gray scale image to be displayed on a monitor for viewing by the radiologist and the technologist.

Displayed CT images can be manipulated with digital image processing software to perform such processing as windowing, image reformatting, and 3D image visualization.

Three-Dimensional Imaging in Radiology

3D imaging is gaining widespread attention in radiology (Beigelman-Aubry et al, 2005; Dalrymple et al, 2005; Neuman and Meyers, 2005; Seeram, 2004; Shekhar et al, 2003). Already 3D imaging is used in CT, MRI, and other imaging modalities with the goal of providing both qualitative and quantitative information from images to facilitate and enhance diagnosis.

The general framework for 3D imaging is shown in Figure 3-28. Four major steps are shown: data acquisition, creation of what is referred to as 3D space (all voxel information is stored in the computer), processing for 3D image display, and finally, 3D image display. Digital processing can

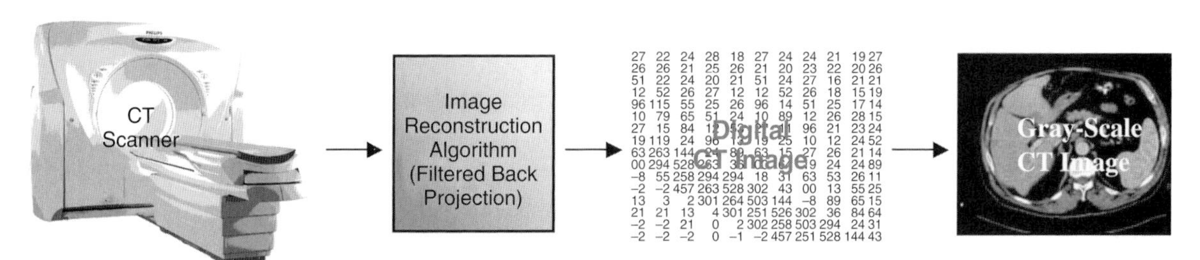

FIGURE 3-27 A conceptual overview of CT imaging. Image reconstruction is performed by the filtered back projection. See text for further explanation.

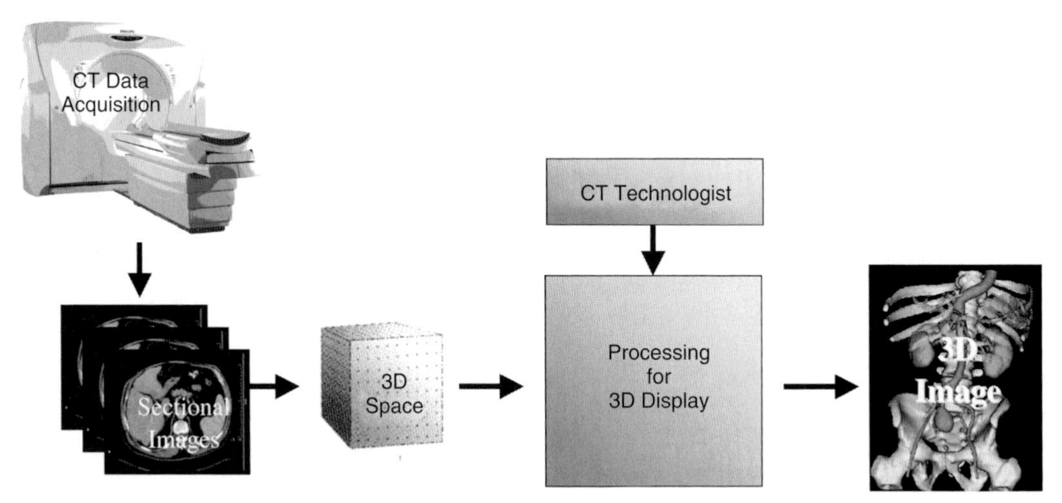

FIGURE 3-28 The general framework for 3D imaging. Four major steps are shown: data acquisition, creation of what is referred to as 3D space, processing for 3D image display, and finally 3D image display. Digital processing can allow the observer to view all aspects of 3D space, a technique referred to as 3D visualization. (Image courtesy Philips Medical Systems.)

allow the observer to view all aspects of 3D space, a technique referred to as 3D visualization. The application of 3D visualization techniques in radiology is referred to as 3D medical imaging.

Dr. Jayaram from the Department of Radiology at the University of Pennsylvania, an expert in 3D imaging, notes that there are four classes of 3D imaging operations: preprocessing, visualization, manipulation, and analysis. Because the visualization operations are now quite popular in digital imaging departments using CT and MRI scanners, it is noteworthy to highlight the major ideas of at least two 3D visualization techniques, surface rendering and volume rendering. Rendering is the final step in 3D image production. It is a computer program used to transform 3D space into simulated 3D images to be displayed on a two-dimensional computer screen.

Two classes of rendering techniques are used in radiology: surface rendering and volume rendering. *Surface rendering* is a simple procedure in which the surface of an object is created using contour data and shading the pixels to provide the illusion of depth. It uses only 10% of the data in 3D space and does not require a great deal of computation. *Volume rendering*, on the other hand, is a much more sophisticated technique. Volume rendering uses all the data in 3D space to provide additional information by allowing the observer to view more details inside the object, as is clearly illustrated in Figure 3-28. It also requires more computational power.

Applications of these rendering techniques are in several areas, including imaging the craniomaxillofacial complex, musculoskeletal system, the central nervous system, and cardiovascular, pulmonary, gastrointestinal, and genitourinary systems. 3D imaging is now popular in CT angiography (Fishman et al, 2006) and magnetic resonance angiography.

3D medical imaging uses stand-alone workstations featuring very powerful computers capable of a wide range of processing functions, including virtual reality imaging (VRI).

Virtual Reality Imaging in Radiology

VRI requires sophisticated digital image processing methods to facilitate the perception of 3D anatomy from a set of two-dimensional images

(Huang, 2004; Kalender, 2005; Seeram, 2004). The vast amount of data collected by multislice CT scanners, for example, provides the opportunity to develop VRI imaging applications in radiology.

Virtual reality is a branch of computer science that immerses the users in a computer-generated environment and allows them to interact with 3D scenes. One common method that uses virtual reality concepts is virtual endoscopy. Virtual endoscopy is used to create inner views of tubular structures.

Virtual endoscopy involves a set of systematic procedures to be followed. These include data acquisition (careful selection of scan parameters in collecting data from the patient), image preprocessing (to optimize images before they are processed), 3D rendering, using both surface and volume rendering, and finally, image display, and analysis. Two examples of software tools available for interactive image assessment, include Philip's Voyager and General Electric's 3D Navigator (advanced visualization packages to allow the user to perform real-time navigation of structures using a "fly through" within and around tubular anatomy in the same manner a real endoscope is used. 3D imaging and VRI will be described in detail in a later chapter.

IMAGE PROCESSING HARDWARE

A basic image processing system consists of several interconnected components (Fig. 3-29). The major components are the ADC, image storage, image display, image processor, host computer, and DAC.

- *Data acquisition:* In Figure 3-29, the video camera is the data acquisition device. In CT this would be represented by the x-ray tube and detectors and the detector electronics.
- *Digitizer:* As can be seen in Figure 3-29, the analog signal is converted into digital form by the digitizer, or ADC.
- *Image memory:* The digitized image is held in storage for further processing. Several components are connected to the image store and provide input and output. The size of this memory depends on the image. For example, a 512 × 512 × 8 bit image requires a memory of 2,097,152 bits.
- *DAC:* The digital image held in the memory can be displayed on a television monitor. However, because monitors work with analog

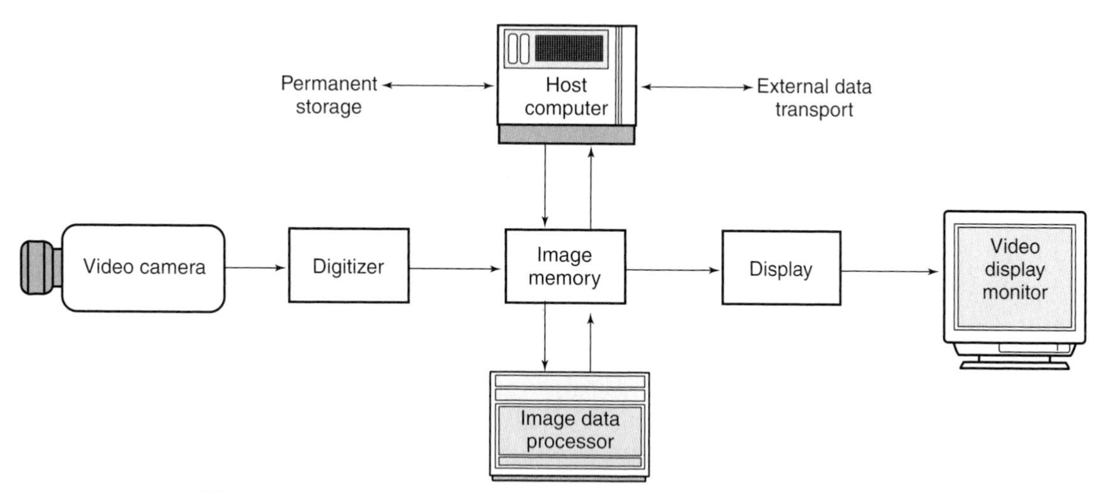

FIGURE 3-29 The essential hardware components of a generalized digital image processing system.

signals, it is necessary to convert the digital data to analog signals with a DAC.

- *Internal image processor:* This processor is responsible for high-speed processing of the input digital data.
- *Host computer:* In digital image processing, the host computer is a primary component capable of performing several functions. For example, the host computer can read and write the data in the image store and provide for archival storage on tape and disk storage systems. The host computer plays a significant role in applications that involve the transmission of images to another location, such as medical imaging.

CT AS A DIGITAL IMAGE PROCESSING SYSTEM

A number of imaging modalities in radiology use image processing techniques, including digital radiography and fluoroscopy, nuclear medicine, MRI, ultrasonography, and CT. The future of digital imaging is promising in that a wide variety of applications have received increasing attention, such as 3D imaging (Seeram and Seeram, 2008). The major image-processing operations in medical imaging that are now common in the radiology department are presented in Table 3-2.

The basic components of a digital imaging system were illustrated in Figure 1-28. As a digital image processing system, CT fits into this scheme. In addition, similar steps in image digitization can be applied to the CT process, as follows:

1. First, divide the picture into pixels. In CT, the slice of the patient is divided into small regions called *voxels* (volume element) because the dimension of depth (slice thickness) is added to the pixel. The patient is scanned as the x-ray tube moves around the patient.
2. Next, sample the pixels. In CT, the voxels are sampled when x rays pass through them. This measurement is performed by detectors. The signal from the detector is in analog form and must be converted into digital form before it can be sent to the computer for processing.

TABLE 3-2 Common Digital Image Processing Operations Used in Diagnostic Digital Imaging Technologies

Digital Imaging Modality	Common Image Processing Operations
CT	Image reformatting, windowing, region of interest, magnification, surface and volume rendering, profile, histogram, collage, image synthesis
MRI	Windowing, region of interest, magnification, surface and volume rendering, profile, histogram, collage, image synthesis
Digital subtraction angiography/digital fluoroscopy	Analytic processing, subtraction of images out of sequence, gray-scale processing, temporal frame averaging, edge enhancement, pixel shifting
Computed radiography/digital radiography	Partitioned pattern recognition, exposure field recognition, histogram analysis, normalization of raw image data, gray-scale processing (windowing), spatial filtering, dynamic range control, energy subtraction, etc.

From Seeram E: Digital image processing, *Radiol Technol* 75:435-455, 2004. Reproduced by permission.

3. The final step is quantization. In CT, the analog signal is also quantized and changed into a digital array for input into the computer. The digital data resulting from quantization are processed by the computer through a series of operations or techniques to modify the input image. In CT, the digital data are also subject to several processing algorithms so the output image can be displayed in a form suitable for human observation.

IMAGE PROCESSING: AN ESSENTIAL TOOL FOR CT

Image postprocessing and its associated techniques such as data visualization, computer-aided detection, and image data set navigation have recently been identified as major research areas in the transformation of medical Imaging (Andriole and Morin, 2006). Image postprocessing methods in CT are intended to enhance the diagnostic interpretation skills of the radiologist. Several examples of these methods include image reformatting to display axial images in the coronal, sagittal, and oblique views, maximum intensity and minimum intensity projections, curved reformatting, shaded surface display (SSD) and virtual reality, and physiologic imaging tools such as image fusion and CT perfusion. These methods will be described in detail in later chapters.

Digital image processing is now an essential tool in the CT and PACS environment, and already technologists and radiologists are actively involved in using the tools of image postprocessing, such as the digital image processing operations and techniques outlined in this chapter. Training programs for both technologists and radiologists are also beginning to incorporate digital image processing as part of their curriculum (Seeram and Seeram, 2008). A suggested list of topics for a course on image processing in CT would be the chapter outline at the beginning of this chapter. These topics can be expanded beyond the content of this chapter.

REFERENCES

Andriole KP, Morin R: Transforming medical imaging—the first SCAR TRIP Conference. *J Digital Imaging* 19:6-16, 2006.

Baxes GA: *Digital image processing: principles and applications*, New York, 1994, John Wiley.

Beigelman-Aubry D et al: Multi-detector row CT and post-processing techniques in the assessment of lung diseases. *Radiographics* 25:1639-1652, 2005.

Castleman KR: *Digital image processing*, Englewood Cliffs, NJ, 1996, Prentice Hall.

Dalrymple NG et al: Introduction to the language of three-dimensional imaging with multi-detector CT, *Radiographics* 25:1409-1428, 2005.

Erickson BJ: Irreversible compression of medical images, *J Digital Imaging* 15:5-14; 2002.

Fishman EK et al: Volume rendering versus maximum intensity projection in CT angiography: what works best, when, and why, *Radiographics* 26:905-922, 2006.

Huang HK: *PACS and imaging informatics: basic prinicples and applications*, Englewood Cliffs, NJ, 2004, John Wiley.

Kalender WA: *Computed tomography*, Munich, 2005, Publicis MCD Werbeagentur Verlag.

Lindley CA: *Practical image processing in C*, New York, 1991, John Wiley.

Luiten AL: Digital: discrete perfection. *Medicamundi* 40: 95-100, 1995.

Marion A: *Introduction to image processing*, London, 1991, Chapman and Hall.

Neuman J, Meyers M: *Volume intensity projection: a new post-processing techniques for evaluating CTA*, Netherlands, 2005, Philips Medical Systems.

Pooley RA et al: Digital fluoroscopy, *Radiographics* 21: 521-534, 2001.

Seeram E: *Computed tomography—physical principles, clinical applications and quality control*, Philadelphia, 2001, WB Saunders.

Seeram E: Digital image processing, *Radiol Technol* 75: 435-455, 2004.

Seeram E: Irreversible compression in digital radiology, *Radiography* 12:45-59, 2006.

Seeram E: Using irreversible compression in digital radiology: a preliminary study of the opinions of radiologists. Progress in Biomedical Optics and Imaging–Proceedings of the SPIE, San Diego, Calif, July 2006.

Seeram E, Seeram D: Image postprocessing in digital radiology: a primer for technologists, *Journal of Medical Imaging and Radiation Sciences* 39:23-41; 2008.

Seibert JA: Digital image processing: basics. In Balter S, Shope TB, editors: *A categorical course in physics: physical and technical aspects of angiography and interventional radiology*, Oak Brook, Ill, 1995, Radiological Society of North America.

Chapter 4

Physical Principles of Computed Tomography

Chapter Outline

The information presented in a computed tomography (CT) image differs from a conventional radiographic image in several respects. The most obvious is that CT shows cross-sectional (transaxial) views of patient anatomy. In addition, CT shows three-dimensional (3D) images that are computer generated (digital image after processing) with use of the transaxial data set (Fig. 4-1). Other significant differences in CT imaging will become apparent in the following chapters. In this presentation of the physical principles of CT, a review of conventional tomography and the limitations of radiography is helpful to understand the CT image.

LIMITATIONS OF RADIOGRAPHY AND TOMOGRAPHY

In both radiography and tomography, x rays pass through the patient and are absorbed in different ways by the body's tissues. For example, because bone is denser, it absorbs more x rays than do the less-dense soft tissues. This differential absorption is contained in the x-ray beam that passes through the patient and is recorded on radiographic film or a radiographic digital detector, such as a computed radiography imaging plate, for example.

Limitations of Film-Based Radiography

The major shortcoming of radiography is the superimposition of all structures on the film, which makes it difficult and sometimes impossible to distinguish a particular detail (Fig. 4-2). This is especially true when structures differ only slightly in density, as is often the case with some tumors and their surrounding tissues. Although multiple views such as laterals and obliques can be taken to localize a structure, the problem of superimposition in radiography still persists.

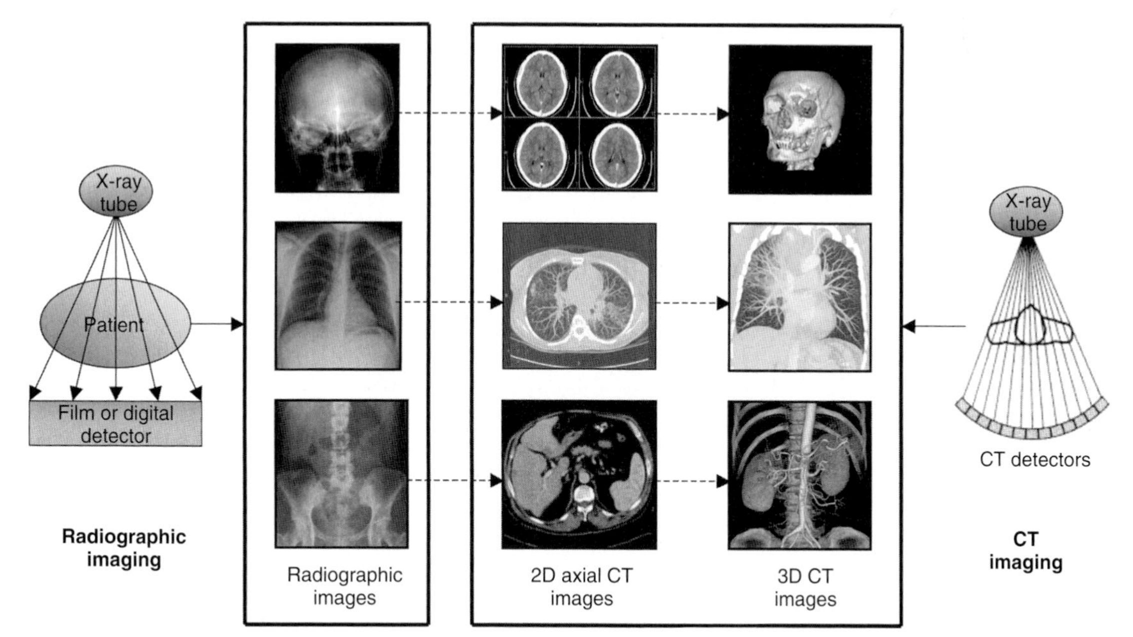

FIGURE 4-1 The most conspicuous difference between conventional radiographic imaging and CT imaging is that CT shows cross-sectional or transaxial anatomy, that can be subject to digital postprocessing operations to produce 3D images. (3D CT images courtesy Philips Medical Systems.)

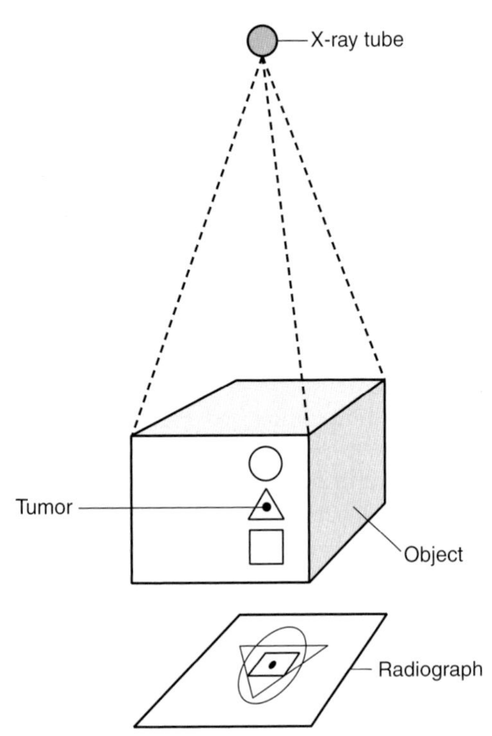

FIGURE 4-2 The major shortcoming of radiography is that the superimposition of all structures on the radiograph makes it difficult to discriminate whether the tumor is in the circle, triangle, or square. (From Seeram E: *Computed tomography technology*, Philadelphia, 1982, WB Saunders.)

A second limitation is that radiography is a qualitative rather than quantitative process (Fig. 4-3). It is difficult to distinguish between a homogeneous object of nonuniform thickness and a heterogeneous object (Fig. 4-3 includes bone, soft tissue, and air) of uniform thickness (Marshall, 1976).

Limitations of Conventional Tomography

The problem of superimposition in radiography can be somewhat overcome by conventional tomography (Bocage, 1974; Vallebona, 1931). The most common method of conventional tomography is sometimes referred to as *geometric tomography* to distinguish it from CT (Fig. 4-4). When the x-ray tube and film are moved simultaneously in opposite directions, unwanted sections can be blurred while the desired layer or section is kept in focus.

The immediate goal of tomography is to eliminate structures above and below the focused section, or the focal plane. However, this is difficult to achieve, and under no circumstances can all unwanted planes be removed. The limitations of tomography include persistent image blurring that cannot be completely removed, degradation of image contrast because of the presence of scattered radiation created by the open geometry of the x-ray beam, and other problems resulting from film-screen combinations.

In addition, both radiography and tomography fail to adequately demonstrate slight differences in subject contrast, which are characteristic of soft tissue. The differences for soft tissues such as human fat, water, human cerebrospinal fluid, human plasma, monkey pancreas, monkey white matter, monkey gray matter, monkey liver, monkey muscle, and human red blood cells are 0.194, 0.222, 0.227, 0.227, 0.230, 0.230, 0.235, 0.236, 0.238, and 0.246, respectively (Ter-Pogossian et al, 1974). Radiographic film is not sensitive enough to resolve these small differences because typical film-screen combinations used today can only discriminate x-ray intensity differences of 5% to 10%.

The limitations of radiography and tomography result in the inability of film to image very small differences in tissue contrast. In addition, contrast cannot be adjusted after it has been recorded on the film. Digital imaging modalities such as CT, for example, can alter the contrast to suit the needs of the human observer (radiologists and technologists) by use of various digital image postprocessing techniques (see Chapter 3).

Enter CT

The goal of CT is to overcome the limitations of radiography and tomography by achieving the following (Hounsfield, 1973):

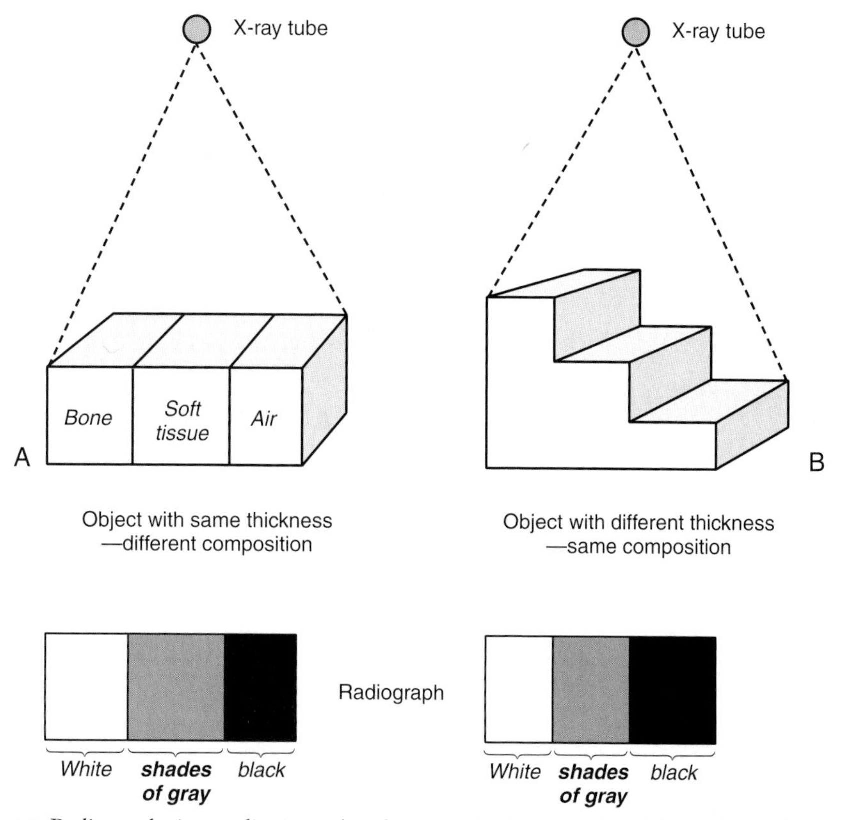

FIGURE 4-3 Radiography is a qualitative rather than quantitative procedure. Two radiographs can appear the same although the two objects, **A** and **B**, are entirely different. (From Seeram E: *Computed tomography technology*, Philadelphia, 1982, WB Saunders.)

1. Minimal superimposition
2. Improved image contrast
3. The recording of very small differences in tissue contrast

The basic methodological approach to these three tasks is shown in Figure 4-5. A few important points can be noted from this figure, as follows:

1. A beam of x rays is transmitted through a specific cross-section of the patient. This procedure removes the problem of superimposition of structures above and below the specific cross-section or slice of tissue.
2. The beam of x rays is highly collimated into a thin beam (a very narrow beam) that only passes through the cross-section of tissue to be imaged. This procedure is intended to minimize scatter production and therefore improve the contrast of the image.
3. When the x-ray beam passes through the patient, it strikes special electronic detectors positioned opposite the x-ray tube. These detectors are quantitative and can measure very small differences in tissue contrast. (However, the film-screen detector in radiography is considered a qualitative detector and cannot record these small differences.) In addition, the analog signals from the electronic detectors are first converted into digital data and are subsequently processed by a digital computer that uses special algorithms to reconstruct an image of the cross-section.

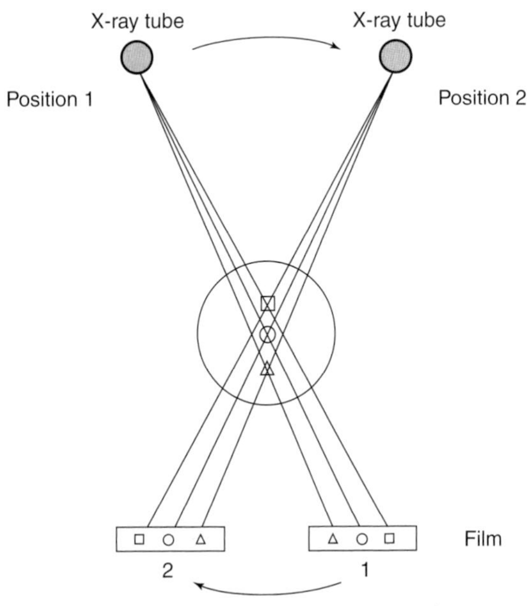

FIGURE 4-4 Basic principles of conventional tomography. The x-ray tube and film move simultaneously and in opposite directions to ensure that the desired section (○) of the patient is imaged by blurring out structures above (□) and below (△) the plane of interest (○). (From Seeram E: *Computed tomography technology*, Philadelphia, 1982, WB Saunders.)

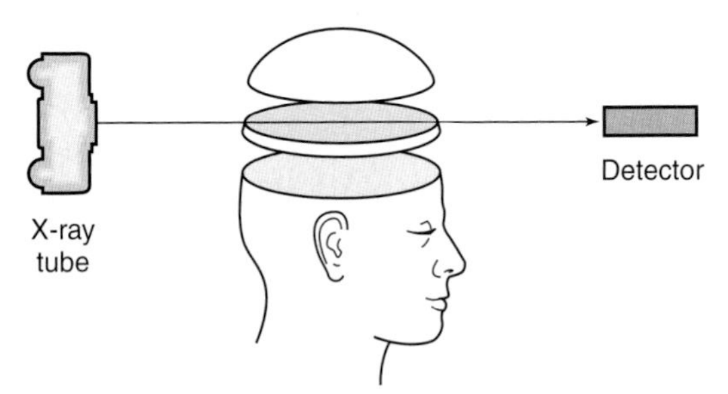

FIGURE 4-5 In CT a thin beam is transmitted through a specific cross-section, striking special detectors opposite the x-ray tube.

PHYSICAL PRINCIPLES

CT can be described in terms of physical principles and technological considerations. The physical principles involve physics and mathematical concepts to understand the way the image is produced, and the technological considerations involve the practical implementation of scientific and engineering principles such as computer science and technology. The physical principles and technology of CT include the three processes referred to in Chapter 1: data acquisition, data processing, and image display, storage, and communication. This section discusses each process in basic terms; they are described in more detail in later chapters.

Data Acquisition

Data acquisition refers to the systematic collection of information from the patient to produce the CT image. The two methods of data acquisition are slice-by-slice data acquisition and volume data acquisition (Fig. 4-6).

In conventional slice-by-slice data acquisition, data are collected through different beam geometries to scan the patient. Essentially, the x-ray tube rotates around the patient and collects data from the first slice. The tube stops, and the patient moves into position to scan the next slice. This process

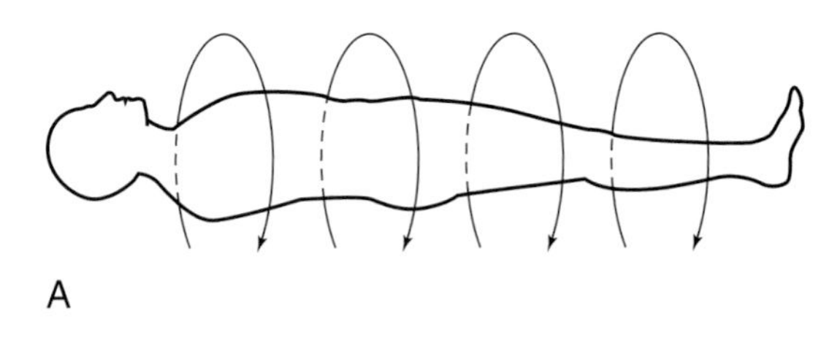

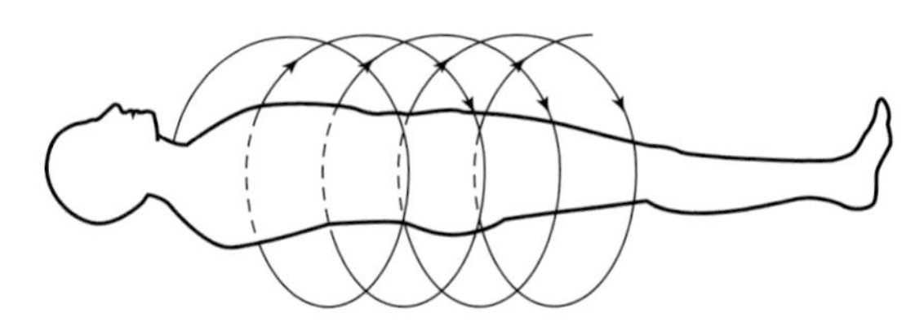

FIGURE 4-6 A, Conventional slice-by-slice CT data acquisition. **B,** Volume CT data acquisition.

continues until all slices have been individually scanned.

In volume data acquisition, a special beam geometry referred to as *spiral* or *helical geometry* is used to scan a volume of tissue rather than one slice at a time (see Fig. 4-6). In spiral/helical CT, the x-ray tube rotates around the patient and traces a spiral/helical path to scan an entire volume of tissue while the patient holds a single breath. This method generates a single slice per one revolution of the x-ray tube and is often referred to as a single-slice spiral/helical CT (SSCT). To improve the volume coverage speed performance of SSCT, multislice spiral/helical CT (MSCT) has become available for faster imaging of patients. MSCT scanners generate multiple slices per one revolution of the x-ray tube. For example, MSCT scanners can now generate 4, 8, 16, 32, 40, or 64 slices per revolution of the x-ray tube. The most recent MSCT scanner commercially available for clinical imaging of patients (at the time of writing this chapter) is the 64-slice MSCT scanner. Additionally, in 2007, an MSCT scanner that can produce 320 slices per revolution of the x-ray tube became commercially available.

The first step in data acquisition is scanning (Fig. 4-7). During scanning, the x-ray tube and detectors rotate around the patient to collect views (intensity readings). The detectors measure the radiation transmitted through the patient from various locations. As a result, relative transmission values (Hounsfield, 1973) or attenuation measurements (Sprawls, 1995) can be calculated as follows:

$$\text{Relative transmission} = \text{Log}\,\frac{\text{Intensity of x-rays at the source }(I_0)}{\text{Intensity of x-rays at the detector }(I)}$$

The relative transmission values are sent to the computer and stored as raw data.

A large number of transmission measurements are needed to reconstruct the CT image. In general, several hundred views are obtained. Each view is composed of a number of rays, and the total

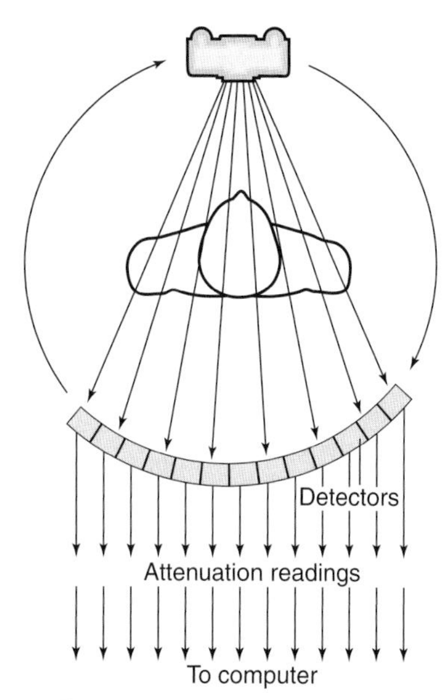

FIGURE 4-7 During scanning, the x-ray tube and detectors rotate around the patient to collect views.

transmission measurements for each scan is given by the following relationship (Sprawls, 1995):

$$\text{Total number of transmission measurements} = \text{Number of views} \times \text{Number of rays in each view}$$

Radiation Attenuation

The problem in CT is to determine the attenuation in the tissues and use this information to reconstruct an image of the slice of tissue. The solution to this problem is complex and involves physics, mathematics, and computer science. This book takes a fundamental approach to the problem and its solution. The study begins with an understanding of attenuation of radiation in general and attenuation in CT in particular.

Attenuation is the reduction of the intensity of a beam of radiation as it passes through an object—some photons are absorbed, but others are scattered. Attenuation depends on the electrons per gram, atomic number, tissue density, and radiation energy used. In addition, because there are two types of radiation beams (homogeneous and heterogeneous), a study of how each of these beams is attenuated is important to understand the problem in CT. Attenuation in CT depends on the effective atomic density (atoms/volume), the atomic number (Z) of the absorber, and the photon energy.

In a homogeneous beam, all the photons have the same energy, whereas in a heterogeneous beam the photons have different energies. A homogeneous beam is also referred to as a *monochromatic* or *monoenergetic beam*, and a heterogeneous beam is referred to as a *polychromatic beam*.

When Hounsfield invented the CT scanner, he used a homogeneous beam (Fig. 4-8) in his initial experiments because such a beam satisfies the requirements of the Lambert-Beer law, an exponential relationship that describes what happens to the photons as they travel through the tissues according to the following attenuation:

$$I = I_0 e^{-\mu x} \tag{4-1}$$

where I is the transmitted intensity, I_0 is the original intensity, x is the thickness of the object, e is Euler's constant (2.718), and μ is the linear attenuation coefficient.

The goal of CT is to calculate the linear attenuation coefficient μ, which indicates the amount of attenuation that has occurred. Therefore it is a quantitative measurement with a unit of per centimeter (cm^{-1})—hence the term *linear* (Bushong, 2004; Kalender, 2005).

The equation $I = I_0 e^{-\mu x}$ can be solved to find the value of μ:

$$\begin{aligned} I &= I_0 e^{-\mu x} \\ I/I_0 &= e^{-\mu x} \\ \ln I/I_0 &= -\mu x \\ \ln I_0/I &= \mu x \\ \mu &= (1/x)\cdot(\ln I_0/I) \end{aligned} \tag{4-2}$$

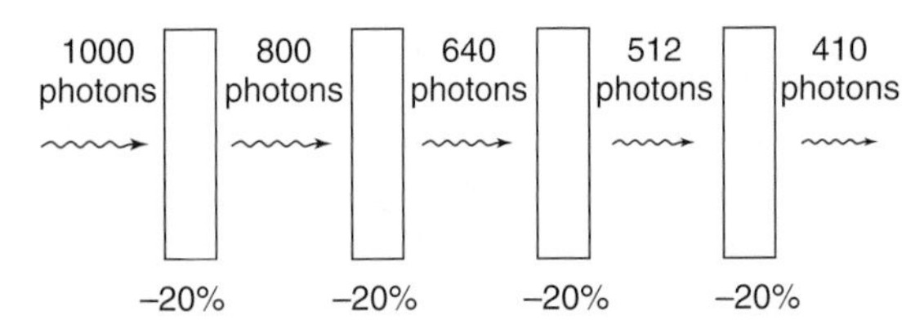

FIGURE 4-8 Attenuation of a homogeneous beam of radiation through water. The absorber is 1 cm of water.

where *ln* is the natural logarithm. In CT, the values of I and I_0 are known (these are measured by the detectors), and x is also known. Hence μ can be calculated.

Figure 4-8 shows the attenuation of a homogeneous beam of radiation. Each section of the absorber attenuates the beam by equal amounts; that is, each 1-cm section removes 20% of the photons remaining in the beam. The initial beam intensity of 1000 photons is reduced to 410 photons. In other words, the quantity of photons is reduced. In a homogeneous beam the quality of the beam, or beam energy, does not change. If the starting beam energy is 88 kiloelectron volts (keV), the transmitted photons all have an energy of 88 keV.

In the early experiments conducted by Hounsfield, the radiation was from a gamma source and the attenuation was that of a homogeneous beam. One problem he encountered was that it took too long to scan and produce an image, and therefore he substituted a beam produced by a conventional x-ray tube. This beam is a heterogeneous beam of radiation that consists of a range of energies. The attenuation of a heterogeneous or polychromatic beam is somewhat different from that of a homogeneous beam, and therefore Hounsfield had to make several assumptions and adjustments to determine the linear attenuation coefficients.

During the attenuation of a heterogeneous beam (Fig. 4-9), as the beam passes through equal thicknesses of material, the attenuation is not exponential but rather both the quantity and quality of the photons change. In Figure 4-9, the initial quantity

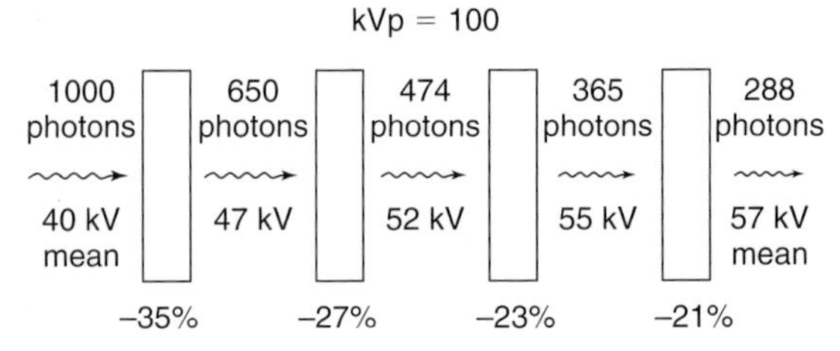

FIGURE 4-9 Attenuation of a heterogeneous beam of radiation through water.

of photons is 1000 with a mean beam quality (energy) of 40 kilovolts (kV). Each block of water removes different quantities of photons, and the mean energy of the transmitted photons increases to 57 kV. The first centimeter of water attenuates more photons than subsequent 1-cm blocks of water. Also, the lower-energy photons are absorbed, which allows the higher-energy photons to pass through. As a result, the penetrating power of the photons increases and the beam becomes harder.

The equation $I = I_0e^{-\mu x}$ applies only to a homogeneous beam. It then follows that in CT, which is based on the use of a heterogeneous beam, it is necessary to make the heterogeneous beam approximate a homogeneous beam to satisfy the equation.

It was stated earlier that attenuation is the result of absorption and scattering. X rays can be attenuated because of the photoelectric effect, or they can be attenuated and scattered by the Compton effect. The total attenuation is then given by

$$I = I_0e^{-(\mu p + \mu c)x} \tag{4-3}$$

where μ_p is the linear attenuation coefficient that results from photoelectric absorption, and μ_c is the linear attenuation coefficient that results from the Compton effect.

The photoelectric effect occurs mainly in tissues with a high atomic number, Z (such as bone, contrast medium) and occurs minimally in some soft tissues and substances with a lower Z. The Compton effect occurs in soft tissues, and differences in density result in differences in Compton interactions. In addition, the photoelectric effect depends on the beam energy (kilovolts); however, the Compton effect is less likely to dominate as the beam energy increases and "the energy dependence is not nearly as dramatic as it is with the photoelectric effect" (Morgan, 1983).

Equation 4-2, like Equation 4-1, holds true only for a homogeneous beam of radiation. Because a heterogeneous beam is used in CT, how is the linear attenuation coefficient determined in CT? The concern is with the number of photons, N, that pass through the tissue during scanning, rather than with the intensity, I. Equation 4-1 can therefore be expressed as

$$N = N_0e^{-\mu x} \tag{4-4}$$

where N is the number of transmitted photons, N_0 is the number of photons entering the tissue (incident photons), x is the thickness of the tissue, μ is $\mu_p + \mu_c$ (linear attenuation coefficients of the tissue), and e is the base of the natural logarithm.

Equation 4-3 applies to a homogenous block of tissue. However, a slice of tissue in the patient through which the radiation passes is not homogeneous because the tissue is composed of several different substances. In this case, the slice is divided into a number of small regions, "each characterized by its own linear attenuation coefficient" (Morgan, 1983). This can be shown as

$$N_0 \rightarrow \boxed{\mu_1}\boxed{\mu_2}\boxed{\mu_3}\boxed{\mu_4}\boxed{\mu_5}\ //\ \boxed{\mu_n} \rightarrow N$$

In this situation, the linear attenuation coefficients can be determined as follows:

$$N = N_0e^{-(\mu_1 + \mu_2 + \mu_3 + \mu_4 + \mu_5 \cdots + \mu_n)x} \tag{4-5}$$

Data Acquisition Geometries

The way that the x-ray tube and detectors are arranged to collect transmission measurements describes the data acquisition geometry of the CT system. Two types of geometries are illustrated in Figure 4-10. In Figure 4-10, *A*, the x-ray tube and detectors are coupled and rotated 360 degrees around the patient to collect transmission measurements by using a fan beam of radiation. In Figure 4-10, *B*, the x-ray tube rotates 360 degrees around the patient and is positioned inside a stationary ring of detectors. The radiation beam also describes a fan. It is interesting to note that the geometry shown in Figure 4-10, *A*, has become commonplace in modern CT scanners.

Data Processing

Data processing essentially constitutes the mathematical principles involved in CT. Data processing

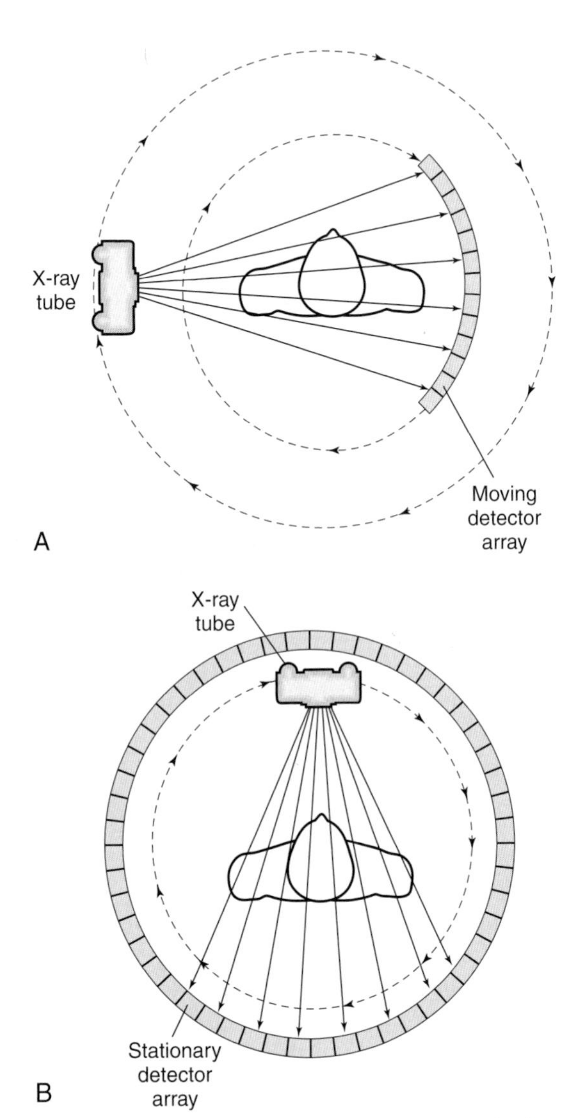

FIGURE 4-10 Two data acquisition geometries. **A,** Continuous rotation. **B,** Stationary detectors.

is basically a two-step process (Fig. 4-11). First, the raw data (data received from the detectors) undergo some form of preprocessing, in which corrections are made and some reformatting of the data occurs. This is necessary to facilitate the next step in data processing, image reconstruction. In this step, the scan data, which represent attenuation readings, are converted into a digital image characterized by CT numbers (Fig. 4-12).

Conversion of the attenuation readings into a CT image is accomplished by mathematical procedures referred to as *reconstruction algorithms.* These algorithms include simple back-projection, iterative methods, and analytic methods. For MSCT scanners that offer 16 and 64 slices per revolution of the x-ray tube, other reconstruction algorithms referred to as cone-beam algorithms are used (Kalender, 2005). These algorithms are described further in Chapter 6. After data processing, the reconstructed image is displayed for viewing and subsequently sent for storage or communicated through the picture archiving and communication system (PACS) to remote sites for review by other physicians (Fig. 4-13).

CT Numbers

As shown in Figure 4-12, each pixel in the reconstructed image is assigned a CT number. CT numbers are related to the linear attenuation coefficients (μ) of the tissues that comprise the slice (Table 4-1) and can be calculated as follows:

$$\text{CT number} = \frac{\mu_t - \mu_w}{\mu_w} \cdot K \qquad (4\text{-}6)$$

where μ_t is the attenuation coefficient of the measured tissue, μ_w is the attenuation coefficient of water, and K is a constant or contrast factor.

The value of K determines the contrast factor, or scaling factor. In the first EMI scanner, the value of K was 500, which resulted in a contrast scale of 0.2% per CT number. The CT numbers obtained with a contrast factor of 500 were referred to as *EMI numbers.* Later, the contrast factor was doubled to give a factor of 1000, and the CT numbers obtained with this factor are referred to as the *Hounsfield (H) scale.* The H scale expresses μ more precisely because the contrast scale is now 0.1% per CT number. (Both the H and EMI scales are shown in Fig. 4-14.) CT numbers are established on a relative basis with the attenuation of water as a reference. Thus the

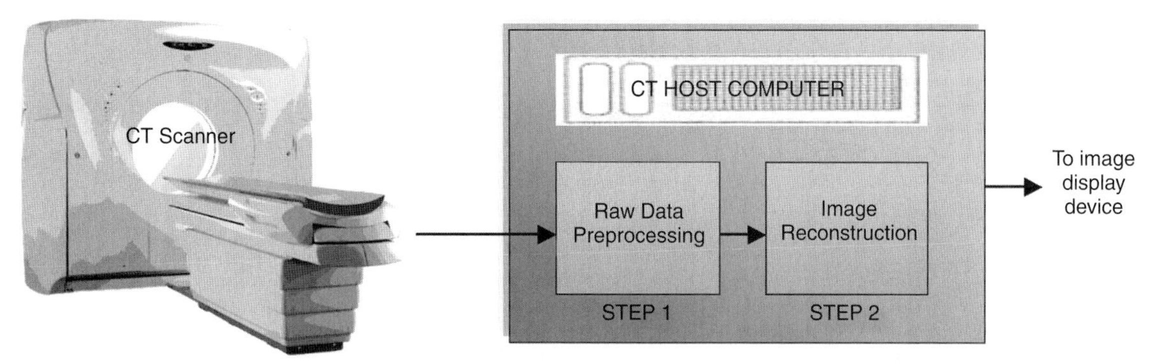

FIGURE 4-11 The two major data processing steps in CT.

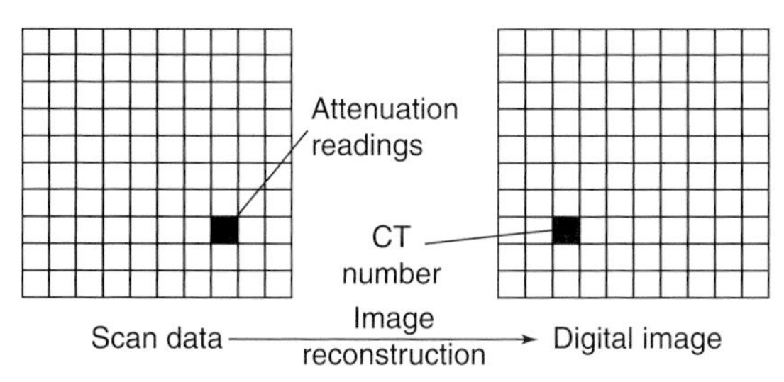

FIGURE 4-12 Data acquired by scanning an object measures beam penetration. A digital image is created by converting these data into CT numbers.

CT number for water is always 0, whereas those for bone and air are +1000 and −1000, respectively, on the H scale. An elaboration of the H scale for several tissues is illustrated in Figure 4-15. Note the range of CT numbers for water, air, fat, kidney, pancreas, blood, and liver.

The computer calculates the CT numbers, which can be printed as a numerical image (Fig. 4-16). This image must be converted into a gray-scale image because it is more useful to the radiologist than is a numerical printout. To facilitate this conversion, brightness levels that correspond with the CT numbers must be established (Fig. 4-17). In Figure 4-17, the upper +1000) and lower −1000) limits of the scale represent white and black, respectively. All other values represent various shades of gray.

CT and Energy Dependence

The linear attenuation coefficient (μ) is affected by several factors, including the energy of the radiation. For example, the linear attenuation coefficients for water at 60, 84, and 122 keV are 0.206, 0.180, and 0.166, respectively. It then follows that

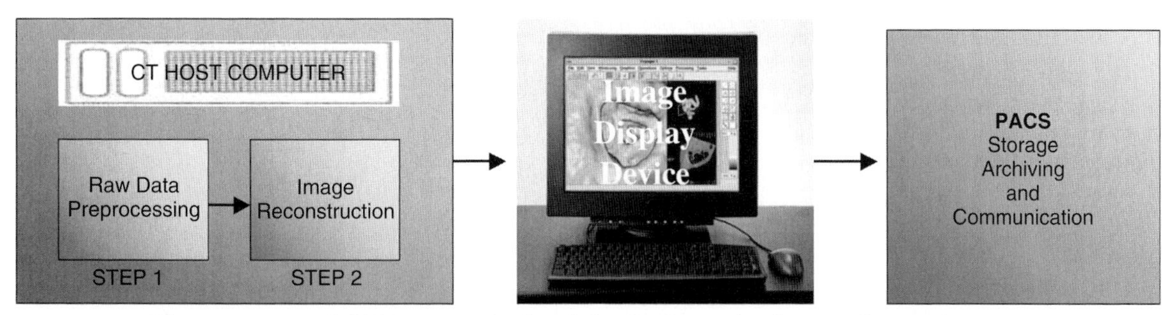

FIGURE 4-13 The reconstructed CT image is displayed for viewing and subsequently sent for storage or communicated by the PACS to physicians at remote sites.

TABLE 4-1 Linear Attenuation Coefficients for Various Body Tissues*

Tissues	Linear Attenuation Coefficient (cm^{-1})
Bone	0.528
Blood	0.208
Gray matter	0.212
White matter	0.213
Cerebrospinal fluid	0.207
Water	0.206
Fat	0.185
Air	0.0004

*At 60 keV.

photon energy also affects CT numbers because they can be calculated on the basis of the attenuation coefficients by the equation

$$\ln I_0/I = \int \mu(E, x)\, dx \qquad \text{(4-7)}$$

In this summation equation, *E* represents the photon energy and demonstrates that the attenuation coefficient changes with the beam energy.

In the original CT scanner, CT numbers were calculated on the basis of 73 keV, which is the effective energy of a 230 peak kilovolt beam after passing through 27 cm of water (Zatz, 1981). At 73 keV, the linear attenuation coefficient for water is 0.19 cm^{-1}. For example, if the linear attenuation coefficients for bone and water are 0.38 and 0.19 cm^{-1}, respectively, and the scaling factor (K) of the scanner is 1000, the CT numbers for bone and water can be calculated:

$$CT_{bone} = \frac{\mu_{bone} - \mu_{water}}{\mu_{water}} \cdot K$$

$$= \frac{0.38 - 0.19}{0.19} \cdot 1000$$

$$= \frac{0.19}{0.19} \cdot 1000$$

$$= 1000$$

Thus the CT number for bone is 1000.

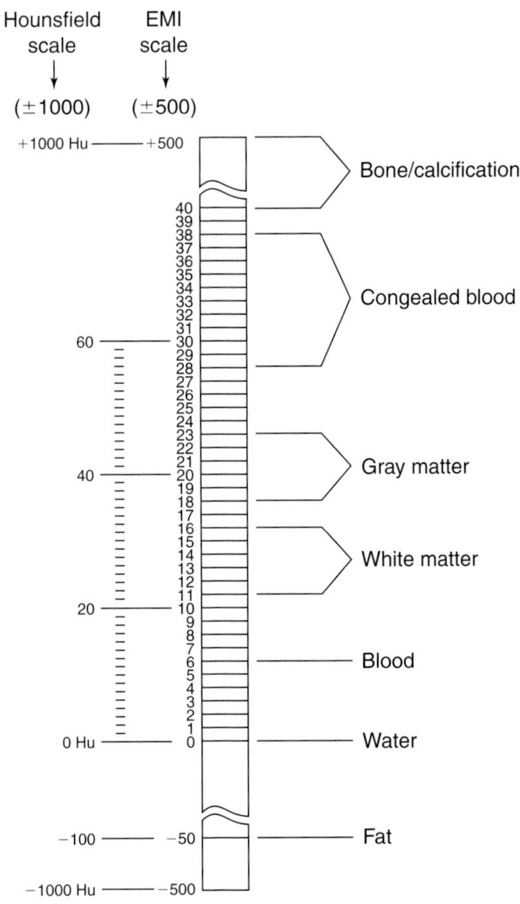

FIGURE 4-14 Distribution of CT numbers on the Hounsfield and EMI scales. (From Seeram E: *Computed tomography technology*, Philadelphia, 2001, WB Saunders.)

$$CT_{water} = \frac{\mu_{water} - \mu_{water}}{\mu_{water}} \cdot K$$

$$= \frac{0.19 - 0.19}{0.19} \cdot 1000$$

$$= \frac{0}{0.19} \cdot 1000$$

$$= 0$$

Thus the CT number for water is 0.

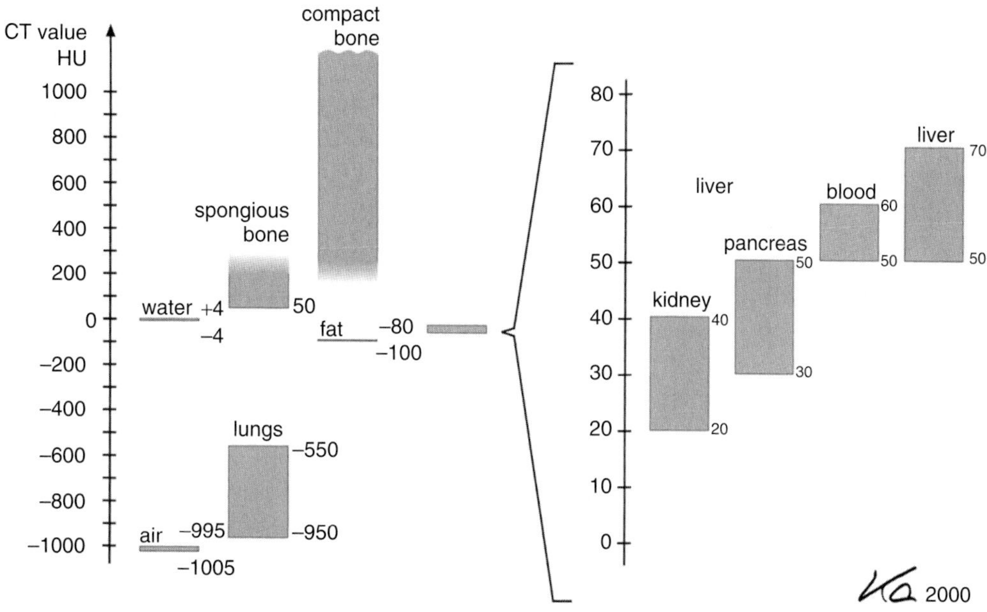

FIGURE 4-15 An elaboration of the Hounsfield scale for several tissues not shown in Figure 4-14. (From Kalender WA: *Computed tomography*, ed 2, Erlangen, Germany, 2005, Publicis Kommunikations Agentur Gmbh; © 2005 by Publicis Kommunikations Agentur GmbH, GWA, Erlangen, Germany. Reproduced by permission.)

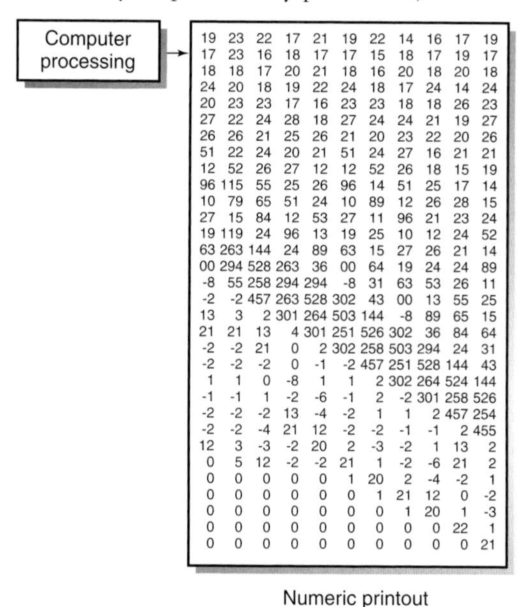

FIGURE 4-16 Appearance of the CT image after computer processing. This is a numerical printout of the processed image.

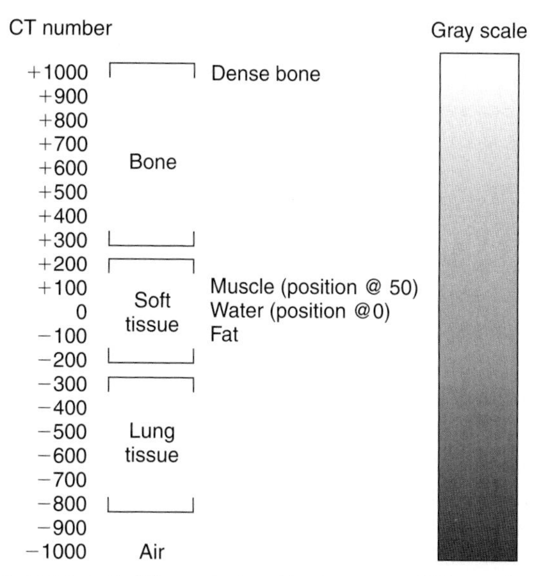

FIGURE 4-17 The relationship between CT number and the brightness level.

In CT, a high-kilovolt technique (about 120 kV) is generally used for the following reasons:

1. To reduce the dependence of attenuation coefficients on photon energy
2. To reduce the contrast of bone relative to soft tissues
3. To produce a high radiation flux at the detector

These reasons are important to ensure optimum detector response (e.g., to reduce artifacts caused by changes in skull thickness, which can conceal small changes in attenuation in soft tissues and to minimize artifacts resulting from beam-hardening effects).

CT numbers may vary because of their energy dependence. It is therefore essential that the CT system ensure the accuracy and reliability of these numbers because the consequences can be disastrous and might lead to a misdiagnosis. The system incorporates a number of correction schemes to maintain the precision of the CT numbers.

Image Display, Storage, and Communication

The third and final step in the CT process involves image display, storage, and communication. After the CT image has been reconstructed, it exits the computer in digital form (see Figs. 4-12 and 4-16). This must be converted to a form that is suitable for viewing and meaningful to the observer (Seeram, 1982).

Display Device

The gray-scale image is displayed on a television monitor (Cathode ray tube [CRT]) or liquid crystal display, which is an essential component of the control or viewing console (see Fig. 4-13). In the display and manipulation of gray-scale images for diagnosis, it is important to optimize image fidelity (i.e., the faithfulness with which the device can display the image). This is influenced by physical characteristics such as luminance, resolution, noise, and dynamic range. These topics are beyond the scope of this chapter.

Resolution, however, is an important physical parameter of the gray-scale display monitor and is related to the size of the pixel matrix, or matrix size. The display matrix can range from 64 × 64 to 1024 × 1024, but high-performance monitors can display an image with a 2048 × 2048 matrix (Dwyer, et al, 1992).

Windowing

The CT image is composed of a range of CT numbers (e.g., +1000 to −1000, for a total of 2000 numbers) that represent varying shades of gray (see Fig. 4-17). The range of numbers is referred to as the *window width* (WW), and the center of the range is the *window level* (WL) or *window center* (C). Both the WW and WL are located on the control console. These controls can alter the image contrast and brightness. With a WW of 2000 and a WL of 0, the entire gray scale is displayed and the ability of the observer to perceive small differences in soft tissue attenuation will be lost because the human eye can perceive only about 40 shades of gray (Castleman, 1994).

The process of changing the CT image gray scale in this way is referred to as *windowing* (Fig. 4-18). Although the WW controls the image contrast, the WL or C controls the image brightness. As can be seen in Figure 4-18, as the WL or C increases the image goes from white (bright) to dark (less bright); and the image contrast changes for different values of WWs. The image contrast is optimized for the anatomy under study, and therefore specified values of WW and WL or C must be used during the initial scanning of the patient. Note that in Figure 4-18 three windows are shown: the bone window (optimized for imaging bone), the mediastinal window (optimized for imaging the mediastinal structures), and the lung window (optimized for imaging the lungs). Windowing is described in detail in a later chapter.

Format of the CT Image

The original clinical CT images were composed of an 80 × 80 matrix for a total of 6400 pixels.

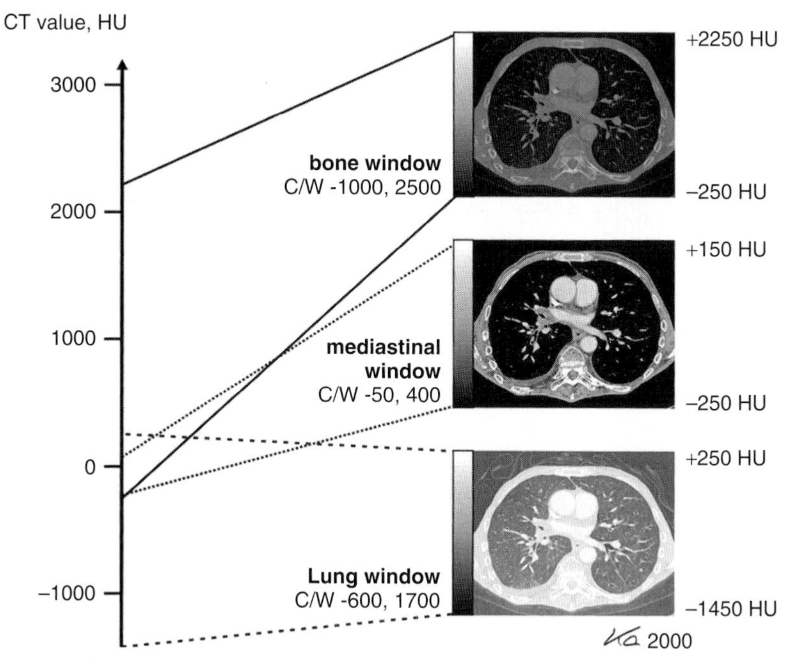

FIGURE 4-18 Windowing is a digital image postprocessing operation intended to alter the image contrast (a function of the WW) and the image brightness (a function of the window center, C, or WL, as it is often referred to). (From Kalender WA: *Computed tomography*, ed 2, Erlangen, Germany, 2005, Publicis Kommunikations Agentur GmbH; 2005 by Publicis Kommunikations Agentur GmbH, GWA, Erlangen, Germany. Reproduced by permission.)

The size of the matrix is chosen by the technologist before the CT examination and depends on the anatomy under study. The technologist must select the field of view (FOV) or reconstruction circle, which is a circular region from which the transmission measurements are recorded during scanning. This region is specifically referred to as the *scan FOV*.

During data collection and image reconstruction, a matrix is placed over the scan FOV to cover the slice to be imaged. In general, a technologist can select the FOV appropriate to the examination within three to four scan FOVs.

Because the slice to be scanned has the dimension of depth, the pixel is transformed into a voxel, or volume element. The radiation beam passes through each voxel and a CT number is then generated for each pixel in the displayed image. The display FOV can be equal to or less than the scan FOV.

The pixel size can be computed from the FOV and the matrix size through the following relationship:

$$\text{Pixel size, } d = \text{field of view/matrix size}$$

For example, if the reconstruction circle (FOV) is 25 cm and the matrix size is 512^2, the pixel size can be determined as follows:

$$\begin{aligned}\text{Pixel size} &= 25 \cdot 10 \text{ mm}/512\\ &= 250 \text{ mm}/512\\ &= 0.488 \text{ mm}\\ &= 0.49 \text{ mm}\\ &= 0.5 \text{ mm}\end{aligned}$$

The pixel size generally ranges from 1 to 10 mm on most scanners. Thus voxel size depends not

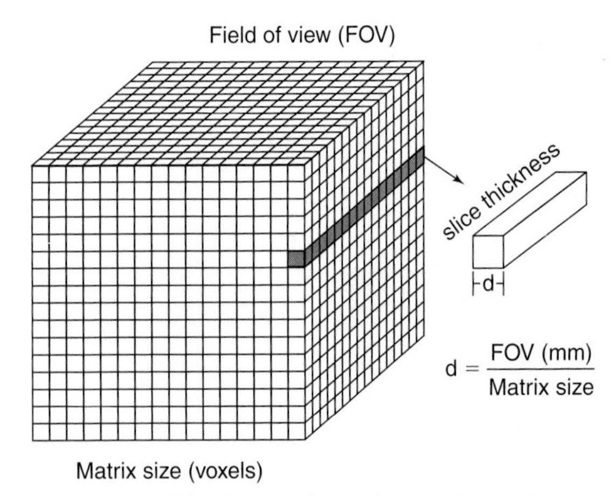

FIGURE 4-19 Voxel size depends on slice thickness, matrix size, and FOV.

only on the thickness of the slice but also on the matrix size and the FOV (Fig. 4-19). When the voxel dimensions of length, width, and height are equal, that is, describe a perfect cube, the imaging process is referred to as *isotropic imaging* (see Chapters 1 and 12).

Finally, each pixel in the CT image can have a range of gray shades. The image can have 256 (2^8), 512 (2^9), 1024 (2^{10}), or 2048 (2^{11}) different gray-scale values. Because these numbers are represented as bits, a CT image can be characterized by the number of bits per pixel. CT images can have 8, 9, 10, 11, or 12 bits per pixel. The image therefore consists of a series of bit planes referred to the *bit depth* (Fig. 4-20) (Seibert, 1995). The numerical value of the pixel represents the brightness of the image at that pixel position. A 12-bits-per-pixel CT image would represent numbers ranging from −1000 to 3095 for a total of 4096 (2^{12}) different shades of gray (Barnes and Lakshminarayanan, 1989).

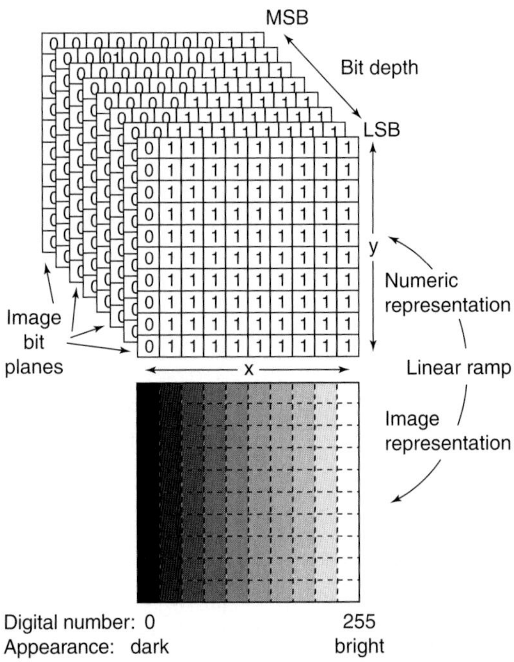

FIGURE 4-20 Representation of the digital image as a stack of bit planes. Encoding of the least significant bit (LSB) to the most significant bit (MSB) as bit planes is shown. The corresponding gray-scale image indicates digital value and brightness relationships. (From Seibert JA: Digital image processing basics. In Balter S, Shope TB, editors: *RSNA categorical course in physics: physical and technical aspects of angiography and interventional radiology*, Oak Brook, Ill, 1995, RSNA.)

TECHNOLOGICAL CONSIDERATIONS

The ultimate goal of a CT scanner is to produce high-quality CT images with minimal radiation dose and physical discomfort to the patient. Whether this is achieved depends on the design of the CT system, which influences the performance of the system's components. In this section, *design* refers to the technology necessary to produce a CT image.

The technology of a CT scanner encompasses a number of subsystems (Fig. 4-21). The major subsystems are described briefly to demonstrate the flow of data through the system.

Data Flow in a CT Scanner

The subsystems shown in Fig. 4-21 include the x-ray tube, power supply, and cooling system; beam

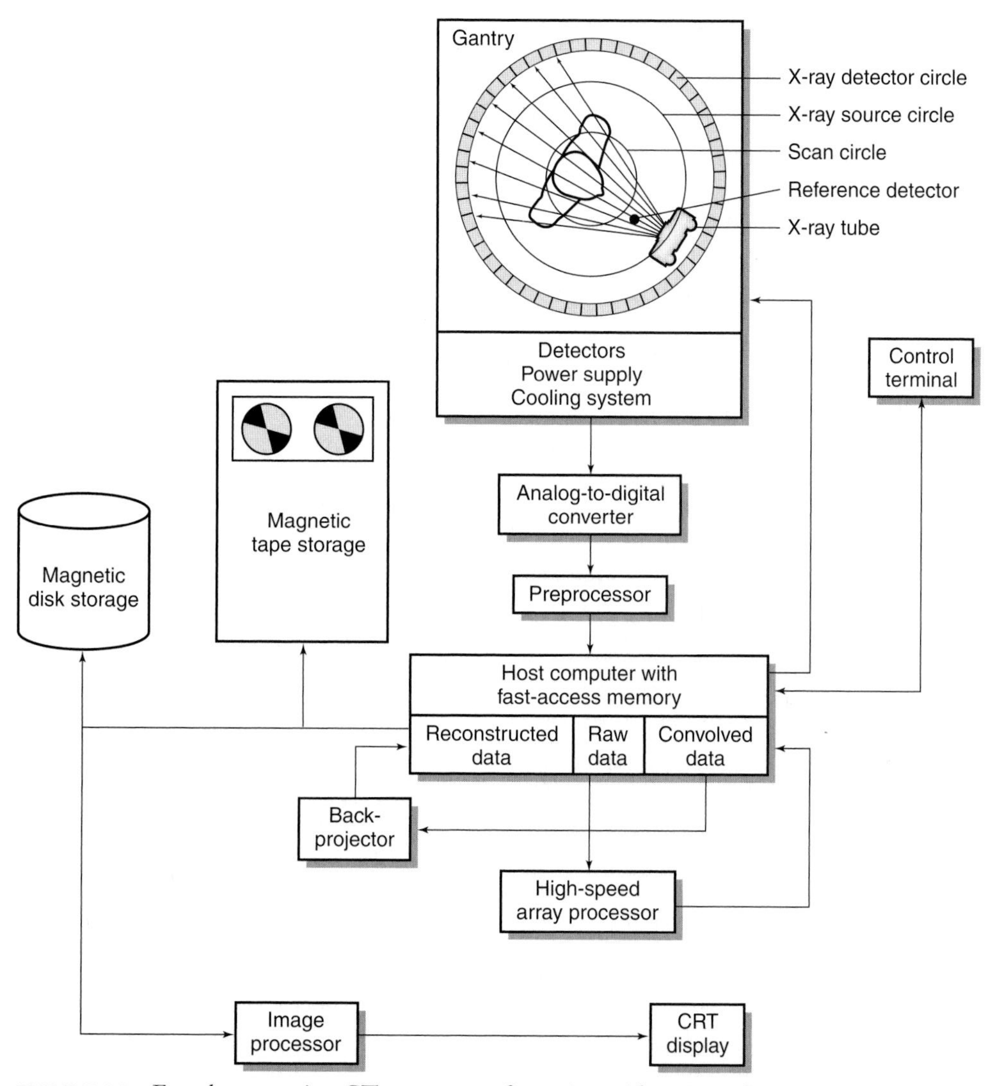

FIGURE 4-21 Fourth-generation CT scanner configuration with major subsystems. (From Huang HK: *PACS and imaging informatics*, Englewood Cliffs, NJ, 2004, John Wiley.)

geometry, defined by collimators and characterized by tube scanning motion; detectors, detector electronics, preprocessors, host computer with fast-access memory, high-speed array processors, digital image processor, storage, display, and system control.

The flow of data from Figure 4-21 is summarized in Figure 4-22. The language that describes some of the events (e.g., *convolution* and *back-projection*) is explained further in subsequent chapters.

Sequence of Events

The events represented in the data flow are as follows:

1. The x-ray tube (and detectors) rotate around the patient, who is positioned in the gantry aperture for the CT examination. This step is characterized by the beam geometry and method of scanning and involves the passage

of x-rays through the patient. The x-ray beam is highly collimated by prepatient collimators.

2. The radiation is attenuated as it passes through the patient. The transmitted photons are measured by two sets of detectors, a reference detector, which measures the intensity of radiation from the x-ray tube, and another set that records x-ray transmission through the patient.
3. The transmitted beam and reference beam are both converted into electrical current signals that are amplified by special circuits. This is followed by logarithmic amplification, in which the relative transmission readings (I_0/I) are changed into attenuation (μ) and thickness (x) data through the use of Equation 4-2:

$$\mu = \frac{1}{x} \ln I_0/I$$

4. Before the data are sent to the computer, they must be converted into digital form. This is done by the analog-to-digital converters, or *digitizers*. Steps 2, 3, and 4 constitute the second step in the data acquisition process.
5. Data processing begins. The digital data undergo some form of preprocessing, which includes corrections and reformatting. "Some of the corrections to the data will include subtraction of the air reference detector signal to normalize the attenuation data, obtaining local averages of detectors to determine if any detectors are outside a predetermined standard deviation which help locate bad detectors, and corrections due to dead time losses (i.e., detection response time losses) by the individual detectors" (Huang, 2004). The data are now referred to as *reformatted raw data*. Additional data corrections are performed on the data by using computer software.
6. As shown in Figure 4-22, convolution is performed on the data by the array processors.
7. The specific reconstruction algorithm then reconstructs an image of the internal anatomic structures under examination.

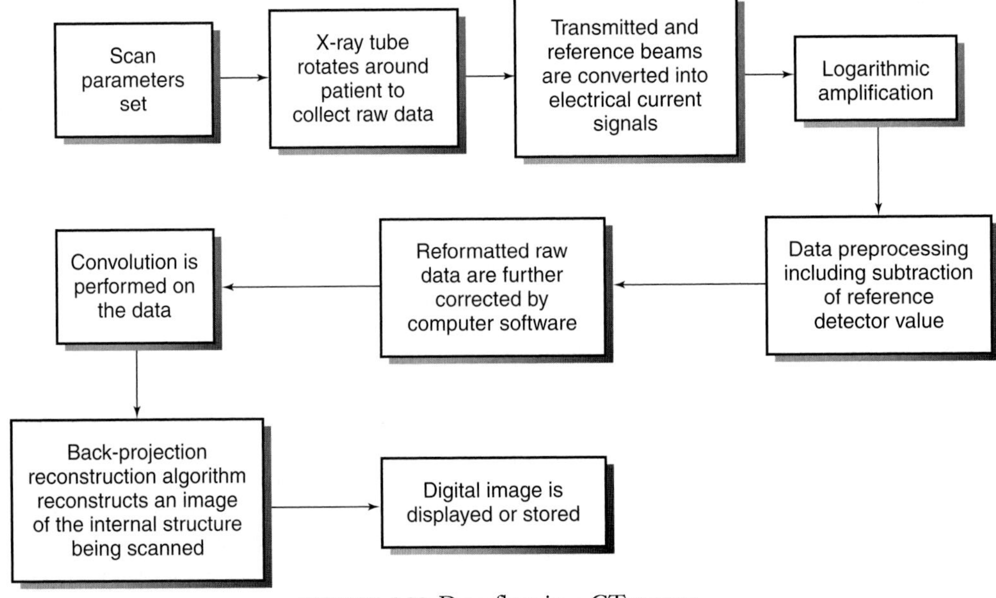

FIGURE 4-22 Data flow in a CT system.

8. The reconstructed image can then be displayed or stored on magnetic or optical tape or disks.
9. The image processor shown in Figure 4-21 allows the performance of various digital image postprocessing operations on the displayed image (Seeram and Seeram, 2008). Figure 4-21 does not show the digital-to-analog converter, a component positioned between the image processor and the CRT display or between the host computer and control terminal, which has a CRT display unit.
10. The control terminal is usually an operator's control console, which completely controls the CT system.

ADVANTAGES AND LIMITATIONS OF CT

Advantages

The main advantages of CT stem from the fact that the technique overcomes the limitations of radiography and conventional tomography. Compared with radiography and conventional tomography, CT offers the following advantages:

1. Excellent low-contrast resolution is possible because (1) a highly collimated beam is used to take an image of a cross-sectional slice of the patient and (2) more sensitive radiation detectors (compared with film-screen or digital radiography detectors) are used to measure the radiation transmitted through the slice. CT offers the best low contrast resolution compared with radiography, nuclear medicine, and ultrasonography. For example, the contrast resolution (in millimeters at 0.5% difference) for CT is 4 compared to 10, 10, and 20 for radiography, ultrasonography, and nuclear medicine, respectively. It is interesting to note here that the contrast resolution (mm at 0.5% difference) for magnetic resonance imaging (MRI) is 1 (Bushong, 2003).
2. By changing the WW and WL settings in image windowing, the contrast scale of the image can be varied to suit the needs of the observer (Seeram, 2004; Seeram and Seeram, 2008).
3. With spiral/helical volume data acquisition, CT scanning in spiral/helical geometry has overcome several limitations of conventional start-stop acquisition. Its advantages include volume data acquisition in a single breath rather than slice-by-slice acquisition, improvements in 3D imaging, multiplanar image reformatting, and other applications, such as continuous imaging, CT angiography, and virtual reality imaging, or CT endoscopy.
4. CT has made available a variety of techniques intended to facilitate the diagnostic process such as xenon CT (the use of inhaled stable xenon to study blood flow), quantitative CT (determination of bone mineral content), dynamic CT (rapid-sequence CT scanning to study physiology), perfusion CT, and high spatial resolution CT scanning to optimize the spatial resolution. In addition, CT can assist in radiation treatment planning. Additionally, CT can be coupled to single-photon emission CT (SPECT) and positron emission tomography (PET) scanners to produce fused SPECT/CT and PET/CT images, in an effort to provide more information about the patient's medical condition.
5. With regard to image manipulation and analysis, the digital nature of the CT image makes it a candidate for digital image processing. Through the application of certain image processing algorithms, the image can be modified to enhance its information content or analyzed to obtain information about the shape and texture of lesions.
6. *3D imaging:* CT now produces 3D images routinely. These images are intended to enhance image information content and improve the diagnostic interpretation skills of the radiologist. 3D imaging is described in detail in Chapter 14.

Limitations

CT is not without its limitations. Compared with radiography and tomography, the following disadvantages can be noted:

1. The spatial resolution (line pairs per millimeter) of CT is "notably poorer" (Hendee and Ritenour, 1992) compared with radiography. For example the spatial resolution for CT is 2. For nuclear medicine, ultrasonography, and MRI, the spatial resolution is 0.1, 0.25, and 2, respectively (Bushong, 2003).
2. The dose in CT is generally higher for similar anatomical regions.
3. In CT, it is difficult to image anatomic regions in which soft tissues are surrounded by large amounts of bone, such as the posterior fossa, spinal cord, pituitary, and the interpetrous space (Oldendorf and Oldendorf, 1991). The imaging process may create artifacts that may obscure diagnosis.
4. The presence of metallic objects on the patient produces streak artifacts on CT images. CT also creates other artifacts not common to radiography.

By no means have these limitations hindered the development of CT or restricted its use. In fact, they have opened avenues for problem solving and research. At present, CT continues to be a useful diagnostic tool in medicine, and more and more research is under way to improve the performance of CT scanners (Kalender, 2005; Mori et al, 2006; Mutic et al, 2004).

REFERENCES

Barnes GT, Lakshminarayanan AV: Computed tomography: physical principles and image quality considerations. In Lee JT et al, editors: *Computed tomography with MRI correlation*, ed 2, New York, 1989, Raven Press.

Bocage EM: Patent No. 536, 464, Paris. Quoted in Massiot J: History of tomography, *Medicamundi* 19:106-115, 1974.

Bushong S: *Magnetic resonance imaging—physical and biological principles*, ed 3, St Louis, 2003, Mosby.

Castleman KR: *Digital image processing*, ed 2, Englewood Cliffs, NJ, 1994, Prentice-Hall.

Dwyer SJ et al: Performance characteristics and image fidelity of gray-scale monitors, *Radiographics* 12: 765-772, 1992.

Hendee WR, Ritenour ER: *Medical imaging physics*, ed 3, St Louis, 1992, Mosby.

Hounsfield GH: Computerized transverse axial scanning (tomography), I: description of the system, *Br J Radiol* 46:1016-1022, 1973.

Huang HK: *PACS and imaging informatics*, Englewood Cliffs, NJ, 2004, John Wiley.

Kalender W: *Computed tomography—fundamentals, system technology, image quality, applications*, Erlangen, 2005, Publicis Corporate Publishing.

Marshall CH: Principles of computed tomography, *Postgrad Med* 59:105-109, 1976.

Morgan CL: *Basic principles of computed tomography*, Baltimore, 1983, University Park Press.

Mori S et al: Comparison of patient doses in 256-slice CT and 16-slice CT scanners, *Br J Radiol* 79:56-61, 2006.

Mutic S et al: Quality assurance for computed tomography simulators and computed tomography simulation process: report of the AAPM Radiation Therapy Committee Task Group No 66, *Med Phys* 30: 2762-2792, 2004.

Oldendorf W, Oldendorf W Jr: *MRI primer*, New York, 1991, Raven Press.

Seeram E: *Computed tomography technology*, Philadelphia, 2001, WB Saunders.

Seeram E: Digital image processing, *Radiol Technol* 75:435-455, 2004.

Seeram E, Seeram D: Image postprocessing in digital radiology: a primer for technologists, *Journal of Medical Imaging and Radiation Sciences* 39:23-41, 2008.

Seibert JA: Digital image processing basics. In Balter S, Shope TB, editors: *RSNA categorical course in physics: physical and technical aspects of angiography and interventional radiology*, Oak Brook, Ill, 1995, Radiological Society of North America.

Sprawls P: *Physical principles of medical imaging*, ed 2, Rockville, Md, 1995, Aspen.

Ter-Pogossian MM et al: The extraction of the yet unused wealth of information in diagnostic radiology, *Radiology* 113:515-520, 1974.

Vallebona A: Radiography with great enlargement (microradiography) and a technical method for radiographic dissociation of the shadow, *Radiology* 17:340-341, 1931.

Zatz LM: Basic principles of computed tomography scanning. In Newton TH, Potts DG, editors: *Radiology of the skull and brain*, St Louis, 1981, Mosby.

Data Acquisition Concepts

Chapter Outline

BASIC SCHEME FOR DATA ACQUISITION

In computed tomography (CT), transmission measurements, or projection data, are systematically collected from the patient. Several schemes are available for such data collection, each based on a specific "geometrical pattern of scanning" (Villafana, 1987).

Data acquisition refers to the method by which the patient is scanned to obtain enough data for image reconstruction. *Scanning* is defined by the beam geometry, which characterizes the particular CT system and also plays a central role in spatial resolution and artifact production.

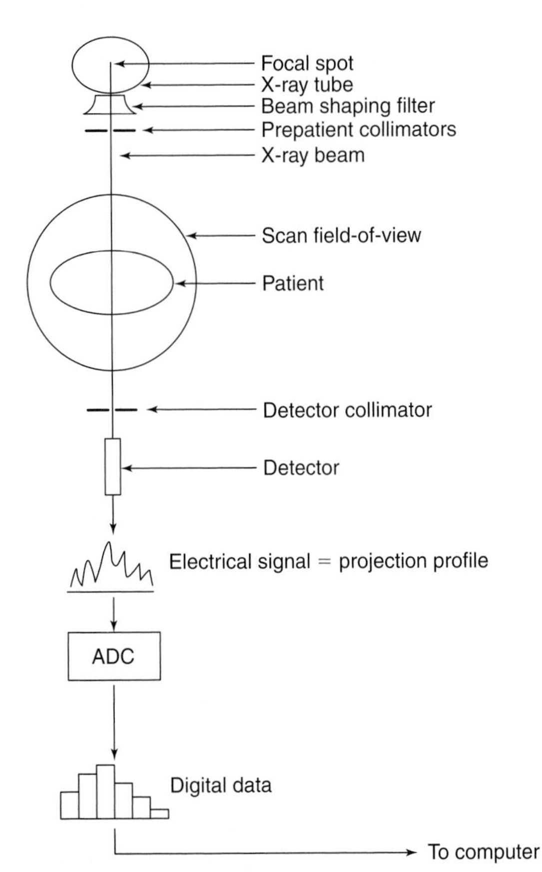

FIGURE 5-1 Basic data acquisition scheme in CT.

Two elements in a basic scheme for data acquisition (Fig. 5-1) are the beam geometry and the components comprising the scheme. *Beam geometry* refers to the size, shape, and motion of the beam and its path, and *components* refer to those physical devices that shape and define the beam, measure its transmission through the patient, and convert this information into digital data for input into the computer.

The following points should be noted from Figure 5-1:

1. The x-ray tube and detector are in perfect alignment.
2. The tube and detector scan the patient to collect a large number of transmission measurements.
3. The beam is shaped by a special filter as it leaves the tube.
4. The beam is collimated to pass through only the slice of interest.
5. The beam is attenuated by the patient and the transmitted photons are then measured by the detector.
6. The detector converts the x-ray photons into an electrical signal (analog data).
7. These signals are converted by the analog-to-digital converter (ADC) into digital data.
8. The digital data are sent to the computer for image reconstruction.

Terminology

Consider the first data acquisition scheme used by Hounsfield and others early in the development of CT (Fig. 5-2). The x-ray tube and detector move across the object or patient in a straight line, or translate, to collect several transmission measurements. After the first translation, the tube and detector rotate by 1 degree to collect more measurements. This sequence is repeated until data are collected for at least 180 degrees for one slice of the anatomy. Scanning also includes the movement of the patient through the gantry to scan the next slice. This sequence is repeated until all slices have been scanned.

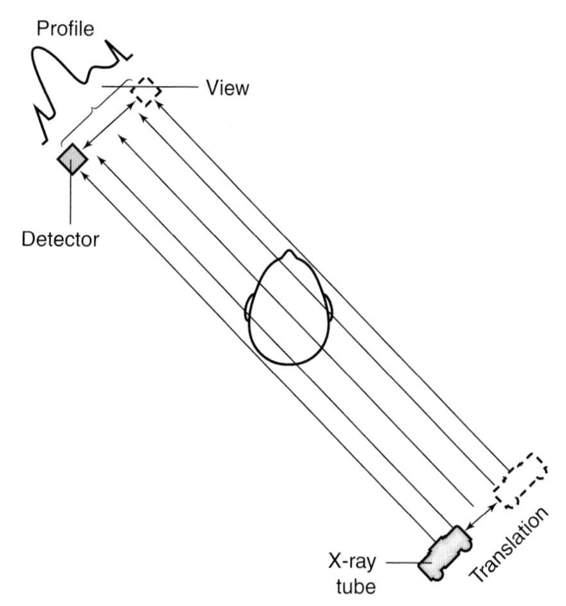

FIGURE 5-2 In CT, a *ray* is the part of the x-ray beam that falls onto one detector. A *view* is a collection of these rays for one translation across the object. The view generates what is called a *profile*.

The x-ray beam that emanates from the tube consists of several rays. In CT, a *ray* is the part of the beam that falls on one detector. In Figure 5-2, the line from the x-ray tube to the detector is considered a single ray, and a collection of these rays for one translation across the object constitutes a *view*.

Projection data are collected by the detector because each ray is attenuated by the patient and subsequently transmitted and projected on the detector. The detector in turn generates an electrical signal, which represents a signature of the attenuation as the ray moves across the slice. This signal represents a profile. Although a view generates a profile, a ray generates only a small part of the profile. In addition, each transmission measurement is referred to as a *data sample*.

The production of a CT image of one slice of the anatomy requires a large set of data samples taken at different locations to satisfy the image reconstruction process. The total number of data samples (DS_{total}) per scan is given by the following expression:

$$DS_{total} = \text{number of detectors} \cdot \text{number of data samples per detector} \quad (5\text{-}1)$$

or

$$DS_{total} = \text{number of data samples per view} \cdot \text{number of views} \quad (5\text{-}2)$$

DATA ACQUISITION GEOMETRIES

Three primary types of acquisition geometries are parallel beam geometry, fan beam geometry, and CT scanning in spiral geometry, which is the most recently developed geometry. As a result, a simple categorization of CT equipment has evolved based on the scanning geometry, scanning motion, and number of detectors, as follows (Fig. 5-3):

1. First-generation scanners were based on the parallel beam geometry and translate-rotate scanning motion.
2. Second-generation scanners were based on the fan beam geometry and translate-rotate motion.
3. Third-generation scanners were based on fan beam geometry and complete rotation of the tube and detectors.
4. Fourth-generation scanners were based on fan beam geometry and complete rotation of the x-ray tube around a stationary ring of detectors.
5. Fifth-generation scanners were developed primarily for high-speed CT scanning. These scanners are based on special configurations intended to facilitate very fast scanning.
6. Sixth-generation scanners have multiple x-ray tubes and detectors. These scanners are intended specifically to image moving structures, such as the heart, for example. One such recent scanner is the dual-source CT (DSCT) scanner (McCollough et al, 2007).

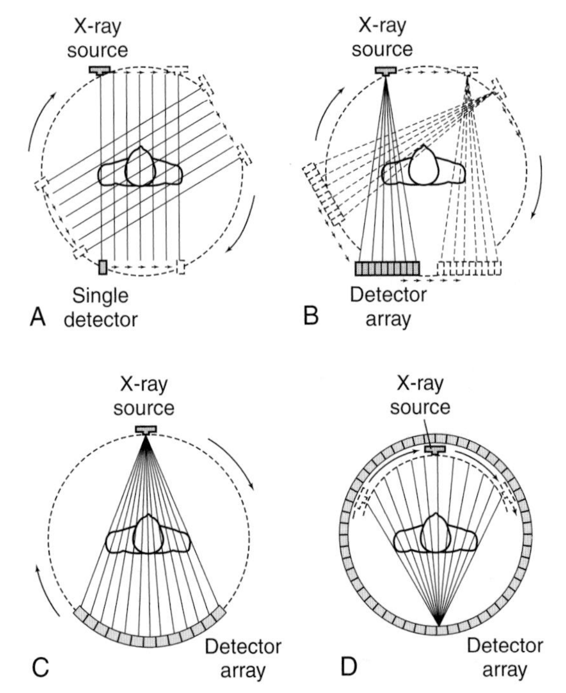

FIGURE 5-3 The geometries of the first four generations of CT scanners. **A,** First generation, parallel beam, translate and rotate. **B,** Second generation, fan beam, translate, and rotate. **C,** Third generation, fan beam, rotate only. **D,** Fourth generation, fan beam, stationary circular detector.

7. Seventh-generation scanners use flat-panel digital area detectors similar to the ones used in digital radiography (Flohr et al, 2005; Kalender, 2005).

First-Generation Scanners

Parallel beam geometry was first used by Hounsfield. The first EMI brain scanner and other earlier scanners were based on this concept.

Parallel beam geometry is defined by a set of parallel rays that generates a projection profile (see Fig. 5-2). The data acquisition process is based on a translate-rotate principle, in which a single, highly collimated x-ray beam and one or two detectors first translate across the patient to collect transmission readings. After one translation, the tube and detector rotate by 1 degree and translate again to collect readings from a different direction. This is repeated for 180 degrees around the patient. This method of scanning is referred to as *rectilinear pencil beam scanning*.

First-generation CT scanners took at least 4.5 to 5.5 minutes to produce a complete scan of the patient, which restricted patient throughput. The image reconstruction algorithm for first-generation CT scanners was based on the parallel beam geometry of the image reconstruction space (a square or circle in which the slice to be reconstructed must be positioned).

Second-Generation Scanners

Second-generation scanners were based on the translate-rotate principle of first-generation scanners with a few fundamental differences, such as a linear detector array (about 30 detectors) coupled to the x-ray tube and multiple pencil beams. The result is a beam geometry that describes a small fan whose apex originates at the x-ray tube. This is the fan beam geometry shown in Figure 5-3, *B*, *C*, and *D*.

Also, the rays are divergent instead of parallel, resulting in a significant change in the image reconstruction algorithm, which must be capable of handling projection data from the fan beam geometry.

In second-generation scanners, the fan beam translates across the patient to collect a set of transmission readings. After one translation, the tube and detector array rotate by larger increments (compared with first-generation scanners) and translate again. This process is repeated for 180 degrees and is referred to as *rectilinear multiple pencil beam scanning*. The x-ray tube traces a semicircular path during scanning.

The larger rotational increments and increased number of detectors result in shorter scan times that range from 20 seconds to 3.5 minutes. In general, the time decrease is inversely proportional to the number of detectors. The more detectors, the shorter the total scan time.

Third-Generation Scanners

Third-generation CT scanners were based on a fan beam geometry that rotates continuously around the patient for 360 degrees (see Fig. 5-3). The x-ray tube is coupled to a curved detector array that subtends an arc of 30 to 40 degrees or greater from the apex of the fan. As the x-ray tube and detectors rotate, projection profiles are collected and a view is obtained for every fixed point of the tube and detector. This motion is referred to as *continuously rotating fan beam scanning*. The path traced by the tube describes a circle rather than the semicircle characteristic of first- and second-generation CT scanners. Third-generation CT scanners collect data faster than the previous units (generally within a few seconds). This scan time increases patient throughput and limits the production of artifacts caused by respiratory motion.

Fourth-Generation Scanners

Essentially, fourth-generation CT scanners feature two types of beam geometries: a rotating fan beam within a stationary ring of detectors and a nutating fan beam in which the apex of the fan (x-ray tube) is located outside a nutating ring of detectors.

Rotating Fan Beam Within a Circular Detector Array

The main data acquisition features of a fourth-generation CT scanner are as follows:

1. The x-ray tube is positioned within a stationary, circular detector array (Fig. 5-4).
2. The beam geometry describes a wide fan.
3. The apex of the fan now originates at each detector. Figure 5-4 shows two fans that describe two sets of views.
4. As the tube moves from point to point within the circle, single rays strike a detector. These rays are produced sequentially during the point's circular travel.
5. Scan times are very short and vary from scanner to scanner, depending on the manufacturer.
6. The x-ray tube traces a circular path.
7. The image reconstruction algorithm is for a fan beam geometry in which the apex of the fan is now at the detector, as opposed to the x-ray tube in the third-generation systems.

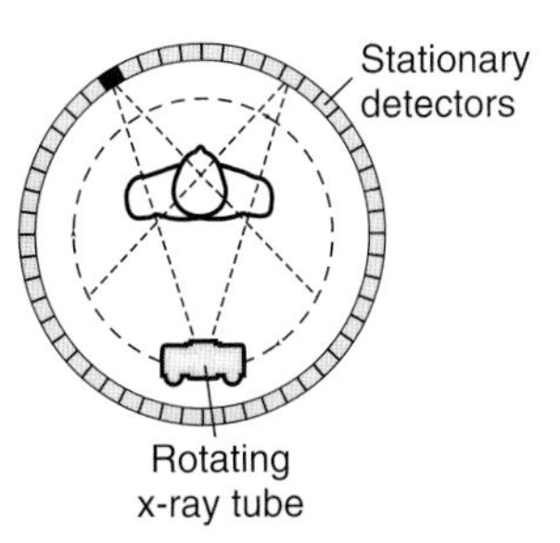

FIGURE 5-4 In a fourth-generation scanner, each detector position gives rise to a fan.

Rotating Fan Beam Outside a Nutating Detector Ring

In this scheme, the x-ray tube rotates outside the detector ring (Fig. 5-5). As it rotates, the detector ring tilts so that the fan beam strikes an array of detectors located at the far side of the x-ray tube while the detectors closest to the x-ray tube move out of the path of the x-ray beam. The term *nutating* describes the tilting action of the detector ring during data collection. Scanners with this type of scanning motion eliminate the poor geometry of other schemes, in which the tube rotates inside its detector ring, near the object. However, nutate-rotate systems are not currently manufactured.

Multislice CT Scanners: CT Scanning in Spiral-Helical Geometry

Scanning in spiral-helical geometry is the most recent development in CT data acquisition. The need for faster scan times and improvements in

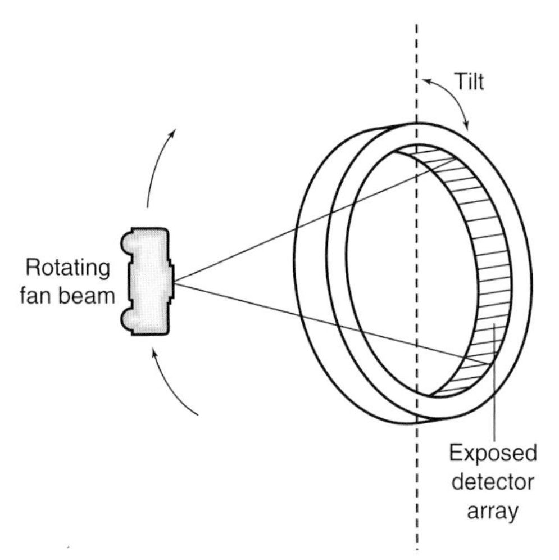

FIGURE 5-5 Rotating fan beam outside a nutating detector ring. *Nutating* refers to how the detector ring tilts to expose an array of detectors to the x-ray beam. Nutate-rotate systems are no longer manufactured.

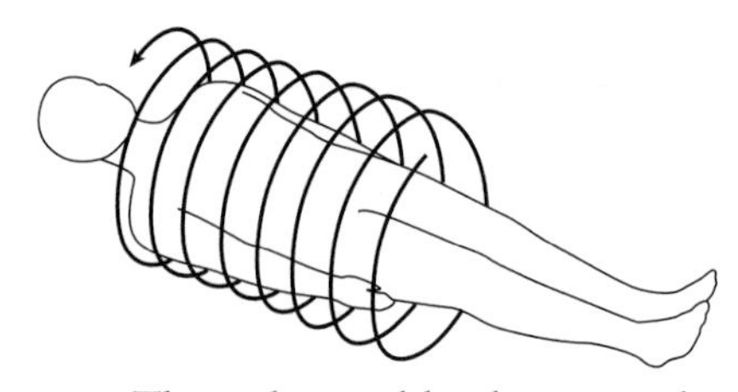

FIGURE 5-6 The path traced by the x-ray tube in CT scanning describes a spiral or helix. These terms are used interchangeably.

three-dimensional (3D) and multiplanar reconstruction have encouraged the development of continuous rotation scanners, or volume scanners, in which the data are collected in volumes rather than individual slices. CT scanning in spiral/helical geometry is based on slip-ring technology, which shortens the high-tension cables to the x-ray tube to allow continuous rotation of the gantry. The path traced by the x-ray tube, or fan beam, during the scanning process describes a spiral (Fig. 5-6) or a helix. The terms *spiral geometry* (Siemens) and *helical geometry* (Toshiba) are commonly and synonymously used to describe the data acquisition

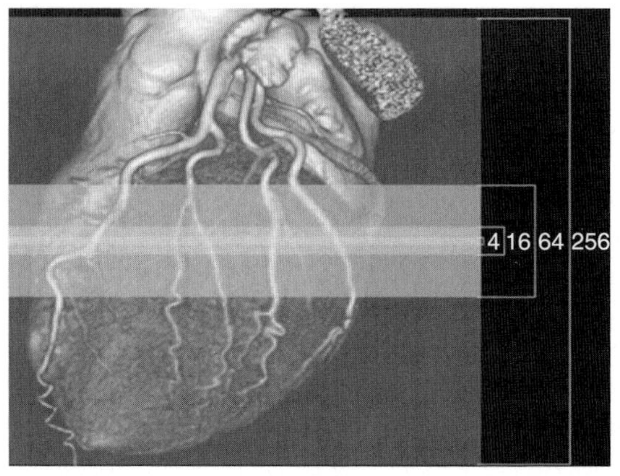

FIGURE 5-7 The 256 prototype CT scanner featuring 256 slices per 360-degree rotation was developed by Toshiba Medical Systems (Japan) for imaging moving structures such as the heart and lungs. One striking feature of this scanner compared with other multislice scanners is that it covers the entire heart in a single rotation. (Courtesy Toshiba America Medical Systems.)

geometry of continuous rotation scanners. This geometry is obtained during the scanning process. As the tube rotates, the patient is transported through the gantry aperture for a single breath hold. Because this results in a volume of the patient being scanned, the term *volume CT* is also used.

Spiral/Helical Geometry Scanners

These systems have evolved through the years from two to eight slices per revolution of the x-ray tube and detectors (360-degree rotation) to 16, 32, 40, 64, and 320 slices per 360-degree rotation. As of 2007, a prototype scanner featuring 256 slices per 360-degree rotation is being developed by Toshiba Medical Systems (Japan) for imaging moving structures such as the heart and lungs. One striking feature of this scanner compared with other multislice scanners is that it covers the entire heart in a single rotation (Fig. 5-7).

An interesting point with respect to scanners capable of imaging 16 or greater slices per 360-degree rotation is that the beam becomes a cone. These systems are therefore based on cone-beam geometries (as opposed to fan-beam geometries) because the detectors are two-dimensional detectors. This means that cone-beam algorithms (as opposed to fan-beam algorithms) are used to reconstruct images. Multislice CT (MSCT) scanner principles and concepts are described in detail in the chapter on MSCT.

Fifth-Generation Scanners

Fifth-generation scanners are classified as high-speed CT scanners because they can acquire scan data in milliseconds. Two such scanners are the electron beam CT scanner (EBCT) (Fig. 5-8) and the dynamic spatial reconstructor (DSR) scanner. In the EBCT scanner, the data acquisition geometry is a fan beam of x rays produced by a beam of electrons that scans several stationary tungsten target rings. The fan beam passes through the patient and the x-ray transmission readings are collected for image reconstruction. The DSR scanner was labeled a high-speed CT scanner capable of producing dynamic 3D images of volumes of the patient. The DSR is now obsolete and is not described further in this book.

The principles and operation of the EBCT scanner were first described by Boyd et al (1979) as a result of research done at the University of California at San Francisco during the late 1970s. In 1983, Imatron developed Boyd's high-speed CT scanner for imaging the heart and circulation (Boyd and Lipton, 1983). At that time, the machine was referred to by such names as the *cardiovascular computed tomography* scanner and the *cine CT* scanner. Today, the machine is known as the *EBCT scanner* (McCollough, 1995). It is expected that more of these machines will be distributed worldwide in the near future. (Siemens Medical Systems will distribute the EBCT scanner under the name "Evolution.")

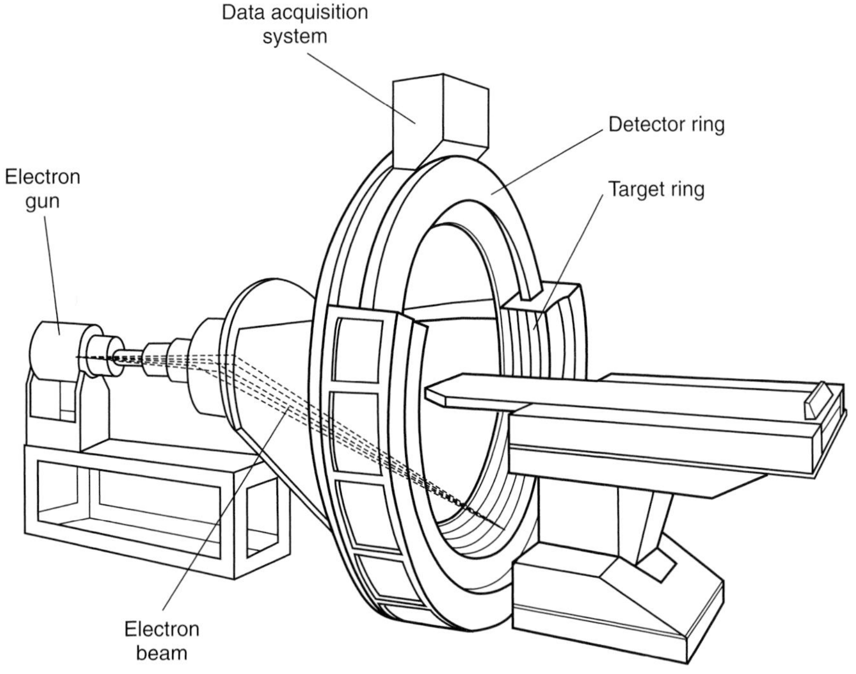

FIGURE 5-8 The essential components of an EBCT scanner. The data acquisition geometry is a fan beam of x rays produced by the electron beam striking the tungsten targets.

The overall goal of the EBCT scanner is to produce high-resolution images of moving organs (e.g., the heart) that are free of artifacts caused by motion. In this respect, the scanner can be used for imaging the heart and other body parts in both adults and children. The scanner performs this task well because its design enables it to acquire CT data 10 times faster than conventional CT scanners.

The design configuration of the EBCT scanner (see Fig. 5-8) is different from that of conventional CT systems in the following respects:

1. The EBCT scanner is based on electron beam technology and no x-ray tube is used.
2. There is no mechanical motion of the components.
3. The acquisition geometry of the EBCT scanner is fundamentally different compared with those of conventional systems.

The basic configuration of an EBCT scanner is shown in Figure 5-8. At one end of the scanner is an electron gun that generates a 130-kilovolt (kV) electron beam. This beam is accelerated, focused, and deflected at a prescribed angle by electromagnetic coils to strike one of the four adjacent tungsten target rings. These stationary rings span an arc of 210 degrees. The electron beam is steered along the rings, which can be used individually or in any sequence. As a result, heat dissipation does not pose a problem as it does in conventional CT systems.

When the electron beam collides with the tungsten target, x rays are produced. Collimators shape the x-rays into a fan beam that passes through the patient, who is positioned in a 47-cm scan field, to strike a curved, stationary array of detectors positioned opposite the target rings.

The detector array consists of two separate rings holding a 216-degree arc of detectors. The first ring holds 864 detectors, each half the size of those in the second ring, which holds 432 detectors (McCollough, 1995). This arrangement allows for the acquisition of either two image slices when one target ring is used or eight image slices when all four target rings are used in sequence.

Each solid-state detector consists of a luminescent crystal and cadmium tungstate (which converts x rays to light) coupled optically with silicon photodiodes (which convert light into current) connected to a preamplifier. The output from the detectors is sent to the data acquisition system (DAS) (see Fig. 5-8).

The DAS consists of analog-to-digital converters, or digitizers, that sample and digitize the output signals from the detectors. In addition, the digitized data are stored in bulk in random access memory (RAM), which can hold data for hundreds of scans in the multislice and single-slice modes. This information is subsequently sent to the computer for processing.

The computer for the EBCT scanner is capable of very fast reconstruction speeds, and image reconstruction is based on the filtered back-projection algorithm used in conventional CT systems.

The EBCT scanner does not have any moving physical parts and, as noted by Flohr et al. (2005), "the EBCT principle is currently not considered adequate for state-of-the-art cardiac imaging or for general radiology applications."

Sixth-Generation Scanners: The Dual Source CT Scanner

The overall goal of the MSCT scanners mentioned previously is to improve the volume coverage speed while providing improved spatial and temporal resolution compared with the older four slices per 360-degree rotation scanner. Although the current 64-slice volume scanners produce better spatial resolution in the order of 0.4 mm isotropic voxels (Flohr et al, 2006; McCollough et al, 2007) and temporal resolution compared with the 16-slice volume CT scanner, they fail to deal effectively with artifacts created in CT angiography (CTA) and the problem of the mechanical forces that need to be addressed in attempting to decrease the rotation time of the x-ray tube and detectors (Flohr et al, 2006). To solve these problems, for example, a new-generation scanner has been introduced. This is the DSCT scanner.

This scanner consists of two x-ray tubes and two sets of detectors that are offset by 90 degrees (Fig. 5-9). The DSCT scanner is designed for cardiac CT imaging because it provides the temporal resolution needed to image moving structures such as the heart. The DSCT scanner will be described further in Chapter 13.

Seventh-Generation Scanners: Flat-Panel CT Scanners

Flat-panel digital detectors similar to the ones used in digital radiography are now being considered for use in CT; however, these scanners are still in the prototype development and are not available for use in clinical imaging. Perhaps they may be labeled seventh-generation CT scanners on the basis of the simple categorization mentioned above.

A flat-panel CT scanner prototype is shown in Figure 5-10. The x-ray tube and detectors are coupled and positioned in the CT gantry. The detector consists of a cesium iodide (CsI) scintillator coupled to an amorphous silicon thin-film transistor (TFT) array. These flat-panel detectors produce excellent spatial resolution but lack good contrast resolution; therefore, they are also being used in angiography to image blood vessels, for example, where the image sharpness is of primary importance. As noted by Flohr et al. (2005), "the combination of area detectors that provide sufficient image quality with fast gantry rotation speed will be a promising technical concept for medical CT systems. The vast spectrum of potential applications may bring about another quantum leap in the evolution of medical CT imaging."

In addition, flat-panel detectors are also being investigated for use in CT of the breast, and currently several dedicated breast CT prototypes are being developed (Glick et al, 2007; Kwan et al, 2007). Breast CT is described further in Chapter 13.

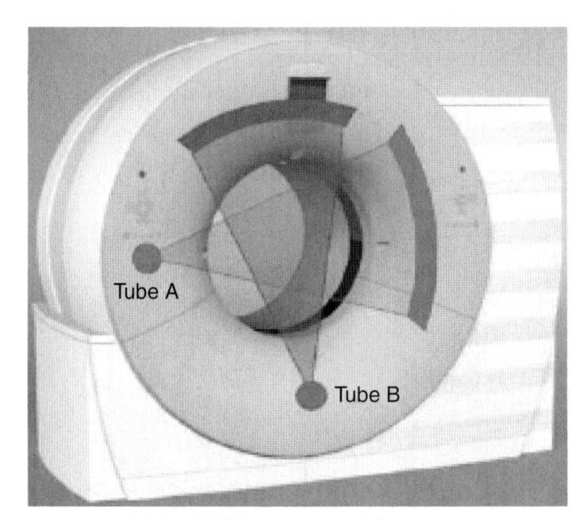

FIGURE 5-9 The DSCT scanner. This scanner consists of two x-ray tubes and two sets of detectors that are offset by 90 degrees and it is particularly designed for cardiac CT imaging. (From Flohr TG et al: First performance evaluation of a dual-source CT [DSCT] system. *Eur Radiol* 16: 256-268, 2006. With kind permission of Springer Science and Business Media.)

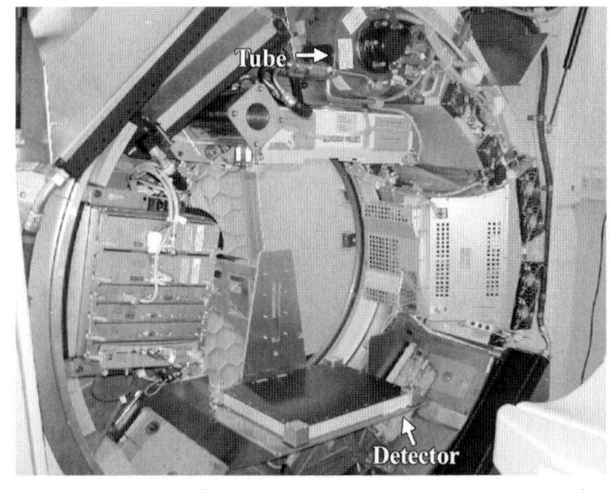

FIGURE 5-10 A flat-panel CT scanner prototype. The x-ray tube and detectors are coupled and positioned in the CT gantry. The detector consists of a CsI scintillator coupled to an amorphous silicon TFT array. (From Flohr TG et al: Multi-detector row CT systems and image reconstruction techniques, *Radiology* 235:756-773, 2005. Reproduced by permission.)

SLIP-RING TECHNOLOGY

Spiral-helical CT is made possible through the use of slip-ring technology, which allows for continuous gantry rotation. Slip rings (Fig. 5-11) are "electromechanical devices consisting of circular electrical conductive rings and brushes that transmit electrical energy across a rotating interface" (Brunnett et al, 1990). Today, CT scanners incorporate slip-ring design and are referred to as *continuous rotation*, *volume CT*, or *slip-ring* scanners. Slip-ring technology is not a new idea, for it has been applied previously in CT. For example, the Varian V-360-3 CT scanner (an old model CT scanner) was based on slip-ring design to achieve continuous rotation of the gantry. Such rotation results in very fast data collection, which is mandatory for certain clinical procedures such as dynamic CT scanning and CTA, for example.

In addition, slip rings not only provide the electrical power to operate the x-ray tube but also transfer the signals from the detectors for input into the image reconstruction computer.

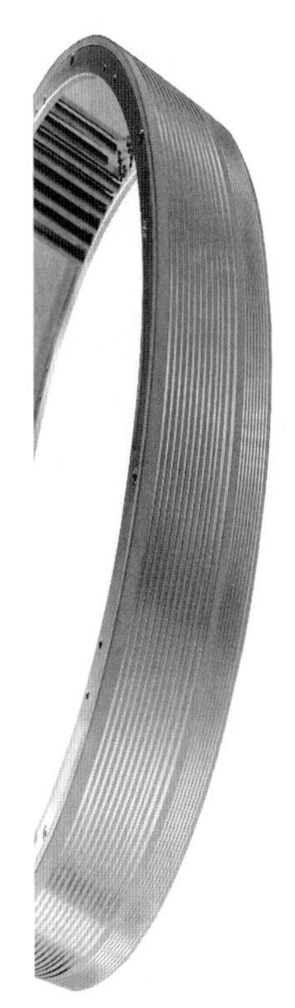

FIGURE 5-11 Conductive rings *(upper strips)* of one slip-ring system. Each strip carries voltage to components such as the generator, x-ray tube, and collimators. (Courtesy Elscint, Hackensack, NJ.)

Design and Power Supply

Two slip-ring designs are the disk (Fig. 5-12) and cylinder. In the disk design, the conductive rings form concentric circles in the plane of rotation. The cylindrical design includes conductive rings positioned along the axis of rotation to form a cylinder (Fig. 5-13). The brushes that transmit electrical power to the CT components glide in contact grooves on the stationary slip ring (Fig. 5-13).

Two common brush designs are the wire brush and the composite brush. The wire brush uses conductive wire as a sliding contact. "A brush consists of one or more wires arranged such that they function as a cantilever spring with a free end against the conductive ring. Two brushes per ring are often used to increase either communication

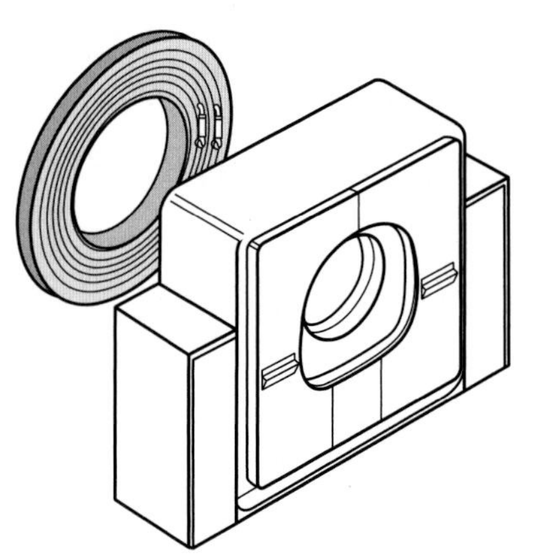

FIGURE 5-12 Slip ring based on the disk design concept. The rings are positioned as concentric circles within the plane of rotation. This is a characteristic design of the Siemens Somatom Plus CT scanner.

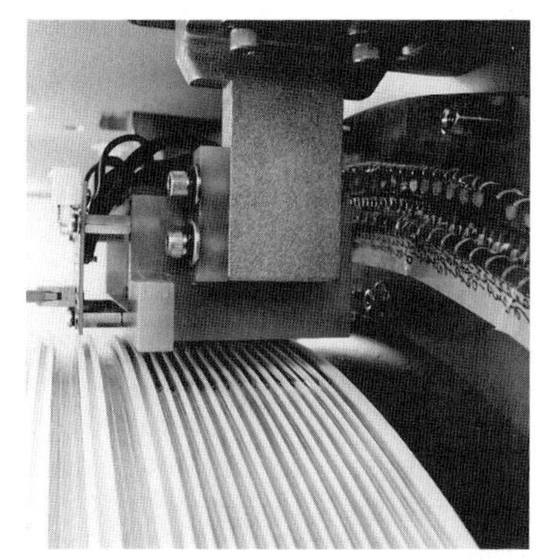

FIGURE 5-13 Slip ring based on the cylindrical design characteristic of the Picker PQ-2000 CT scanner. The brushes glide in contact grooves on the stationary slip ring. (Courtesy Picker International, Cleveland, Ohio.)

reliability or current carrying capacity" (Brunnett et al, 1990). The composite brush uses a block of some conductive material (e.g., a silver-graphite alloy) as a sliding contact. A variety of different spring designs are commonly used to maintain contact between the brush and ring including cantilever, compression, or constant force.

Slip-ring scanners provide continuous rotation of the gantry through the elimination of the long high-tension cables to the x-ray tube used in conventional start-stop scanners, which must be unwound after a complete rotation. In conventional scanners, these cables originate from the high-voltage generator, usually located in the x-ray room. The high-voltage generators of slip-ring scanners are located in the gantry. Scanners with either low-voltage or high-voltage slip rings, based on the power supply to the slip ring, are available (Fig. 5-14).

Low-Voltage Slip Ring

In a low-voltage slip-ring system, 480 alternating (AC) power and x-ray control signals are transmitted to slip rings by means of low-voltage brushes that glide in contact grooves on the stationary slip ring. The slip ring then provides power to the high-voltage transformer, which subsequently transmits

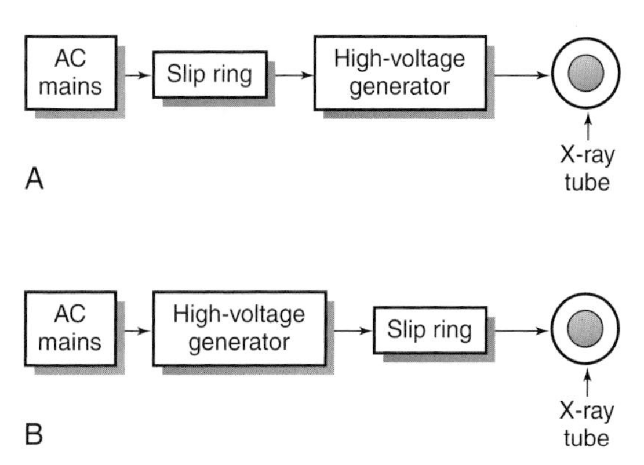

FIGURE 5-14 Basic differences between low-voltage **(A)** and high-voltage **(B)** slip-ring CT scanners in terms of high-voltage power to the x-ray tube.

high voltage to the x-ray tube (see Fig. 5-14, *A*). In this case, the x-ray generator, x-ray tube, and other controls are positioned on the orbital scan frame.

High-Voltage Slip Ring

In a high-voltage slip-ring system (see Fig. 5-14, *B*), the AC delivers power to the high-voltage generator, which subsequently supplies high voltage to the slip ring. The high voltage from the slip ring is transferred to the x-ray tube. In this case, the high-voltage generator does not rotate with the x-ray tube.

Advantages

The major advantage of slip-ring technology is that it facilitates continuous rotation of the x-ray tube so that volume data can be acquired quickly from the patient. As the tube rotates continuously, the patient is translated continuously through the gantry aperture. This results in CT scanning in spiral geometry. Other advantages are as follows:

1. Faster scan times and minimal interscan delays
2. Capacity for continuous acquisition protocols
3. Elimination of the start-stop process characteristic of conventional CT scanners
4. Removal of the cable wraparound process

X-RAY SYSTEM

In his initial experiments, Hounsfield used low-energy, monochromatic gamma ray radiation. He later conducted experiments with an x-ray tube because of several limitations imposed by the monochromatic radiation source, such as the low radiation intensity rate, large source size, low source strength, and high cost. Subsequently, CT scanners were manufactured to function with x-ray tubes to provide the high radiation intensities necessary for clinical high-contrast CT scanning. However, the heterogeneous beam was problematic because it did not obey the Lambert-Beer exponential law (see Equation 4-1).

The components of the x-ray system include the x-ray generator, x-ray tube, x-ray beam filter, and collimators (see Fig. 5-1).

X-Ray Generator

CT scanners use three-phase power for the efficient production of x rays. In the past, generators for CT scanners were based on the 60-Hertz (Hz) voltage frequency, so the high-voltage generator was a bulky piece of equipment located in a corner of the x-ray room. A long high-tension cable ran from the generator to the x-ray tube in the gantry.

CT scanners now use high-frequency generators, which are small, compact, and more efficient than conventional generators. These generators are located inside the CT gantry. In some scanners, the high-frequency generator is mounted on the rotating frame with the x-ray tube; in others it is located in a corner of the gantry and does not rotate with the tube.

In a high-frequency generator (Fig. 5-15), the circuit is usually referred to as a *high-frequency inverter circuit.* The low-voltage, low-frequency current (60 Hz) from the main power supply is converted to high-voltage, high-frequency current (500 to 25,000 Hz) as it passes through the components, as shown in Figure 5-15. Each component changes the low-voltage, low-frequency AC waveform to supply the x-ray tube with high-voltage, high-frequency direct current (DC) of almost constant potential. After high-voltage rectification and smoothing, the voltage ripple from a high-frequency generator is less than 1%, compared with 4% from a three-phase, 12-pulse generator. This makes the high-frequency generator more efficient at x-ray production than its predecessor. The x-ray exposure technique obtained from these generators depends on the generator power output. The power ratings of CT generators vary and depend on the CT vendor; however, typical ratings can range from 20 to 100 kilowatts (kW) (Kalender, 2005). An output capacity of, say, 60 kW will provide a range of kilovolt and milliampere settings, where 80,120 to 140 kV and 20 to 500 milliamperes (mA) with 1-mA increments are typical.

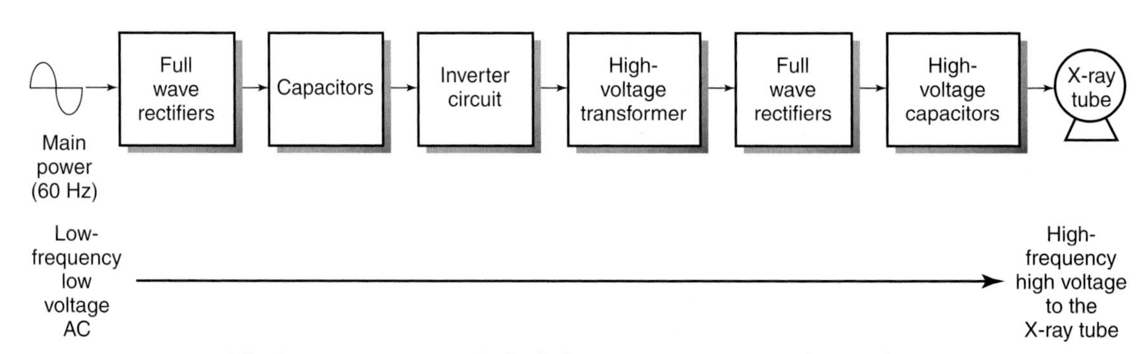

FIGURE 5-15 The basic components of a high-frequency generator used in modern CT scanners.

X-Ray Tubes

The radiation source requirement in CT depends on two factors: (1) radiation attenuation, which is a function of radiation beam energy, the atomic number and density of the absorber, and the thickness of the object, and (2) the quantity of radiation required for transmission. X-ray tubes satisfy this requirement.

First- and second-generation scanners used fixed-anode, oil-cooled x-ray tubes, but rotating anode x-ray tubes have become common in CT because of the demand for increased output (Fig. 5-16). These rotating anode tubes produce a heterogeneous beam of radiation from a large-diameter anode disk with focal spot sizes to facilitate the spatial resolution requirements of the scanner. The disk is usually made of a rhenium, tungsten, and molybdenum (RTM) alloy and other materials with a small target angle (usually 12 degrees) and a rotation speed of 3600 revolutions per minute (rpm) to 10,000 rpm (high-speed rotation).

The introduction of spiral/helical CT with continuous rotation scanners has placed new demands on x-ray tubes. Because the tube rotates continually for a longer period compared with conventional scanners, the tube must be able to sustain higher power levels. Several technical advances in component design have been made to achieve these power levels and deal with the problems of heat generation, heat storage, and heat dissipation. For example, the tube envelope, cathode assembly, anode assembly including

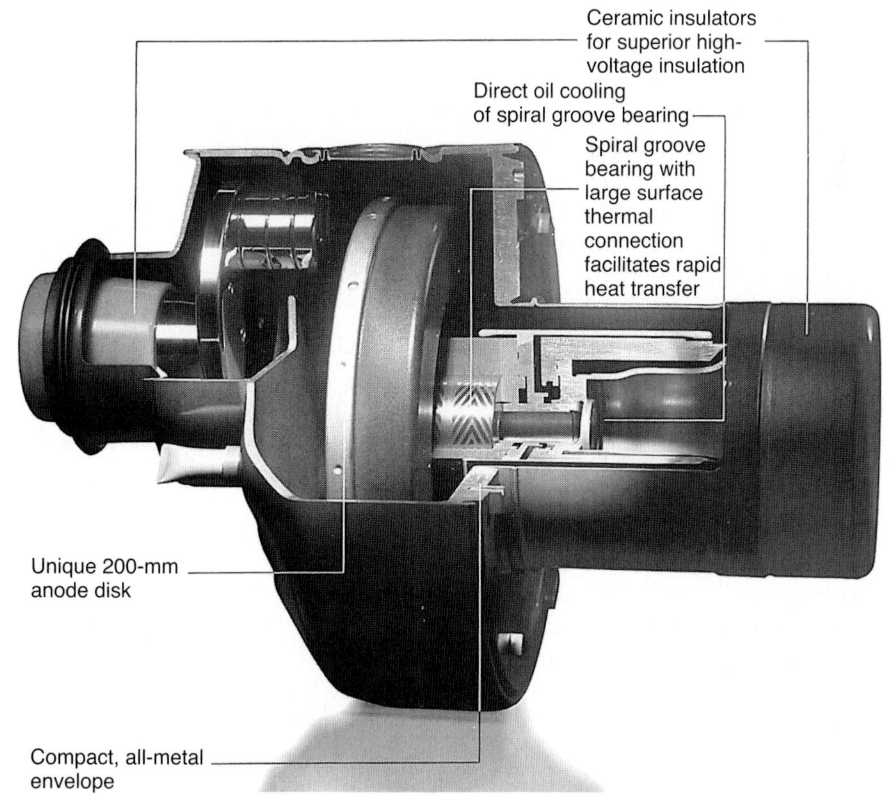

FIGURE 5-16 A modern rotating anode x-ray tube used in CT scanners. (Courtesy Philips Medical Systems, Shelton, Conn.)

anode rotation, and target design have been redesigned (Fox, 1995; Homberg and Koppel, 1997).

The glass envelope ensures a vacuum, provides structural support of anode and cathode structures, and provides high-voltage insulation between the anode and cathode. Internal getters (ion pumps) remove air molecules to ensure a vacuum. Although the borosilicate glass provides good thermal and electrical insulation, electrical arcing results from tungsten deposits on the glass caused by vaporization. Tubes with metal envelopes, which are now common, solve this problem. Ceramic insulators (see Fig. 5-16) isolate the metal envelope from the anode and cathode voltage. Metal envelope tubes have larger anode disks; for example, the tube shown in Figure 5-16 has a disk with a 200-mm diameter compared with the 120- to 160-mm diameter typical of conventional tubes. This feature allows the technologist to use higher tube currents. Heat storage capacity is also increased with an improvement in heat dissipation rates.

The cathode assembly consists of one or more tungsten filaments positioned in a focussing cup. The getter is usually made of barium to ensure a vacuum by the absorption of air molecules released from the target during operation.

The anode assembly consists of the disk, rotor stud and hub, rotor, and bearing assembly. The large anode disk is thicker than conventional disks; the three basic designs are the conventional all-metal disk (Fig. 5-17), the brazed graphite disk, and the chemical vapor deposition (CVD) graphite disk. In conventional tubes, the all-metal disk (see Fig. 5-17, *A*) consists of a base body made of titanium, zirconium, and molybdenum with a focal track layer of 10% rhenium and 90% tungsten. It can transfer heat from the focal track very quickly. Unfortunately, tubes with this all-metal design cannot meet the needs of spiral/helical CT imaging because of their weight.

The brazed graphite anode disk (see Fig. 5-17, *B*) consists of a tungsten-rhenium focal track brazed to a graphite base body. Graphite increases the heat storage capacity because of its high thermal

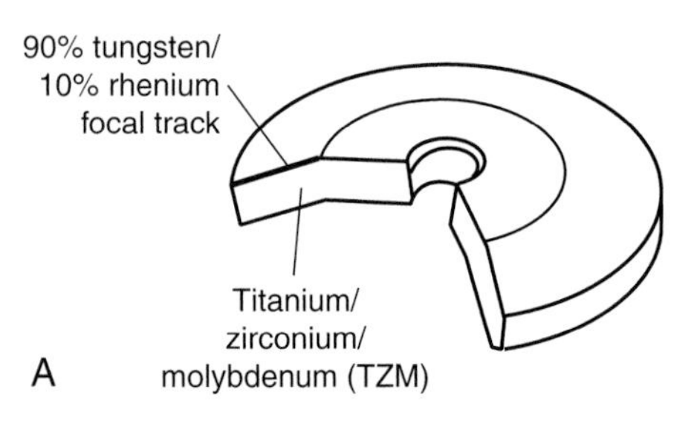

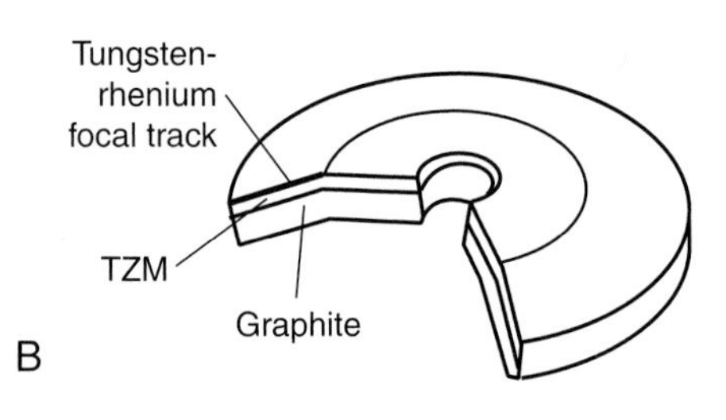

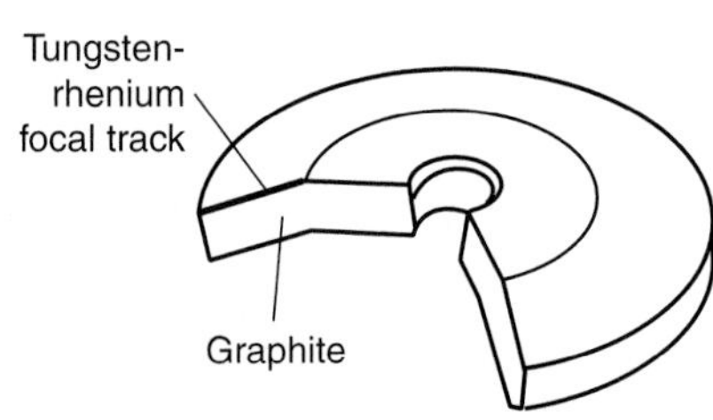

FIGURE 5-17 Three types of disk designs for modern x-ray tubes used in CT scanners: **A,** conventional all-metal disk; **B,** brazed graphite anode disk; and **C,** CVD graphite anode disk.

capacity, which is about 10 times that of tungsten. As noted by Fox (1995), the material used in the brazing process influences the operating temperature of the tube, and the higher temperatures result in higher heat storage capacities and faster cooling of the anode. Tubes for spiral/helical CT scanning are based mostly on this type of design.

The final type of anode design (see Fig. 5-17, *C*) is also intended for use in spiral/helical CT x-ray tubes. The disk consists of a graphite base body with a

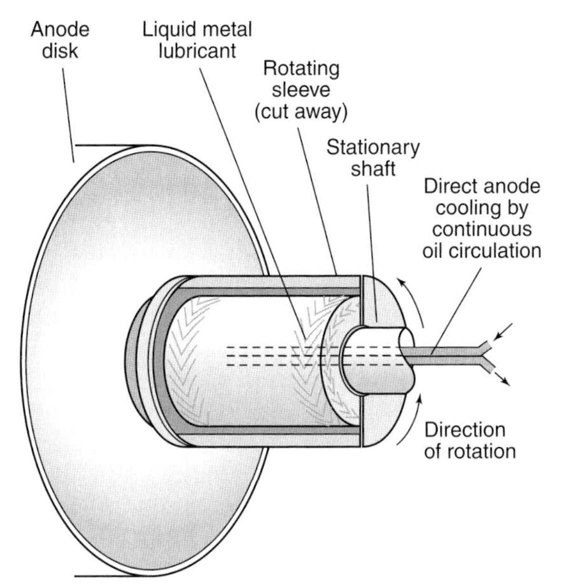

FIGURE 5-18 The anode assembly of a modern x-ray tube used in CT imaging. The main parts of the assembly are the disk, rotor, and bearing assembly that contains liquid metal lubricant.

tungsten-rhenium layer deposited on the focal track by a chemical vapor process. This design can accommodate large, lightweight disks with large heat storage capacity and fast cooling rates (Fox, 1995).

The purpose of the bearing assembly is to provide and ensure smooth rotation of the anode disk. In CT, high-speed anode rotation allows the use of higher loadability. Rotation speeds of 10,000 rpm are possible with increased frequency to the stator windings. Smooth rotation of the disk is possible because of the ball bearings lubricated with silver; however, because ball-bearing technology results in mechanical problems and limits x-ray tube performance, a liquid-bearing method to improve anode disk rotation was introduced (Fig. 5-18).

The stationary shaft of the anode assembly consists of grooves that contain gallium-based liquid metal alloy. During anode rotation, the liquid is forced into the grooves and results in a hydroplaning effect between the anode sleeve and liquid (Homberg and Koppel, 1997). The purpose of this bearing technology is to conduct heat away from the x-ray tube more efficiently than conventional ball bearings with improved tube cooling. Additionally, the liquid bearing technology is free of vibrations and noise.

As noted by Fox (1995), the rotor hub and rotor stud also prevent the transmission of heat from the disk to the bearings. The rotor is a copper cylinder "brazed to an inner steel cylinder with a ceramic coating around the outside to enhance heat radiation" (Fox, 1995).

The working life of the tubes can range from about 10,000 to 40,000 hours, compared with 1000 hours, which is typical of conventional tubes with conventional bearing technology.

An example of the specifications for one type of x-ray tube is listed in Table 5-1.

Straton X-Ray Tube: A New X-Ray Tube for MSCT Scanning

As noted above, the fundamental problem with conventional x-ray tubes is that of heat dissipation and slow cooling rates. Efforts have been made to

Table 5-1 Specifications for the Philips MRC X-Ray Tube

Features	Values
Effective heat storage capacity	26 MHU
Anode storage capacity	8.0 MHU
Maximum cooling rate	1608 kHU/min
Focal spot (IEC)	
Large	1.0 mm × 1.0 mm
Small	0.5 mm × 1.0 mm
Anode diameter	200 mm
Anode rotation speed	105 Hz (6300 rpm)
Target angle	7 degrees
Focus-detector distance	1040 mm
Focus-isocenter distance	570 mm

Courtesy Philips Medical System.

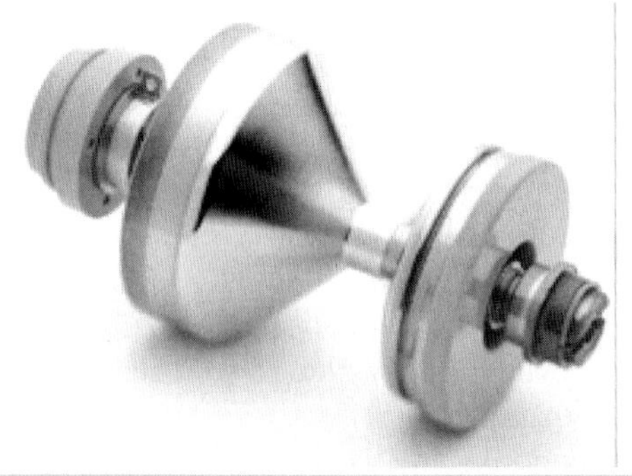

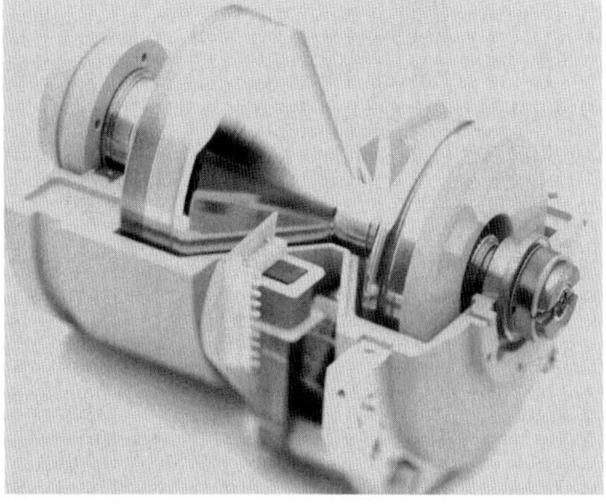

FIGURE 5-19 The Straton x-ray tube, a new x-ray tube for MSCT scanning. See text for further description. (Courtesy of Siemens Medical Solutions, Germany.)

deal with these problems by introducing various designs, such as, for example, large anode disks and the introduction of the compound anode design (RTM disk), which has higher heat storage capacities and cooling rates. Additionally, as gantry rotation times increase, higher milliampere values are needed to provide the same milliamperes per rotation. As the electrical load (milliamperes and kilovolts) increases, faster anode cooling rates are needed. Despite these efforts, the problem of heat transfer and slow cooling rates still persist with MSCT scanners, especially for multiple longer scan times and cardiac CT imaging.

To overcome these problems, a new type of x-ray tube has been introduced for use with MSCT scanners. This unique and revolutionary tube was designed by Siemens Medical Solutions (Siemens AG Medical Solutions, Erlangen, Germany). Because this tube represents a new technology for dealing with the problem of x-ray tube heat in multislice CT scanning and leads to an innovative method of improving image quality in CT, it is described here.

A photograph of the tube is shown in Figure 5-19. As can be seen, it is encased in a protective housing that contains oil for cooling. The tube is compact in design and is much smaller than conventional x-ray tubes described earlier. This size ensures a fast gantry rotation of 0.37 seconds (Kalender, 2005).

The Straton x-ray tube, illustrated in Figure 5-20, has anode and cathode structures, deflection coils, an electron beam, and a motor. The electron beam produced by the filament housed in the cathode assembly is deflected to strike the anode (120-mm diameter) to produce x rays used for imaging. The motor provides the rotation of the entire tube, which is immersed in oil. It is important to note that the anode is in direct contact with the oil, which is forced out of the housing for cooling and subsequently circulates back into the housing. The fact that the anode is in direct contact with the circulating oil results in very high cooling rates of 5.0 MHU/min that results in about 0 MHU anode heat storage capacity. The advantage of this is that high-speed volume scanning is possible with high milliamperes and long exposure times for increasing length of anatomical coverage. A comparison of the design structures of both conventional and the Straton x-ray tubes is illustrated in Figure 5-21.

Another important feature of the Straton x-ray tube relates to the electron beam from the cathode. This beam is deflected to strike the anode at two precisely located focal spots (Fig. 5-22) that vary in sizes. Kalender (2005) reports that the sizes can be 0.6 mm × 0.17 mm, 0.8 mm × 1.1 mm, and 0.7 mm × 0.7 mm. The electron beam alternates at about 4640 times per second to create two separate x-ray beams that pass through the patient

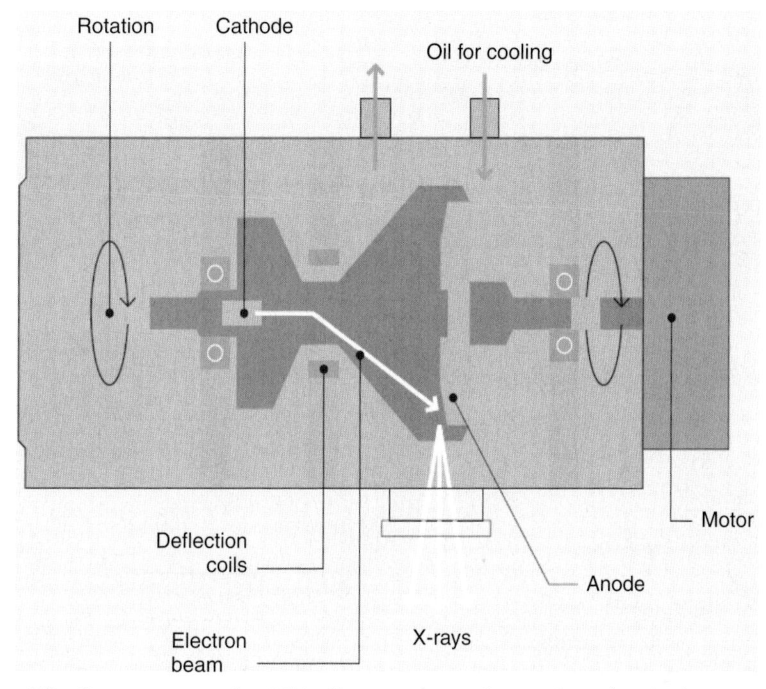

FIGURE 5-20 The Straton x-ray tube. This diagram shows the anode and cathode structures, deflection coils, an electron beam, and a motor. See text for further explanation. (Courtesy of Siemens Medical Solutions, Germany.)

and fall on the detectors. This is described later in the chapter.

Filtration

Radiation from x-ray tubes consists of long and short wavelengths. The original experiments in the development of a practical CT scanner used monochromatic radiation to satisfy the Lambert-Beer exponential attenuation law. However, in clinical CT, the beam is polychromatic. Because it is essential that the polychromatic beam have the appearance of a monochromatic beam to satisfy the requirements of the reconstruction process, a special filter must be used.

In CT, filtration serves a dual purpose, as follows:

1. Filtration removes long-wavelength x-rays because they do not play a role in CT image formation but instead contribute to patient dose. As a result of filtration, the mean energy of the beam increases and the beam becomes "harder," which may cause beam-hardening artifacts.

Recall that the total filtration is equal to the sum of the inherent filtration and the added filtration. In CT the inherent filtration has a thickness of about 3 mm Al-equivalent. The added filtration, on the other hand, consists of filters that are flat or shaped filters made of copper sheets, for example, the thickness of which can range from 0.1 to 0.4 mm (Kalender, 2005)

2. Filtration shapes the energy distribution across the radiation beam to produce uniform beam hardening when x-rays pass through the filter and the object.

In Figure 5-23, the attenuation differs in sections 1, 2, and 3 and the penetration increases in

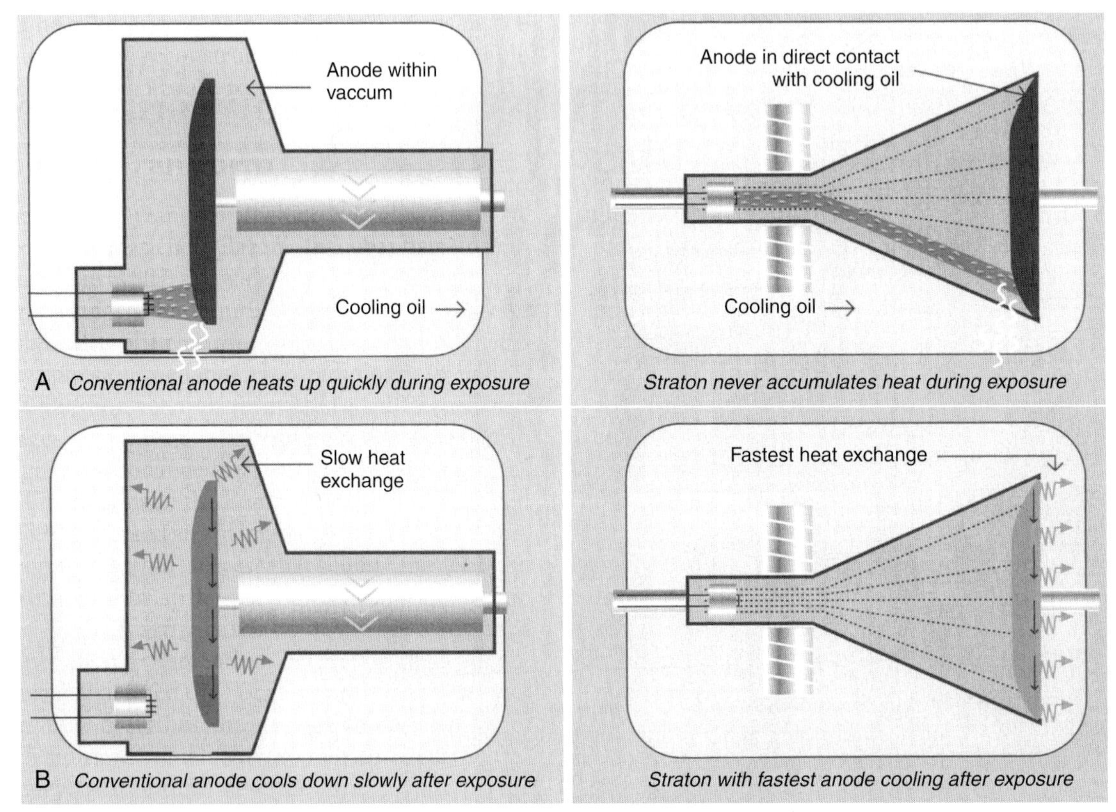

FIGURE 5-21 A comparison of the design structures of both conventional and the Straton x-ray tubes. (Courtesy of Siemens Medical Solutions, Germany.)

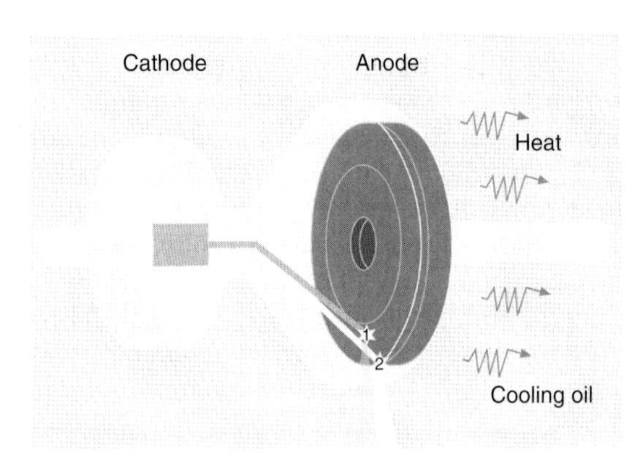

FIGURE 5-22 An important feature of the Straton x-ray tube is that the electron beam from the cathode is deflected to strike the anode at two precisely located focal spots that vary in size. (Courtesy Siemens Medical Solutions, Germany.)

sections 2 and 3. This results from the absorption of the soft radiation in sections 1 and 2 that is referred to as *hardening of the beam.* Because the detector system does not respond to beam-hardening effects for the circular object shown, "the problem can be solved by introducing additional filtration into the beam" (Seeram, 2001). In the original EMI scanner, this problem was solved with a water bath around the patient's head. Today, specially shaped filters conform to the shape of the object (Fig. 5-24). These filters are called shaped filters such as the "bowtie" filter and are usually made of Teflon, for example, a material that has low atomic number and high density, so as not to have a significant impact on beam hardening. The filters are positioned between the x-ray tube and patient, and they shape

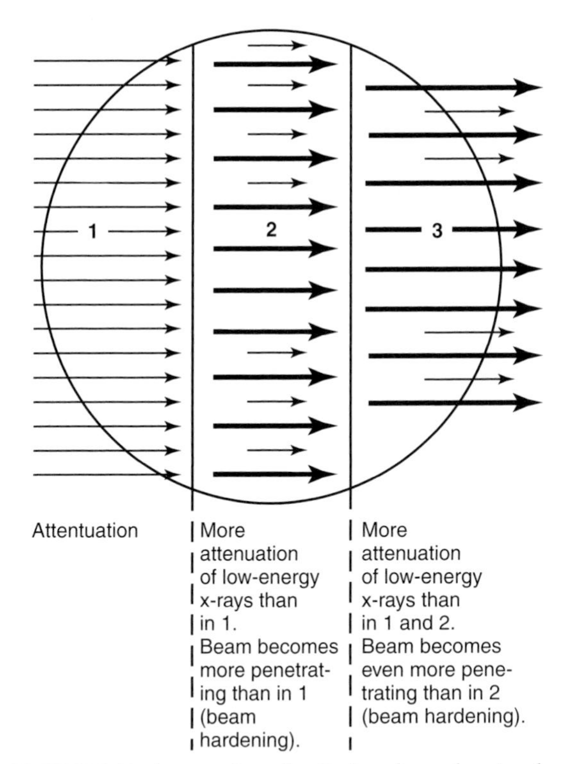

FIGURE 5-23 Attenuation of radiation through a circular object. The beam becomes more penetrating (harder) in section 3 because of differences in attenuation in sections 1 and 2. The heavier arrows indicate less attenuation and more penetrating rays.

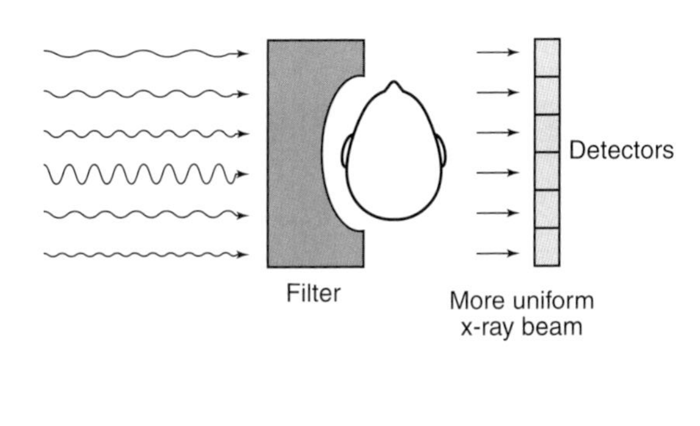

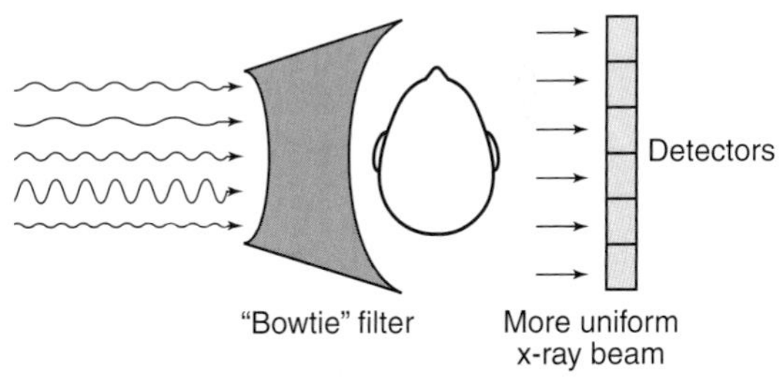

FIGURE 5-24 Two types of beam-shaping filters for use in CT. These filters attenuate the beam so that a more uniform (monochromatic) beam falls onto the detectors. This uniform beam reduces the dynamic range of the electronics (analog-to-digital converters).

the beam to produce more uniformity at the detectors.

Collimation

The purpose of collimation in conventional radiography and fluoroscopy is to protect the patient by restricting the beam to the anatomy of interest only. In CT, collimation is equally important because it affects patient dose and image quality (Fig. 5-25). The basic collimation scheme in CT is shown in Figure 5-25, *A*, with adjustable prepatient and postpatient collimators and predetector collimators. These detectors must be perfectly aligned to optimize the imaging process. This alignment is accomplished with the fixed collimators, not shown in Fig 5-25, *A*.

Prepatient collimation design is influenced by the size of the focal spot of the x-ray tube because of the penumbra effect associated with focal spots. The larger the focal spot, the greater the penumbra and the more complicated the design of the collimators.

In general, a set of collimator sections is carefully arranged to shape the beam, which is proximal to the focal spot. Both proximal and distal (predetector) collimators are arranged to ensure a constant beam width at the detector. Detector collimators also shape the beam and remove scattered radiation. Such removal improves axial resolution as illustrated in Figure 5-25, *B*, in which the golf ball dimples are apparent. The collimator section at the distal end of the collimator assembly also helps define the thickness of the slice to be imaged. Various slice thicknesses are available depending on the type of scanner.

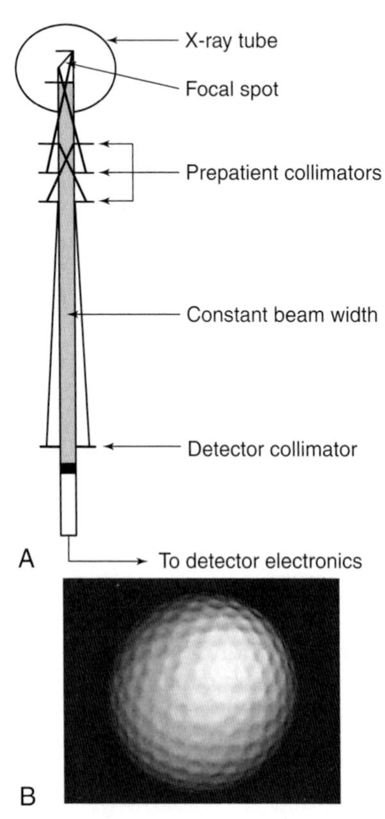

FIGURE 5-25 A, Collimation scheme typical of CT scanning. **B,** The removal of scattered radiation by the two sets of collimators improves the resolution of the golf ball dimples. (Courtesy Shimadzu Medical Systems, Seattle, Wash.)

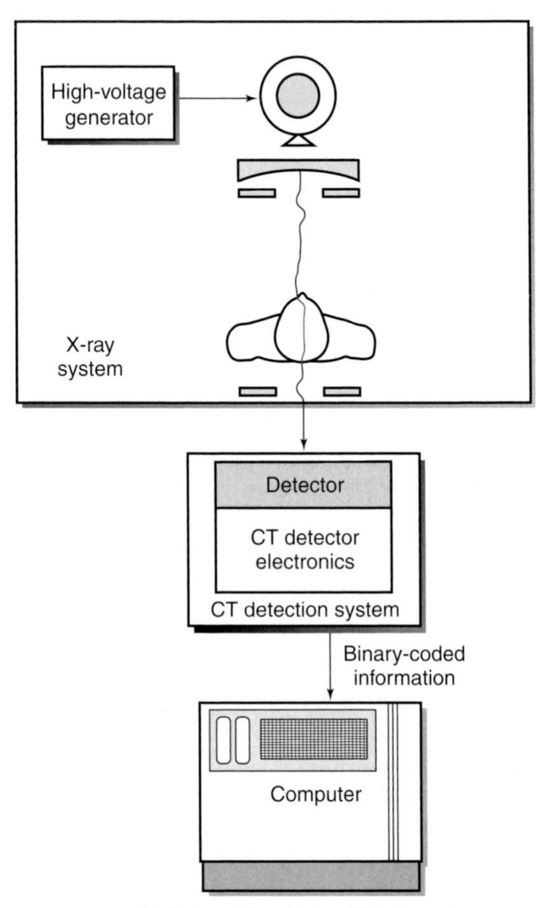

FIGURE 5-26 Relationship of the CT detection system to the x-ray system and computer.

Some scanners incorporate an antiscatter grid to remove radiation scattered from the patient. This grid is placed just in front of the detectors and it is intended to improve image quality.

CT DETECTOR TECHNOLOGY

The position of the CT detection system is shown in Figure 5-26. CT detectors capture the radiation beam from the patient and convert it into electrical signals, which are subsequently converted into binary coded information.

Detector Characteristics

Detectors exhibit several characteristics essential for CT image production; however, only the following are highlighted in this book: efficiency, response time, dynamic range, high reproducibility, stability, and afterglow.

Efficiency refers to the ability to capture, absorb, and convert x-ray photons to electrical signals. CT detectors must possess high capture efficiency, absorption efficiency, and conversion efficiency. *Capture efficiency* refers to the efficiency with which the detectors can obtain photons transmitted from the patient; the size of the detector area facing the beam and distance between two detectors determine capture efficiency. *Absorption efficiency* refers to the number of photons absorbed by the detector and depends on the atomic number, physical density, size, and thickness of the detector face (Seeram, 2001; Villafana, 1987).

Stability refers to the steadiness of the detector response. If the system is not stable, frequent calibrations are required to render the signals useful.

The *response time* of the detector refers to the speed with which the detector can detect an x-ray event and recover to detect another event. Response times should be very short (i.e., microseconds) to avoid problems such as afterglow and detector "pile-up."

The *dynamic range* of a CT detector is the "ratio of the largest signal to be measured to the precision of the smallest signal to be discriminated (i.e., if the largest signal is 1 μA and the smallest signal is 1 nA, the dynamic range is 1 million to 1)" (Parker and Stanley, 1981). The dynamic range for most CT scanners is about 1 million to 1. The total detector efficiency, or dose efficiency, is the product of the capture efficiency, absorption efficiency, and conversion efficiency (Seeram, 2001; Villafana, 1987).

Afterglow refers to the persistence of the image even after the radiation has been turned off. CT detectors should have low afterglow values, such as < 0.01%, 100 milliseconds after the radiation has been terminated (Kalender, 2005).

Types

The conversion of x-rays to electrical energy in a detector is based on two fundamental principles (Fig. 5-27). Scintillation detectors convert x-ray energy into light, and then the light is converted into electrical energy (Fig. 5-27, *A*). Gas ionization detectors convert x-ray energy directly to electrical energy (Fig. 5-27, *B*).

Scintillation Detectors

Scintillation detectors are solid-state detectors that consist of a scintillation crystal coupled to a photodiode tube. When x rays fall onto the crystal, flashes of light, or scintillations, are produced. The light is then directed to the photomultiplier, or PM tube. As illustrated in Figure 5-28, the light from the crystal strikes the photocathode of the PM tube, which then releases electrons. These electrons cascade through a series of dynodes that are

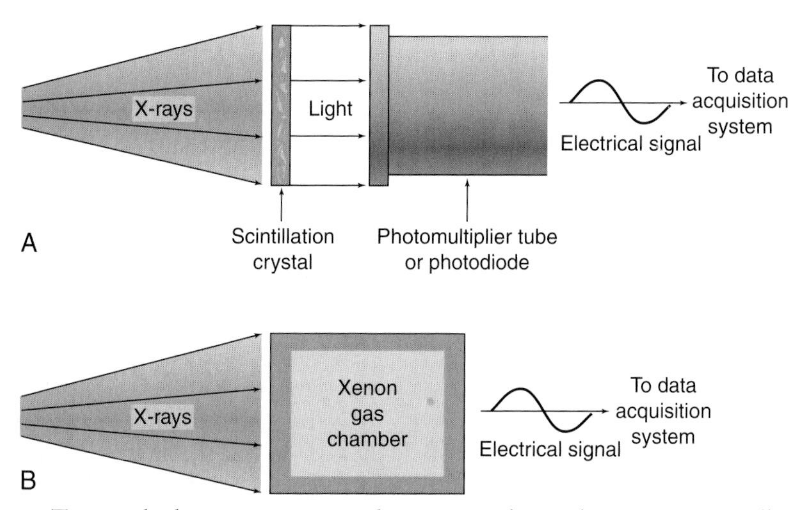

FIGURE 5-27 Two methods to convert x-ray photons into electrical energy. **A,** Scintillation crystal detection and conversion scheme. **B,** Conversion of x rays into electrical energy through gas ionization.

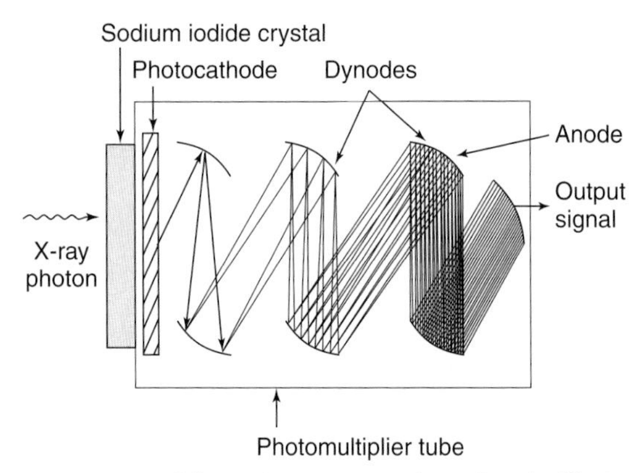

FIGURE 5-28 Schematic representation of a scintillation detector based on the photomultiplier tube.

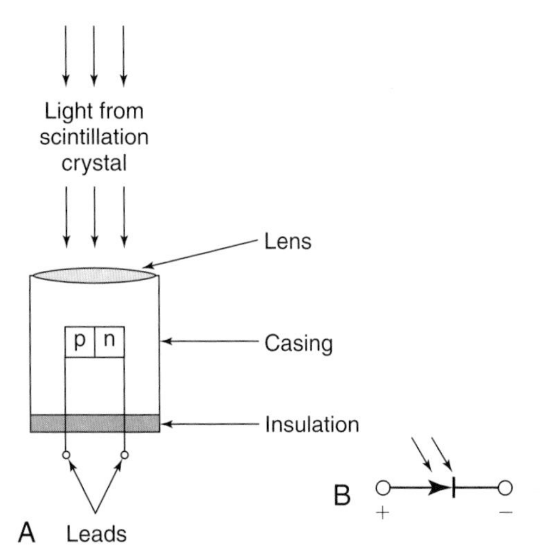

FIGURE 5-29 A, Basic structure of a photodiode. **B,** The electronic symbol of a photodiode.

carefully arranged and maintained at different potentials to result in a small output signal.

In the past, early scanners used sodium iodide crystals coupled to PM tubes. Because of afterglow problems and the limited dynamic range of sodium iodide, other crystals such as calcium fluoride and bismuth germanate were used in later scanners. Today, solid-state photodiode multiplier scintillation crystal detectors are used (Fig. 5-29). The photodiode is a semiconductor (silicon) whose *p-n* junction allows current flow when exposed to light. A lens is an essential part of the photodiode and is used to focus light from the scintillation crystal to the *p-n* junction, or semiconductor junction. When light falls on the junction, electron hole pairs are generated and the electrons move to the *n* side of the junction while the holes move to the *p* side. The amount of current is proportional to the amount of light. Photodiodes are normally used with amplifiers because of the low output from the diode. In addition, the response time of a photodiode is extremely fast (about 0.5 to 250 nanoseconds, depending on its design).

Scintillation materials currently used with photodiodes are cadmium tungstate and a ceramic material made of high-purity, rare earth oxides based on doped rare earth compounds such as yttria and gadolinium oxysulfide ultrafast ceramic (Kalender, 2005). Usually these crystals are optically bonded to the photodiodes. The advantages and disadvantages of these two scintillation materials can be discussed in terms of the detector characteristics described earlier. The conversion efficiency and photon capture efficiency of cadmium tungstate are 99% and 99%, respectively, and the dynamic range is 1 million to 1. On the other hand, the absorption efficiency of the ceramic rare earth oxide is 99%, whereas its scintillation efficiency is three times that of cadmium tungstate.

Gas Ionization Detectors

Gas ionization detectors, which are based on the principle of ionization, were introduced in third-generation scanners. The basic configuration of a gas ionization detector consists of a series of individual gas chambers, usually separated by tungsten plates carefully positioned to act as electron collection plates (Fig. 5-30). When x rays fall on the individual chambers, ionization of the gas (usually xenon) results and produces positive and negative ions. The positive ions migrate to the negatively charged plate, whereas the negative ions are attracted to the positively

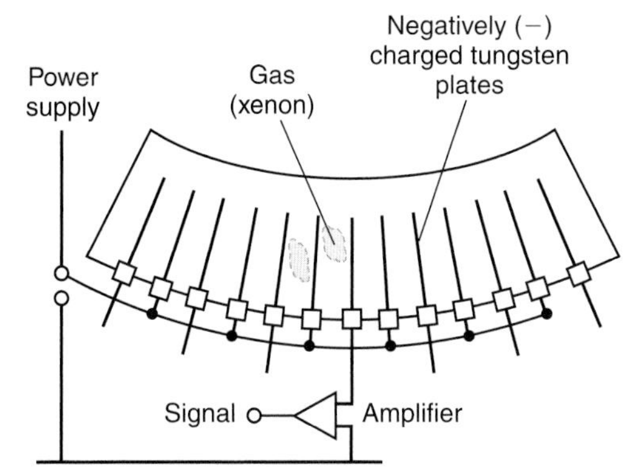

FIGURE 5-30 The basic configuration of a gas ionization detector consists of a series of individual gas chambers separated by tungsten plates.

charged plate. This migration of ions causes a small signal current that varies directly with the number of photons absorbed.

The gas chambers are enclosed by a relatively thick ceramic substrate material because the xenon gas is pressurized to about 30 atmospheres to increase the number of gas molecules available for ionization. Xenon detectors have excellent stability and fast response times and exhibit no afterglow problems. However, their quantum detection efficiency (QDE) is less than that of solid-state detectors. As reported in the past, the QDE is 95% to 100% for crystal solid-state scintillation detectors and 94% to 98% for ceramic solid-state detectors, it is only 50% to 60% for xenon gas detectors (Arenson, 1995). It is important to note that with the introduction of MSCT scanners with their characteristic multirow detector arrays, gas-ionization detectors and fourth-generation CT systems are not used anymore. MSCT scanners are all based on the third-generation beam geometry (rotate-rotate principle) and use solid-state detector arrays (Kalender, 2005).

Multirow/Multislice Detectors

One major problem with single-slice, single-row detectors is related to the length of time needed to acquire data. The dual-slice, dual-row detector system was introduced to increase the volume coverage speed and thus decrease the time for data collection. CT scanners now use multirow detectors to image multislices during a 360-degree rotation. It is important to realize that other terms such as multidetector and multichannel have been used to describe the detectors for MSCT scanners (Douglas-Akinwande et al, 2006).

Dual-Row/Dual-Slice Detectors

In 1992, Elscint introduced the first dual-slice volume CT scanner. The configuration of the dual-row detector system results in faster volume coverage compared with single-row CT systems (Fig. 5-31). This technology uses a dual-row, solid-state detector array coupled with a special x-ray tube based on a double-dynamic focus system. Figure 5-31 also shows the conventional beam geometry (single focal spot, single fan beam, and single detector arc array) and the beam geometry that arises as a result of the dynamic focal spot system. The dynamic focal spot is where the position of the focal spot is switched by a computer-controlled electron-optic system during each scan to double the sampling density and total number of measurements. Twin-beam technology results in the simultaneous scan of two contiguous slices with excellent resolution (Fig. 5-32) because the fan beam ray density and detector sampling are doubled twice, once for each of the two contiguous slices.

Multirow/Multislice Detectors

The goal of multirow/multislice (MR/MS) detectors is to increase the volume coverage speed performance of both single-slice and dual-slice CT scanners. The MR-MS detector consists of one detector with rows of detector elements (Fig. 5-33). A detector with *n* rows will be *n* times faster than its single-row counterpart. MR-MS detectors are solid-state detectors that can acquire 4 to 64 to 320 slices per 360-degree rotation. In addition, the design of these detectors can influence the thickness of the slices.

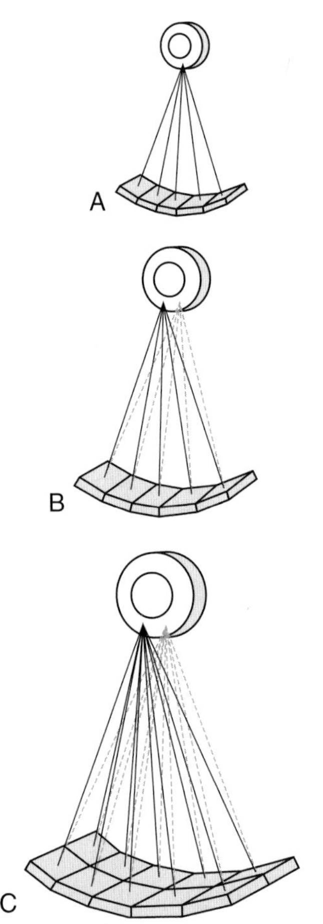

FIGURE 5-31 **A,** Conventional beam geometry with single focal spot, single fan beam, and single-detector arc array. **B,** Twin-beam geometry from Elscint's dynamic focal spot system. **C,** Dual-row, dual-detector system.

An MR/MS detector is an array consisting of multiple separate detector rows. For example, these detector rows can range from two (Elscint dual-row detector) to 64 detector rows that can image simultaneously two to 64 slices, respectively, per 360-degree rotation. It is fairly obvious that the number of slices obtained per 360-degree rotation depends on the number of detector rows. For example, while a 16-detector row scanner can produce 16 images per 360-degree rotation, a 64-detector row scanner will produce 64 slices per 360-degree rotation.

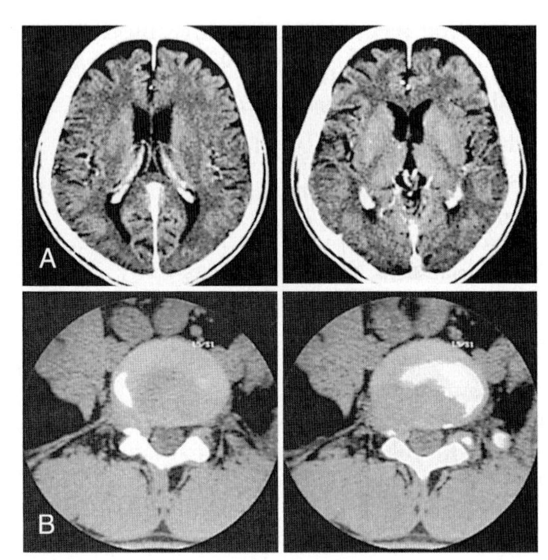

FIGURE 5-32 Two contiguous slices acquired simultaneously for the brain **(A)** and spine **(B).** The brain images are contiguous 10-mm slices and the spine images are contiguous 2.5-mm slices. (Courtesy Elscint, Hackensack, NJ.)

Multirow CT detectors fall into two categories (Fig. 5-34), namely, *matrix array detectors* and *adaptive array detectors* (Dalrymple et al, 2007; Flohr et al, 2005; Kalender, 2005). The matrix array detector (Fig. 5-34, *A*) is sometimes referred to as a fixed array detector, contains channels or cells as they are often referred to, that are equal in all dimensions. Because of this, these detectors are sometimes referred to as being *isotropic* in design, that is, all cells are perfect cubes. The adaptive array detector, on the other hand, is *anisotropic* in design (Kalender, 2005). This means that the cells are not equal but rather they have different sizes (Fig. 5-34, *B*). The overall goal of isotropic imaging is to produce improved spatial resolution in both the longitudinal and transverse planes (Dalrymple et al, 2007).

During scanning, the number of slices and the thickness of each slice are determined by the detector configuration used. This configuration "describes the number of data collection channels and the effective section thickness determined by

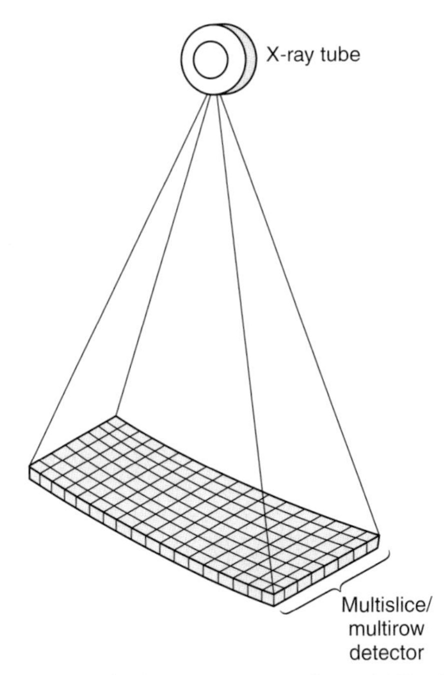

FIGURE 5-33 The basic structure of a multislice/multirow detector used in multislice volume CT scanners.

the data acquisition system settings" (Dalrymple et al, 2007). For the sake of simplicity, the detector configuration for a four-row matrix array detector is illustrated in Figure 5-35. In this example, each detector channel is 1.25 mm and four cells are activated or grouped together to produce four separate images of 1.25-mm thickness per 360-degree rotation. On the other hand, eight cells can be configured to produce four images of 2.5 mm thickness (1.25 mm + 1.25 mm = 2.5 mm) per 360-degree rotation, and so on. Multirow detectors are described further in Chapter 12.

Multirow detectors feature a number of imaging characteristics that are important to the technologist during scanning. These characteristics and specifications are shown in Table 5-2 from one CT vendor.

Area Detectors

As discussed previously, several groups are investigating the use of area detectors for CT imaging

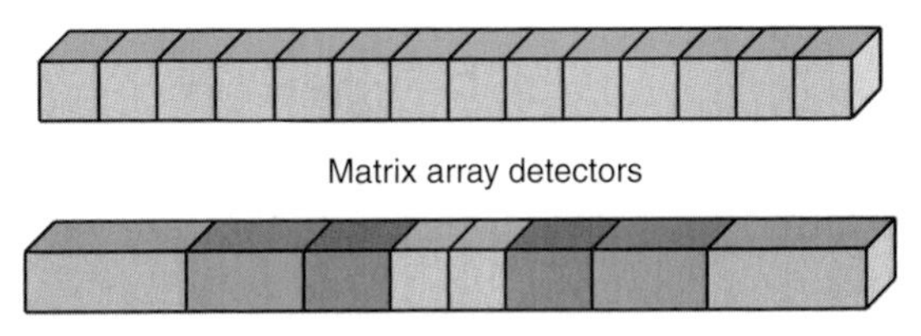

FIGURE 5-34 Multirow CT detectors fall into two categories (see Fig. 5-35), namely, *matrix array detectors* and *adaptive array detectors*. (See text for further explanation.)

and prototypes gave been developed and are currently undergoing clinical testing. Two such CT scanners based on area detector technology are the 256-slice CT scanner prototype (Toshiba Acquilion, Toshiba Medical Systems, Japan) and the flat-panel CT scanner prototypes (one from Siemens Medical Solutions, and another from the Koning Corporation-USA).

The 256-Slice CT Prototype Detector

An illustration of the gantry and detector for this scanner is shown in Chapter 1 (Fig 1-16). The detector is a wide area multirow array detector that has 912 channels × 256 segments and a beam width of 128 mm (four times larger than the third-generation 16-slice Toshiba Acquilion CT Scanner). This wide beam width makes it possible to scan larger volumes such as the entire heart in a single rotation (Mori, 2006, personal communications; Mori et al, 2006). This scanner is described further in Chapter 12.

Flat-Panel Detectors

Flat-panel detectors similar to the ones used in digital radiography are being investigated for use in CT imaging. In this respect, several prototypes have been developed and are currently being evaluated for use in CT imaging. One such prototype is shown in Figure 5-10. Note that the detector is a flat-panel type and is based on the CsI indirect conversion digital radiography detector. More recently, flat-panel detectors are being investigated

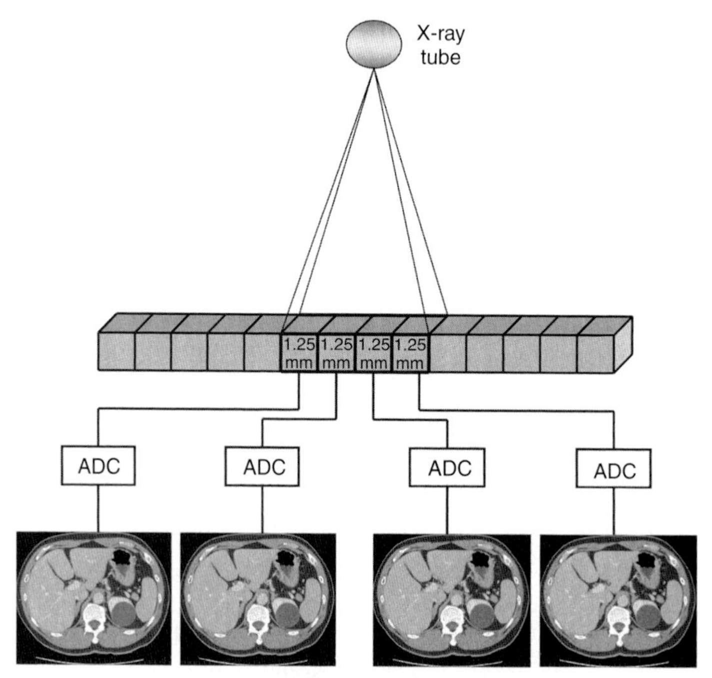

FIGURE 5-35 The detector configuration for a 4-row matrix array detector. In this example, each detector channel is 1.25 mm and four cells are activated or grouped together to produce four separate images of 1.25-mm thickness per 360-degree rotation.

for use in breast CT, and several prototypes are now undergoing clinical testing (Glick et al, 2007; Kwan et al, 2007). Breast CT is described in Chapter 13.

DETECTOR ELECTRONICS

Function

The *data acquisition system* (DAS) refers to the detector electronics positioned between the detector array and the computer (Fig. 5-36). Because the DAS is located between the detectors and the computer, it performs three major functions: (1) it measures the transmitted radiation beam, (2) it encodes these measurements into binary data, and (3) it transmits the binary data to the computer.

Components

The detector measures the transmitted x-rays from the patient and converts them into electrical energy. This electrical signal is so weak that it must be amplified by the preamplifier before it can be analyzed further (Fig. 5-37).

The transmission measurement data must be changed into attenuation and thickness data. This process (logarithmic conversion) can be expressed as follows:

$$\text{Attenuation} = \text{log of transmission} \cdot \text{thickness} \quad \textbf{(5-3)}$$

or

$$\mu_1 + \mu_2 + \mu_3 \ldots \mu_n = \ln I_0/I \cdot 1/x$$

where μ is the linear attenuation coefficient, I_0 is the original intensity, I is the transmitted intensity, and x is the thickness of the object.

Table 5-2 Characteristics and Specifications of Multirow Detectors

Characteristics	Specifications
Material	Solid-state GOS
No. of elements	43,008 86,016 effective with DFS
Dynamic range	1,000,000 to 1
Slip ring	Optical—up to 5.3 Gbps transfer rate
Data sampling rate	Up to 4640 views/revolution/element
Slice collimation	2×0.5 mm, 16×2.5 mm, 32×1.25 mm, 64×0.625 mm
Slice thickness	Spiral mode: 0.67-7.5 mm variable Axial mode: 0.5-12 mm
Scan angles	240, 360, 420 degrees
Scan field of view	250, 500 mm

Courtesy Philips Medical System.
DFS, Dual focal spot; *GOS*, gadolinium oxysufide.

Logarithmic conversion is performed by the logarithmic amplifier, and these signals are subsequently directed to the ADC. The ADC divides the electrical signals into multiple parts—the more parts, the more accurate the ADC. These parts are measured in bits: a 1-bit ADC divides the signal into two digital values (2^1), a 2-bit ADC generates four digital values (2^2), and a 12-bit ADC results in 4096 (2^{12}) digital values. These values help determine the gray-scale resolution of the image. Modern CT scanners use 16-bit ADCs.

The final step performed by the DAS is data transmission to the computer. CT manufacturers have introduced optoelectronic data transmission schemes for this purpose because of the continuous rotation of the tube or detector arc and vast amount of data generated.

Optoelectronics refers to the use of lens and light diodes to facilitate data transmission (Fig. 5-38). Several optical transmitters send the data to the optical receiver array so that at least one transmitter and one receiver are always in optical contact. These receivers and transmitters are light-emitting diodes capable of very high rates of data transmission; 50 million bits per second is common.

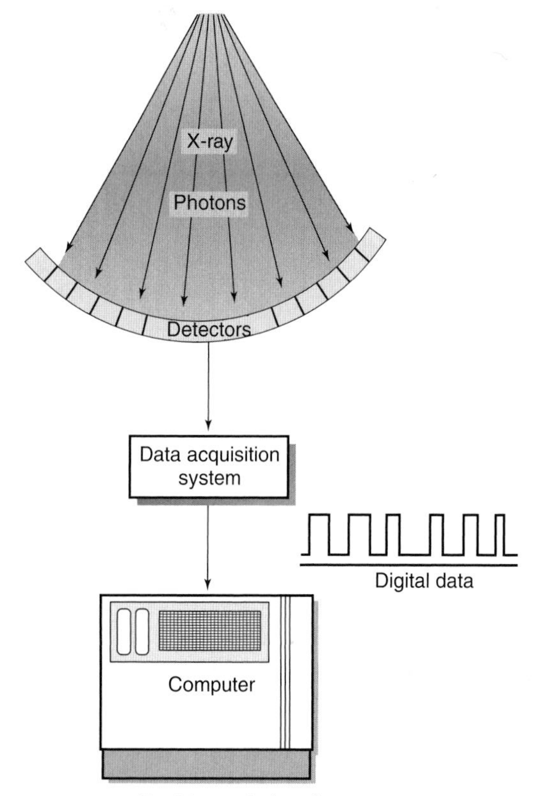

FIGURE 5-36 Position of the data acquisition system in CT.

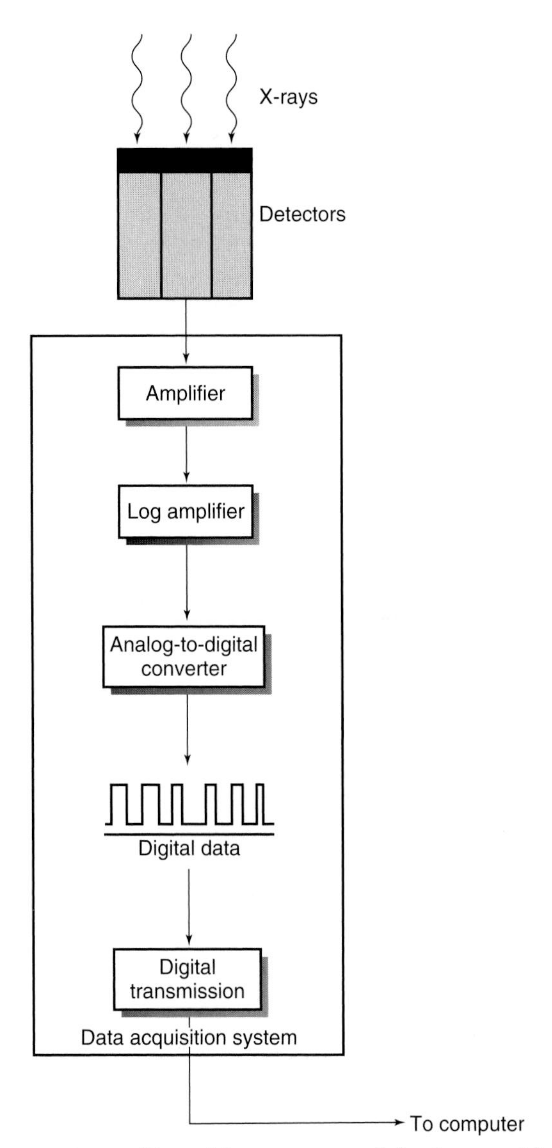

FIGURE 5-37 Essential components of the data acquisition system in CT.

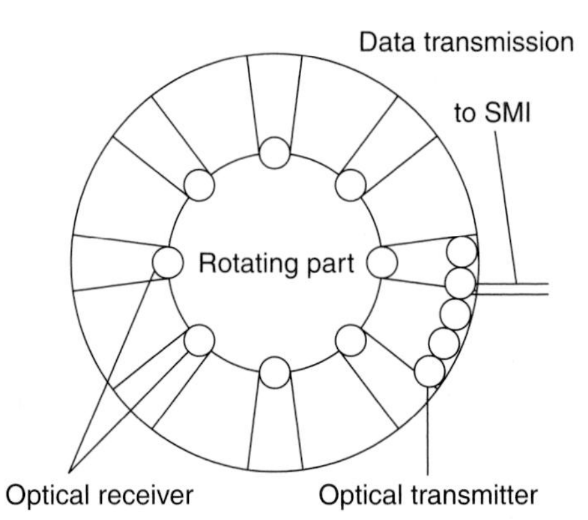

FIGURE 5-38 Optoelectric data transmission. Optical transmitters on the gantry send data to the optical receiver array. At least one transmitter and one receiver are always in optical contact.

DATA ACQUISITION AND SAMPLING

During data acquisition, the radiation beam transmitted through the patient falls on the detectors. Each detector then measures, or samples, the beam intensity incident on it. If enough samples are not obtained, artifacts such as streaking (an aliasing artifact) appear on the reconstructed image. To solve this problem, the following methods have been devised to increase the number of samples available for image reconstruction and to thus improve the quality of the image:

- Slice thickness: The imaging of thin slices helps reduce streaking artifacts related to sampling.
- Closely packed detectors: When the detectors are closely packed, more detectors are available for data acquisition, which ensures more samples per view and an increase in the total measurements taken per scan.
- In the past, *the quarter-shifted detector arc* has been used: In conventional CT systems, the fan beam is composed of the same number of beams and detectors, and the spacing of the beams often causes sampling errors. These errors can be minimized if the detector arc is shifted by one-quarter detector space. The goal of detector shifting is to provide two sets of data that can be individually reconstructed or combined to provide a doubly fine sampling grid so more data are

available for image reconstruction. In the Siemens Somatom Plus scanner, for example, this shifting is accomplished by the flying focal spot (dual focal spot x-ray tube). The same detector is used more than once to provide a large number of discrete measurements, which eliminates the aliasing artifact. This process is referred to as the *multifan measurement technique* (Siemens Medical Systems, 1999).

- The *double-dynamic focus* system used by Elscint in their CT twin scanner was yet another method of increasing detector sampling during data acquisition.

New Sampling Technique: z-Sharp Technology

A more recent innovation is one that involves the use of the Straton x-ray tube described earlier in the chapter. As seen in Figure 5-39, the *z-flying focal spot technique* (referred to as the *z-sharp technology*) provides doubling sampling, where two overlapping slices for each detector row are obtained at the same time per 360-degree rotation. The Siemens Somatom 64 CT scanner, for example, will provide 64 slices for the 32 × 0.6 mm detector array. As noted by Kalender (2005) "the data thus acquired with its 32 × 0.6mm detector present the equivalent to the sampling pattern of a 64 × 0.3mm detector. The data set results are representing 64 overlapping slices of 0.6mm width with a sampling distance of 0.3mm."

The results of double sampling in the z-direction by the *z-flying focal spot* (z-FFS) technique on image quality are illustrated in Figure 5-40. It is clearly apparent that the image is much sharper with the z-FFS (Fig. 5-40, *A*) sampling technique than without the z-FFS (Fig. 5-40, *B*) sampling technique.

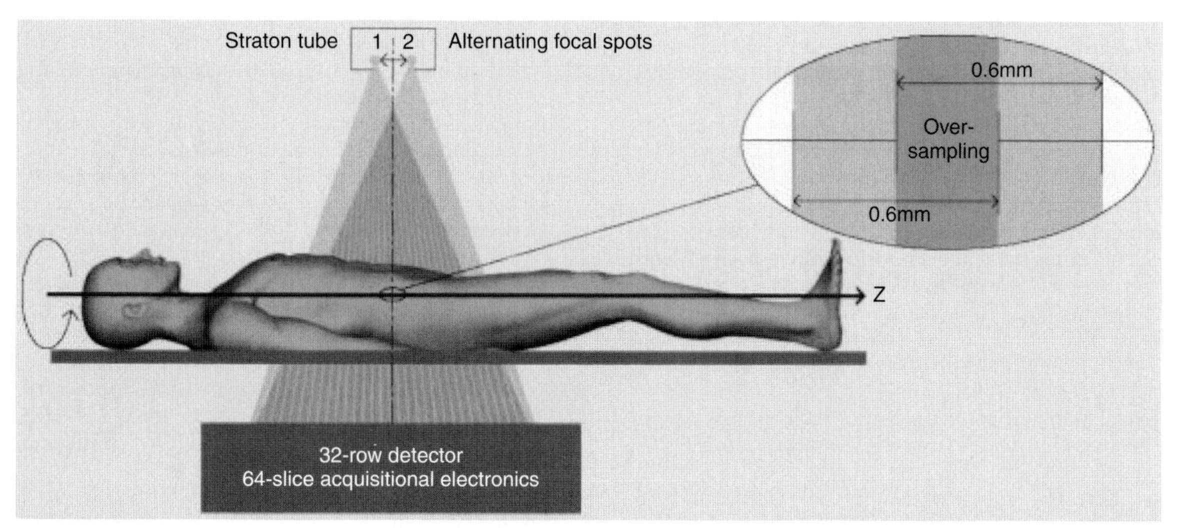

FIGURE 5-39 The *z-flying focal spot technique* (referred to as the *z-sharp technology*) provides doubling sampling, where two overlapping slices for each detector row are obtained at the same time per 360-degree rotation. (Courtesy Siemens Medical Solutions, Germany.)

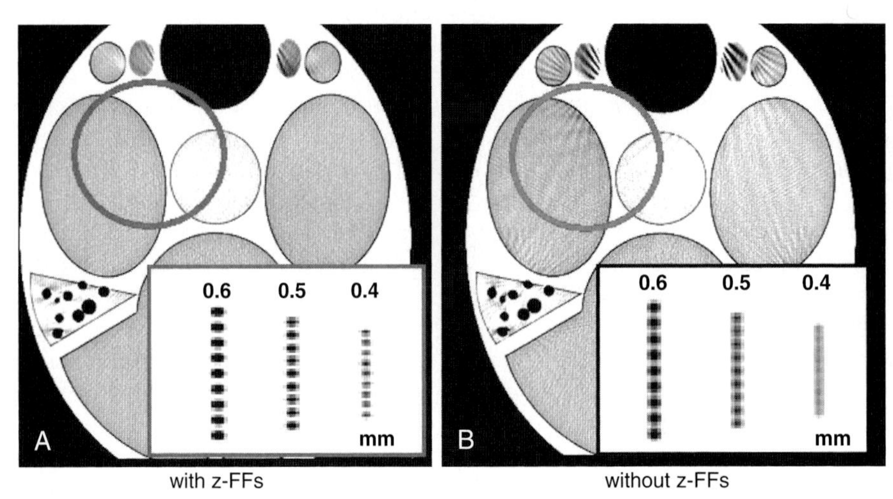

FIGURE 5-40 The results of double sampling in the z-direction by the *z-flying focal spot* (z-FFS) technique on image quality. It is clearly apparent that the image is much sharper with the z-FFS **(A)** sampling technique than without the z-FFS **(B)** sampling technique. (Courtesy Siemens Medical Solutions, Germany.)

REFERENCES

Arenson J: Data collection strategies: gantries and dectectors. In Goldman LW, Fowlkes JB, editors: *Medical CT and ultrasound: current technology and applications*, pp 329-347, College Park, Md, 1995, American Association of Physicists in Medicine.

Boyd DP, Lipton MJ: Cardiac computed tomography, *Proc IEEE* 198:198-307, 1983.

Brunnett CJ et al: *CT design considerations and specifications*, Cleveland, Ohio, 1990, Picker International.

Dalrymple NC et al: Price of isotropy in multidetector CT, *Radiographics* 27:49-62, 2007.

Douglas-Akinwande AC et al: Multichannel CT: Evaluating the spine in postoperative patients with orthopedic hardware, *Radiographics* 26:S96-S110, 2006.

Flohr TG et al: Multi-detector row CT systems and image reconstruction techniques, *Radiology* 235:756-773, 2005.

Flohr TG et al: First performance evaluation of a dual-source CT (DSCT) system, *Eur Radiol* 16:256-268, 2006.

Fox SH: CT tube technology. In Goldman LW, Fowlkes JB, editors: *Medical CT and ultrasound: current technology and applications*, pp 349-357, College Park, Md, 1995, American Association of Physicists in Medicine.

Glick SJ et al: Evaluating the impact of x-ray spectral shape on image quality in flat-panel CT breast imaging, *Med Phys* 34:5-20, 2007.

Homberg R, Koppel R: An x-ray tube assembly with rotating-anode spiral groove bearing of the second generation, *Electromedica* 66:65-66, 1997.

Hupke R et al: Low-dose CT imaging with the new UFC detector, *Electromedica* 66: 56-57, 1997.

Kalender WA: *Computed tomography: fundamentals, system technology, image quality, applications*, ed 2, Erlangen, Germany, 2005, Publicis Corporate Publishing.

Kwan ALC et al: Evaluating the spatial resolution characteristics of a cone-beam breast CT scanner, *Med Phys* 34:275-281, 2007.

McCollough CH: Principles and performance of electron beam CT. In Goldman LW, Fowlkes JB, editors: *Medical CT and ultrasound, current technology and applications*, College Park, Md, 1995, American Association of Physicists in Medicine.

McCollough CH et al: Dose performance of a 64-channel dual-source CT scanner, *Radiology* 243: 775-784, 2007.

Mori S: Personal communication, 2006.
Mori S et al: Comparison of patient doses in 256-slice CT and 16-slice CT scanners, *Br J Radiol* 79:56-61, 2006.
Parker DL, Stanley JH: Glossary. In Newton TH, Potts DG, editors: *Radiology of the skull and brain: technical aspects of computed tomography*, St Louis, 1981, Mosby.
Seeram E: *Computed tomography technology*, Philadelphia, 2001, WB Saunders.
Siemens Medical Systems: *The technology and performance of the Somatom Plus*, Iselin, NJ, 1999, Siemens.
Villafana T: Physics and instrumentation: CT and MRI. In Lee SH, Rao KCVG, editors: *Cranial computed tomography*, New York, 1987, McGraw-Hill.

Image Reconstruction

Chapter Outline

BASIC PRINCIPLES

For the computer to reconstruct an image of the patient by computed tomography (CT), the x-ray tube and detectors must rotate around the patient for at least 180 degrees. In this way, sufficient x-ray transmission values or attenuation data are collected to satisfy the image reconstruction process that builds up an image of acceptable quality. The reconstruction process is based on the use of an algorithm that uses the attenuation data measured by the detectors to systematically build up the image for viewing and interpretation. The sequence of events after the data are collected from the detectors is shown in Figure 6-1. Although the older CT scanners collected data over 180 degrees, present-day CT scanners collect more attenuation data over 360 degrees to generate better-quality images. The image reconstruction algorithms, as they are referred to, are numerous and have been developed and subsequently modified to meet the requirements of the new generation of CT scanners. Understanding these algorithms requires a basic introduction to several concepts, including the Fourier transform, convolution, and interpolation.

The purpose of this chapter is to present a brief nonmathematical description of several image reconstruction algorithms with the goal of impressing on the technologist that the problem in CT is a mathematical one and therefore mathematical solutions are needed to solve the problem. The description will begin with the algorithms used in the earlier conventional CT scanners, followed by a brief introduction to the algorithms used in single-slice spiral/helical CT (SSCT) and multislice spiral/helical CT (MSCT) scanners. The latter is described in more detail in later chapters dealing with SSCT and MSCT scanning principles.

Algorithms

The algorithm is now common in radiology because computers are used in many imaging and nonimaging applications. The word *algorithm* is derived from the name of the Persian scholar, Abu Ja'Far Mohammed ibn Mûsâ Alkowârîzmî, whose textbook on arithmetic (c. 825 CE) significantly influenced mathematics for many years (Knuth, 1977). According to Knuth, an algorithm is "a set of rules or directions for getting a specific output from a specific input. The distinguishing feature of an algorithm is that all vagueness must be eliminated; the rules must describe operations that are so simple and well defined, they can be executed by a machine. Furthermore, an algorithm must always terminate after a finite number of steps."

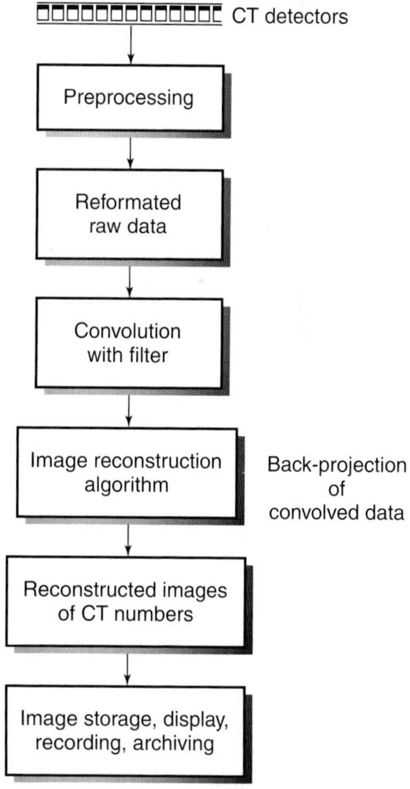

FIGURE 6-1 Sequence of events after signals leave the detectors. The image reconstruction algorithms deal with the mathematics of the CT process.

The solutions to mathematical problems in CT require image reconstruction algorithms, available as computer software to reconstruct the image.

Fourier Transform

The Fourier transform, which was developed by the mathematician Baron Jean-Baptiste-Joseph Fourier in 1807, is widely used in science and engineering. The Fourier transform is a useful analytical tool in mathematics, astronomy, chemistry, physics, medicine, and radiology. In radiology, the Fourier transform is used to reconstruct images of a patient's anatomy in CT and also in magnetic resonance imaging (MRI).

To understand the Fourier transform, Bracewell (1989) presented an analogy with the act of hearing. Incoming sound waves that enter the ear are separated into different signals and intensities. These signals arrive at the brain and are rearranged to produce a perception of the original sound. Bracewell defined the Fourier transform as "a function that describes the amplitude and phases of each sinusoid, which corresponds to a specific frequency. (Amplitude describes the height of the sinusoid; phase specifies the starting point in the sinusoid's cycle.)" In other words, the Fourier transform is a mathematical function that converts a signal in the spatial domain to a signal in the frequency domain.

The Fourier transform divides a waveform (sinusoid) into a series of sine and cosine functions of different frequencies and amplitudes. These components can then be separated. In imaging, when a beam of x rays passes through the patient, an image profile denoted by *f(x)* is obtained. This can be expressed mathematically in the form of the Fourier series as follows:

$$f(x) = a_0/2 + (a_1 \cos x + b_1 \sin x) + (a_2 \cos 2x + b_2 \sin 2x) + (a_3 \cos 3x + b_3 \sin 3x) + \ldots + (a_n \cos nx + b_n \sin nx)$$

The constants—a_0, a_1, b_1, and so on—are called *Fourier coefficients* (Gibson, 1981) and can easily be calculated. Use of these Fourier coefficients makes it possible to reconstruct an image in CT.

Convolution

Convolution is a digital image processing technique to modify images through a filter function (see Chapter 3). "The process involves multiplication of overlapping portions of the filter function and the detector response curve selectively to produce a third function which is used for image reconstruction" (Berland, 1987). (This will become clear in the discussion of the filtered back-projection algorithm.)

Interpolation

Interpolation is used in CT in the image reconstruction process and the determination of slices in spiral/helical CT imaging. Interpolation is a mathematical technique to estimate the value of a function from known values on either side of the function.

> For example, if the speed of an engine controlled by a lever increases from 40 to 50 revolutions per second when the lever is pulled down by 4 cm, one can interpolate from this information and assume that moving it 2 cm gives 45 revolutions per second. This is the simplest method of interpolation, called *linear interpolation*. If known values of one variable, Y, are plotted against the other variable, X, an estimate of an unknown value of Y can be made by drawing a straight line between the two nearest known values.
>
> The mathematical formula for linear interpolation is
>
> $$Y_3 = Y_1 + (X_3 - X_1)(Y_2 - Y_1)/(X_2 - X_1)$$
>
> where Y_3 is the unknown value of Y (at X_3) and Y_2 and Y_1 (at X_2 and X_1) are the nearest known values between which the interpolation is made (Gibson, 1981).

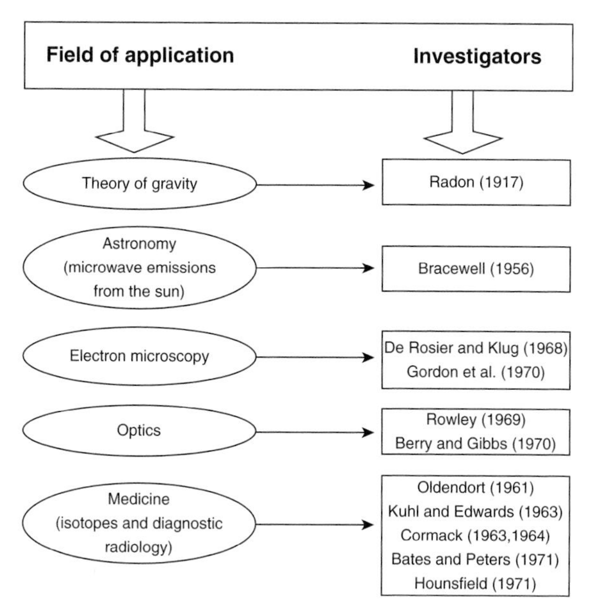

FIGURE 6-2 Fields of application and principal investigators of image reconstruction techniques.

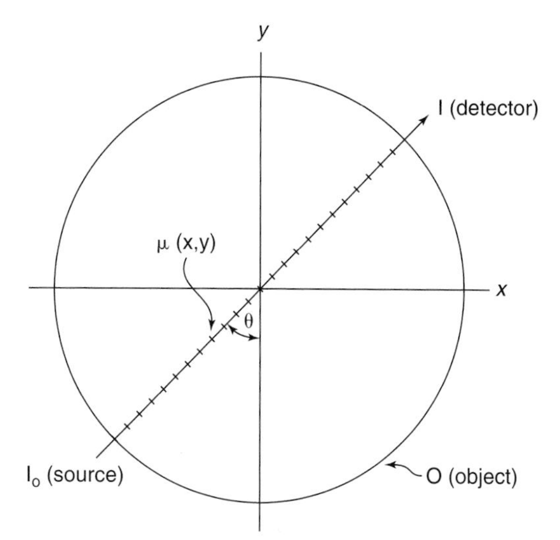

FIGURE 6-3 The total distribution of attenuation coefficients in the object O is $\mu(x,y)$. The problem in CT is to calculate $\mu(x,y)$ from a set of projections specified by the angle θ. I_0 and I represent beam intensities from the source and at the detector, respectively. (From Seeram E: *Computed tomography technology*, Philadelphia, 2001, WB Saunders.)

IMAGE RECONSTRUCTION FROM PROJECTIONS

Historical Perspective

The history of reconstruction techniques dates to 1917 when Radon developed mathematical solutions to the problem of image reconstruction from a set of its projections. He applied these techniques to gravitational problems. These techniques were later used to solve problems in astronomy and optics, but they were not applied to medicine until 1961 (Fig. 6-2).

In his initial work, Hounsfield's images were noisy as a result of his chosen reconstruction technique. Special algorithms (convolution back-projection algorithms) were soon introduced. These algorithms were developed by Ramachandran and Lakshminarayanan (1971) and later used by Shepp and Logan (1974) to improve image quality and processing time.

Problem in CT

Consider an object, O, represented by an x-y coordinate system (Fig. 6-3). The spatial distribution of all attenuation coefficients, μ, is given by $\mu(x,y)$, which varies between points in the object. Suppose a pencil beam of x rays passes through the object along a straight path *(arrow)*, and the intensity of the transmitted beam that falls on the CT detector is I. Then a projection is given by the line integral* of $\mu(x,y)$:

$$I = I_0 \exp\left[-\sum_{\text{Source}}^{\text{Detector}} \mu(x,y)\right] \quad (6\text{-}1)$$

*A *line integral* is the integral (summation of values that are infinitesimally close to each other multiplied by the infinitesimal distance separating the values) of a two-dimensional or three-dimensional object along the point of a line (Parker and Stanley, 1981).

By taking the negative logarithm, Equation 6-1 can be linearized to generate integral equations of the form

$$T_\theta(x) = \ln \frac{I}{I_0} \quad (6\text{-}2)$$

$$\ln \frac{I_0}{I} = \sum_{\text{Source}}^{\text{Detector}} \mu(x, y) \quad (6\text{-}3)$$

where $T_\theta(x)$ is the x-ray transmission at angle θ, which is a measure of the total absorption along the straight line in Figure 6-3. $T_\theta(x)$ is referred to as the *ray sum*, which is the integral of μ(x,y) along the ray.

The computational problem in CT is to find μ(x,y) from the ray sums for a sufficiently large number of beams of known locations that pass through the object, *O*. The beam geometries discussed in Chapter 5 ensure that every point in the object is scanned successively by a large set of ray sums $T_\theta(x)$.

A set of ray sums is referred to as a *projection* (Fig. 6-4), which can be generated as shown in Figure 6-4, as the x-ray tube and detector scan the object simultaneously. The ray *AA′* is equal to $x \cos \theta + y \sin \theta = d$. The projection is given by *P*(θ,d):

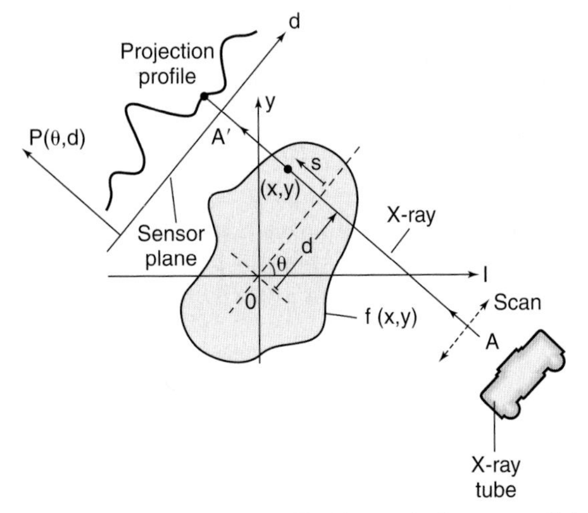

FIGURE 6-4 Projection profile obtained when a parallel beam of x rays scans the object represented by *f*(x,y). (*d* is the distance of the ray *AA′* from the origin *0*).

$$P(\theta, d) = \int_{AA'} f(x,y)ds \quad (6\text{-}4)$$

where *ds* is the differential along the path length *s*.

To understand the meaning of a projection, consider the following case in which a beam of intensity I_{in} enters an object of thickness *x:*

$$I_{in} \rightarrow \boxed{\mu} \rightarrow I_{out}$$
$$\leftarrow x \rightarrow$$

The beam is attenuated according to Lambert-Beer's law, as follows:

$$I_{out} = I_{in}e^{-\mu x} \quad (6\text{-}5)$$

Because x, I_{in}, I_{out}, and e are known, μ can be calculated:

$$\mu = \frac{1}{x} \cdot \log \frac{I_{in}}{I_{out}}$$

The following case represents the situation in the patient:

$$I_{in} \rightarrow \boxed{\mu_1 | \mu_2 | \mu_3 | \ldots\ldots | \mu_n} \rightarrow I_{out}$$

From x-ray tube $\leftarrow x_1 \rightarrow \leftarrow x_2 \rightarrow \leftarrow x_3 \rightarrow \quad \leftarrow x_n \rightarrow$ To the detector

$$I_{out} = I_{in}e^{-(\mu_1 x_1 + \mu_2 x_2 + \mu_3 x_3 + \ldots + \mu_n x_n)} \quad (6\text{-}6)$$

Because $x_1 = x_2 = x_3 \ldots = x_n$,

$$1/x \log I_{in}/I_{out} = \mu_1 + \mu_2 + \mu_3 \ldots + \mu_n \quad (6\text{-}7)$$

The problem in CT is to calculate all values for the μ terms for a large set of projections. Projections can be obtained through both parallel and fan beam geometries (Fig. 6-5). Hounsfield's original CT scanner used parallel beam projections acquired through a 180-degree rotation.

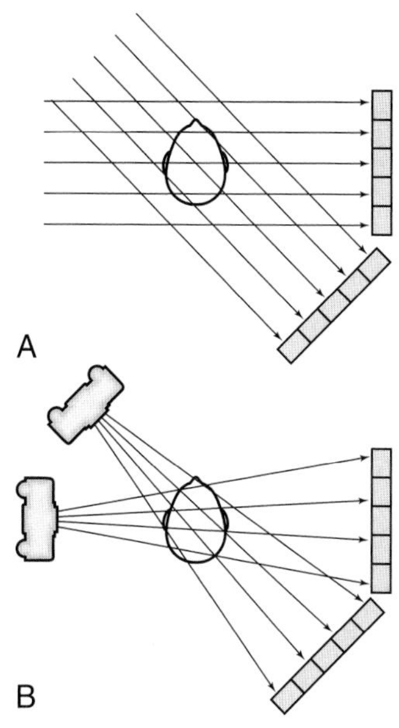

FIGURE 6-5 Beam geometries used in CT to generate projection data. **A,** Parallel beam geometry used in the first CT scanners. **B,** Fan beam geometry was introduced to acquire the projection data faster than parallel beam geometries.

RECONSTRUCTION ALGORITHMS

Image reconstruction from projections involves several algorithms to calculate all the μ terms in Equation 6-7 from a set of projection data. The algorithms applicable to CT include back-projection, iterative methods, and analytic methods.

Back-Projection

Back-projection is a simple procedure that does not require much understanding of mathematics. Back-projection, also called the "summation method" or "linear superposition method," was first used by Oldendorf (1961) and Kuhl and Edwards (1963). Back-projection can be best explained with a graphical or numerical approach.

Consider four beams of x rays that pass through an unknown object to produce four projection profiles P_1, P_2, P_3, P_4 (Fig. 6-6). The problem involves the use of these profiles to reconstruct an image of the unknown object (black dot) in the box. The projected data sets are back-projected (i.e., linearly smeared) to form the corresponding images *BP1*, *BP2*, *BP3*, and *BP4*. The reconstruction involves summing these back-projected images to form an image of the object.

The problem with the back-projection technique is that it does not produce a sharp image of the object and therefore is not used in clinical CT. The most striking artifact of back-projection is the typical star pattern that occurs because points outside a high-density object receive some of the back-projected intensity of that object (Curry et al, 1990).

Back-projection can also be explained with the following 2 × 2 matrix:

	I_0 ↓	I_0 ↓	
I_0 →	μ_1	μ_2	$x \rightarrow I_1$
I_0 →	μ_3	μ_4	$x \rightarrow I_2$
	←x→ ↓ I_3	←x→ ↓ I_4	

Four separate equations can be generated for the four unknowns, μ_1, μ_2, μ_3, and μ_4:

$$I_1 = I_0 e^{-(\mu_1+\mu_2)x}$$
$$I_2 = I_0 e^{-(\mu_3+\mu_4)x}$$
$$I_3 = I_0 e^{-(\mu_1+\mu_3)x}$$
$$I_4 = I_0 e^{-(\mu_2+\mu_4)x}$$

A computer can solve these equations very quickly.

A numerical example might help to give some insight into the calculations involved. Consider an object divided into four squares (2 × 2 matrix with four pixels), as shown on the follwing page.

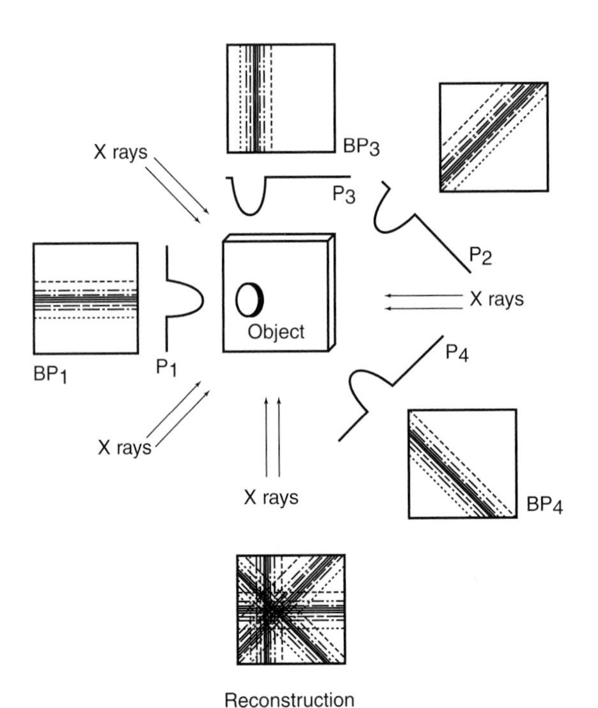

FIGURE 6-6 Graphic representation of the back-projection reconstruction technique.

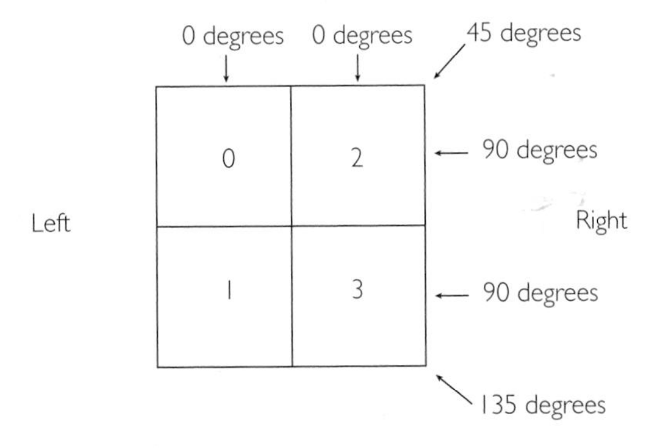

Four projections are collected at four different known locations: 0, 45, 90, and 135 degrees.

To start, data are collected for four projections: 0, 45, 90, and 135 degrees.

1. The ray sum for the 0-degree projection on the left side is 1 (0 + 1).
2. The ray sum for the 0-degree projection on the right side is 5 (2 + 3).
3. The ray sums for the 45-degree projection are 0, 3 (2 + 1), and 3.
4. The ray sum for the 90-degree projection on the upper row is 2 (2 + 0).
5. The ray sum for the 90-degree projection on the lower row is 4 (3 + 1).
6. The ray sums for the 135-degree projection are 2, 3 (3 + 0), and 1.

These projection data—1, 5, 0, 3, 3, 2, 4, 2, 3, and 1—are then used systematically as defined by the algorithm to reconstruct the original image.

1. First guess: Place the data from the 0-degree projections into the matrix to obtain the first guess:

1 (0 + 1)	5 (2 + 3)
1 (0 + 1)	5 (2 + 3)

2. Second guess: Add the data from the 45-degree projections to the value of each square in the first guess:

1 (0 + 1)	8 (5 + 3)
4 (1 + 3)	8 (5 + 3)

3. Third guess: Add the data from the 90-degree projections to the value of each square in the second guess:

3 (1 + 2)	10 (8 + 2)
8 (4 + 4)	12 (8 + 4)

4. Fourth guess: Add the data from the 135-degree projections to the value of each square in the third guess:

6 (3 + 3)	12 (10 + 2)
9 (8 + 1)	15 (12 + 3)

The next step is to obtain the original matrix, as follows:

1. Subtract a constant value 6 (obtained by summing the values in the original matrix—$0 + 1 + 2 + 3 = 6$) from each square in the fourth guess:

0 (6 − 6)	6 (12 − 6)
3 (9 − 6)	9 (15 − 6)

2. Now reduce the preceding matrix to a simple ratio. By using the obvious common divisor, 3, the following is obtained:

0 (0 / 3)	2 (6 / 3)
1 (3 / 3)	3 (9 / 3)

This is the original 2×2 matrix.

Iterative Algorithms

Another approach to image reconstruction is based on iterative techniques. "An iterative reconstruction starts with an assumption (for example, that all points in the matrix have the same value) and compares this assumption with measured values, makes corrections to bring the two into agreement, and then repeats this process over and over until the assumed and measured values are the same or within acceptable limits" (Curry et al, 1990).

Techniques include the simultaneous iterative reconstruction technique, the iterative least-squares technique, and the algebraic reconstruction technique (Brooks and Di Chiro, 1976; Gordon and Herman, 1974). These techniques differ in the application of corrections to subsequent iterations. The algebraic reconstruction technique was used by Hounsfield in the first EMI brain scanner (Hounsfield, 1972) and is detailed here.

Consider the following numeric illustration:

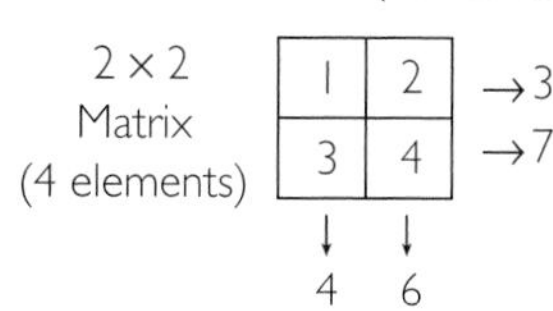

1. Initial estimate: Compute the average of four elements and assign it to each pixel, that is, $1 + 2 + 3 + 4 = 10$; $10/4 = 2.5$

New projection data sets
(horizontal ray sums)

2.5	2.5	→ 5
2.5	2.5	→ 5

2. First correction for error (original horizontal ray sums minus the new horizontal ray sums divided by 2) = (3−5)/2 and (7−5)/2 = −2/2 and 2/2 = −1.0 and 1.0:

(2.5 − 1) 1.5	(2.5 − 1) 1.5
(2.5 + 1) 3.5	(2.5 + 1) 3.5

3. Second estimate:

1.5	1.5
3.5	3.5
↓ 5	↓ 5

new projection data sets
(vertical ray sums)

4. Second correction for error (original vertical ray sums minus new vertical ray sums divided by 2) = (4−5)/2 and (6−5)/2 = −1.0/2 and +1.0/2 = −0.5 and +0.5:

(1.5 − 0.5) 1	(1.5 + 0.5) 2
(3.5 − 0.5) 3	(3.5 + 0.5) 4

The final matrix solution is thus

1	2
3	4

Today these techniques are not used in commercial scanners because of the following limitations:

1. It is difficult to obtain accurate ray sums because of quantum noise and patient motion.
2. The procedure takes too long to generate the reconstructed image because the iteration can be done only after all projection data sets have been obtained.
3. To produce a "true" image, there should be more projection data sets than pixels. Therefore diagonal projection data sets are taken to eliminate ambiguity.

Analytic Reconstruction Algorithms

Analytic reconstruction algorithms were developed to overcome the limitations of back-projection and iterative algorithms and are used in modern CT scanners. Two analytic reconstruction algorithms are the Fourier reconstruction algorithm and filtered back-projection.

Filtered Back-Projection

Filtered back-projection is also referred to as the *convolution method* (Fig. 6-7). The projection profile is filtered or convolved to remove the typical starlike blurring that is characteristic of the simple back-projection technique.

The steps in the filtered back-projection method (Fig. 6-7, *B*) are as follows:

1. All projection profiles are obtained.
2. The logarithm of the data is obtained.
3. The logarithmic values are multiplied by a digital filter, or convolution filter, to generate a set of filtered profiles.
4. The filtered profiles are then back-projected.
5. The filtered projections are summed and the negative and positive components are therefore canceled, which produces an image free of blurring.

Fourier Reconstruction

The Fourier reconstruction process is used in MRI but not in modern CT scanners because it requires more complicated mathematics than does the filtered back-projection algorithm.

A radiograph can be considered an image in the spatial domain; that is, shades of gray represent various parts of the anatomy (e.g., bone is white and air is black) in space. With the Fourier transform, this spatial domain image—the radiograph represented by the function *f(x,y)*—can be transformed into a frequency domain image represented by the function *F(u,v)*. This frequency domain image consists of a range of high to low frequencies. In addition, this image can be retransformed into a spatial domain image with the inverse Fourier transform (Fig. 6-8).

There are several advantages to this transformation process. First, the image in the frequency domain can be manipulated (e.g., edge enhancement or smoothing) by changing the amplitudes of the frequency components. Second, a computer can perform those manipulations (digital image processing). Third, frequency information can be used to measure image quality through the point spread function, line spread function, and modulation transfer function (Huang, 1999).

The Fourier slice theorem states that the Fourier transform of the projection of an object at angle θ is equal to a slice of the Fourier transform of the object along angle θ (Fig. 6-9).

The Fourier reconstruction consists of the following steps (Fig. 6-10):

1. The object to be scanned is represented by the function *f(x,y)*.
2. Projection data are obtained from the object. A projection data set for at least a 180-degree rotation is required for adequate reconstruction. These projections represent a spatial domain image.
3. Each projection is transformed into the frequency domain by the Fourier transform. This image must be converted into a clinically useful image.

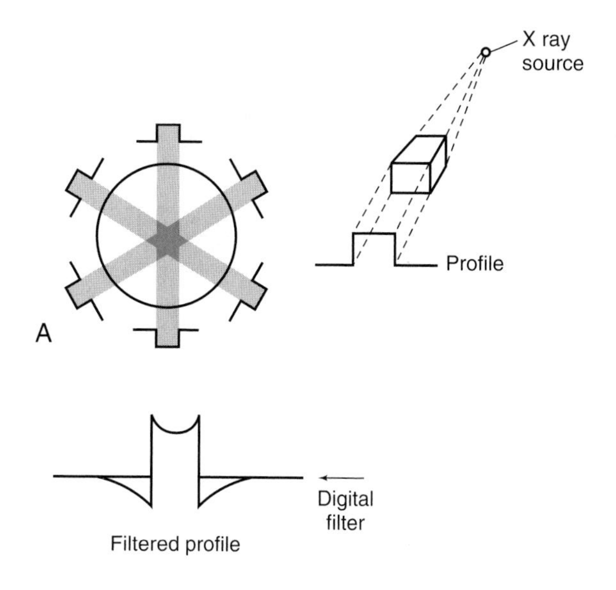

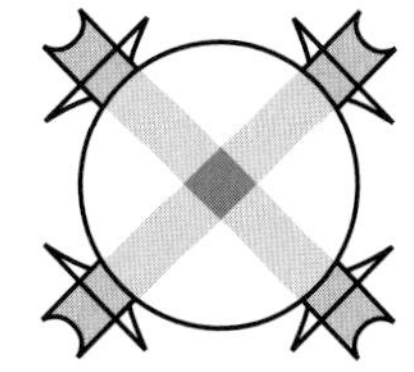

FIGURE 6-7 Back-projection and filtered back-projection techniques used in CT. **A,** Back-projection results in an unsharp image. **B,** Filtered back-projection uses a digital filter (a convolution filter) to remove this blurring, which produces a sharp image.

4. Because CT scanners use a fast Fourier transform developed specifically for digital implementation, the frequency domain image must be placed on a rectangular grid (see Fig. 6-10). This is accomplished by interpolation. The fast Fourier transform requires that the pixels in the grid array be 2, 4, 8, 16, 32, 64, 128, 256, 512, 1024, and so on.
5. Finally, the interpolated image is transformed into a spatial domain image of the object through an inverse Fourier transform operation.

The Fourier reconstruction technique does not use any filtering because interpolation produces a

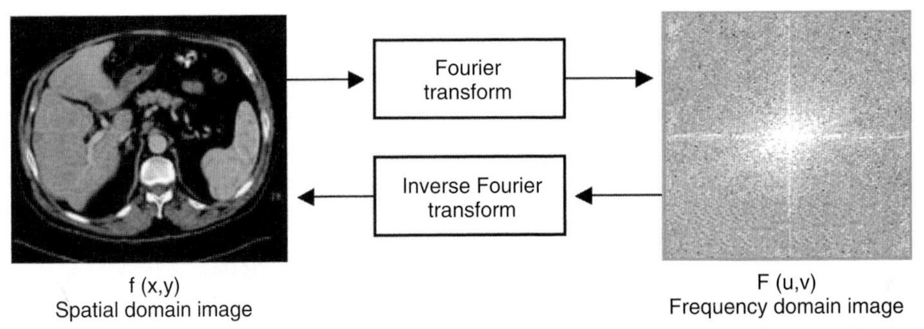

FIGURE 6-8 Radiograph of an image represented in the spatial domain by the function f(x,y). This can be transformed to an image in the frequency domain $F(u,v)$ with use of the Fourier transform. In addition, $F(u,v)$ can be retransformed into f(x,y) with use of the inverse Fourier transform.

similar result. Also, the two-dimensional (2D) interpolation process may introduce artifacts if it is not conducted accurately; therefore it is not used in CT.

TYPES OF DATA

Figure 6-11 shows the data evolution from acquisition, reconstruction, and image display. Four data types are measurement data, raw data, filtered raw data or convolved data, and image data or reconstructed data.

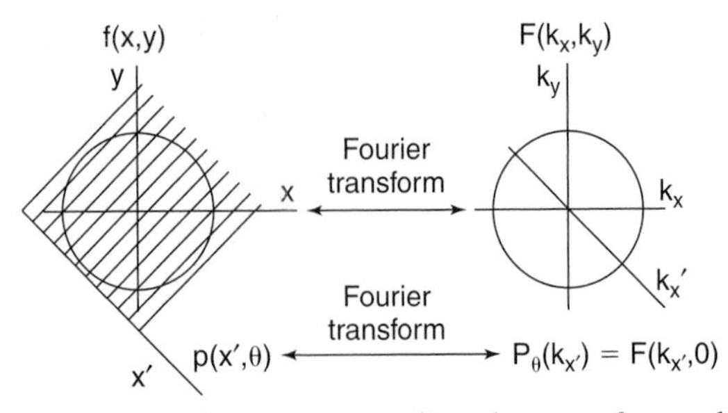

FIGURE 6-9 The projection slice theorem forms the basis of Fourier reconstruction mathematics. The Fourier transform of the projection with respect to x',$P_\theta(k_x)$ is equal to a slice of the Fourier transform $F(k_x,k_y)$ in the θ direction.

Measurement Data

Measurement data, or scan data, arise from the detectors. This data set is subject to preprocessing to correct the measurement data before the image reconstruction algorithm is applied. Such corrections are necessary because of errors in the measurement data from beam hardening, adjustments for bad detector readings, or scattered radiation. If these errors are not corrected, they will cause poor image quality and generate image artifacts.

Raw Data

Raw data are the result of preprocessed scan data and are subjected to the image reconstruction algorithm used by the scanner. These data can be stored and subsequently retrieved as needed.

Convolved Data

The image reconstruction algorithm used by current CT scanners is the filtered back-projection algorithm, which includes both filtering and back-projection. Raw data must first be filtered with a mathematical filter, or kernel. This process is also referred to as the *convolution technique*. Convolution improves image quality through the removal of blur (Fig. 6-12). Figure 6-12, *A*, shows the degree of blurring present in an image before convolution. Figure 6-12, *B*, demonstrates image sharpening after convolution. Convolution kernels can only be applied to the raw data.

Image Data

Image data, or reconstructed data, are convolved data that have been back-projected into the image matrix to create CT images displayed on a monitor. Various digital filters are available to suppress noise and improve detail (Fig. 6-13). Figure 6-13 shows the relationship between image noise and image detail of a standard algorithm, a smoothing algorithm, and an edge enhancement algorithm.

The standard algorithm is usually used before the previous algorithms, especially when a balance between image noise and image detail is mandatory. Smoothing algorithms (Fig. 6-14) reduce image noise and show good soft tissue anatomy; they are used in examinations where soft tissue discrimination is important to visualize very low contrast structures. Edge enhancement algorithms emphasize the edges of structures and improve detail but create image noise (see Fig. 6-14). They are used in examinations in which fine detail is important, such as inner ear, bone structures, thin slice, and fine pulmonary structures.

IMAGE RECONSTRUCTION IN SINGLE-SLICE SPIRAL/HELICAL CT

The image reconstruction algorithms previously described apply to single-slice conventional CT. In single-slice spiral/helical CT (SSCT), the same filtered back-projection algorithm is used with an additional consideration. Because the patient moves continuously through the gantry for a 360-degree rotation, the reconstructed image will be blurred and therefore interpolation is necessary before the filtered back-projection is used. A planar section must first be computed from the

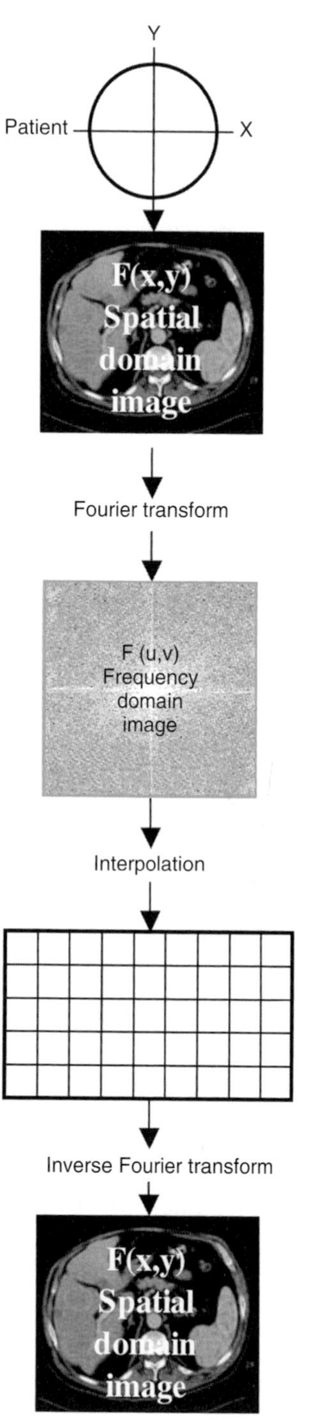

FIGURE 6-10 Steps involved in Fourier reconstruction.

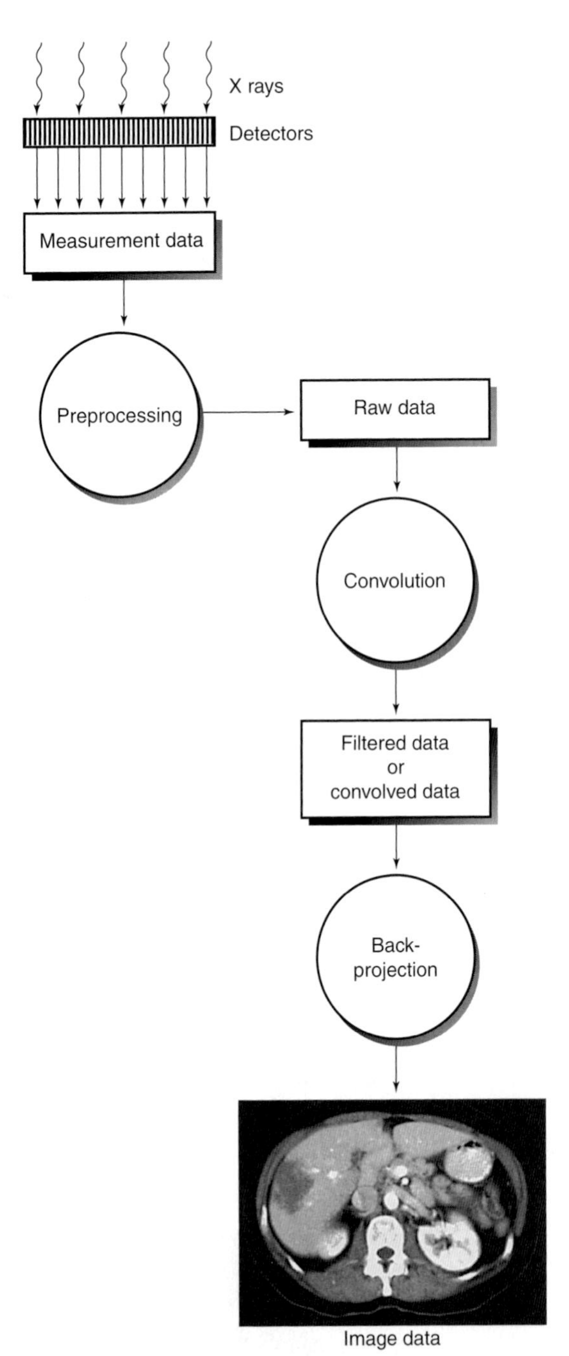

FIGURE 6-11 The evolution of data in CT, from acquisition to image display on a monitor.

volume data set by using interpolation, after which images are generated with various interpolation algorithms. A more comprehensive description of these algorithms is presented in Chapter 11.

IMAGE RECONSTRUCTION IN MULTISLICE SPIRAL/HELICAL CT

A notable difference between SSCT and multislice spiral/helical CT (MSCT) is that the latter uses multiple detector rows that cover a larger volume at an increased speed and therefore require new algorithms. In general, for CT scanners with four detector rows, MSCT algorithms have been developed to allow for the reconstruction of variable slice thicknesses and address the problems of increased volume coverage and speed of the patient table. This is made possible by spiral/helical scanning with interlaced sampling, longitudinal interpolation, and fan-beam reconstruction with the filtered back-projection algorithm. These three major steps are described further in Chapter 12.

The new generation of MSCT scanners (those with 16 and greater detector rows) require modified image reconstruction algorithms. These algorithms are very complex and beyond the scope of this textbook; however, a few foundational concepts relating to these algorithms are introduced in the next section and further elaborated in Chapter 12, which deals specifically with MSCT principles and concepts.

CONE-BEAM ALGORITHMS FOR THE NEW GENERATION OF MULTISLICE CT SCANNERS

As noted in the chapter so far, a number of image reconstruction algorithms have been developed for conventional "stop-and-go" (or "step-and-shoot")

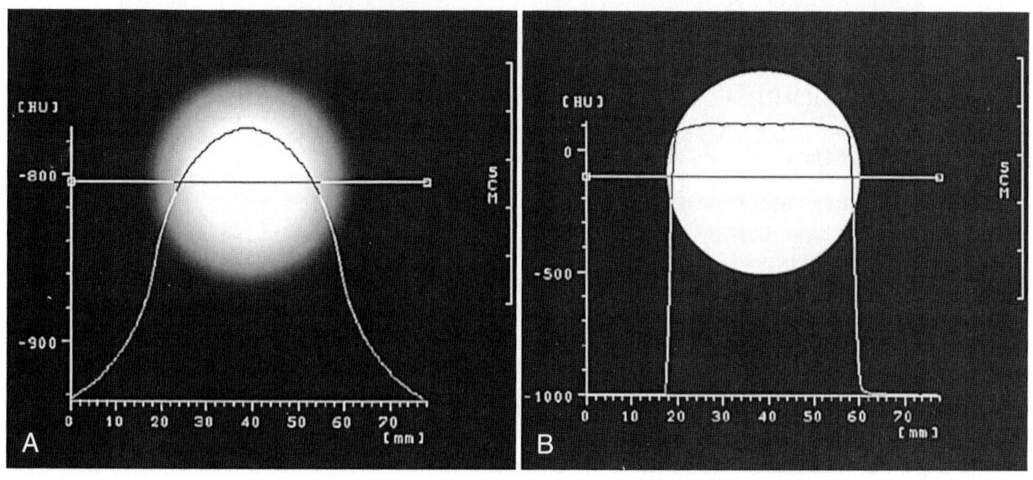

FIGURE 6-12 The effect of convolution on image quality in CT. **A,** The image is back-projected without convolution. **B,** The data set has been convolved before back-projection. (Courtesy Siemens Medical Systems, Iselin, NJ.)

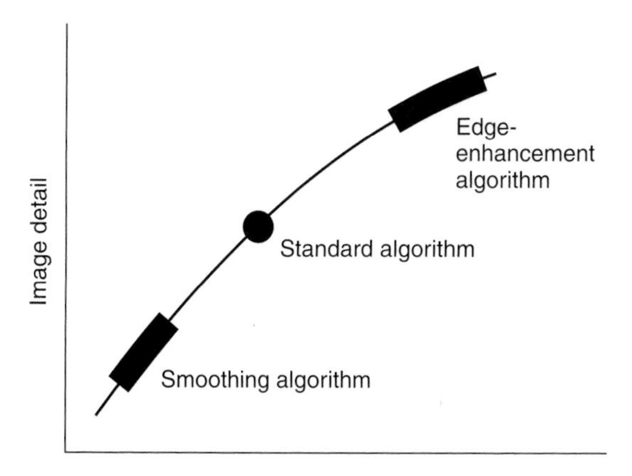

FIGURE 6-13 The relationship between image detail and image noise for three digital filters in CT. Although edge enhancement algorithms provide good detail compared with smoothing algorithms, they also result in more noise. Smoothing algorithms reduce the image noise at the expense of detail but show good soft tissue structures.

CT scanners, SSCT scanners, and MSCT scanners with four detector rows.

The types of image reconstruction algorithms and the specific beam geometries characteristic of the new CT scanners are several and are described further in Chapters 11 and 12. Although conventional CT scanners use pencil beam and small fan-beam geometries with the filtered back-projection image reconstruction algorithm, SSCT scanners use wide fan-beam geometries. The image reconstruction algorithm in this case is based on interpolation followed by filtered back-projection. MSCT scanners with four detector rows use a wider fan-beam geometry (compared with SSCT scanners), and therefore use a 2D reconstruction with interpolation and z-filtering, known as z-interpolation algorithms (Chen et al, 2003).

The algorithms for the SSCT and MSCT with four detector rows are referred to as spiral/helical fan-beam approximation algorithms (Hsieh, 2000; Hu, 1999, 2001) simply because they are based on the fan-beam geometry. According to Hein et al (2003), the fan-beam approximation algorithm "assumes that the source, detector, and slice of interest lie in the same plane, and that the projection of the slice of interest falls on a single detector row. This approximation is valid for small cone angles associated with one to four slice systems." The cone angle is associated with what has been referred to as *cone-beam geometry* (Flohr et al, 2005).

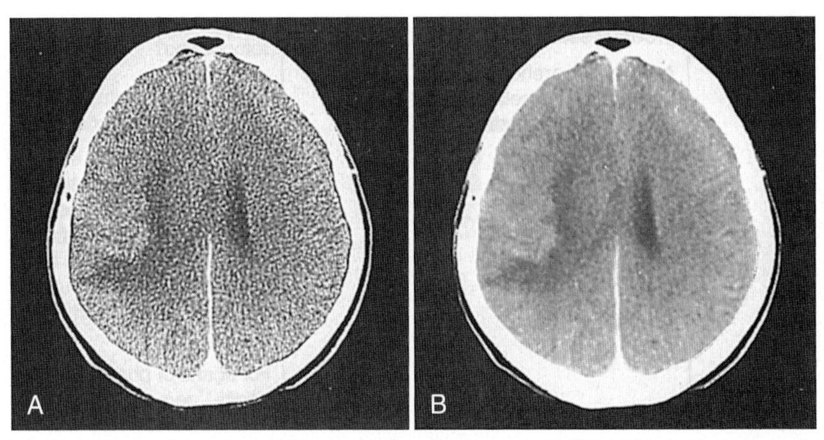

FIGURE 6-14 The effect of two digital filters on the appearance of the CT image. **A,** An edge enhancement filter is used and more image noise is apparent. **B,** A smoothing digital filter is used and results in reduced image noise and good soft tissue discrimination. (Courtesy Siemens Medical Systems, Iselin, NJ.)

Cone-Beam Geometry

For a four-detector row MSCT scanner, the beam divergence from the x-ray tube to the outer edges of the detectors increases as shown in Figure 6-15. Such a beam is called a cone beam. Within the cone beam, the rays that will be measured by the detectors are tilted at an angle relative to the central plane (plane perpendicular to the long axis of the patient, the z-axis). This angle is called the cone angle.

As the number of detector rows increases from four to 16 to 64, the cone angle becomes larger. The larger cone angles cause problems where the beam divergence along the z-axis becomes greater. This will result in the plane of interest (planar section of slice of interest) being projected onto several detector rows (Hein et al, 2003). This situation generates inconsistent data that will lead to artifacts called cone-beam artifacts, such as streaking and density changes, both of which will have a negative effect on image quality.

Cone-Beam Algorithms

Fan-beam approximation algorithms require that the data be consistent, that is, the x-ray beam from the tube to the detector, and the section being imaged must be in the same plane. This is no longer the case for large cone angles characteristic of MSCT systems with larger than four detector rows. The fan-beam approximation algorithms are not very accurate for use with the new generation of MSCT scanners, and therefore other image reconstruction algorithms are needed. These algorithms are called cone-beam algorithms, and they have been developed to eliminate the cone-beam artifacts mentioned above. One such popular algorithm is the adaptive multiple plane reconstruction algorithm (Bruening and Flohr, 2003).

Essentially, several cone-beam algorithms have become available for use with the new generation of MSCT scanners, and they basically fall into two classes; exact cone-beam algorithms and approximate cone-beam algorithms (Kalender, 2005). These algorithms are described further in the chapter dealing specifically with MSCT scanners because the terminology for these new MSCT scanners is an important requirement for understanding cone-beam algorithms.

THREE-DIMENSIONAL ALGORITHMS

The applications of three-dimensional (3D) imaging are rapidly increasing (Calhoun et al, 1999;

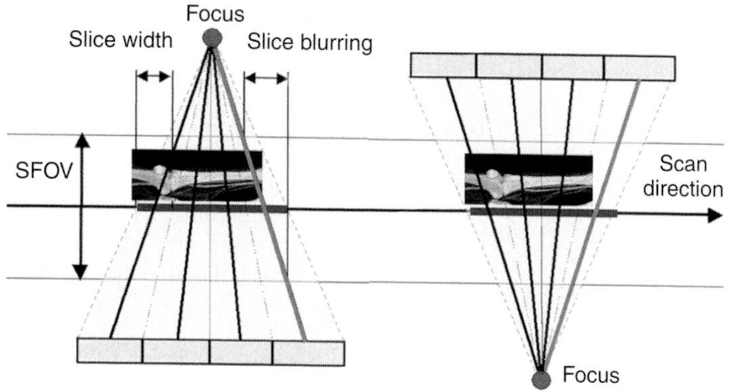

FIGURE 6-15 Diagram shows geometry of four-section CT scanner demonstrating the cone-angle problem: measurement rays are tilted by the so-called cone angle with respect to the center plane. Left and right: Two view angles from sequential scan that are shifted by 180 degrees so that positions of x-ray tube and detector are interchanged. With single-section CT, identical measurement values would be acquired. With multidetector row CT, different measurement values are acquired. *SFOV*, Scan field of view. (From Flohr TG et al: Multi-detector row CT systems and image reconstruction techniques, *Radiology* 235:756-773, 2005. Reproduced by permission of the Radiological Society of North America and the authors.)

Cody, 2002; Dalrymple et al, 2005; Fishman et al, 2006; Logan, 2001; Udupa, 1999; Udupa and Herman, 2000). 3D imaging uses 3D surface and volumetric reconstruction. The algorithms for 3D imaging are based on those used in computer graphics and visual perception science. An algorithm for surface display (Fig. 6-16) is based on at least two processes, preprocessing and display, and consists of the following operations: interpolation, segmentation, surface formation, and projection (Cody, 2002; Udupa and Herman, 2000). 3D algorithms allow the user to "interactively visualize, manipulate, and measure large 3D objects on general purpose workstations" (Dalrymple et al, 2005; Fishman et al, 2006; Udupa and Herman, 2000).

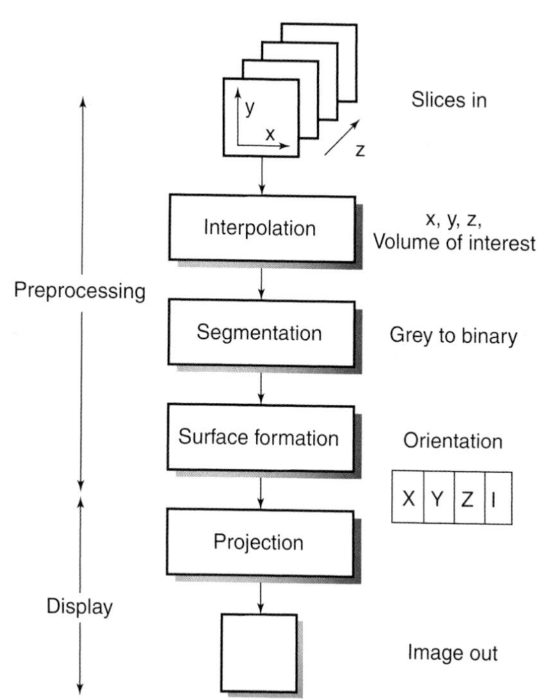

FIGURE 6-16 A generalized algorithm for surface display of three-dimensional images from a CT scanner.

REFERENCES

Berland LL: *Practical CT: technology and techniques*, New York, 1987, Raven Press.

Bracewell R: The Fourier transform, *Sci Am* 260:86-95, 1989.

Brooks RA, Di Chiro G: Principles of computer assisted tomography (CAT) in radiographic and radioisotopic imaging, *Phys Med Biol* 21:689-732, 1976.

Bruening R, Flohr T: *Protocols for multislice CT—4 and 16 row applications*, New York, 2003 Springer Verlag.

Calhoun PS et al: Three-dimensional volume rendering of spiral CT data: theory and method, *Radiographics* 19:745-764, 1999.

Chen L et al: General surface reconstruction for cone beam multislice spiral computed tomography, *Med Phys* 30:2804-2812, 2003.

Cody DD: AAPM/RSNA physics tutorial for residents: topics in CT. Image processing in CT, *Radiographics* 22:1255-1268, 2002.

Curry TS III et al: *Christensen's physics of diagnostic radiology*, ed 4, Philadelphia, 1990, Lea & Febiger.

Dalrymple NC et al: Introduction to the language of three-dimensional imaging with multidetector CT, *Radiographics* 25:1409-1428, 2005.

Fishman EK et al: Volume rendering versus maximum intensity projection in CT angiography: what works best, when, and why, *Radiographics* 26: 905-922, 2006.

Flohr TG et al: Multi-detector row CT systems and image reconstruction techniques, *Radiology* 235: 756-773, 2005.

Gibson C, editor: *The Facts on File dictionary of mathematics*, New York, 1981, Facts on File.

Gordon R, Herman GT: Three-dimensional reconstruction from projections: a review of algorithms, *Int Rev Cytol* 38:111-123, 1974.

Hein I et al: Feldkamp-based cone beam reconstruction for gantry-tilted helical multislice CT, *Med Phys* 30: 3233-3242, 2003.

Hounsfield GH: *A method of and apparatus for examination of a body by radiation such as x or gamma radiation*, London, British Patent Office, Patent No. 1283915, 1972.

Huang HK: *PACS: basic principles and applications*, New York, 1999, Wiley-Liss.

Kalender WA: *Computed tomography: fundamentals, system technology, image quality, applications*, Erlangen, 2005, GWA.

Knuth DE: Algorithms, *Sci Am* 236:63-80, 1977.

Kuhl DE, Edwards RQ: Image separation radioisotope scanning, *Radiology* 80:653-661, 1963.

Logan L: Seeing the future in three dimensions, *Radiol Technol* 15:483-487, 2001.

Oldendorf WH: Isolated flying spot detection radiodensity discontinuities displaying the internal structural pattern of a complex object, *IEEE Trans Biomed Eng BME* 8:68-72, 1961.

Parker JA: *Image reconstruction in radiology*, Boca Raton, Fla, 1991, CRC Press.

Parker DL, Stanley JH: Glossary. In Newton TH, Potts DG, editors: *Glossary Radiology of the skull and brain: technical aspects of computed tomography*, St Louis, 1981, Mosby.

Ramachandran GN, Lakshminarayanan AV: Three-dimensional reconstructions from radiographs and electron micrographs: application of convolution instead of Fourier transforms, *Proc Natl Acad Sci U S A* 68:2236-2240, 1971.

Seeram E: *Computed tomography technology*, Philadelphia, 2001, WB Saunders.

Shepp LA, Logan BF: The Fourier reconstruction of a head section, *IEEE Trans Nucl Sci* 21:21-43, 1974.

Udupa JK: Three-dimensional visualization and analysis methodologies: a current perspective, *Radiographics* 19:783-803, 1999.

Udupa JK, Herman GT: *3D imaging in medicine*, Boca Raton, 2000, CRC Press.

BIBLIOGRAPHY

Cho ZH, Ahn IS: Computer algorithms for the tomographic image reconstruction with x-ray transmission scans, *Comput Biomed Res* 8:8-25, 1975.

Fishman EK et al: Three-dimensional imaging, *Radiology* 181:321-337, 1991.

Gabor HT: *Image reconstruction from projections*, New York, 1980, Academic Press.

Kalender WA et al: Single-breath-hold spiral volumetric CT by continuous patient translation and scanner rotation, *Radiology* 173:414-419, 1989.

Strong AB et al: Applications of three-dimensional display techniques in medical imaging, *J Biomed Eng* 12: 233-238, 1990.

Chapter 7

Basic Instrumentation

Chapter Outline

CT SCANNER—BASIC EQUIPMENT CONFIGURATION

The basic equipment configuration for computed tomography (CT) is illustrated in Figure 7-1. Three major systems are the imaging system, the computer system, and the image display, recording, storage, and communication system. Figure 7-2 shows an earlier unit with the associated major system components.

The three major systems are housed in separate rooms, as follows:

1. The imaging system is located in the scanner room.
2. The computer system is located in the computer room.
3. The display, recording, and storage system is located in the operator's room.

Today, CT scanners are typically housed in similar physical spaces that contain the three system components identified in Figure 7-2.

The purpose of the imaging system is to produce x rays, shape and filter the x-ray beam to pass through only a defined cross-section of the patient, detect and measure the radiation passing through the cross-section, and convert the transmitted photons into digital information. The major components of the imaging system are the x-ray tube and generator, collimators, filter, detectors, and detector electronics. The x-ray tube and generator are responsible for x-ray production. The radiation beam that emanates from the tube is filtered through a specially designed filter that protects the patient from low-energy rays and ensures beam uniformity at the detectors. The collimators help define the slice thickness and restrict the x-ray beam to the cross-section of interest. The detectors capture the x-ray photons and convert them into

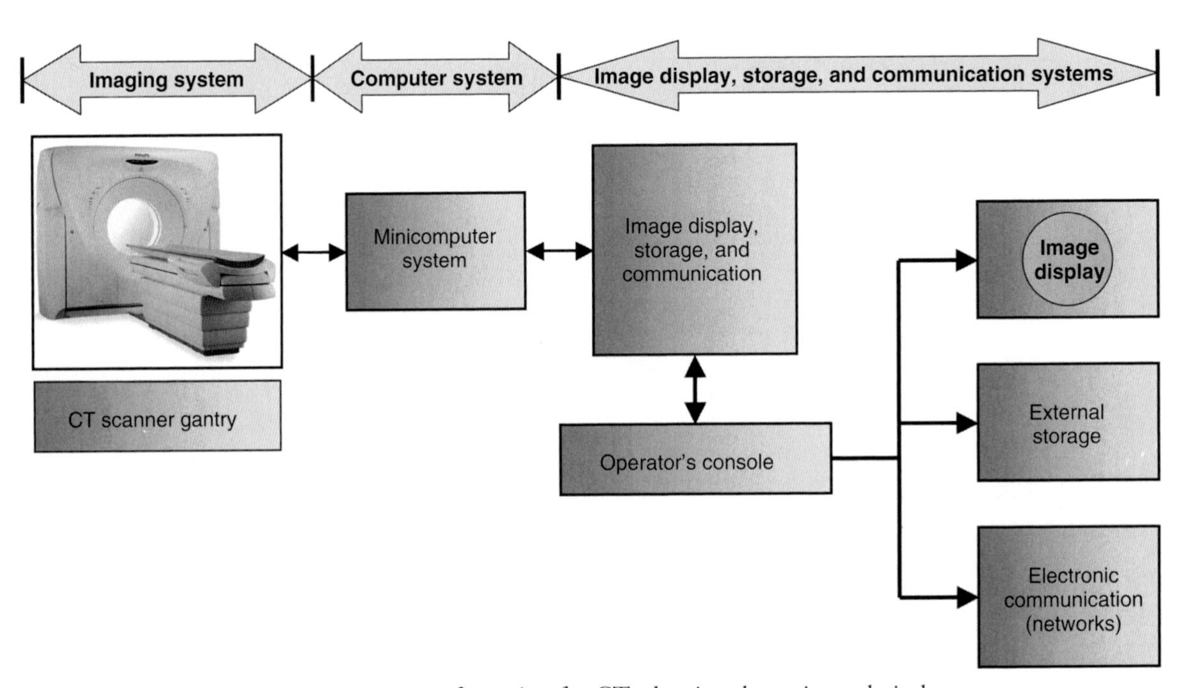

FIGURE 7-1 Basic equipment configuration for CT, showing the major technical components.

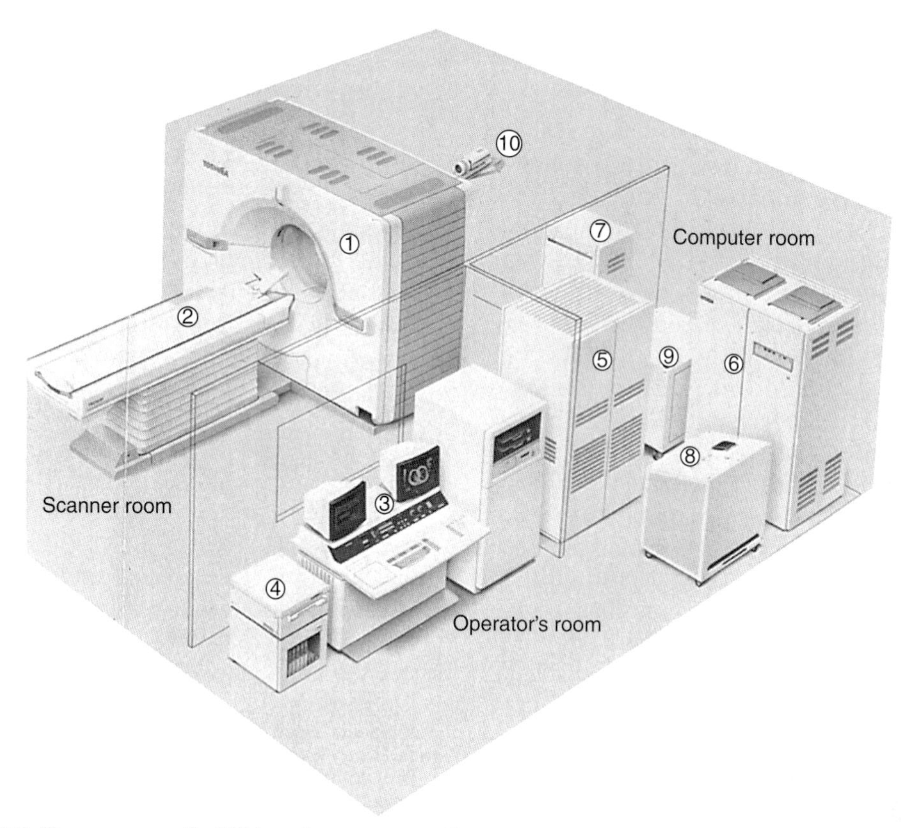

FIGURE 7-2 Components of a CT imaging system. *1*, Gantry; *2*, patient couch; *3*, integrated console; *4*, optical disk system including cassette storage; *5*, high-speed processor system; *6*, x-ray high-voltage generator; *7*, couch control unit; *8*, system transformer I; *9*, system transformer II; *10*, patient observation system. (Courtesy Toshiba America Medical Systems, Tustin, Calif.)

electrical signals (analog information); the detector electronics, or data acquisition system (DAS), converts this information into digital data.

The computer system receives the digital data from the DAS and processes it to reconstruct an image of the cross-sectional anatomy. In addition, the computer system performs image manipulation and various image processing operations such as windowing, image enhancement, image enlargement and measurements, multiplanar reconstruction, three-dimensional (3D) imaging, and quantitative measurements.

The computer system generally includes input-output devices, central processing units, array processors, interface devices, back-projector processors, storage devices, and communications hardware. The computer system also includes software that allows each hardware component to perform specific tasks. For example, the software enables scanning procedures to be created and activated from an input device and extensive image display and analysis functions such as image pan and zoom, image annotation, multiple image display, windowing, reverse video, image rotation, collage and sagittal-coronal display. Computer hardware and software are described in detail in Chapter 2.

The purpose of the image display, recording, storage, and communication system is as follows:

1. To display the output digital image from the computer in a form meaningful to the observer or diagnostician. CT images are now displayed on flat panel monitors or on cathode ray tube (CRT) monitors. These are highlighted subsequently.
2. To provide a hard copy of the image on a recording medium that provides for a permanent copy of the reconstructed image and accommodates the preference of the radiologist during diagnostic interpretation. Today, film images are no longer available and radiologists now have to make the primary diagnosis from a display monitor in the total digital imaging department.
3. To facilitate the storage and retrieval of digital data to address the problems of film storage and archiving and the environmental concerns of film manufacturing, consumption, and disposal. The filmless imaging department now stores images in the picture archiving and communication system (PACS), briefly described in Chapter 2.
4. To communicate images, diagnostic reports, and patient demographic data in an electronic communications network environment such as PACS and radiology information systems.

IMAGING SYSTEM

The imaging system comprises several components housed in the gantry that work together to acquire an image from the patient. The gantry and patient table or couch are often referred to as the *scanner* (Fig. 7-3).

Gantry

The gantry is a mounted framework that surrounds the patient in a vertical plane. It contains a rotating scan frame onto which the x-ray generator, x-ray tube, and other components are mounted.

The gantry houses imaging components (Fig. 7-4) such as the slip rings, x-ray tube, high-voltage generator, collimators, detectors, and the data acquisition system.

The x-ray tubes of slip-ring scanners require high instantaneous power and therefore have larger anodes with a typical diameter of 5 inches or more. Some CT scanners may incorporate an on-board oil-to-air heat exchanger to assist in cooling the x-ray tube during operation.

The generator in the gantry is usually a small, solid-state, high-frequency generator mounted on

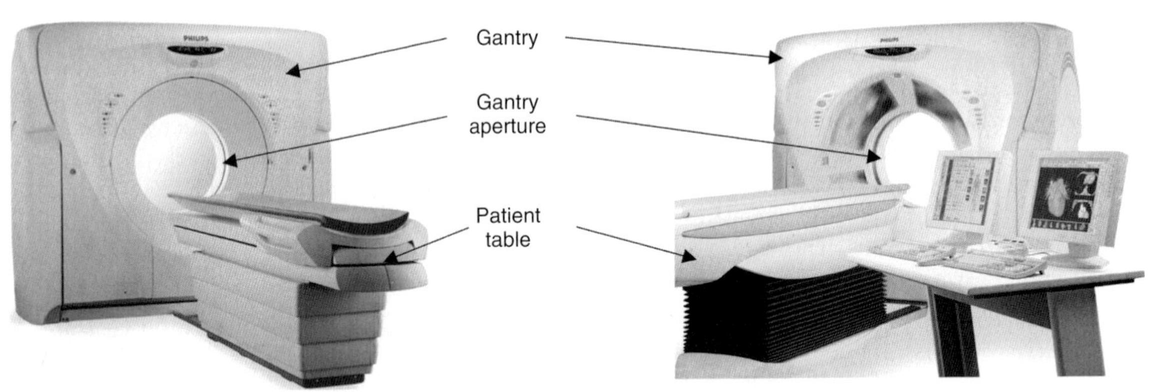

FIGURE 7-3 The external appearance of a CT scanner, showing the gantry, the gantry aperture, and the patient table. (Courtesy Philips Medical Systems.)

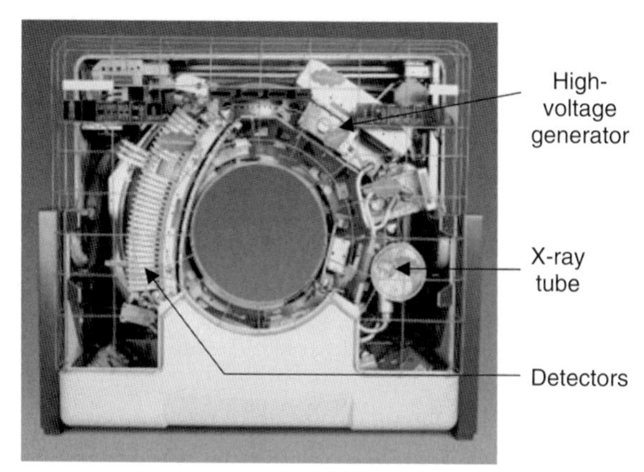

FIGURE 7-4 The gantry houses imaging components such as the x-ray tube and generator, slip rings, collimators, detectors, and detector electronics. (Courtesy Philips Medical Systems.)

the rotating scan frames. Because it is located close to the x-ray tube, only a short high-tension cable is required to couple the x-ray tube and generator. This design eliminates external x-ray control cabinets and long high-tension cables as was typical of the older CT imaging systems.

The power ratings of generators typically range from 30 to 60 kilowatts, depending on the scanner. These ratings enable a large selection of exposure techniques (values such as 80, 100, 120, 130, and 140 kilovolts and about 20 to 500 milliamperes [mA], in 1-mA increments, are not uncommon).

Gantry cooling is a prime consideration because the ambient air temperature affects several components. In the past, air conditioners were placed in the gantry. Modern cooling systems circulate ambient air from the scanner room throughout the gantry.

Two important features of the gantry are the gantry aperture and gantry tilting range. The gantry aperture is the opening in which the patient is positioned during the scanning procedure (Fig. 7-5). The technologist can approach the patient from both the front and back of the gantry. Most scanners have a 70-cm aperture that facilitates patient positioning and helps provide access to patients in emergency situations.

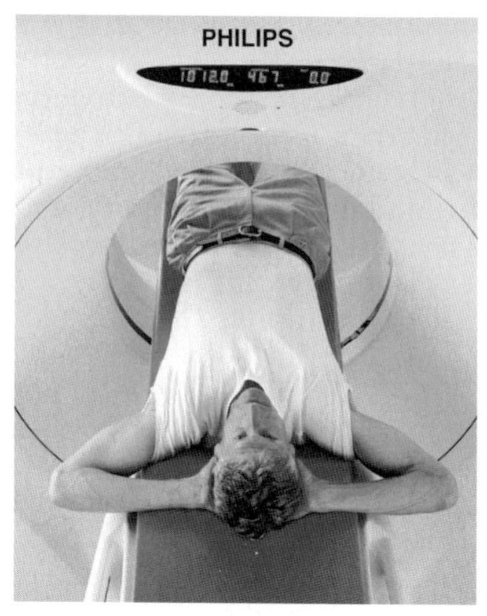

FIGURE 7-5 The gantry aperture is the opening in the gantry in which the patient is positioned for the examination. The diameter of the aperture shown is 700 mm. (Courtesy Philips Medical Systems.)

The CT gantry must be capable of tilting (Fig. 7-6) to accommodate all patients and clinical examinations. The degree of tilt varies between systems, but ±12 to ±30 degrees in 0.5-degree increments is somewhat standard. The gantry also includes a set of laser beams to aid patient positioning. Other gantry characteristics include

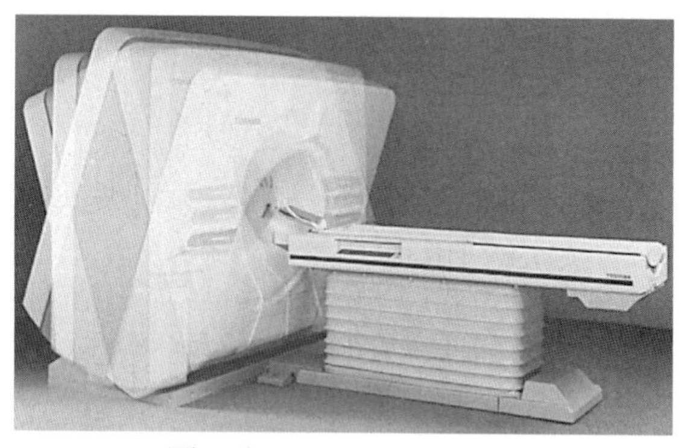

FIGURE 7-6 The tilting range of the gantry. (Courtesy Toshiba America Medical Systems, Tustin, Calif.)

scan control panels (controls gantry tilt and patient table elevation, for example), scan control box (controls emergency stop, intercom, and scan enable and pause functions, for example), slice position indicator, radiation indicator, and intercom systems with multilingual autovoice to facilitate communication with the patient in one of several languages.

Patient Table

The patient couch, or patient table, provides a platform on which the patient lies during the examination (see Fig. 7-3). The couch should be strong and rigid to support the weight of the patient. Additionally, it should provide for safety and comfort of the patient during the examination.

The couch consists of a support referred to as the *table top*, which floats and rests on a pedestal. The couch top is usually made of carbon fiber composites because they have low absorption and provide excellent vibration damping features and meet the strength requirements necessary to take images of heavy patients. The technologist has ample room between the gantry and table for patient access and positioning (Fig. 7-7). The pedestal houses the mechanical and electrical components that facilitate vertical and horizontal couch movements. The vertical movement should provide a range of heights to make it easy for patients to mount and dismount the table (Fig. 7-8). This feature is especially useful in the examination of geriatric, trauma, and pediatric patients. Horizontal or longitudinal couch movements should enable the patient to be scanned from head to thighs without repositioning (Fig. 7-9).

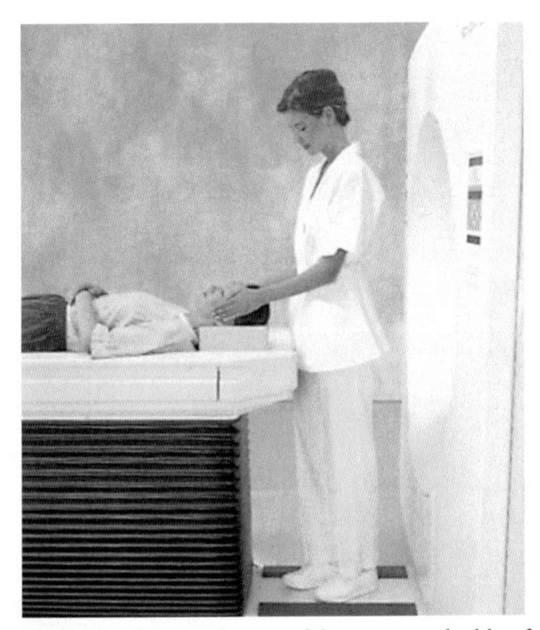

FIGURE 7-7 A design feature of the gantry and table of a CT scanner that facilitates both access to and positioning of the patient. (Courtesy Siemens Medical Solutions USA, Inc.)

Box 7-1 lists the table characteristics for one CT system.

CT COMPUTER AND IMAGE PROCESSING SYSTEM

Processing Architectures and Hardware

The computer system in CT belongs to the class of minicomputers (see Chapter 2). The two most important characteristics of the CT computer system are a large storage capacity and fast and efficient processing of various kinds of data.

Various computer architectures for CT have been developed to accommodate fast image reconstruction and other image processing functions such as image manipulation and visualization software. For example, the evolution of computer architectures for CT scanners first used pipeline processing architectures (Fig. 7-10), followed by the use of parallel and distributed processing architectures (Fig. 7-11) as the processing and clinical application tasks became more sophisticated. The basis for these architectures depends on the way that the computer assigns various tasks (e.g., preprocessing raw data, convolution, back-projection, and visualization tasks such as 3D imaging, CT

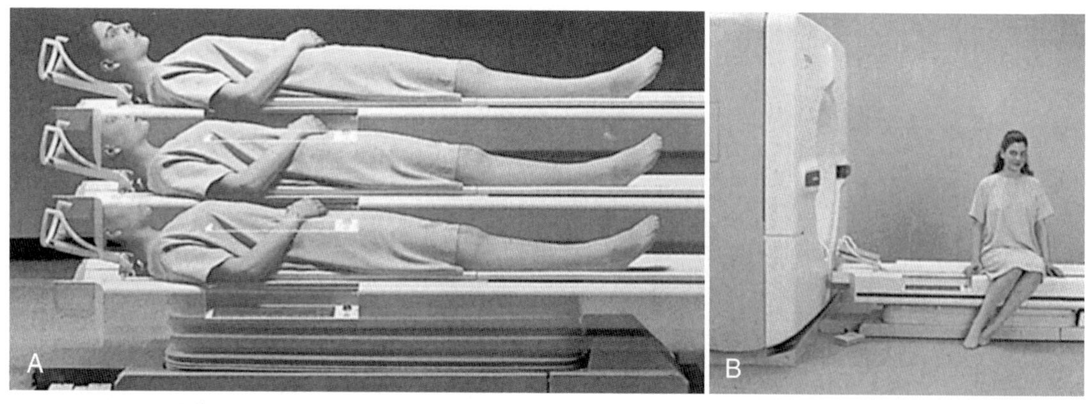

FIGURE 7-8 The vertical movement of the couch can provide a range of heights **(A)** and allow the patient to mount and dismount the table with little effort **(B).** (Courtesy Toshiba America Medical Systems, Tustin, Calif.)

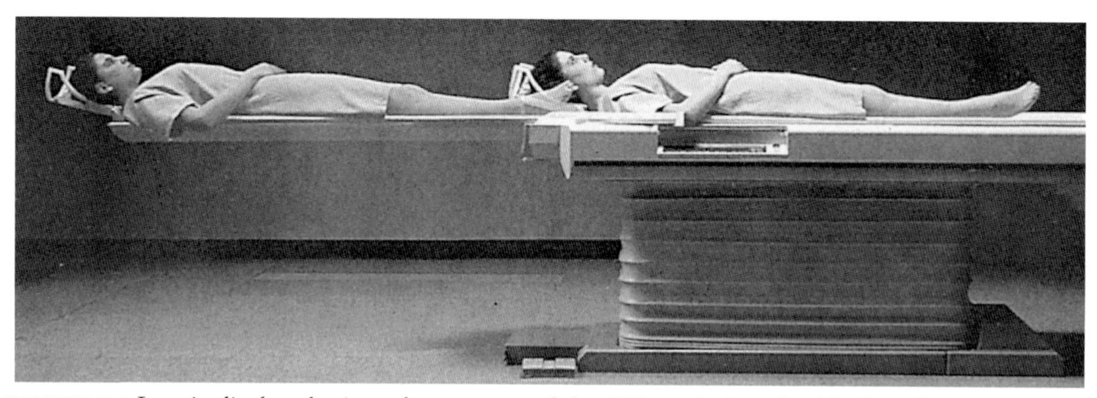

FIGURE 7-9 Longitudinal or horizontal movement of the CT couch *(top)* should allow the patient to be scanned from head to thigh without repositioning. (Courtesy Toshiba America Medical Systems, Tustin, Calif.)

Box 7-1 *Characteristics of the Brilliance Computed Tomography Scanner Table*

Longitudinal Motion
Stroke: 1900 mm
Scannable range: 1620 mm
Speed: 0.5-143 mm/second
Position accuracy: ±0.25 mm

Vertical Motion
Range: 526-1040 mm, 1.0 inch
Speed: 2.5-50 mm/second

Table Load Capacity
204 kg (450 pounds) with full accuracy

Floating Table Top
Carbon-fiber table top with foot pedal and hand control for easy positioning and quick release

Courtesy Philips Medical Systems.

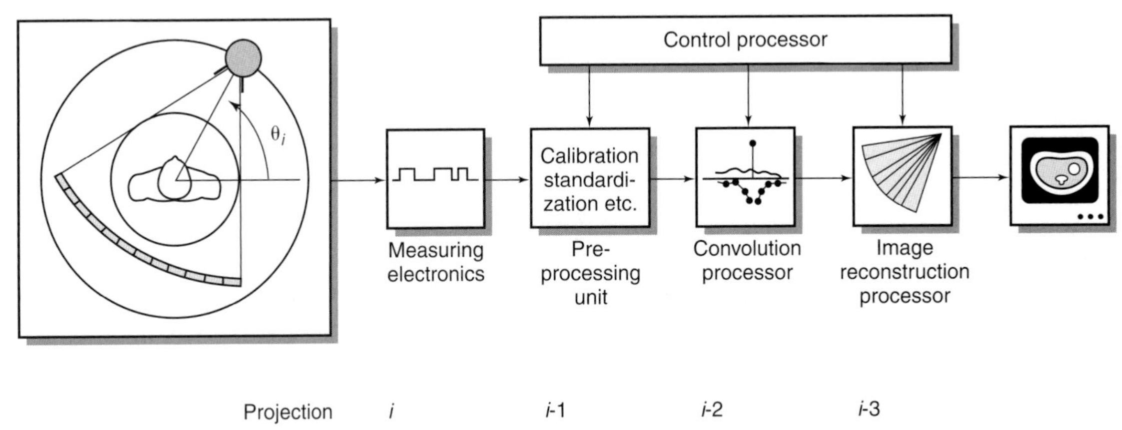

FIGURE 7-10 A historical illustration of a computer configuration of the Siemens Somatom whole-body CT scanner with pipeline processing. The reconstruction steps of preprocessing, convolution, and basic projection are assigned to separate processors. (From Dümmling K: 10 years of computed tomography: a retrospective view, *Electromedica* 52:13-28, 1984.)

angiography, and virtual reality imaging) to the numerous processors in its electronic circuits.

An important component of computer processing architectures for CT and magnetic resonance imaging is the array processor, which is a dedicated electronic circuit capable of the high-speed calculations needed in CT. Array processors feature key elements such as speed, power, flexibility, and expandability. To accommodate these elements, the array processor architecture may consist of the following:

- Multiple dedicated processors (voxel processor) and storage to accommodate high-speed data acquisition such as spiral/helical imaging and two-dimensional (2D), 3D, and four-dimensional image reconstruction, storage, display, and recording
- Dedicated image storage and independent manipulation of data including raw spiral/helical data.
- The Digital Imaging and Communications in Medicine (DICOM) network is the standard for connectivity in radiology. It allows multimodality and multivendor equipment to connect electronically to facilitate data and image communications. DICOM functionality includes, for example, Service Class User and Service Class Provider; DICOM Print; Query/Retrieve; Storage Commitment; and Modality Worklist, to mention only a few.

Scanner Control and Image Reconstruction

The operator must be able to communicate with the system to enable scanning, which may be activated through keyboard commands or a touch screen. In the case of the touch screen, the operator can select prestored protocols, modify protocol parameters, or select the sharp, smooth, or standard algorithm, depending on the CT examination. PC interfaces that use a mouse and drop-down Windows-based menus are increasingly becoming common.

Image Display and Manipulation

A wide range of image display and manipulation techniques is afforded by the CT software. Software is highlighted in a following subsection.

Operating Systems

Operating systems are programs that control the hardware components and the overall operation

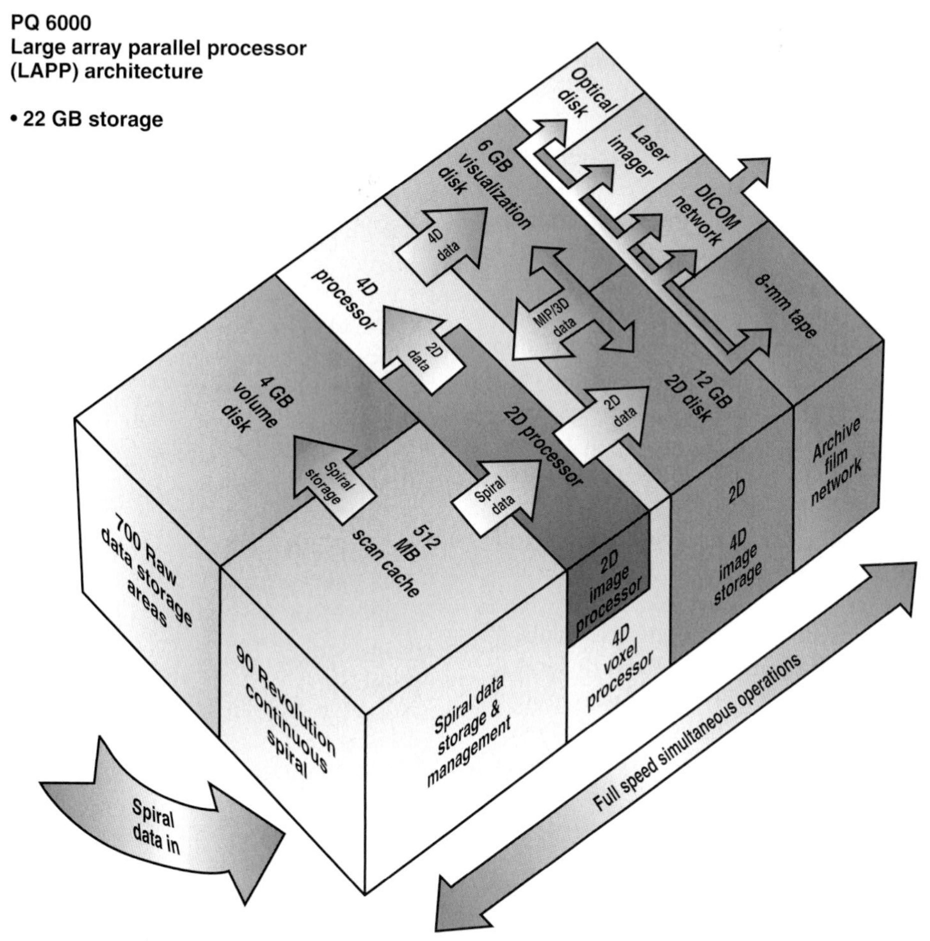

FIGURE 7-11 The Picker PQ 6000 CT Imaging System is based on a large-array parallel processor architecture. (Courtesy Picker International, Cleveland, Ohio.)

of the computer; they also enable the computer to run other programs. The operating system consists of a major program called the *supervisor*, which resides in primary memory and controls all other portions of the operating system. CT computers often use interleaved processing techniques such as multitasking, multiprocessing, and multiprogramming, which allow computers to process several programs almost simultaneously and thus increase the number of jobs the computer can handle at any given time. In addition, the system runs rapidly and efficiently. The operating system used in some CT systems is UNIX compatible and facilitates multiuser and multitasking capabilities. Microsoft Windows NT and XP operating systems have become commonplace in CT scanning.

CT Software

CT software is a special topic in itself that is beyond the scope of this book. It should be noted, however, that the software for CT has been evolving rapidly as more and more clinical applications are made possible by multislice CT scanners that can provide 16 to 64 or more slices per revolution of the tube and detectors.

CT software can be placed in one of three categories, namely, reconstruction software, preprocessing software, and image postprocessing software. Reconstruction software, which builds up the image from the raw data collected from the detectors, consists of very sophisticated algorithms with thousands of lines of coding. Preprocessing software, on the other hand, performs corrections on the data collected from the detectors before the data are sent to the reconstruction computer. Beam-hardening corrections and corrections for bad detector readings are examples of these corrections. Finally, image postprocessing software operates on reconstructed images displayed for viewing to facilitate diagnostic interpretation. For example, a list of what has been popularly referred to as visualization and analysis software is shown in Box 7-2. This software can be placed into two categories: basic and advanced image visualization and analysis tools.

Box 7-3 provides a brief description of several image visualization and analysis software tools. These include tools such as the CT viewer, multiplanar reformation (MPR), maximum or minimum intensity projection (MIP), 3D surface-shaded display reconstruction, Relate Slice, Master Cut, and custom image filters.

Finally Box 7-4 briefly describes several other tools, such as 3D small volume analysis, quantitative CT angiography (Q-CTA), combine images, and CT time lapse. Additionally, advanced clinical applications tools such as CT/MR Fusion, functional CT, brain perfusion, and virtual colonoscopy are briefly described.

Box 7-2 *Examples of Visualization and Image Analysis Software Tools from One Computed Tomography Vendor*

Volume rendering
Brain perfusion
ViewForum
Cardiac review
Cardiac CT angio
Cardiac CT LV/RV function
Calcium scoring
CT endoscopy
Real-time MPR
Dental planning
DICOM remote viewer
Image fusion
Advanced vessel analysis (AVA)
General reporting
Application reporting
Lung nodule assessment (LNA)
MasterCut
Stent planning
RelateSlice
Bone removal
Slab viewer
Combine images
CT perfusion
3D shaded surface display
Custom image filters
Maximum or Minimum Intensity Projection (MIP)
Multi-Planar Reconstruction
Q-BMAP II bone mineral analysis
Quantitative CTA (Q-CTA)
CT viewer
Rapid view remote reconstruction
3-D small volume analysis
CT time lapse
LNA reporting
Stereotaxis
Stenosis analysis
Bone mineral analysis
CT/MR Fusion
Endo 3D

Courtesy Philips Medical Systems.

IMAGE DISPLAY, STORAGE, RECORDING, AND COMMUNICATIONS

Image Display

A display device for CT is generally a black-and-white or color monitor (Fig. 7-12). These can be CRT flat display or liquid crystal display flat-panel

Box 7-3 *Brief Description of Several Image Visualization and Analysis Software Tools from One Computed Tomography Vendor*

Features

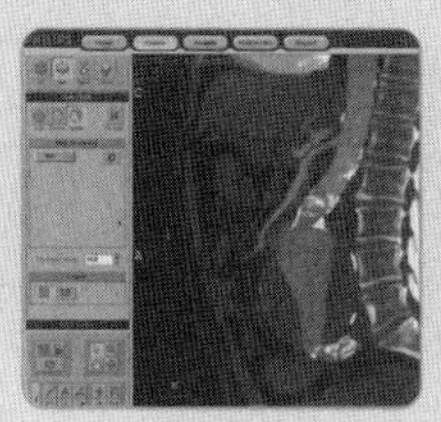

CT Viewer

A powerful and easy to use general viewing environment with Slab, Planar, Endoscopy and Volume review modes that utilize any rendering technique (Volume Rendering, Minimum & Maximum MIP; Volume Intensity Projection (VIP); and Average modes) for rapid inspection of large volume CT datasets.

- Slab inspection mode allows user to rotate around any structure such as an aneurysm, while keeping area of interest in view

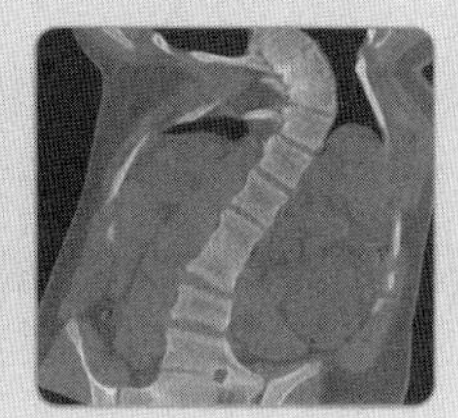

MPR- Multiplanar Reformation

Real-time reformation of axial images into any user-defined plane - coronal, sagittal or general oblique – or curved plane. Interactive and friendly user interface is provided. The user defines the number of planes, their position, orientation, thickness and spacing and the reformatted image is displayed in real-time. Zoom, pan, leaf and window are available.

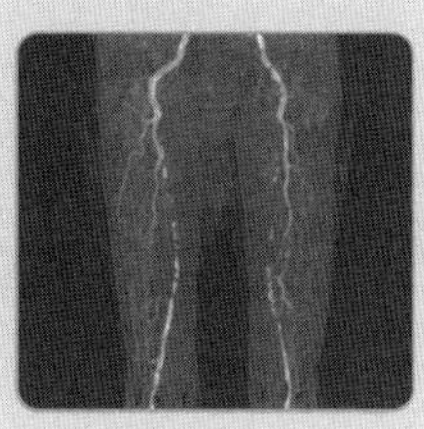

Maximum or Minimum Intensity Projection (MIP)

CT and MR Angiography Maximum Intensity Projection (MIP) images, from a volumetric set of images, can be quickly reconstructed to demonstrate enhanced vascular structures. The projection images can be interactively generated in any arbitrary viewing angle, and can be windowed, zoomed and panned.

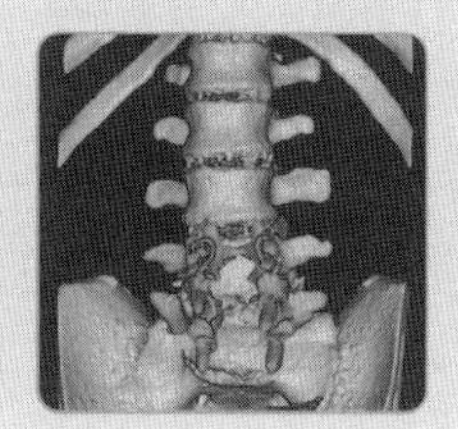

3-D SSD Reconstruction

Provides fast reconstruction of three-dimensional images of up to 15 different tissues or organs and easy to understand presentation of complex anatomy. Real-time manipulation of 3-D images includes zoom, pan, rotation around any axis, and cutting of the organs with a user-defined viewing aperture to expose underlying tissues. Making a tissue transparent enables viewing of underlying organs.

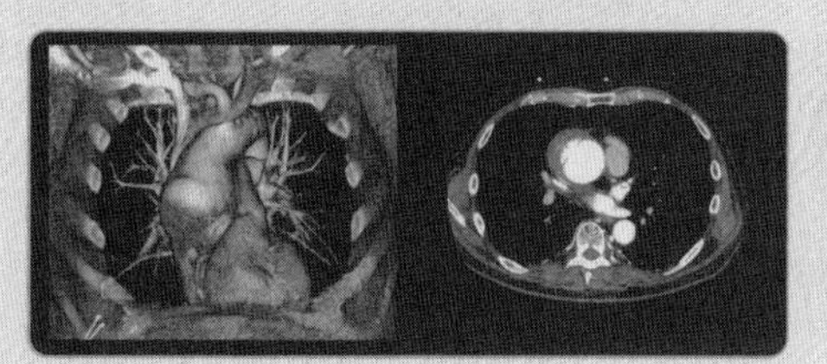

RelateSlice™

Displays corresponding 2-D axial information of areas identified on volume-rendered, MIP or virtual endoscopy images.

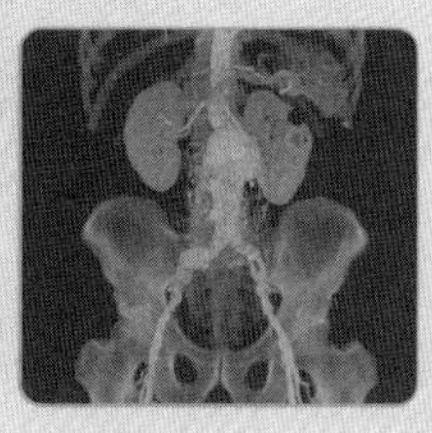

MasterCut™

Defines MPR curved cuts along vascular structures on MIP or volume-rendered images for panoramic and cross-sectional views.

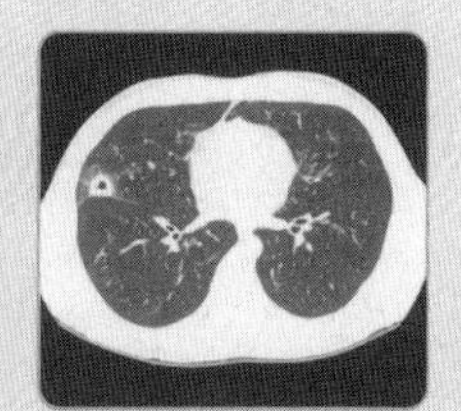

Custom Image Filters

Automated real-time image enhancement or smoothing, defined for up to three independent density ranges such as lung, soft tissue and bone.

Courtesy Philips Medical Systems.

Box 7-4 *Several Other Image Visualization and Analysis Software Tools from One Computed Tomography Vendor, Including Tools for Advanced Clinical Applications*

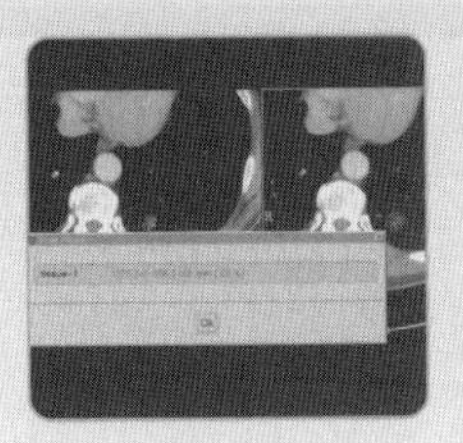

3-D Small Volume Analysis

Enables tumor or nodule characterization with respect to growth rates within the 3-D application. This tool uses automatic segmentation to help in identifying a solitary nodule or tumor (early staging of lung cancer) and measures volumetric parameters such as nodule volume, long axis, and short axis for follow-up purposes.

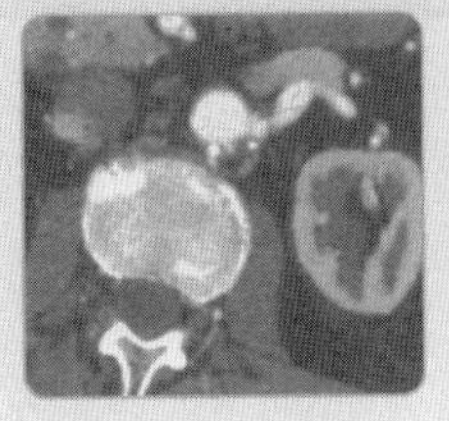

Quantitative CTA (Q-CTA)

Q-CTA is a tool kit for taking quantitative measurements of anatomic structures, including vasculature from the 2-D, 3-D or 4-D Angio volume-rendered image. This is accomplished by semi-automatically defining the dimensions of the vessel.

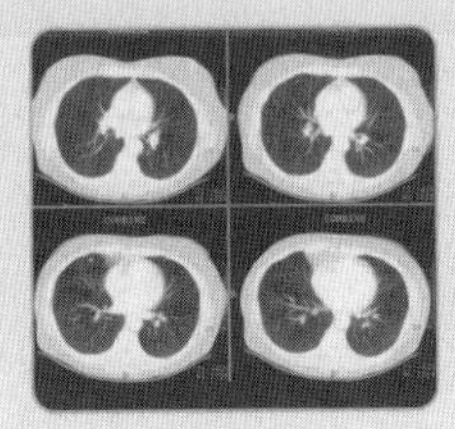

Combine Images

Post processing function enabling linear combination of axial images. Used for filming and reviewing thick slices from thin slice acquisitions, helping to manage large datasets. Does not require raw data or office processing.

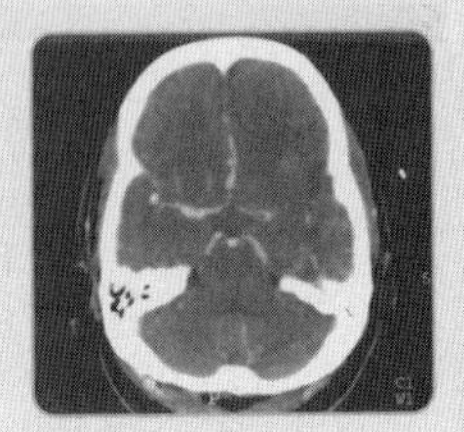

CT Time Lapse

Graphic display of CT pixel values vs. time is available for analysis of uptake and perfusion of contrast media with time.

Advanced Clinical Applications

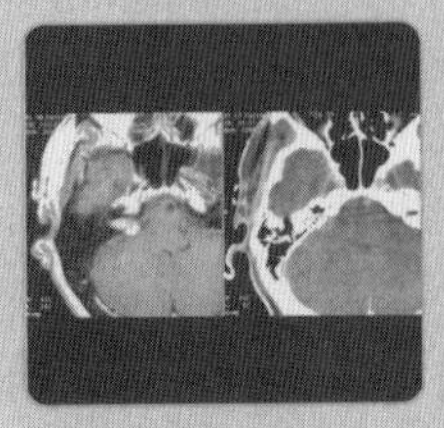

CT/MR Fusion™*

Allows for the three-dimensional coregistration of studies acquired in different modalities (CT and MR) or in the same modality at different times or with different scan conditions.

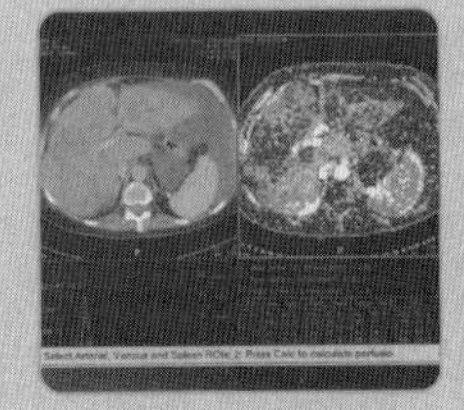

Functional CT*

Delivers whole organ liver perfusion. Capable of evaluating tumor perfusion to improve your ability to characterize known lesions. Provides both arterial and portal perfusion measurements for whole liver or single location liver studies.

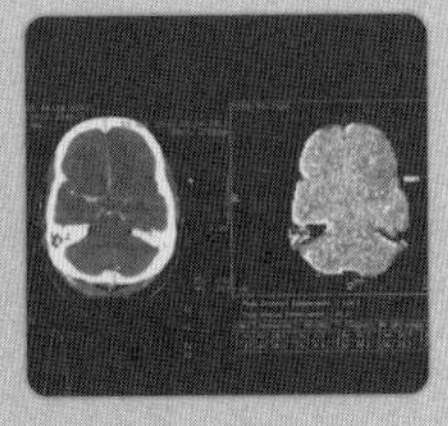

Brain Perfusion*

Brain Perfusion delivers quantifiable brain perfusion results to evaluate the acute or chronic stroke patient. This technique is further enhanced by extended coverage of 40mm and new acquisition techniques. With its powerful clinical tools, including large coverage and low dose imaging, the brain perfusion application allows users to evaluate tissue perfusion for improved characterization of known or suspected lesions.

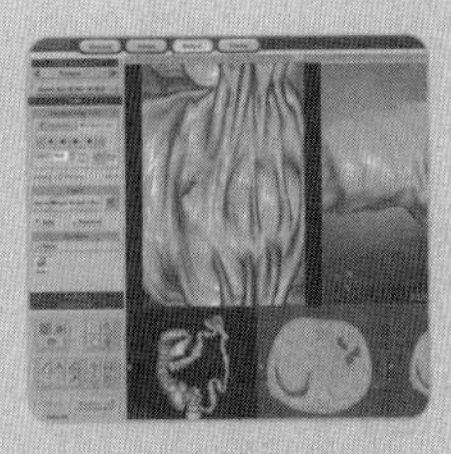

Virtual Colonoscopy*

Provides many exclusive features to improve time-to-diagnosis and significantly increase clinical confidence such as real-time Filet View mode to view 100% of colon surface and MIP colonoscopy view display for identifying contrast-enhanced lesions such as polyps, tumors, or even inflammatory disease.

Courtesy Philips Medical Systems.

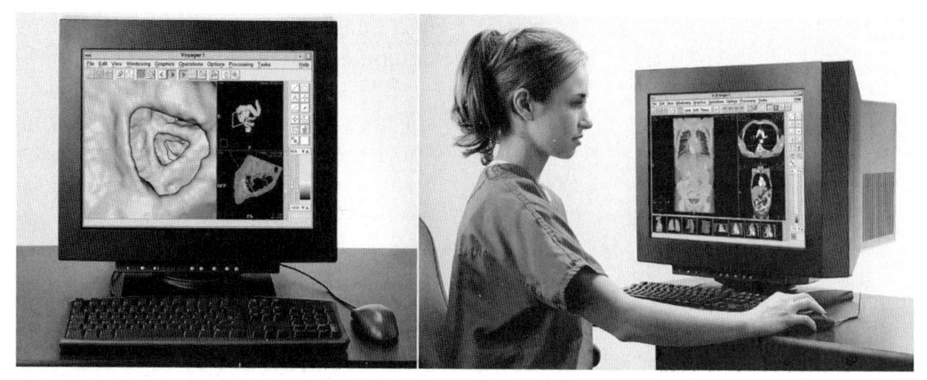

FIGURE 7-12 A typical CT workstation showing the image monitor and keyboard for image display and data entry, respectively. (Courtesy Philips Medical Systems.)

display devices. Although images are usually displayed in gray scale, nonimage data such as text fields, patient data, and option selections can be displayed in color.

The image display system includes such features as the display matrix, pixel size, bit depth, CT value scale, gray scale, image monitor and the number of lines, selectable window width and window center, single and double windows, and highlighting. CT manufacturers provide detailed specifications for each of these features.

Image Storage

Data are stored in digital form to preserve the wide dynamic range of images, including the capability for image processing and intensity transformations, and to decrease the possibility of lost records and reduce the space needed for archiving.

Digital images are stored in 2D pixel arrays; each pixel point is represented by a number of bits that determine how many gray levels can be represented by a particular pixel. CT image size varies according to the anatomy being examined. A typical CT image has a matrix size of 512 × 512 × 8 bytes (12 bits). In this case, each has a gray-level range of 512 (2^8) to 4096 (2^{12}).

A CT image of 512 × 512 × 2 bytes (16 bits) would require 0.5 megabytes (MB) of storage. If the CT examination contains about 50 images, then 25 MB of storage are needed. If 50 examinations are performed in one day, then 1.25 gigabytes (GB) of storage are needed.

Storage devices for CT include magnetic tape and disks, digital videotape, optical disks, and optical tape. It is interesting to note that the capacity of an optical disk simply is so much more than that of magnetic tapes. This is clearly illustrated in Figure 7-13 from the early days of image storage discussions. Today, compact disk (CD) writers can be used for archiving CT images as well.

The type of storage devices used, their respective storage capacities, and the typical number of images that can be stored on each device will be different depending on the manufacturer.

Laser Recording System

In the past, the requirements for hard copy recording of CT images were a major consideration during CT imaging because the images were used for diagnostic interpretation. The requirements were broad gray-scale contrast resolution to enable the perception of subtle differences in tissue contrast and high spatial resolution to detect boundaries of different tissues.

Laser image recording systems were used to meet these requirements. Although multiformat

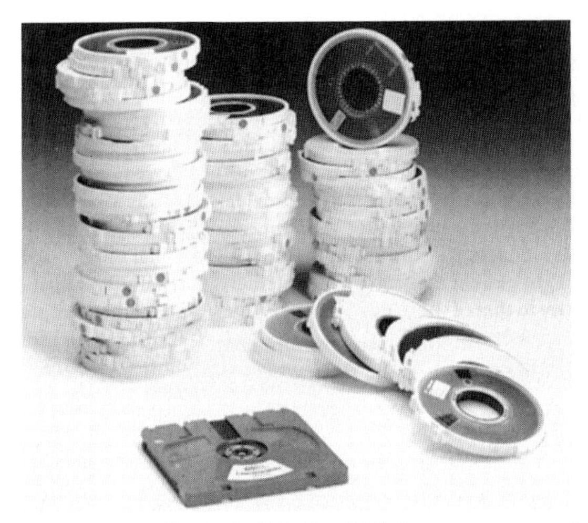

FIGURE 7-13 Optical disk for CT image storage. A single disk can hold the equivalent of 70 magnetic tapes. (From Alexander J, Krumme HJ: Somatom Plus: new perspectives in computerized tomography, *Electromedica* 56:50-56, 1988.)

video cameras were popular in the past, laser cameras, or laser imagers replaced the video camera technology.

Two types of lasers were used for film recording in CT: solid-state laser diodes and gas lasers such as helium-neon (He-Ne), helium, cadmium, argon, carbon dioxide, and nitrogen. The He-Ne laser is the simplest and most reliable gas laser. The solid-state laser typical of the 3M laser imaging systems has a wavelength of 820 nanometers (nm), but the He-Ne laser has a wavelength of 633 nm. Both systems use infrared-sensitive films (820 nm) and He-Ne laser films sensitive to the 633-nm wavelength beam.

Today laser printing on film is obsolete and is not described further in this book.

Communications

Communications refers to electronic networking or connectivity by using a local-area or wide-area network. Connectivity ensures the transfer of data and images from multivendor and multimodality equipment according to the DICOM standard.

CT scanners must support various network speeds such as 10/100/1000 megabits per second and Ethernet switching for very fast image transfer. CT scanners now feature full implementation of the DICOM communication protocol that allows connectivity to various scanners and workstations in the digital radiology department.

CT CONTROL CONSOLE

CT control consoles have evolved into what is commonly referred to as the integrated console. The multimedia concept allows the operator full control of the physical system (e.g., gantry control) and allows for real-time processing such as multiplanar reformatting, 3D manipulation, zoom, and pan. The integrated console controls the entire system and enables the operation of various functions.

Typically, an integrated console consists of the following components:

- Floating keyboard: Important components include alphanumerical and special function keys, the trackball or mouse, and window controls.
- Touch panel: The touch panel allows system parameters such as scan setup and control parameters to be actuated without typed keyboard commands.
- Window controls: Window controls include the window width and window level controls, which alter picture contrast. *Window width* refers to the range of CT numbers. *Window level* is the center of the range.
- Image display: CT images are displayed on monitors for viewing and manipulation by the operator before the final image is communicated to the PACS.
- High-capacity optical disk drive and CD writer: A 9.1-GB erasable optical disk drive is not uncommon.
- Control functions: Various automated functions such as autoarchive, autowindow, and

autovoice are featured on CT control consoles. These allow the technologist to devote more time to the scanning procedure and the needs of the patient.

OPTIONS AND ACCESSORIES FOR CT SYSTEMS

Options

A number of options, both hardware and software, are currently available for CT scanners. The hardware options, for example, may include optical disks, optical cartridge tape, remote diagnostic stations, independent workstations, and so forth.

Software options (see Box 7-4) include packages for bone mineral analysis, dynamic scan, 3D image reconstruction, volumetric MPR, evaluation of regional cerebral blood flow (xenon CT), perfusion CT, dental CT, and networking.

Accessories

Accessories support and provide excellent immobilization of the patient to enhance the overall efficiency of the CT examination. These accessories include pediatric cradles, arm and leg supports, elevated and flat head holders, table mattresses, side rails, table extenders, knee supports, head pillows with hand rests, axial and coronal head holders, and radiation therapy table tops, to mention only a few.

OTHER CONSIDERATIONS

Modular Design Concept

The modular design concept is intended to simplify the upgrading of scanners. The hardware modular design concept features detector modules, analog-to-digital conversion cards, tubes, generators and subassemblies, memory boards, array processors, back-projectors, display camera interfaces, and network interface boards. Software modules allow for the easy modification, updating, and revision of software packages to meet the demands of the clinical environment.

Operating Modes of the Scanner

A modern CT scanner can operate in a variety of modes to meet the requirements of various clinical examinations. Typical operating modes include routine scan mode and rapid or dynamic scan mode. Various spiral/helical scan modes such as overlap scan, skip scan, and tilt scan are available to suit the needs of the examination (Fig. 7-14).

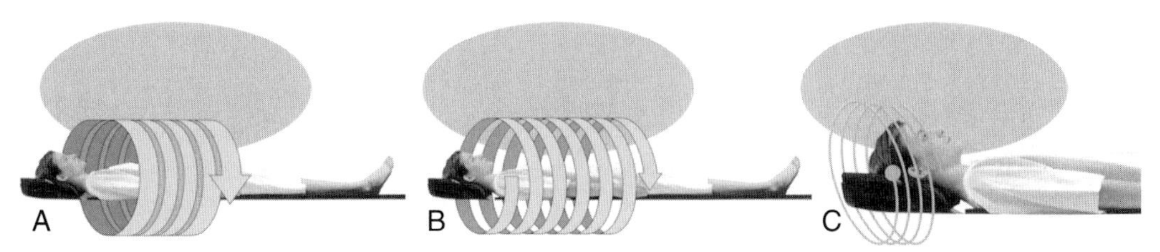

FIGURE 7-14 Three scan modes for spiral/helical CT scanning. Each scan mode includes Overlap Scan, which is useful to make high-quality 3D images. Skip Scan can be used to scan a wide area in a short amount of time. Tilt Scan is used with various gantry tilts. **A,** High-quality 3D images: overlap scan. **B,** Short time/wide range scan: skip scan. **C,** According to head OM line: tilt scan. (Courtesy Shimadzu Medical Systems, Seattle, Wash.)

Room Layout for CT Equipment

The room layout for CT scanners varies among institutions and depends on the particular type of scanner. A typical room layout (Fig. 7-15) includes at least three sections or rooms to house different components of the scanner, as follows:

1. The scanning room houses the gantry and patient couch. This room should be large enough to accommodate gurneys and emergency equipment.
2. The computer room generally houses the host computer and other peripheral computing equipment.
3. The control room houses the control console and film recording equipment.

Equipment Specifications

The acquisition of a CT scanner is an interesting experience, and the CT technologist should take advantage of the opportunity to participate in such an activity. The CT department or purchasing committee generally informs the vendor of the necessary equipment specifications. In addition, vendors will have equipment specifications available for review.

In general, several major technical specifications and features of a CT scanner to be considered are as follows:

1. The x-ray generator: both physical and operating parameters
2. The x-ray tube and detectors: heat storage capacity and cooling rates of the tube; the

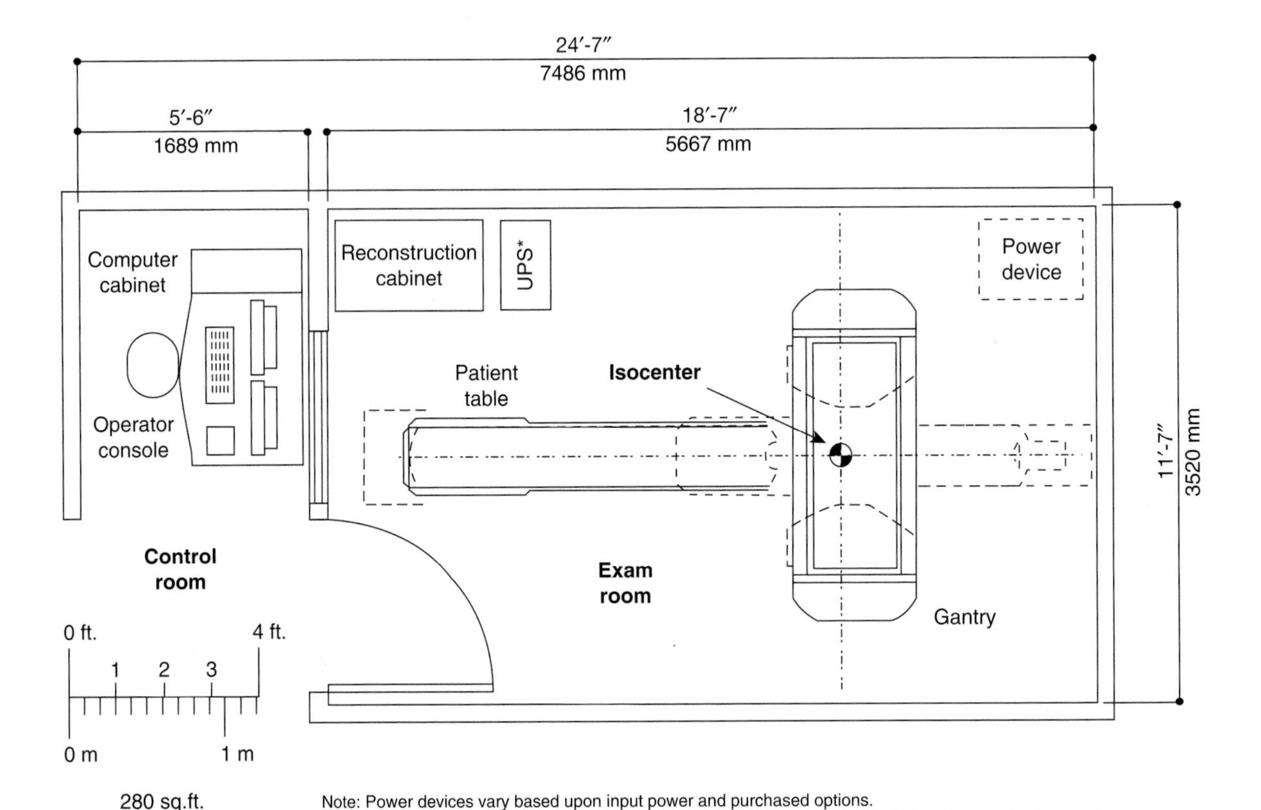

FIGURE 7-15 Typical room layout for CT scanning equipment. (Courtesy Philips Medical Systems.)

type, quantum detection, and conversion efficiencies of detectors
3. Scanning gantry: aperture size, tilting range, and laser positioning aids and controls
4. Patient couch: movement characteristics and strength of the couch top
5. Operator's console: characteristics of the display monitor, keyboard, and touch panel control; general ergonomics and storage considerations
6. Physician's console: hardware and software
7. Computer hardware: the main central processing unit, operating system, and storage device type and capacity
8. Computer software: image reconstruction, display, visualization, and analysis packages
9. Workstations: both hardware and software
10. Accessories
11. Quality control equipment; includes phantoms for quality control and radiation dose measurements

BIBLIOGRAPHY

Alexander J, Krumme HJ: Somatom Plus: new perspectives in computerized tomography,. *Electromedica* 56: 50-56, 1988.

Fugita K et al: Advanced computer architecture for CT, *Radiology* S:63, 1992.

Philips Medical Systems: *Brilliance™ CT-64 channel configuration*, The Netherlands, 2007, Global Information Center.

Siemens Medical Solutions: *CT SOMATOM Sensation, SOMATOM Emotion, and SOMATOM Spirit—product data*, Malvern, Pa, 2007, Siemens Medical Solutions USA.

Toshiba America Medical Systems: *Aquilion 64 CT scanner*, Tustin, Calif, 2007, Toshiba America Medical Systems.

Image Postprocessing and Visualization Tools

Chapter Outline

Image postprocessing and visualization techniques belong to the domain of digital image processing (see Chapter 3). Image postprocessing has become an integral part of the operation of the computed tomography (CT) department. Today, more and more techniques are available for modifying the original reconstructed image displayed for viewing by the technologist and interpretation by the radiologist.

The purpose of this chapter is to elaborate on several image postprocessing techniques now used routinely in CT, the purpose of which is to allow the observer to manipulate or change the image quality characteristics such as brightness and contrast, for example, to enhance diagnostic interpretation of images. In this respect, the operations are essentially postprocessing digital operations intended to display the acquired axial images in other two-dimensional (2D) formats, such as, for example, sagittal, coronal, and oblique images, and three-dimensional (3D) image displays such as surface-shaded displays (SSD), projection displays (maximum and minimum intensity projections), and volume-rendered (VR) images. Additionally, 3D rendered images can be used to generate another technical application referred to as virtual reality imaging (Kalender, 2005). This chapter also includes an overview of basic and advanced visualization tools integrated into the CT imaging system.

IMAGE POSTPROCESSING

Definition

Image postprocessing refers to the use of various techniques (image processing software or algorithms) that modify the reconstructed images displayed for viewing and interpretation by an observer. The observer uses these operations or techniques to change the overall appearance of the displayed image to enhance the visualization of structures in the image. For example, observers can change other image characteristics such as brightness and contrast to suit their viewing needs. One very important point to note about these postprocessing operations is that they do not produce more information content. As a result, "the information content in the processed image is always less than or equal to that in the original image" (Glen et al, 1981).

Techniques

Image processing operations such as point, local, and global processing operations or techniques are described in Chapter 3. Essentially, these operations fall into two categories: linear and nonlinear. Linear techniques include such processes as image smoothing and image enhancement, for example; nonlinear techniques are concerned with gray-scale manipulation, in which the gray scale of the image can be modified with different algorithms. This chapter discusses nonlinear techniques.

One such common algorithm of interest used in CT routinely by technologists and radiologists alike is based on a point processing technique (see Chapter 3) referred to as *gray-level mapping*. Gray-level mapping is also popularly referred to as "contrast enhancement," "contrast stretching," "histogram modification," "histogram stretching," or "windowing." Because windowing is the most common image-processing technique used in CT, it is described in detail in the next section. Furthermore, image postprocessing will use the axial image data set stored in the computer to produce new 2D and 3D images. As mentioned above, although the 2D images are reformatted images such as coronal, sagittal, and oblique images, 3D images are displayed as maximum and minimum intensity images, SSD images, and VR images. 3D imaging will be described in detail in Chapter 14.

WINDOWING

The CT image is reconstructed from projection data collected from the patient. The result of

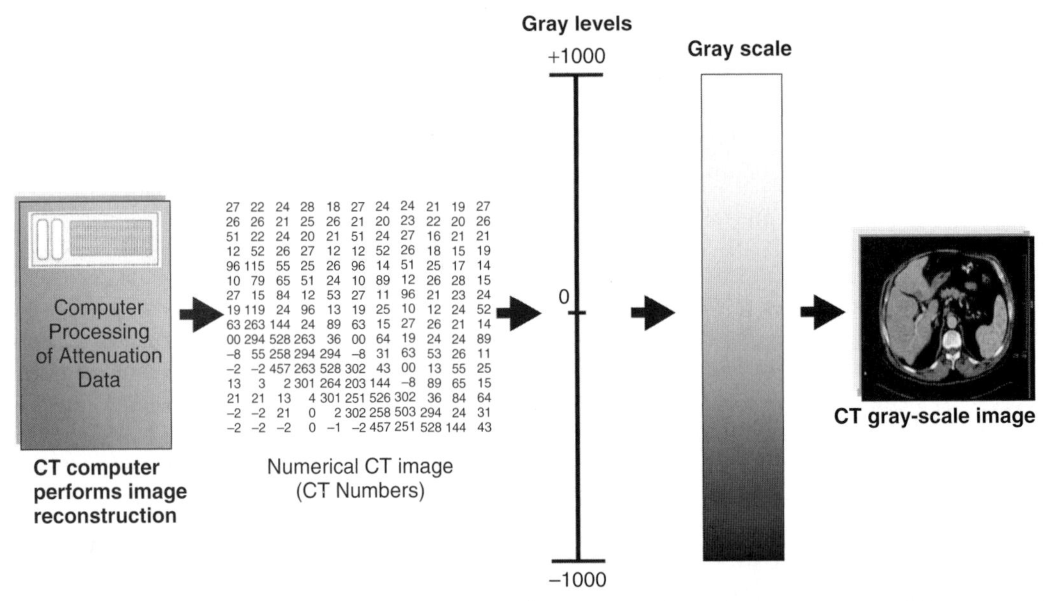

FIGURE 8-1 The computer processes attenuation data collected from the patient to generate CT numbers. These numbers represent a numerical image (digital image) that is subsequently converted into a gray-scale image that is displayed for viewing by an observer. This image is now subject to digital image postprocessing, such as windowing, for example.

image reconstruction is a numerical image. This image must be changed into a gray-scale image for observation by technologists and radiologists. The process is outlined graphically in Figure 8-1. The numerical image consists of a range of CT numbers (gray levels), and these numbers are converted into gray scale, with the lower numbers being assigned black and the higher numbers being assigned white (see Chapter 4).

Windowing refers to a method by which the CT image gray scale can be manipulated with the CT numbers of the image (Seeram, 2005; Seeram and Seeram, 2008). The operator (or observer) can alter these numbers to optimize the demonstration of the different structures as shown in Figure 8-2. Through the manipulation of CT numbers of the various tissues, the picture can be changed to show soft tissues and dense structures such as bone.

The picture contrast and brightness are easily changed with two control mechanisms: the window width and the window level, respectively.

Window Width and Window Level

Definitions

By definition, the range of the CT numbers in the image is referred to as the *window width* (WW). It determines the maximum number of shades of gray that can be displayed on the CT monitor. The *window level* (WL) is defined as the center or midpoint of the range of CT numbers (Fig. 8-3). In the case of Figure 8-3, the WW is 2000 (1000 + 1000), the WL is 0, and the number of shades of gray assigned is 256.

When the WW and WL are changed, the image contrast and brightness can be optimized to suit the viewing needs of the observer. "Specifically, a large window width indicates that there is a relatively long gray scale or a large block of CT numbers that will be assigned some value of gray. Thus, the transition zone between the lower CT numbers portrayed as black and the higher

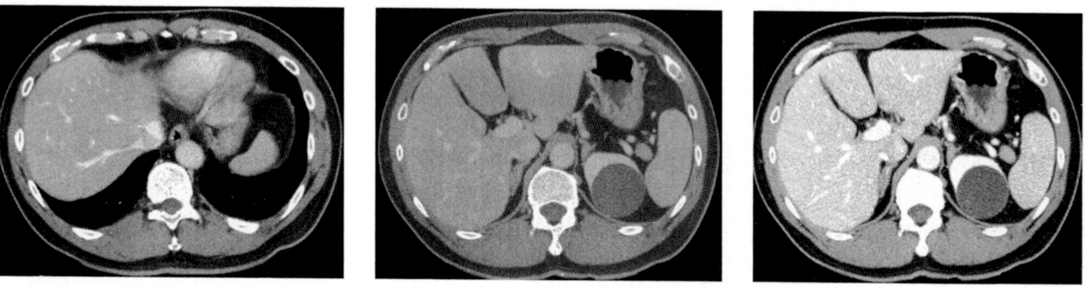

FIGURE 8-2 Different structures of the abdomen can be optimized for viewing through windowing, a digital image postprocessing technique that can be used to manipulate the gray-scale image by using the CT numbers that comprise the image.

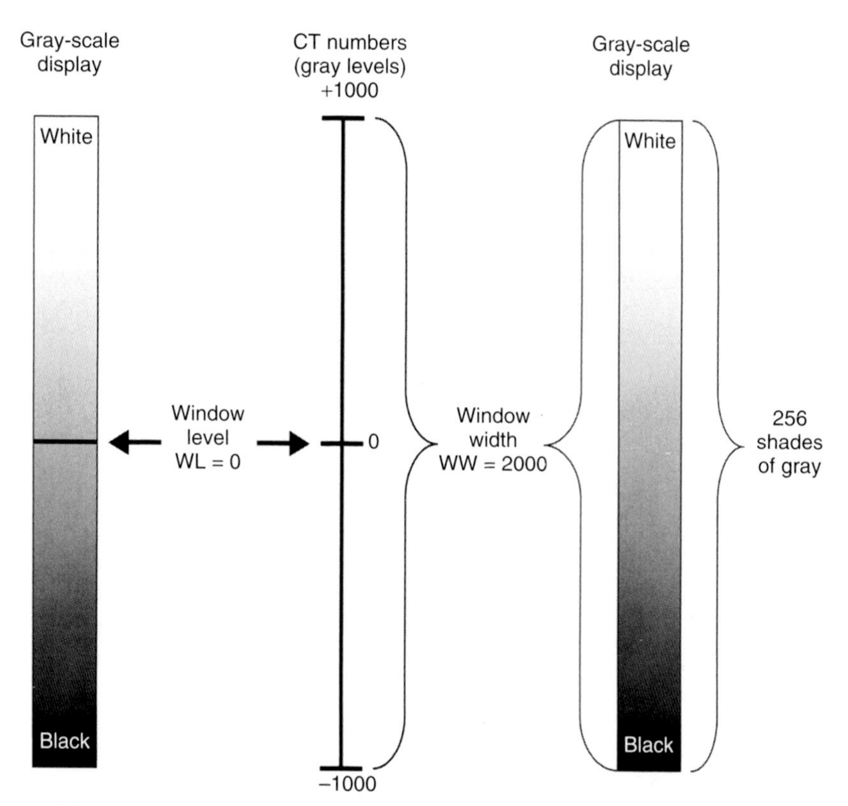

FIGURE 8-3 The concepts of WW and WL and corresponding gray levels and gray scale. While the WW is the range of the CT numbers that make up an image, the WL is defined as the center of the range of numbers.

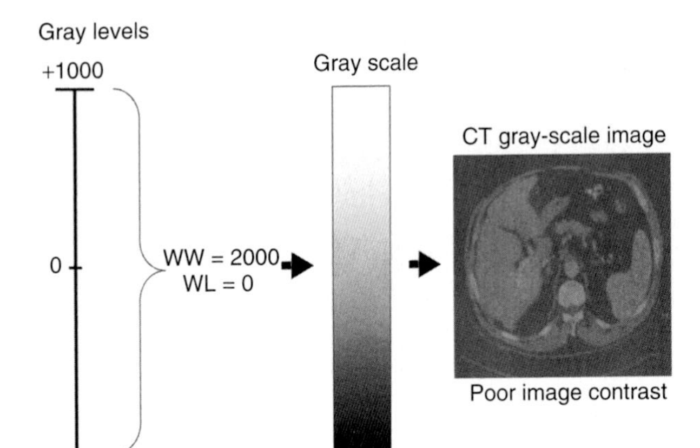

FIGURE 8-4 The effect of a wide WW on the image gray scale. In this case wide WW of 2000 produces an image with poor contrast. The WL is set at 0.

CT numbers portrayed as white will be large. A narrow window width implies that the transition from black to white will take place over a relatively few CT numbers" (Morgan, 1983). Figure 8-4 illustrates the effect of a wide WW (WW = 2000) on the image gray scale, and Figure 8-5 shows the effect of using a narrow WW (WW = 1000) on image gray scale to optimize image contrast. As shown in Figure 8-5, *A*, the upper and lower limits of the gray levels can be calculated by using the values of the WW and WL through the following relationships:

- The upper gray level value = WL + WW ÷ 2
- The lower gray level = WL − WW ÷ 2

Manipulating Window Width and Window Level

A graphic illustration of the effect of different WW and WL settings is shown in Figure 8-6. For ease of explanation and simplicity, a WW of 2000 and a WL of 0 will be used here. In Figure 8-6, *A*, the CT numbers range from +1000 for bone to −1000 for air. In this case, the WW is 2000; that is, there are 1000 CT numbers above 0 and another 1000 numbers below 0. The midpoint of the range (WL) is 0; this is referred to as a *reference point* because it represents water. Air, which is assigned a CT number of −1000, is also considered a reference point.

In Figure 8-6, *B*, the WW is 200 and the WL is 0. At this setting, all CT numbers greater than +100 appear white and those less than −100 appear black, whereas those between +100 and −100 appear as shades of gray.

In Figure 8-6, *C*, the WW is 200 and the WL is +40. CT numbers less than −60 appear black, those greater than +140 appear white, and those between +140 and −60 appear as shades of gray.

In Figure 8-6, *D*, the WW is 400 and the WL is 0. All CT numbers greater than +200 appear white, those less than −200 appear black, and those between +200 and −200 appear as shades of gray. If the entire range of CT numbers (the entire WW) is displayed, rather than a portion of the range, "small differences in attenuation between soft tissues will be obscured" (Zatz, 1984).

It is important to note that the CT number range varies among scanners. Although the range for some CT scanners varies from −1000 to +3095 Hounsfield units (HU) (4095 CT numbers), the range for other scanners may be −2048 to +6143 HU (8191 CT numbers). The tissue gray scale is stretched out with white at one end, black at the other, and shades of gray in between. The gray scale changes as the WW is expanded or narrowed. For bone structures, the WW must include the higher CT numbers on the scale. For structures that contain air, the WW moves

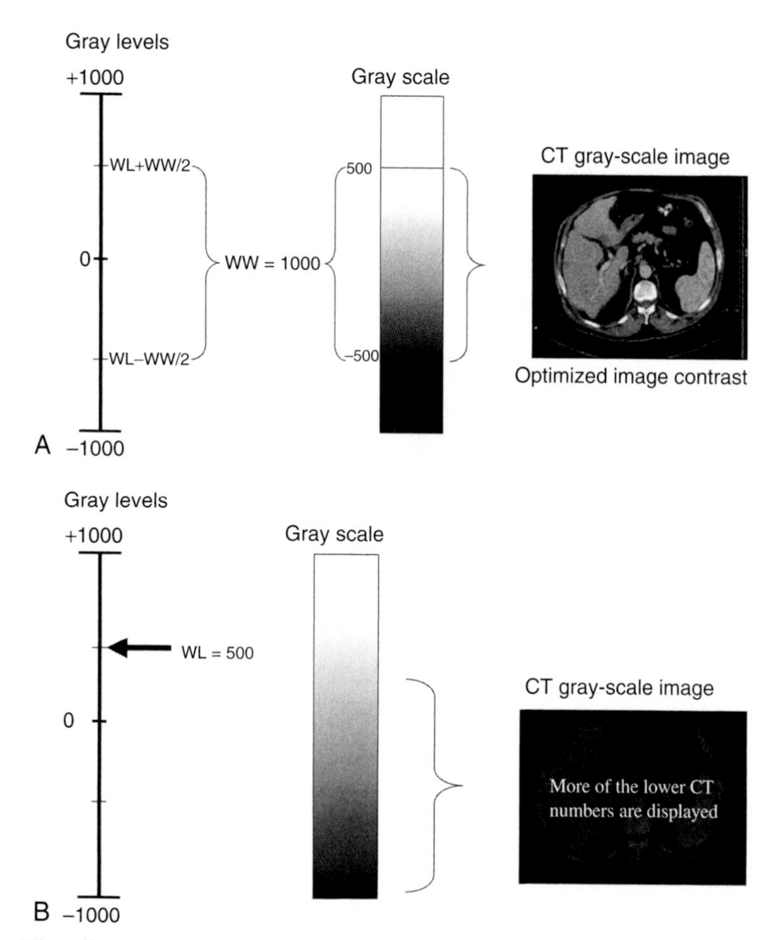

FIGURE 8-5 The effect of a narrow WW on image gray scale. In this case the WW of 1000 produces an image with optimized image contrast compared with a WW of 2000, as shown in Figure 8-4. The WL is set at 0. Although the upper limit of the gray scale is calculated by the relationship WL + WW/2 (0 + 1000/2 = 500), the lower limit of the scale is equal to WL – WW/2 (0 – 1000/2 = –500).

toward the lower CT numbers on the scale. Similarly, the WL can fall anywhere on the scale, depending on the structures of interest (Fig. 8-7). An example of the effect of WW and WL adjustment on the appearance of the CT image is shown for the thorax (Fig. 8-8).

In his discussion of the proper use of WW and WL in clinical CT, Berland (1987) noted the following:

1. Wide windows (400 to 2000 HU) should be used to encompass tissues of greatly differing attenuation within the image. For example, body scans are usually filmed at 350 to 600 HU to encompass the attenuation numbers of fat, fluid, and muscle. Lung and bone are filmed at 1000 to 2000 HU to include air spaces and vessels for lungs and cortex and marrow for bone.

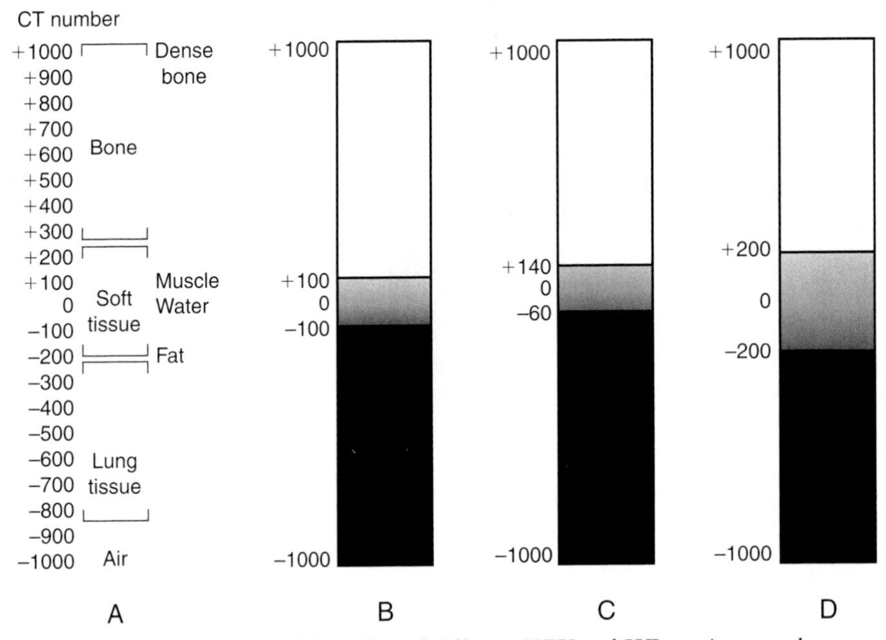

FIGURE 8-6 Graphic illustration of the effect of different WW and WL settings on the appearance of the CT image.

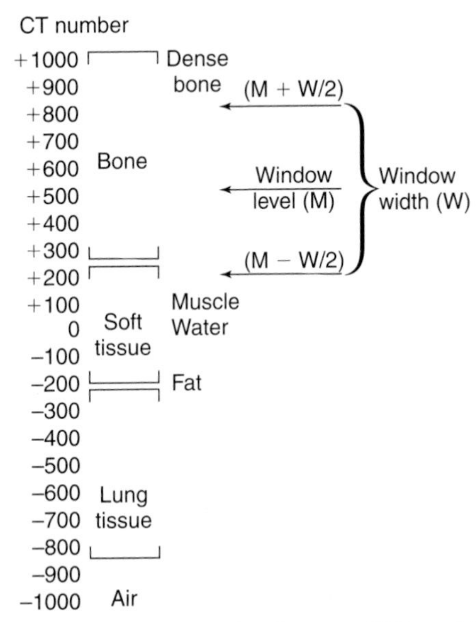

FIGURE 8-7 The relationship between WL and WW. These windows can be moved along the scale to optimize images of particular structures

2. Narrow windows (50 to 350 HU) should be used to display soft tissues within structures that contain different tissues of similar densities. For example, brain may be displayed at 80 to 150 HU to show differences between gray and white matter. Liver may be viewed at 100 to 250 HU to highlight liver metastases. The effect of both wide and narrow window widths on image appearance is shown in Figure 8-9.
3. Levels should be centered near the average attenuation of the tissues of interest. For example, attenuation body scans may be viewed at a level of 0 to 60 HU because fat has attenuation numbers from –60 to –100 HU, whereas the attenuation numbers of muscle and organs may range from 60 to 150 HU with intravenous contrast. Lung is viewed at a level of –600 to –750 HU.

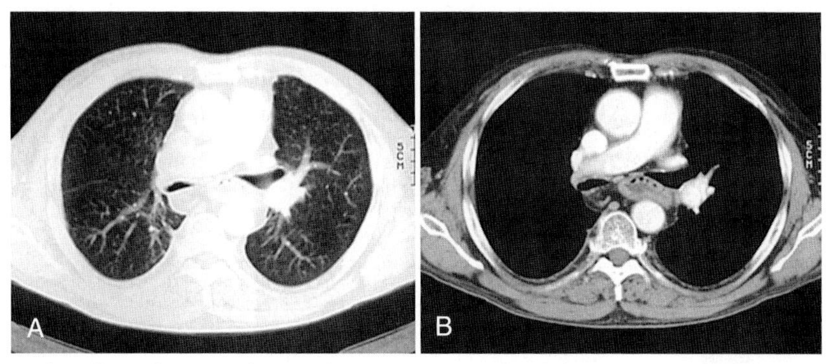

FIGURE 8-8 The effect of WW and WL adjustments on image appearance. **A,** A lung WW of 1500 HU and a WL of −530 HU are used. **B,** Soft tissue window width of 500 HU and a window level of +40 HU are used. (Courtesy Siemens Medical Systems.)

Effect of Window Width on Image Contrast

In general, the viewer can alter the contrast of the CT image by changing the WW. A graphic illustration is shown in Figure 8-10. When the WW is large (wide WW), the three different structures—the lung, liver (soft tissues), and pelvis (bone)—have the same gray tone (*bottom of diagram*). With a narrow WW, there is very sharp contrast to the point where the lungs appear black, bone appears white, and the liver is shown as gray tones. Finally, image contrast is optimized with the use of a medium WW (*middle of diagram*).

The effect of different WW settings (603, 499, 249, and 95) on an abdominal CT image with a fixed WL (+40) is clearly shown in Figure 8-11. The following conclusions may be drawn:

1. As the WW increases, the contrast decreases (Fig. 8-11, *A*).
2. As the WW decreases, the contrast becomes greater. The image appears totally black and white with a WW of 95 (Fig. 8-11, *D*).

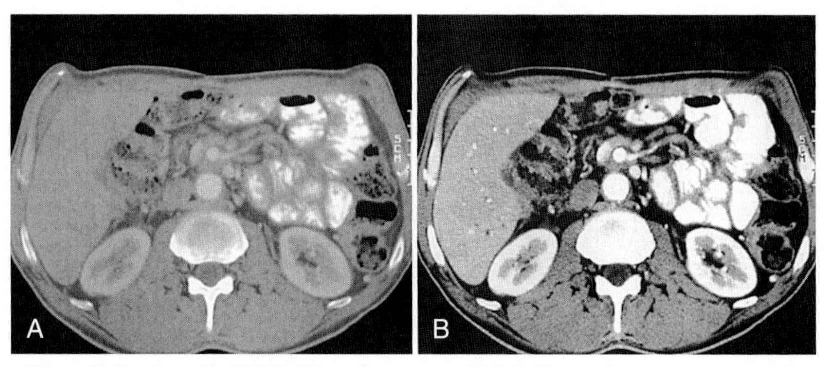

FIGURE 8-9 The effect of a wide WW **(A)** and a narrow WW **(B)** on the appearance of the CT image. (Courtesy Siemens Medical Systems.)

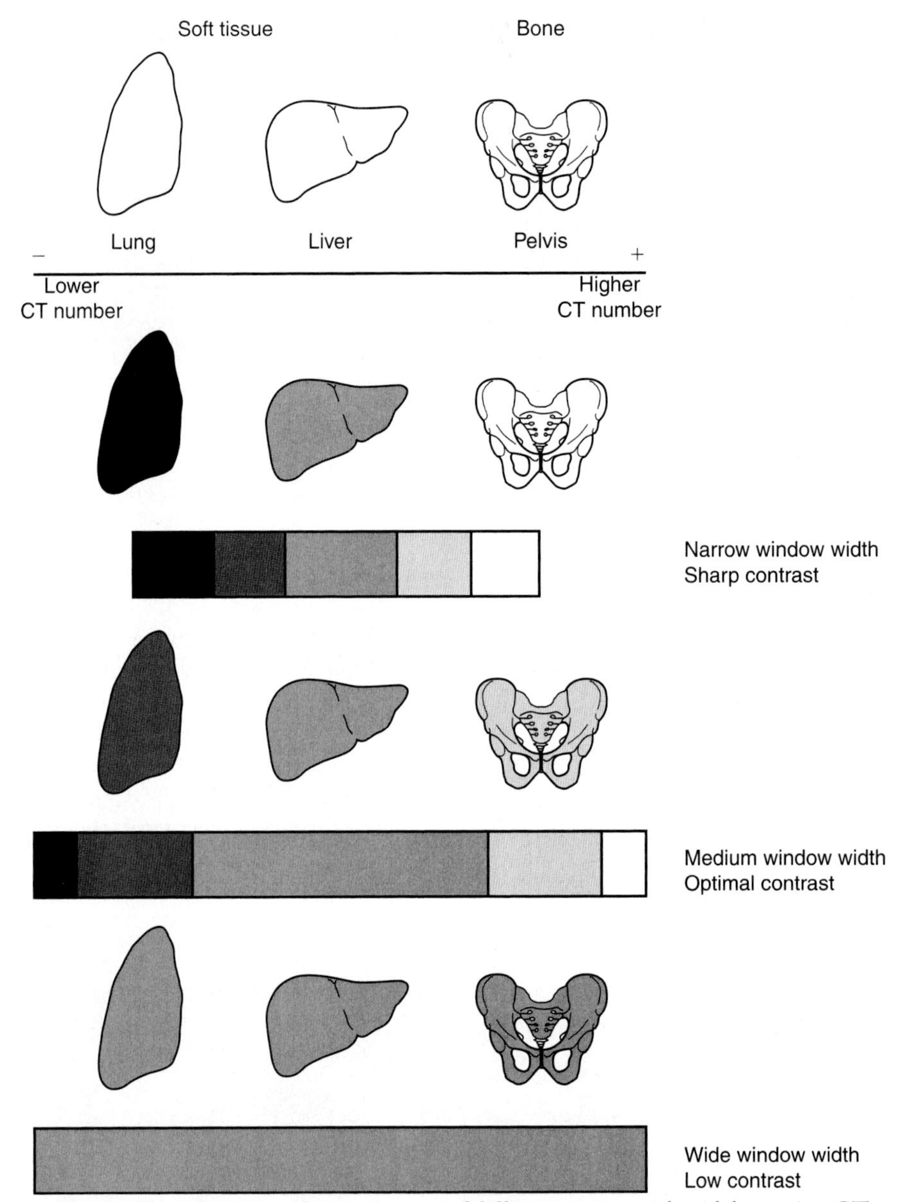

FIGURE 8-10 The effect of WW on the appearance of different organs with widely varying CT numbers.

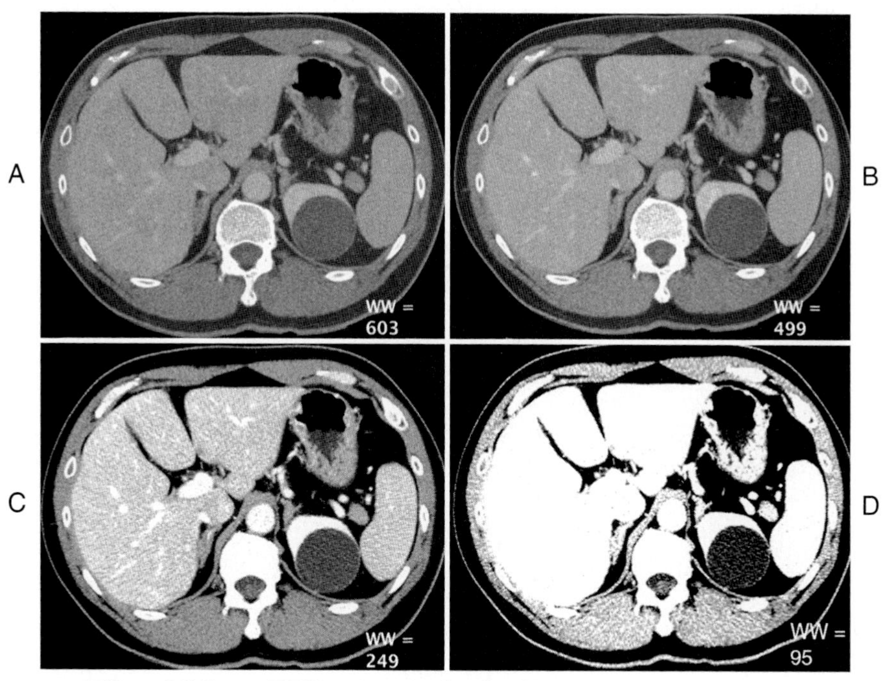

FIGURE 8-11 Effect of different WW settings (with a fixed WL = +40) on image contrast with a fixed WL setting. As WW decreases from 603 **(A)**, 499 **(B)**, 249 **(C)**, to 95 **(D)**, contrast improves.

3. Contrast is optimized with medium WW settings and is probably best (depending on the observer's subjective impression) when the image is recorded with a WW of 499 for the optimization of certain abdominal structures (Fig. 8-11, *B*).

Effect of Window Level on Image Brightness

Recall Figure 8-3, which shows the WL as the CT number in the middle of the WW and represents the medium gray scale. As graphically illustrated in Figure 8-12, when the WL is centered on the lungs (lower CT numbers), the image display is optimized for that structure, and the liver (soft tissue) and pelvis (bone) are displayed as white. On the other hand, when the WL is centered on the pelvis (higher CT numbers), the image display is optimized for the pelvis, and the lungs and liver appear black. Finally, with the WL centered on the liver (middle CT numbers), the pelvis appears white, and the liver is optimized for viewing.

The effects of different WL settings (with fixed WW) on the display of images of the abdomen are shown in Figure 8-13. As the WL decreases from +248 to −106, the picture changes from black (Fig. 8-13, *A*) to white (Fig. 8-13, *D*). A graphic illustration of this effect is clearly apparent in Figure 8-14. As the WL moves toward the higher CT numbers (generally white), more CT numbers with lower values (generally black) are displayed. In addition, as the WL moves toward the lower CT numbers, more CT numbers with higher values are displayed, and the image looks white.

Preset Windows

Preset windows are available on scanners to optimize windowing. For example, a double (dual) window display will facilitate the simultaneous display of two different density ranges. Both windows

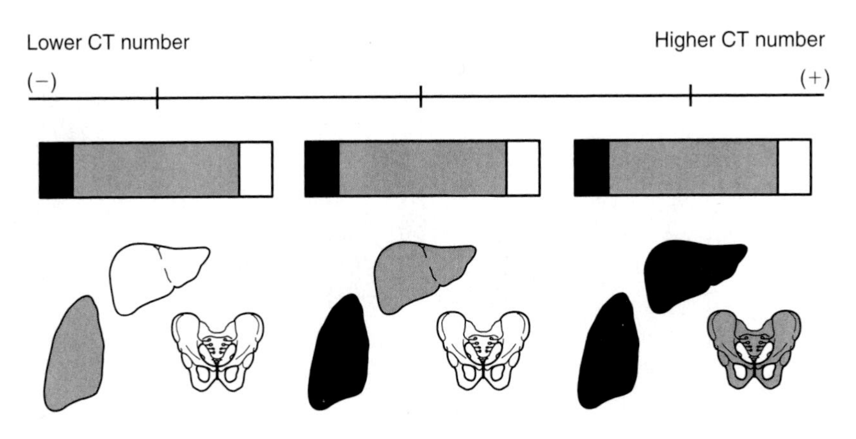

FIGURE 8-12 Graphic illustration of the effect of WL on gray-tone appearance of different organs.

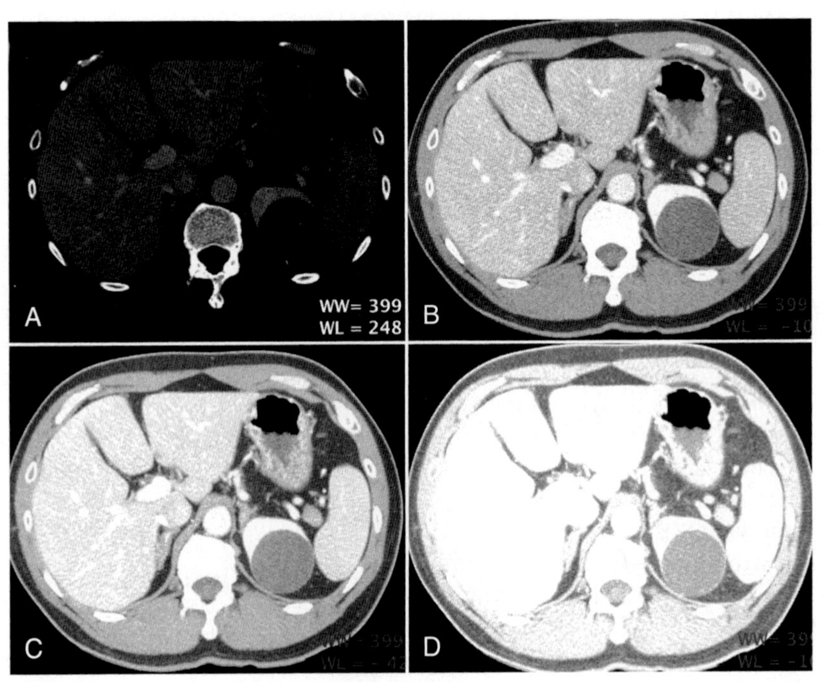

FIGURE 8-13 Effect of different WL settings on image display with a fixed WW. As the WL decreases from +248 to −106, the picture changes from black **(A)** to white **(D)**.

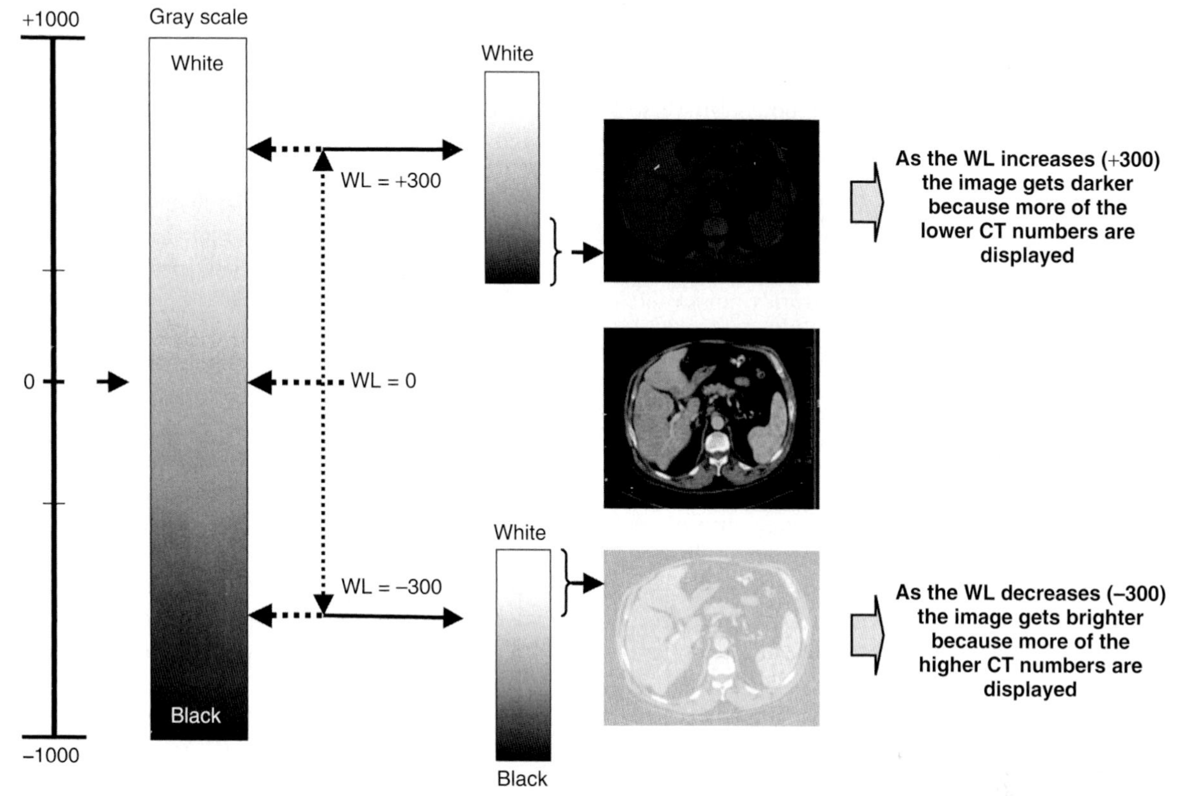

FIGURE 8-14 Graphic illustration of this effect (Fig. 8-13). As the WL moves toward the higher CT numbers (generally white), more CT numbers with lower values (generally black) are displayed. In addition, as the WL moves toward the lower CT numbers, more CT numbers with higher values are displayed, and the image looks white.

have different window widths and window levels (Fig. 8-15). Although a single window setting displays one anatomic region, a double (or dual) window display provides well-defined contours to separate two different anatomic areas (Fig. 8-16).

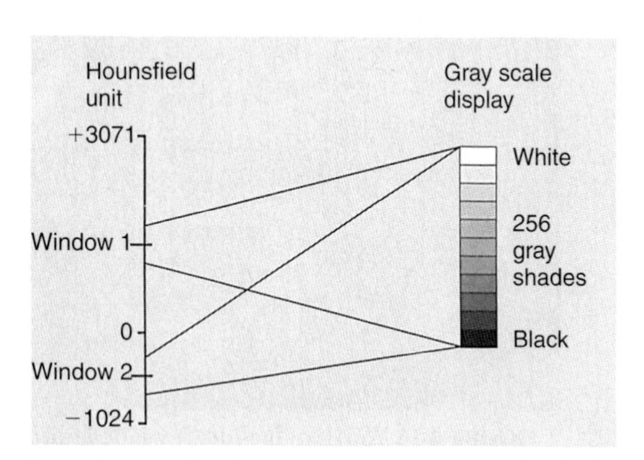

FIGURE 8-15 The fundamental principles of the double (dual) window setting. (Courtesy Siemens Medical Systems, Iselin, NJ.)

TWO-DIMENSIONAL IMAGE PROCESSING: CT IMAGE REFORMATTING TECHNIQUES

Multiplanar Reconstruction

Multiplanar reconstruction or multiplanar reformation (MPR), sometimes referred to as *image reformatting* or *image reformation* (not to be confused with image reconstruction), is a computer program that can create coronal, sagittal, and paraxial images from a stack of contiguous transverse axial scans (Fig. 8-17).

The sagittal image defines a plane that passes through an anatomical region from anterior to posterior and divides the body into right and left sections; the coronal image defines a plane that passes through the body region from right to left (or left to right), dividing the region into anterior and posterior sections. The paraxial image, on the other hand, defines a plane that cuts through the coronal and sagittal planes in the longitudinal direction of an anatomical region.

Irregular, oblique, and other views can also be generated. The irregular view (e.g., linear or curved) can be reconstructed from a stack of contiguous transverse images (Fig. 8-18). The oblique view can be reconstructed with at least three arbitrarily definable points in different transverse images (Fig. 8-19).

In the conceptual framework to generate these images (Fig. 8-20), the voxel on the left represents the information contained and stored in a specific volume of tissue. In reformatting, the computer program uses any set of points to build an image of the selected plane. Mackay (1984) has noted the following:

> Suppose in the figure that the first image computed and stored was the left-hand face of the cube, followed by the plane parallel to it with the number 2, after which the third set of projections would be collected to form the parallel plane containing the number 3, and so on. All the points in the cube would gradually be accumulated and stored in the computer, and it is convenient to think of the position of the storage of a number as corresponding to the position of a point in the cube. Any of the original planes could be displayed by "calling up" the number representing the points in that plane and producing a proportional brightness on the oscilloscope screen at the corresponding position. On the screen instead could be displayed the dots shown at the center section [of Fig. 8-20]. On the lower left of the screen

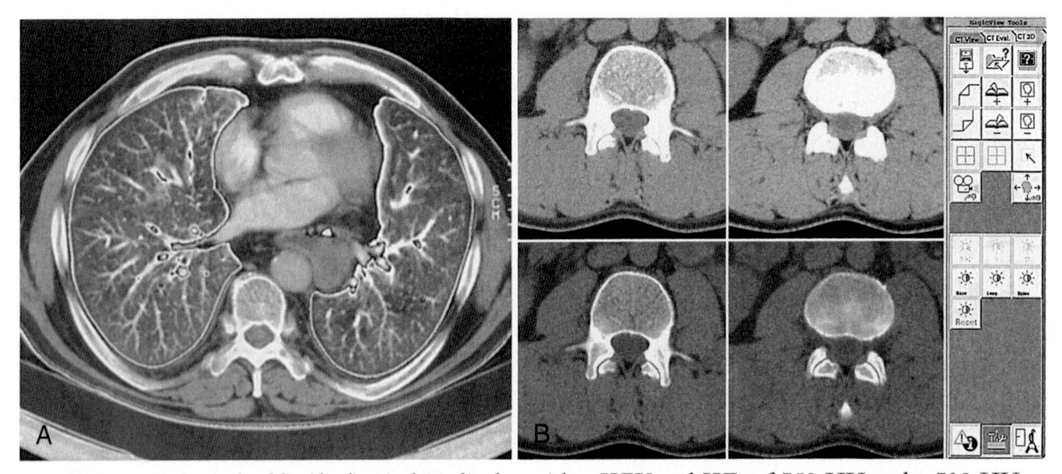

FIGURE 8-16 **A,** A double (dual) window display with a WW and WL of 750 HU and −730 HU, respectively, with a WW and a WL of 500 HU and 35 HU, respectively. **B,** Dual windows allow the observer to view bone and soft tissue windows of the same images simultaneously. (Courtesy Siemens Medical Systems, Iselin, NJ.)

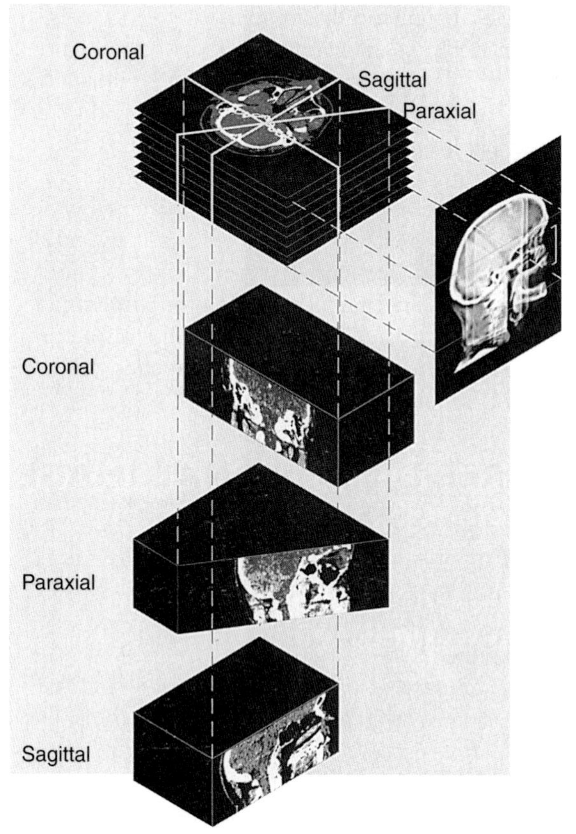

FIGURE 8-17 Multiplanar reconstruction involves the use of a computer program to reformat sagittal, paraxial, and coronal views from a stack of contiguous transverse axial images. (Courtesy Siemens Medical Systems, Iselin, NJ.)

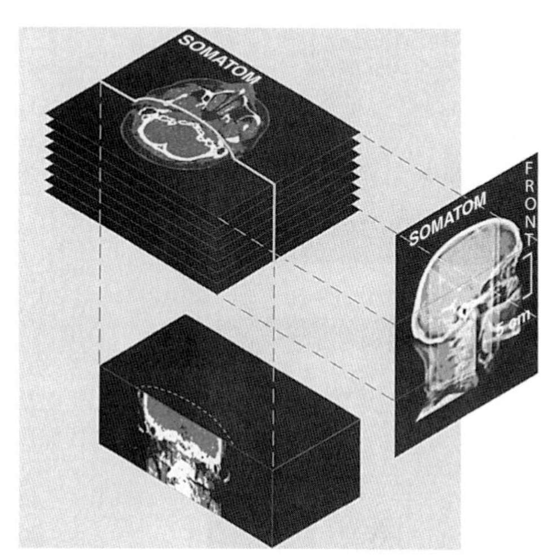

FIGURE 8-18 Irregular views can be created through multiplanar reconstruction techniques using the images from a stack of contiguous transaxial slices. (Courtesy Siemens Medical Systems, Iselin, NJ.)

would be displayed the point designated (1, B, a), which came from the first section, for example. Next to it would be displayed a point from the bottom of the second section and in one increment from the right side, and so on. By sequentially calling up all the points located inward one increment from the right face of the cube one can display a section through the subject perpendicular to all the planes that were originally scanned. In the display one can instead move to the left one increment from each successive step inward to a new line on the television screen; this results in the display of a

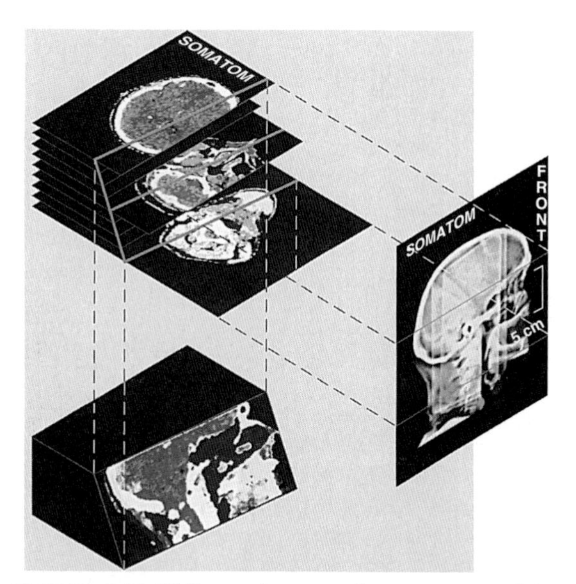

FIGURE 8-19 Oblique views can be reconstructed by multiplanar reconstruction techniques using definable points in different transaxial slices. (Courtesy Siemens Medical Systems, Iselin, NJ.)

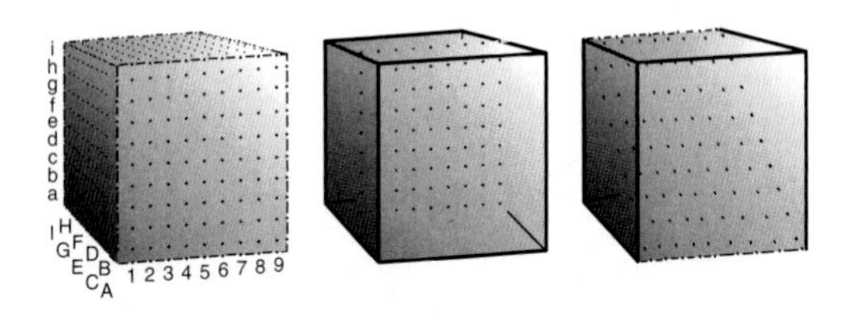

FIGURE 8-20 A conceptual framework for generating reformatted images in CT.

plane at an angle through the body as shown in the right-hand part of the figure. It should be clear that from this array of computed data one can display any section through the volume. Often the sections across a subject are more widely spaced than are the lines across the section in making the original projections, in which case the resolution in a tilted display will not be the same up and down as across the image.

There are both advantages and disadvantages to reformatted images (see following box). Major advantages include the following:

1. To enable the visualization of specific structures such as the optic nerves and lesions in relation to surrounding structures.
2. To determine the true extent of lesions or fractures and to help localize lesions and intra-articular bone fragments or foreign bodies.

Reformatted Images

Advantages

- Enables visualization of specific structures in relation to surrounding structures
- Determines extent of lesions or fractures
- Helps to localize lesions, bone fragments, or foreign bodies

Disadvantages

- Loss of image detail

One major disadvantage of MPR relates to image quality. Image detail is not as good as that obtained in transaxial images. The reformatted image quality depends on the quality of the axial images, and it is therefore important that the patient does not move or breathe during the scanning procedure. In addition, the plane thickness affects image detail; thus thick planes result in blurring and loss of structural detail. Today, multislice CT scanners capable of isotropic imaging (see Chapter 12) solve these problems because all dimensions of the voxel are equal, that is, the voxel is a perfect cube.

THREE-DIMENSIONAL IMAGE PROCESSING

Three-Dimensional Imaging: An Overview

3D imaging in CT belongs to a class of digital image processing referred to as image synthesis (see Chapter 3). Image synthesis operations "create images from other images or non-image data. These operations are used when a desired image is either physically impossible or impractical to acquire, or does not exist in a physical form at all" (Baxes, 1994). Synthesis operations include image reconstruction techniques (see Chapter 6) that are the basis for CT and magnetic resonance (MR) images and 3D visualization techniques that are based on computer graphics technology. Special software gathers information from the transaxial scan data to display 3D images on a 2D television screen.

A thorough description of 3D CT imaging is not within the scope of this chapter. The concepts are elaborated in Chapter 14. It is important, however, to introduce some of the language of 3D imaging here.

3D imaging is gaining widespread attention in radiology (Calhoun et al, 1999; Choplin et al, 2004; Cody, 2002; Dalrymple et al, 2005; Fatterpekar et al, 2006; Fishman et al, 2006; Kalender, 2005; Lell et al, 2006; Seeram, 2001; Seeram, 2005;

Seeram and Seeram, 2008; Udupa, 1999). Already 3D imaging is used in CT, MR imaging, and other imaging modalities with the goal of providing both qualitative and quantitative information from images to facilitate and enhance diagnosis.

The general framework of 3D imaging (Fig. 8-21) includes four major steps: data acquisition, creation of what is referred to as 3D space (all voxel information is stored in the computer), processing for 3D image display, and, finally, 3D image display. Images can be displayed as projection images such as maximum intensity projection (MIP) and minimum intensity projection images (MinIP), SSD images, VR images, and finally virtual reality images. The principles of the generation of each of these are elaborated in Chapter 14.

Digital image postprocessing can allow the observer to view all aspects of 3D space, a technique referred to as 3D visualization. The application of 3D visualization techniques in radiology is referred to as 3D medical imaging. Basic and advanced visualization tools in 3D medical imaging are highlighted later.

Dr. Jayaram Udupa, an expert in 3D imaging from the Department of Radiology at the University of Pennsylvania, notes that there are four classes of 3D imaging operations: preprocessing, visualization, manipulation, and analysis. For example, as noted by Dr. Udupa, visualization operations are intended "to create renditions from a given set of scenes or objects that facilitate the visual perception of object information." These four classes of operations are described further in Chapter 14.

VISUALIZATION TOOLS

Visualization tools such as windowing are computer programs that provide the observer-diagnostician with additional information to facilitate diagnosis. Visualization tools range from basic to advanced.

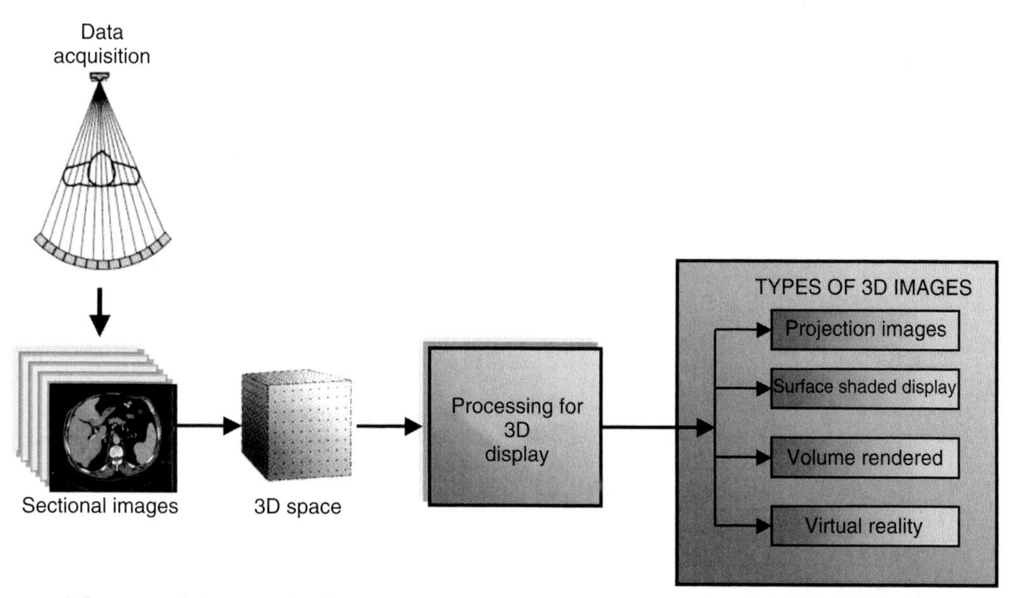

FIGURE 8-21 The general framework of 3D imaging includes four major steps: data acquisition, creation of what is referred to as 3D space, digital image processing for 3D image display, and finally, 3D image display. As noted, several different types of 3D images can be displayed to suit the needs of the observer.

Basic Tools

Basic visualization tools are basic computer programs integrated into the CT system with the following capabilities (Fig. 8-22):

1. Multiple imaging and multiple windows (Fig. 8-22, *A*)
2. Image magnification (Fig. 8-22, *B*)
3. Evaluation of geometric characteristics such as distances and angles (Fig. 8-22, *C*)
4. Superimposition of coordinates on the image to provide a reference for biopsies (Fig. 8-22, *D*)
5. Highlighting, in which the pixels in certain regions of the image can be made to appear brighter (Fig. 8-22, *E*)
6. CT histogram, which is a plot of the pixel values as a function of the frequency with which each value occurs. This can be done for the entire image or a portion of the image, as defined by the region of interest (ROI) (Fig. 8-22, *F*).
7. ROI statistics, which allow for statistical calculations such as the mean and standard deviation within the ROI
8. ROI transfer, whereby the ROI can be transferred from slice to slice
9. Split imaging, in which an image can be split into two detailed thin slices, and fused imaging, in which two contiguous thin slices can be fused into a single thick slice

Optional software packages are also available for dental CT applications, dynamic CT, networking, workstations, and 3D imaging.

Advanced Tools

Advanced visualization tools require powerful computer workstations with advanced image processing capabilities and increased memory to handle the vast amount of data used in various visualization techniques. An example of one such workstation is shown in Figure 8-23. Currently, a wide variety of advanced visualization tools are commercially available, as follows:

- 3D visualization tools allow the user to render various 3D images from the axial data set. 3D rendering falls into three categories: SSD (surface rendering), VR, and MIP and MinIP.
- Computed tomography angiography (CTA) is a relatively new technique based on volume scanning principles. CTA is an application of 3D imaging and is becoming more popular in the examination of the circulatory system. Examples of CTA visualization tools include four-dimensional (4D) angio, vessel tracking, skull removal, and multiple target volume.
- In 4D angio, the fourth dimension is opacity instead of time. 4D angio is based on VR technology. Changes in the opacity values of various tissues enable the observer to simultaneously visualize bone, soft tissues, and vascular structures; therefore both foreground and background structures are visible. 4D angio is useful and it is preferred over conventional MIP techniques for the visualization of aortic aneurysms, renal arteries, stents, and carotid bifurcation. Target volume MIP allows the user to render only a selected volume of data and does not require segmentation techniques.
- The vessel tracking tool allows the user to produce a set of MPR images (batches), including curved MPR images, for the entire vessel. The skull removal tool facilitates the subtraction of bones of the skull from the CTA image and allows the observer to visualize very detailed images of the vessels and soft tissues.
- MPR tools display all types of MPR images from the axial data set in the axial, coronal, sagittal, and oblique planes, as described earlier in this chapter.
- Interactive visualization tools offer the following features in any 3D rendering mode:

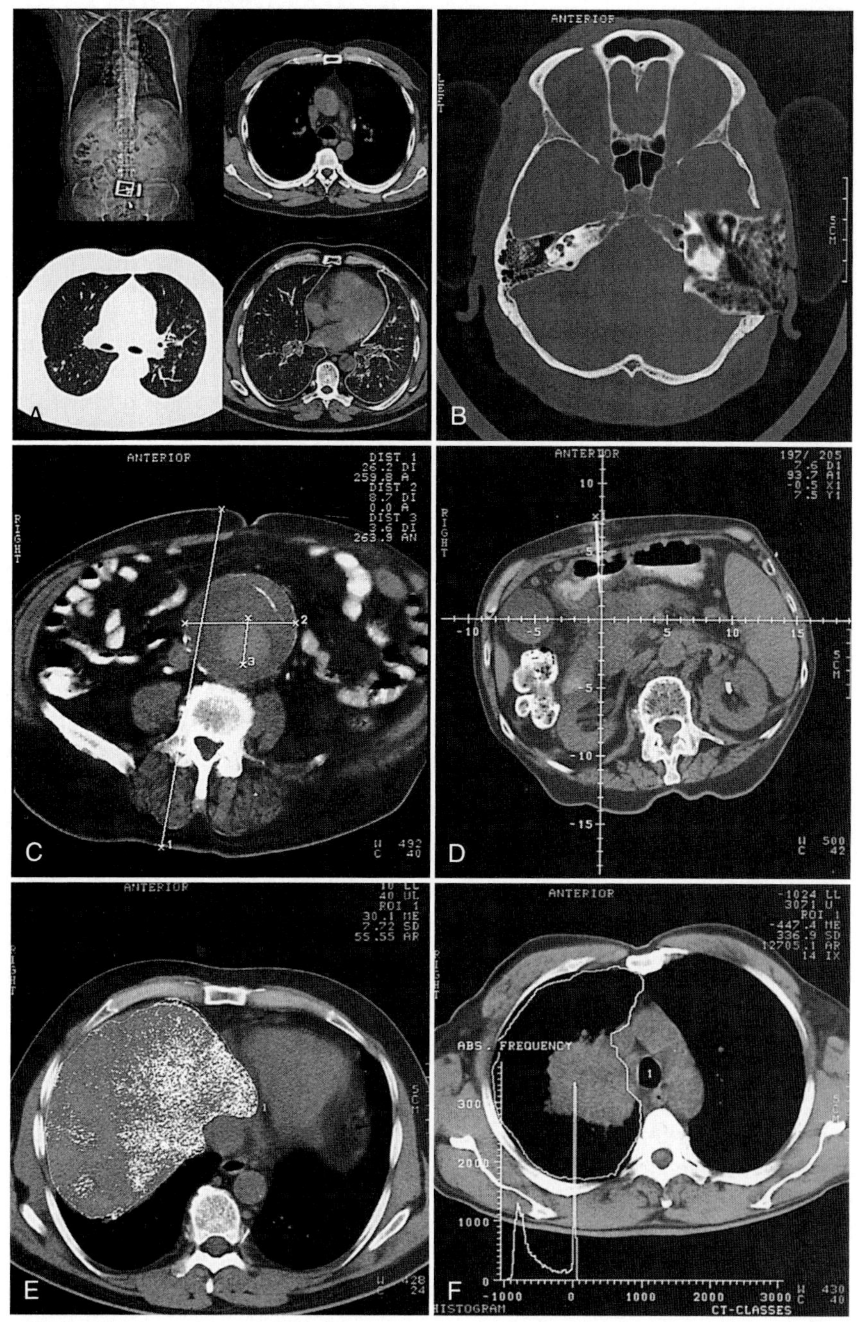

FIGURE 8-22 Other computer programs for CT are capable of the following: **A,** Multiple imaging and windows; **B,** image magnification; **C,** measurement of distances; **D,** superimposition of coordinates on the image; **E,** highlights; and **F,** histogram. (Courtesy Siemens Medical Systems, Iselin, NJ.)

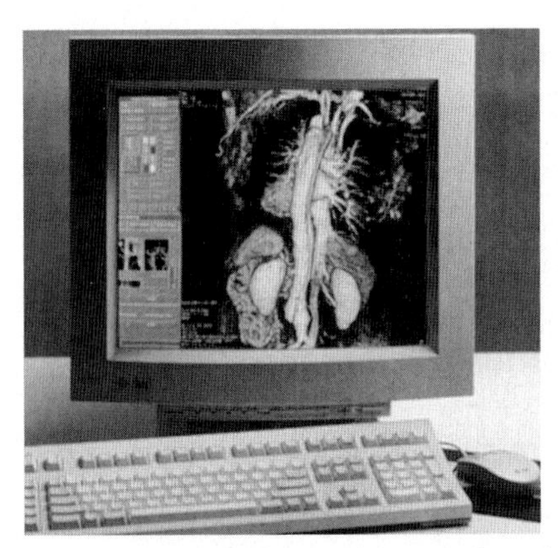

FIGURE 8-23 Example of a workstation for advanced image processing. (Courtesy Philips Medical Systems.)

window/level adjustment, volume of interest adjustment, scan information display, movie creation and playback, split screen presentation, zoom, and measurements.

- Cine visualization tools allow the user to view a large set of images very quickly.
- Advanced quantitative measurement tools facilitate measurements such as distances, angles, areas, mean, standard deviation, minimum and maximum voxel values, density value in HU, density histogram for a particular ROI, and volume of 3D objects.
- Multimodality image fusion tools allow the user to combine images from a wide variety of imaging modalities such as CT, MR imaging, positron emission tomography, and single-photon emission computed tomography to facilitate diagnosis of tumor localization and quantification, surgical planning, and oncology planning.
- Virtual reality visualization tools include Voyager and 3D Navigator. These tools create 3D and 4D images of tubular structures such as the colon and bronchi and allow the user to "fly through" the images of hollow organs in a technique referred to as *CT virtual endoscopy*, which is gaining widespread attention in radiologic imaging.

ADVANCED VISUALIZATION AND ANALYSIS WORKSTATIONS

Hardware Components

Hardware components include the central processing unit, various processors, and data and image storage devices. The host computer of an advanced visualization and analysis workstation can be a Sun SPARC (Sun Microsystems) or a Silicon Graphics platform with varying amounts of random access memory depending on the cost of the system. The operating system of both platforms is the UNIX multitasking system, which provides optimum speed and system response. In addition, these workstations feature various microprocessors to improve data processing.

The monitor of the workstation must provide good image quality and offer a maximum luminance of at least 50 foot-lamberts (American College of Radiology, 2006). These monitors are usually cathode ray tubes or flat-panel displays with at least 2.5 K × 2 K pixel resolution and should be capable of a wide range of display formats. The keyboard is a full alphanumerical keyboard with function, archiving, and display keys. Additionally, a mouse can be used to communicate with the computer.

Data and image storage devices include hard disks and magnetic tape. The storage capacity of these media varies depending on the system.

Connectivity

Connectivity, or networking, is an important feature of current workstations because of the trend toward filmless radiology departments through the implementation of picture archiving and communication systems, radiology information systems, and hospital information systems (see Chapter 2).

The transfer of data and images to and from the CT scanner and workstations is an essential component of connectivity. Such transfer must comply with industry standards for electronic communications between different imaging modalities and devices from multiple vendors. One such standard is the Digital Imaging and Communications in Medicine (DICOM), and workstations for CT, MR imaging, and other imaging modalities must be DICOM compliant.

REFERENCES

American College of Radiology: *ACR technical standard for digital image data management*, Reston, Va, 2006, American College of Radiology.

Baxes GA: *Digital image processing: principles and applications*, New York, 1994, John Wiley.

Berland LL: *Practical CT: technology and techniques*, New York, 1987, Raven Press.

Cody D: Image processing in CT, *Radiographics* 22: 1255-1268, 2002.

Dalrymple NC et al: Introduction to the language of three-dimensional imaging with multidetector CT, *Radiographics* 25: 1409-1428, 2005.

Fatterpekar GM et al: Role of 3D CT in the evaluation of the temporal bone, *Radiographics* 26: S117-S132, 2006.

Fishman EK et al: Volume rendering versus maximum intensity projection in CT angiography: what works best, when and why? *Radiographics* 26: 905-921, 2006.

Glen W et al: Image manipulation and pattern recognition. In Newton TH, Potts DG, editors: *Radiology of the skull and brain: technical aspects of computed tomography*, St Louis, 1981, Mosby.

Kalender W: *Computed tomography: fundamentals, system technology, image quality, applications*, Erlangen, 2005, Publicis Corporate Publishing.

Lell MM et al: New techniques in CT angiography, *Radiographics* 26: S45-S62, 2006.

Mackay RS: *Medical images and displays*, New York, 1984, John Wiley.

Morgan CL: *Basic principles of computed tomography*, Baltimore, 1983, University Park Press.

Seeram E: *Computed tomography technology*, Philadelphia, 2001, WB Saunders.

Seeram E: Digital image processing, *Radiol Technol* 76: 435-452, 2005.

Seeram E, Seeram D: Image postprocessing in digital radiology: a primer for technologists, *Journal of Medical Imaging Radiation Sciences* 39:23-43, 2008.

Zatz LM: Basic principles of computed tomography scanning. In Newton TH, Potts DG, editors: *Radiology of the skull and brain: technical aspects of computed tomography*, St. Louis, 1984, Mosby.

Image Quality

Jiang Hsieh

Chapter Outline

In general, the image quality of a computed tomography (CT) scanner can be described by several key performance parameters: high-contrast spatial resolution, low-contrast resolution, temporal resolution, CT number uniformity and accuracy, noise, and artifacts. These parameters are influenced not only by the CT system performance but also by the operator's selection of protocols such as x-ray tube voltage (in kilovolts [kV]), tube current (in milliamperes [mA]), slice thickness, helical pitch, reconstruction parameters, and scan speed. As often is the case of a real-life problem, tradeoffs have to be made between image quality, dose to the patient, system limitations, patient conditions, and clinical indications. Over the years, many studies have been conducted to understand such tradeoffs (Barnes and Lakshminarayan, 1981; Blumenfeld and Glover, 1981; Hanson, 1981; Hsieh, 2003; Kalender and Polacin, 1995; McCollough and Zink, 2000; Morgan, 1983; Pfeiler et al, 1976; Robb and Mortin, 1991). Clearly, tradeoff decisions between various performance parameters are not as straightforward as would be hoped. Although the design of CT scanners has been evolved significantly over the years to minimize the complexity of parameter selection, even state-of-the-art scanners still depend, in various degrees, on the experience of the operator to produce optimal image quality.

Given the limited scope of this chapter, it is impossible to discuss all factors that affect the image quality of a CT scanner, let alone the tradeoffs among these factors. Instead, only the most important performance parameters are the focus, and, whenever possible, some of the common factors that influence the CT performance and phantoms used to perform quantitative measurements are briefly discussed. Because of the wide availability of the helical/spiral and multislice/volumetric CT scanners in recent years, their specific characteristics and requirements are incorporated into the discussion of each topic, rather than being isolated in a separate section.

HIGH-CONTRAST SPATIAL RESOLUTION

High-contrast spatial resolution of a CT scanner describes the scanner's ability to resolve closely placed objects that are significantly different from their background. Historically, spatial resolution was defined and measured predominately within the scanning plane. With the popularity of the multislice/volumetric helical CT, however, the cross-plane resolution becomes just as important.

In-Plane Spatial Resolution

Definition and Measurements

The in-plane resolution is specified in terms of line pairs per centimeter (lp/cm) or line pairs per millimeter (lp/mm). A line pair is a pair of equal-sized black-white bars. Therefore, a bar pattern representing 10 lp/cm is a set of uniformly spaced combshaped bars with 0.5-mm wide teeth. Because the CT acquisition and reconstruction process is band limited (high-frequency contents are suppressed or eliminated), the reconstructed image of a bar pattern is a blurred version of the original object, as illustrated in Figure 9-1. The edges of the bars are softened, and the magnitude of the bar pattern is reduced. If the peak-to-valley magnitude of the original object is normalized as unity, the reconstructed peak-to-valley is smaller. For example, in Figure 9-1, at 1 lp/cm spatial frequency, the reconstructed peak-to-valley magnitude is 0.88; at 2 lp/cm, the magnitude is 0.59, and so on. In general, the magnitude reduces as the frequency (lp/cm) of the bar pattern increases. If the spatial frequency is plotted as a function of the image fidelity, a smooth curve is obtained (Fig. 9-2). This is often referred to as the modulation transfer function (MTF) of the system. MTF can be used to compare the performance of different CT systems. For example, scanner A can image 5.2 lp/cm at

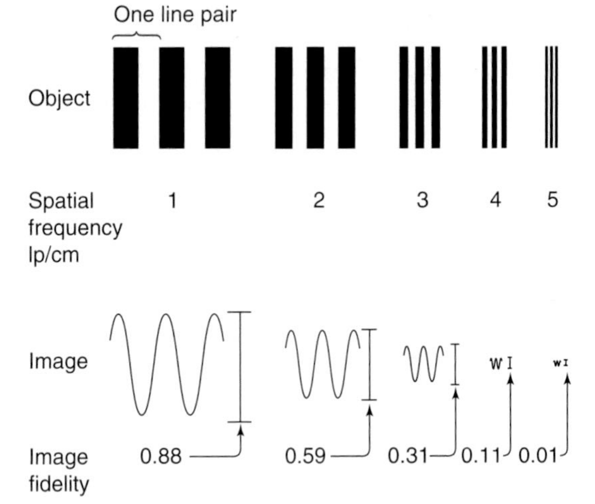

FIGURE 9-1 A bar pattern (object) consists of line pairs (lp, one line pair equals one bar plus one space). The number of line pairs per unit length is called the spatial frequency. Large objects have a low spatial frequency, whereas small objects have a high spatial frequency.

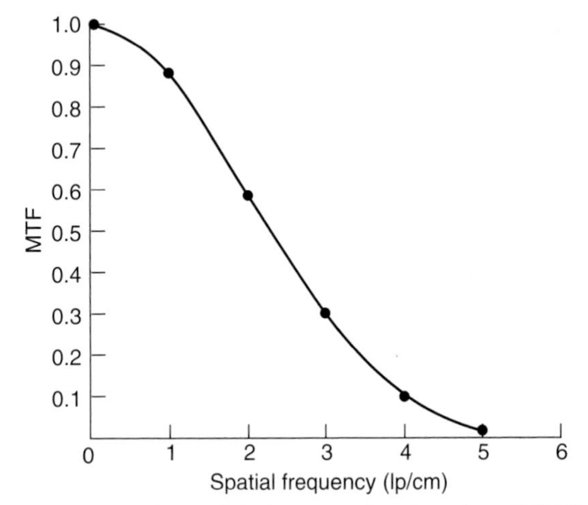

FIGURE 9-2 A modulation transfer function (MTF) curve obtained from the data given in Figure 9-1.

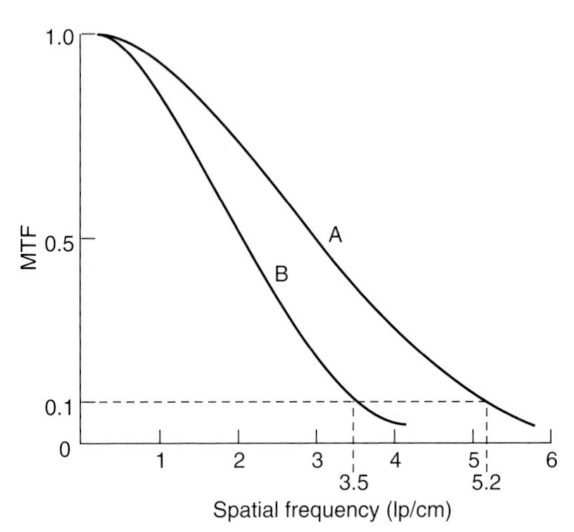

FIGURE 9-3 MTF curves for two CT scanners.

0.1 MTF compared with scanner B, which can only image 3.5 lp/cm at 0.1 MTF (Fig. 9-3). This simply means that scanner A has a better spatial resolution capability than scanner B.

An ideal system would have a flat MTF curve, a unity response independent of frequency. Such a system ensures that the object can be reproduced exactly. For practical systems, however, the frequency response falls off quickly as the frequency increases. Three points on the MTF curve are of particular interest: 50%, 10%, and 0%. The 50% MTF refers to the frequency at which the magnitude of the MTF curve drops to 50% of its peak value. Similarly, the 10% and 0% MTF refer to the frequencies at which the MTF drops to 10% and 0% of the peak value. Various phantoms have been designed specifically to measure the MTF of the system. For example, the Catphan High Resolution Insert contains high-density metal bar patterns ranging from 1 to 21 lp/cm, as shown in Figure 9-4.

Alternatively, the MTF of a system can be derived from the point spread function (PSF) of the system (Hsieh, 2003). PSF is defined as the system response to a Dirac delta function. If the scanned object is a high-density thin wire placed perpendicular to the scanning plane, and as long as the diameter of the wire is significantly smaller than the resolution of the system, the wire can be considered as a Dirac delta function. The reconstructed image of such wire is then simply the PSF of the system. By definition, MTF is related to PSF by the magnitude of the Fourier transform. As an illustration, Figure 9-5 depicts a GE

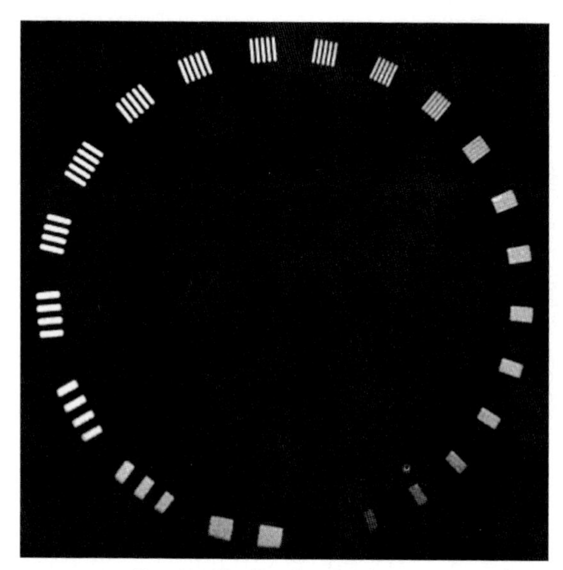

FIGURE 9-4 Image of a Catphan high-resolution insert. Bar patterns range from 1 lp/cm to 21 lp/cm.

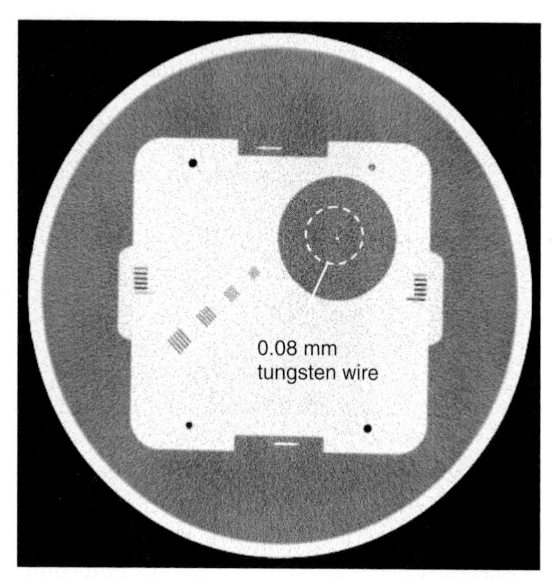

FIGURE 9-5 Image of a GE Performance phantom. A thin tungsten wire is submerged in water for MTF measurement.

Performance Phantom with a 0.08-mm diameter tungsten wire submerged in water. If we isolate the wire portion of the image and remove its background (Fig. 9-6, *A*) and take the Fourier transform of this image (Fig. 9-6, *B*), the MTF of the CT system can be obtained by averaging the frequency domain image over 360 degrees, as shown by the curve in Figure 9-6.

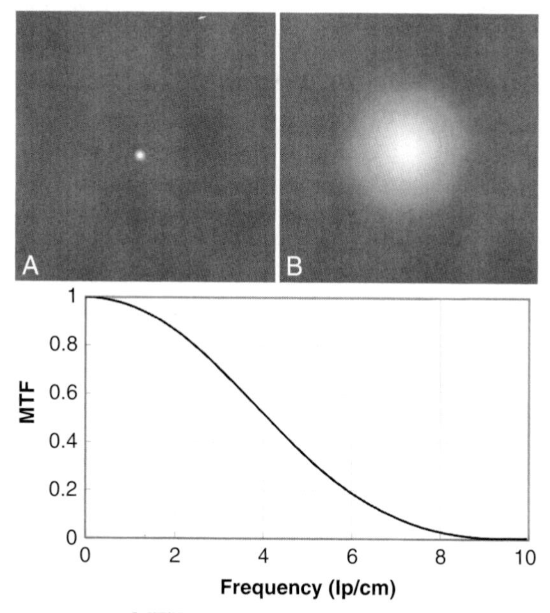

FIGURE 9-6 MTF measurement with a thin wire. **A,** A tungsten wire reconstructed with standard algorithm to approximate PSF. **B,** Magnitude of the Fourier transform of the PSF image. The MTF curve is averaged over 360 degrees.

Factors Affecting Resolution

Many factors affect the in-plane spatial resolution. The most dominating factors are the x-ray focal spot size and shape, detector cell size, scanner geometry, and sampling frequency. Although these factors are largely determined by CT manufacturers, operators do have limited control. For example, most CT scanners have more than one x-ray focal spot to account for an increased tube loading. By properly selecting the x-ray tube current, an operator has the option to use either the small spot (lower tube current, higher spatial resolution) or the large spot (higher tube current, lower spatial resolution).

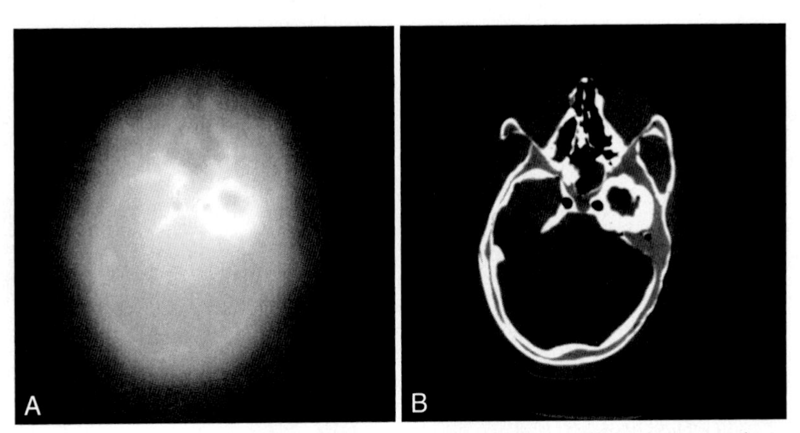

FIGURE 9-7 Images of a head phantom to illustrate the impact of the convolution process. **A,** Reconstructed with back-projection only. **B,** Reconstructed with filtered back-projection.

The in-plane resolution is also strongly influenced by the reconstruction algorithm. Chapter 6 indicates that image reconstruction involves two mathematical procedures: convolution and back-projection. Essentially, if the projection profiles are back-projected without correction, blurring results (Fig. 9-7, *A*). To sharpen the image, a convolution process (a ramp filter) is applied to modify the frequency contents of the projection before back-projection (Fig. 9-7, *B*). The convolution algorithm, or kernel, affects the appearance of image structures. Convolution algorithms have been developed for each anatomic-specific application. In general, these algorithms are applied to emphasize soft tissue (standard algorithm) and bone (bone algorithm). The former is applied to the mid brain, pancreas, adrenal, or any soft tissue region, and the latter is applied to bony structures such as the inner ear and extremities. As an illustration, two images in Figure 9-8 are reconstructed from the same scan data with two different reconstruction kernels. Figure 9-8, *A*, was reconstructed with a standard kernel and Figure 9-8, *B*, with a bone kernel. It is clear that the bone kernel produces a much sharper image (higher spatial resolution) as demonstrated by the

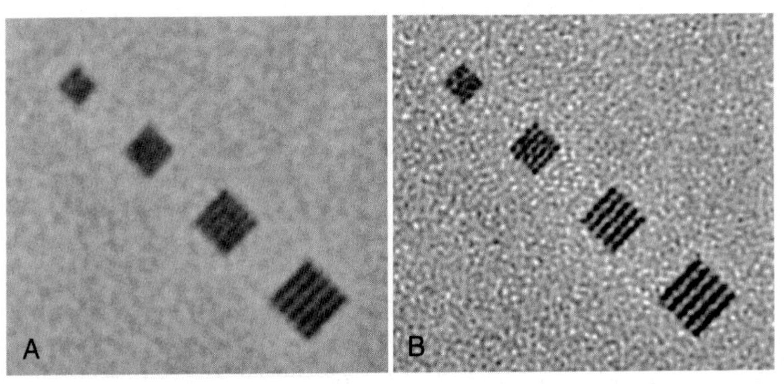

FIGURE 9-8 Impact of the selection of reconstruction kernel on spatial resolution. **A,** Reconstructed with a standard kernel. **B,** Reconstructed with a bone kernel.

bar patterns. It is also worth pointing out that increased noise often accompanies the spatial resolution improvement. Similar clinical examples are given in Figure 9-9, where a lung scan was reconstructed with a standard (*A*) and a lung kernel (*B*).

Another parameter that affects the spatial resolution is the reconstruction field of view (FOV). On the basis of the Nyquist sampling theory, the sampling interval (pixel size) has to be sufficiently small to support the reconstruction and visualization of small objects. The pixel size is related to FOV by the following equation:

$$\text{Pixel size} = \frac{\text{FOV}}{\text{Matrix size}} \tag{9-1}$$

For a 50-cm FOV at a matrix size of 512 × 512, the pixel size is 0.98 mm (500 mm/512). If the FOV is reduced to 10 cm, the pixel size is 0.20 mm. (This is often referred to as targeting.) To illustrate the impact of pixel size, Figure 9-10 depicts images reconstructed with the same projection dataset at two different FOVs. Both Figures 9-10, *A* and *B*, were reconstructed with a 50-cm FOV. The reconstructed image was then interpolated in image space to a 10-cm FOV to produce Figure 9-10, *B*. Figure 9-10, *C*, was reconstructed directly to 10-cm FOV. Note that for the 10-cm target-reconstructed image, all bar patterns are clearly visible, whereas even the fourth largest bar pattern is barely visible for the reconstructed images with 50-cm FOV.

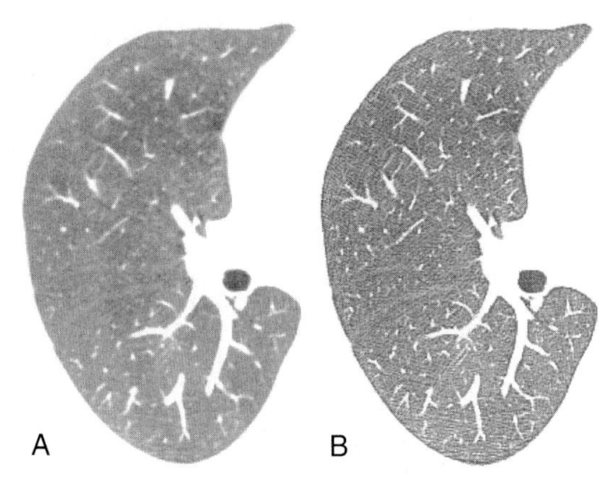

FIGURE 9-9 A patient chest scan reconstructed with different kernels. **A,** Standard algorithm. **B,** Lung algorithm.

Cross-Plane Spatial Resolution

The introduction of helical/spiral and multislice/volumetric CT has fundamentally changed the way many radiologists view CT images. Historically, CT images were always viewed one slice at a time. New technologies have enabled radiologists to view images in three dimensions by using

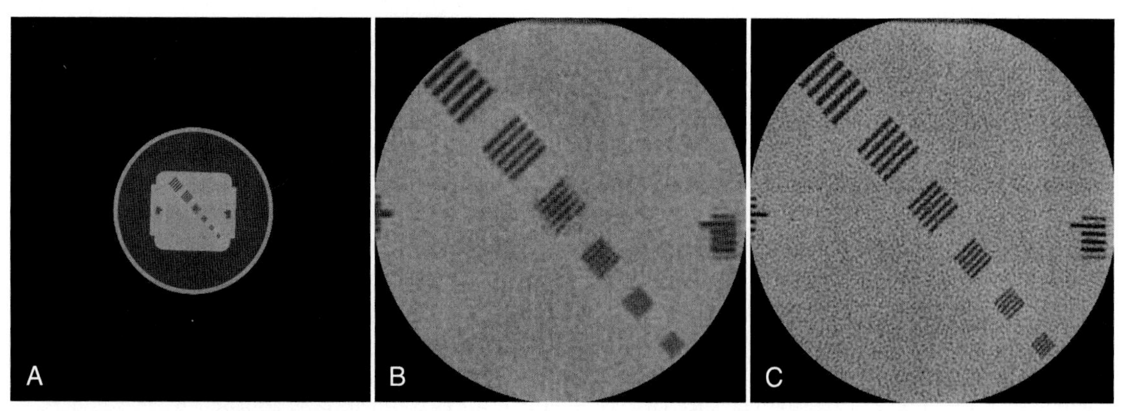

FIGURE 9-10 Images reconstructed with different FOVs. **A,** Reconstructed with 50-cm FOV. **B,** Reconstructed with 50-cm FOV and interpolated to 10-cm FOV. **C,** Targeted reconstruction to 10-cm FOV.

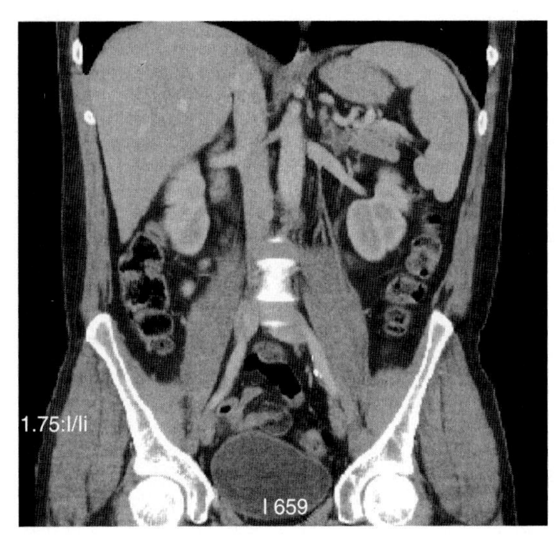

FIGURE 9-11 Coronal view of a patient study scanned on a LightSpeed scanner.

multiplanar reformat (MPR), maximum-intensity-projection (MIP), or volume rendering (VR). One such example is shown in Figure 9-11, where a coronal view of a patient study is displayed. It is difficult to tell from the image alone whether the data were acquired slice by slice or directly in the coronal plane. This demonstrates that the spatial resolution of the state-of-the-art scanner is nearly isotropic.

Improved cross-plane spatial resolution also reduces artifacts caused by partial volume averaging. Figure 9-12 presents a comparison of the spatial resolution afforded by two slices of different thicknesses. Thin slice imaging of lung "is currently the most accurate noninvasive tool for evaluation of lung structure" (Mayo, 1991).

Cross-plane spatial resolution is traditionally described by the slice sensitivity profile (SSP). Similar to the in-plane resolution, SSP represents the system response to a Dirac delta function. In practice, the Dirac delta function is often approximated by an object whose thickness is significantly smaller than the slice thickness of the system. For example, researchers use a small bead or a thin disk to perform SSP measurement. The disk is placed perpendicular to the z-axis and a series of scans are collected to construct the SSP. In many cases, the SSP curve itself is replaced by two numbers: the full width at half-maximum (FWHM) and the full width at tenth-maximum (FWTM). Definitions of FWHM and FWTM are illustrated in Figure 9-13, where FWHM represents the distance between two points on the SSP curve whose intensity is 50% of the peak and FWTM

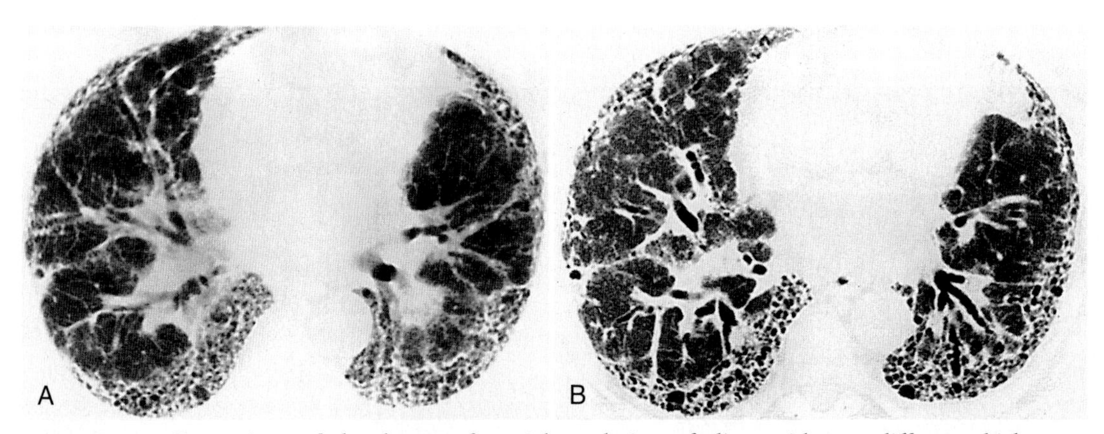

FIGURE 9-12 Comparison of the degree of spatial resolution of slices with two different thicknesses. The spatial resolution of the thinner slice **(B)** taken with 1.5-mm collimation is apparent when compared with the image of the slice taken with 10-mm collimation **(A)**. (From Mayo JR: High-resolution computed tomography, *Radiol Clin North Am* 29:1043-1048, 1991.)

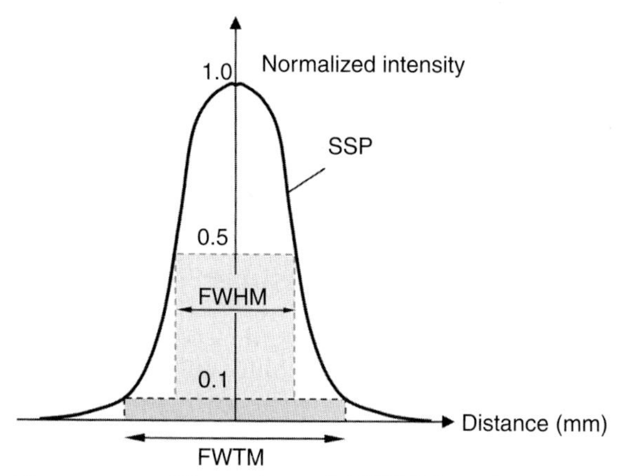

FIGURE 9-13 Illustration of FWHM and FWTM. FWHM represents the distance between two points on the SSP curve whose intensity is 50% of the peak. FWTM represents the distance between two points on the SSP whose intensity is 10% of the peak.

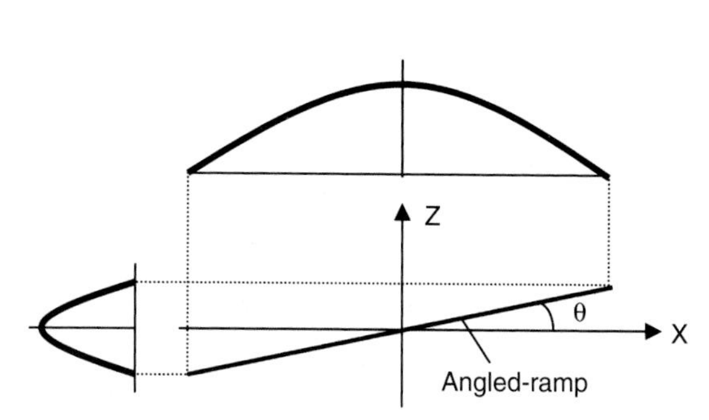

FIGURE 9-14 Illustration of measurement of slice-sensitivity profile by a shallow-angled slice ramp. The slice ramp is projected onto the x-y plane during reconstruction. A magnified version of the SSP is produced.

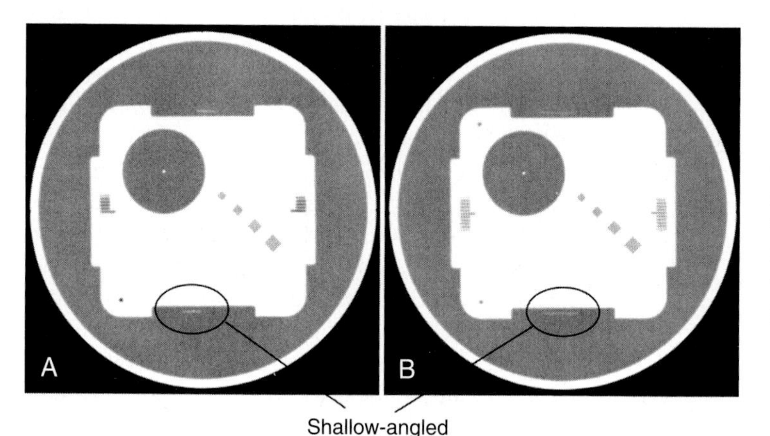

FIGURE 9-15 Illustration of the use of slice ramp to measure SSP. **A,** Acquired with 5-mm slice thickness in step-and-shoot mode. **B,** Acquired with 10-mm slice thickness in step-and-shoot mode.

represents the distance between two points on the SSP whose intensity is 10% of the peak.

A more convenient method of measuring SSP is to use a shallow-angled slice ramp (Goodenough et al, 1977; Hsieh, 2001). A line or thin strip is placed at a shallow angle with respect to the x-y plane. During the scan, the line or thin strip is projected onto the x-y plane, as shown in Figure 9-14. On the basis of simple trigonometry, the SSP in z is magnified by a factor, $1/\tan(\theta)$, where θ is the angle of the strip formed with the x-y plane. When θ is small, the magnification factor is large. For example, Catphan phantom uses a 23-degree ramp to produce a 2.4-fold enlargement in the measured SSP. Therefore, the FWHM of the system, Z_{FWHM}, can be calculated from the FWHM measurement of the wire in the reconstructed image, W_{FWHM}, by:

$$Z_{FWHM} = W_{FWHM} \times 0.42 \tag{9-2}$$

For illustration, Figure 9-15 shows a GE Performance phantom scanned with a 5-mm and a 10-mm detector aperture in a step-and-shoot mode. It is clear from the figure that the image of the slice ramp is twice as wide for the 10-mm case as for the 5-mm, indicating a linear relationship between the width of the reconstructed wire and the thickness of the slice. It is also clear that a significant reduction in contrast is observed for the 10-mm case as a result of the partial volume effect.

It should be noted that once the SSP is obtained, MTF can be calculated in a straightforward fashion by taking the Fourier transform of the SSP. As the spatial resolutions in all orientations become isotropic, it is more convenient and reasonable to specify both the in-plane and cross-plane resolution in a similar fashion, such as MTF.

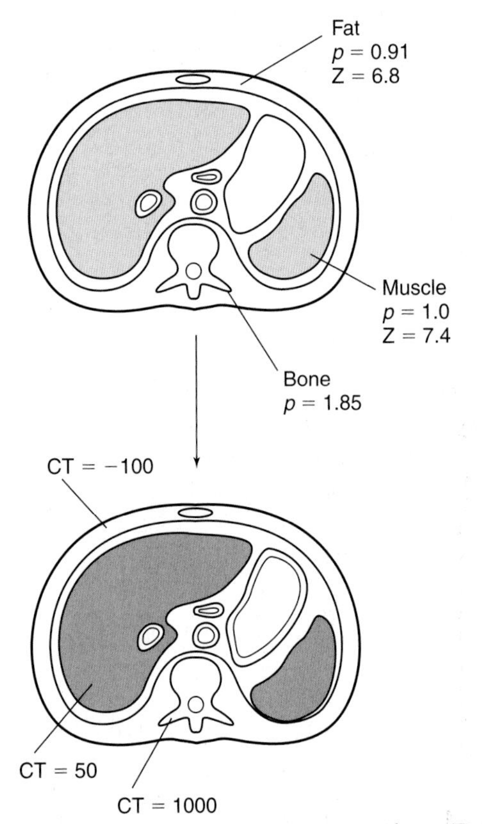

FIGURE 9-16 Densities *(p)* and atomic numbers *(Z)* for three types of tissue. When they are imaged by CT, excellent low-contrast resolution is obtained. (From Bushong S: *Radiologic science for technologists*, ed 9, St Louis, 2009, Mosby.)

LOW-CONTRAST RESOLUTION

Definition and Measurements

One of the key advantages of CT over conventional radiography is its ability to observe low-contrast objects whose density is slightly different from the background. In CT, this is sometimes referred to as the *sensitivity of the system* (Hounsfield, 1978). To understand low-contrast resolution, consider three tissues of different densities and atomic number (Z), as shown in Figure 9-16. If these tissues were imaged by conventional radiography, the obtained image would have shown good contrast between bone and soft tissue (muscle and fat) only. The values of the density and Z for muscle and fat are too close to be clearly distinguished by radiography, and they appear as "soft tissue shadows." The contrast between bone with a Z of 13.8 and soft tissue with a Z of 7.4 is apparent because of the significant difference between the densities and Z of these two tissues. CT, on the other hand, can image tissues that vary only slightly in density and atomic number. Although radiography can discriminate a density difference of about 10% (Curry et al, 1990), CT can detect density differences from 0.25% to 0.5%, depending on the scanner (Hsieh, 2003).

Low-contrast resolution can be measured with phantoms that contain low-contrast objects of different sizes. The low-contrast performance or low-contrast detectability (LCD) of the scanner is typically defined as the smallest object that can be visualized at a given contrast level and dose. For illustration, Figure 9-17 shows a low-contrast portion of a Catphan. There are three sets of discs with contrast of 0.3%, 0.5%, and 1.0%, and the sizes of the discs are 2 mm, 3 mm, 4 mm, 5 mm, 6 mm, 7 mm, 8 mm, 9 mm, and 15 mm. In CT, the contrast level is specified in terms of the percent linear attenuation coefficient. A 1% contrast means that the mean CT number of the object differs from its background by 10 Hounsfield units (HU).

Factors That Affect Low-Contrast Detectability

From the definition of LCD, it can easily be concluded that the visibility of an object depends not only on its size but also on its contrast (intensity difference) to the background. This is easily demonstrated with the Catphan. Note that the three sets of objects are of matching sizes. The discs located from the 10 o'clock to 2 o'clock positions are more easily visualized than the ones that are located from the 2 to 6 o'clock positions. The difference in contrast between these two sets is 7 HU. The figure also illustrates the impact of the object size on the LCD. As the object size decreases, the confidence level of identifying a 0.3% disc decreases.

The LCD definition also implies that an object's visibility is highly influenced by the presence of noise. To demonstrate this effect, the low-contrast portion of a GE Performance Phantom was scanned with two different tube currents: 200 mA and 50 mA; the reconstructed images are shown in Figure 9-18. All other acquisition parameters were kept the same. The noise for the 50-mA scan is a factor of two higher compared with the 200-mA case (one fourth of the dose). For the 200-mA scan, all four low-density holes are clearly identifiable, whereas the smallest hole is obscured by the noise for the 50-mA scan.

Many factors affect the noise level in the reconstructed images. Some of them can be controlled by the operator, and others are outside the operator's reach. The parameters under operator control include x-ray tube voltage (in kV), tube current (in mA), scan speed (in seconds), helical pitch, and slice thickness. The selection of the parameters, however, is not straightforward. For example, by increasing the tube current, a noise reduction, better LCD, can be achieved.

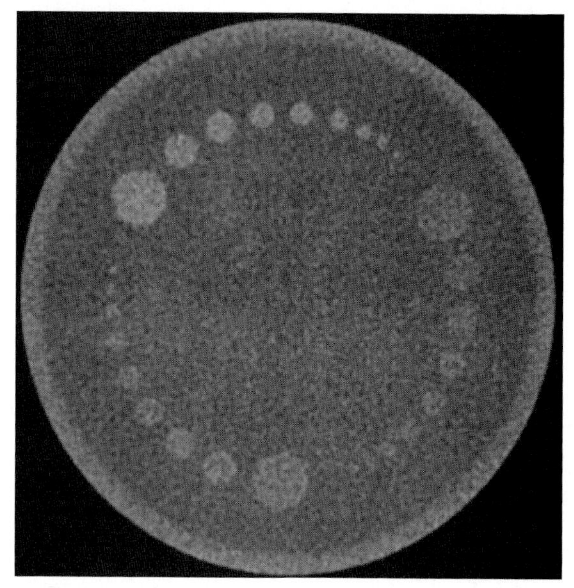

FIGURE 9-17 Image of a low-contrast portion of the Catphan phantom.

However, increased tube current translates to a higher dose to the patient and, potentially, runs the risk of a tube cooling (forced delay during scans to prevent the tube from overheating).

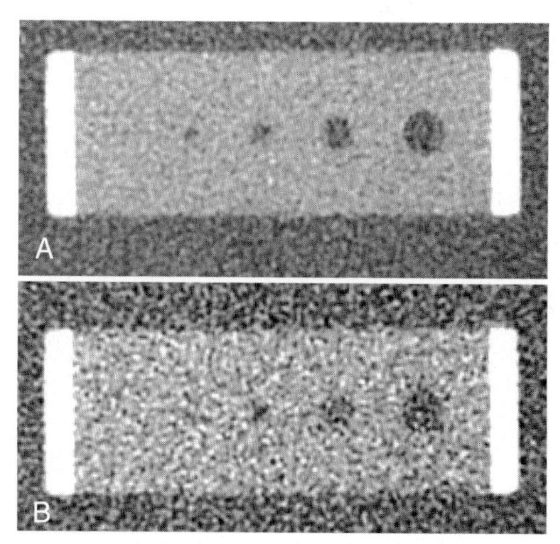

FIGURE 9-18 Illustration of the impact of noise to low-contrast detectability. **A,** Acquired with 200 mA and standard algorithm. **B,** Acquired with 50 mA and standard algorithm.

Similarly, although the use of a higher tube voltage (kV) results in improved x-ray photon statistics (therefore lower noise in the image), the quality of the x-ray beam is somewhat compromised because the visibility of low-contrast objects depends on the presence of low-energy photons, which are disproportionally less for the higher tube voltage. Consequently, LCD may not improve or degrade with an increased kV. The same applies to the selection of slice thickness. Although, in general, an image with a thicker slice contains more x-ray photons (less noise), the partial volume effect can reduce the visibility of smaller objects. This is illustrated in Figure 9-19, where the low-contrast portion of the GE Performance Phantom was reconstructed with 3.75-mm and 7.5-mm slice thickness. Because the phantom is made of a thin plate (less than 1 mm in thickness), a thicker slice produces a larger partial volume effect and reduces the contrast of the object. As a result, although the noise is reduced with the 7.5-mm thickness, the LCD of the low-density objects is reduced as well.

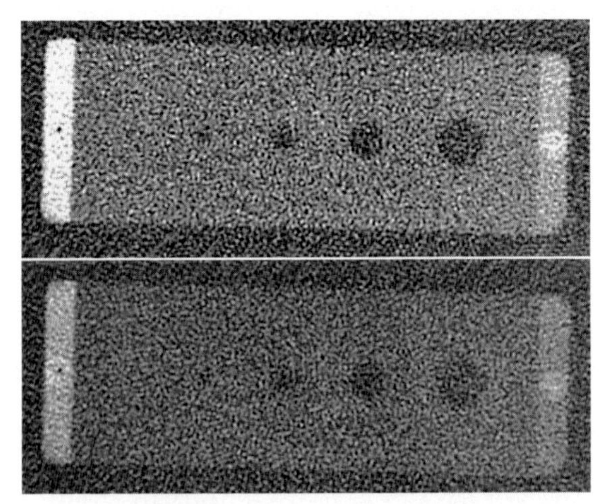

FIGURE 9-19 Illustration of the impact of slice thickness, at 3.75 mm *(top)* and 7.5 mm *(bottom)*.

TEMPORAL RESOLUTION

Temporal resolution is an indication of a CT system's ability to freeze motions of the scanned object. An oversimplified analogy is the "shutter" speed of a camera. When a photo is taken at a sports event, a higher shutter speed should be used to reduce the blurring effects caused by the moving athletes. The awareness and importance of the temporal resolution for CT scanners has increased significantly in recent years thanks to cardiac imaging. Because the heart motion is continuous and often irregular, cardiac imaging is one of the most challenging clinical applications for CT.

Factors That Affect Temporal Resolution

There are several methods that improve a CT scanner's ability to freeze the cardiac motion. The most straightforward way to reduce or eliminate the motion impact is to increase the scan speed. The state-of-the-art third-generation multislice scanners are capable of rotating at speeds of 0.3 to 0.4 seconds per gantry rotation. Considering the size of a typical CT gantry (1 meter), and the weight of the components on the rotating side (hundreds of pounds), the centrifugal force is huge. One attempt to overcome the mechanical difficulty is the use of an electron-beam scanner in which high-speed electrons are deflected by the specially designed magnetic field so that x-ray photons are generated along an arc surrounding the patient. Because there is no moving part for such a scanner, scan speeds as high as 33 milliseconds can be achieved.

It should be noted that even at the speed of 33 milliseconds, it is insufficient to completely freeze the cardiac motion. Therefore all third-generation CT scanners also rely on reconstruction algorithms that use less than a full rotation of projection data for reconstruction (Parker, 1982). The most commonly used algorithm is the so-called half-scan algorithm in which the projection dataset in the view range of 180 degrees plus fan angle are used. For typical CT scanner geometries, this represents a 220-degree, or roughly 40%, improvement in terms of temporal resolution. To further improve the temporal resolution of the scanner, multisector reconstruction is also used in which the 220 degrees of projection data are acquired over multiple cardiac cycles (Hsieh, 2003). Typically, the dataset is uniformly divided over these heart cycles to optimize the performance. Because of the limited scope of this chapter, the details are not discussed.

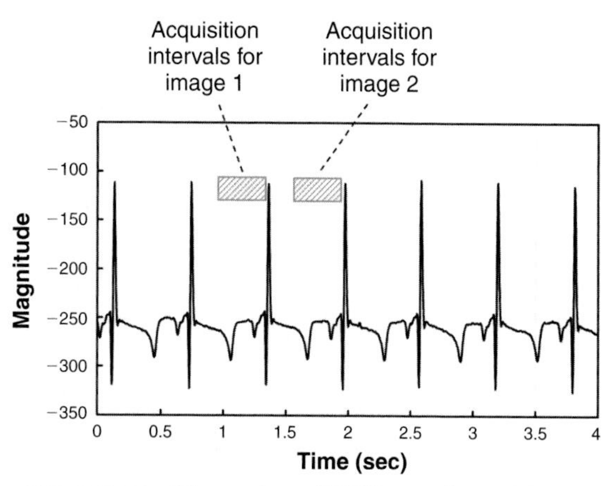

FIGURE 9-20 Illustration of ECG-gated acquisition.

Techniques to Reduce Motion Impact

A technique used by all CT vendors incorporates a physiological gating device for cardiac imaging (Hsieh et al, 1999; Kachelriess et al, 2000). Although this approach does not improve the temporal resolution of the scanner, it helps to minimize the heart motion. In a typical cardiac motion cycle, there are quiescent time periods in which the heart is in a relatively motionless state. These correspond to the diastole and systole phases of the heart. Therefore if the data acquisition takes place during these time periods, fewer motion artifacts can be expected. This can be accomplished by synchronizing the data acquisition and reconstruction with an electrocardiographic (ECG) signal, as shown in Figure 9-20. This can be performed either retrospectively or prospectively. The advantage of a prospective gating is the reduction in x-ray dose to the patient. The x-ray tube can be shut off during the non–data acquisition periods to minimize the x-ray exposure. The disadvantage of the prospective gating is its reliance on the regularity of the heart motion because the data acquisition timing for the current cardiac cycle is predicted on the basis of previous heart cycles. For compromise, x-ray tube current modulation is often used in practice in which the x-ray tube current is reduced to a fraction of the peak current during the nonquiescent time periods. It provides a balance between patient dose and image quality. To illustrate the impact of ECG gating, Figure 9-21 depicts two reconstructed cardiac images, with and without the proper ECG gating. Motion artifact reduction with ECG gating is obvious.

For cardiac imaging, there is another important factor that affects the image quality: coverage. Note that all the commercially available CT scanners today cannot cover the entire heart (12 to 16 cm) in a single rotation. Consequently, the heart volume has to be scanned over multiple heart cycles, with each cycle covering a subsection of the heart. Superb temporal resolution only ensures that within each subsection the motion-induced image degradation is kept to a minimum. It does not guarantee, however, that the heart is in exactly the same state from one subsection to the next. This is determined mainly by the consistency of the heart motion from cycle to cycle. Studies have shown that the probability of a stable heart rate decreases quickly as the total data acquisition time increases. The total data acquisition time is determined by the gantry speed, helical pitch, and detector coverage. For the same gantry speed and helical pitch, a larger detector-coverage translates

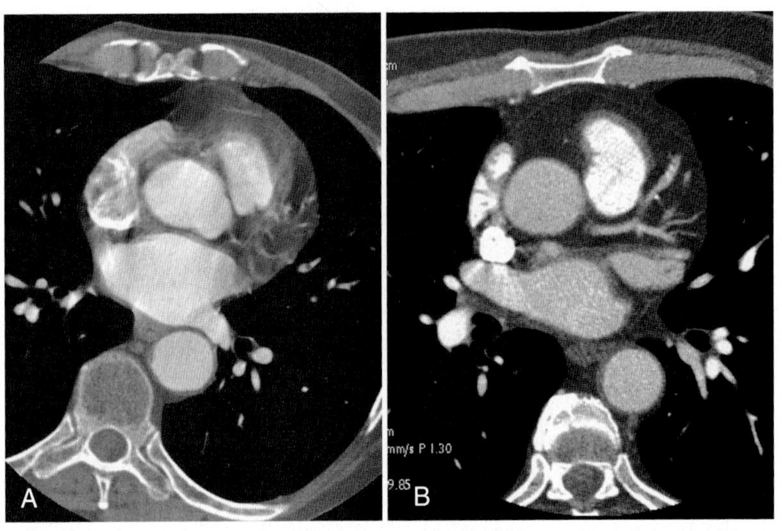

FIGURE 9-21 Impact of ECG gating in cardiac imaging. **A,** Nongated cardiac acquisition. **B,** ECG-gated acquisition.

to a faster study time and, in turn, an improved probability of a consistent cardiac volume. Figure 9-22 shows a reformatted image of a heart vessel with phase misregistration. The vessel looks discontinuous and can lead to misdiagnosis.

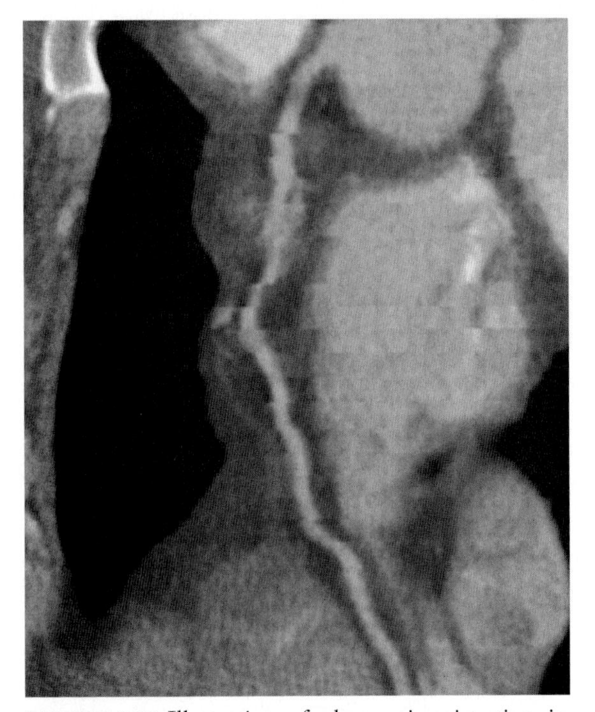

FIGURE 9-22 Illustration of phase misregistration in cardiac imaging.

CT NUMBER ACCURACY AND UNIFORMITY

Accuracy and Linearity

The CT number is related to the attenuation coefficient of the object by the following equation:

$$\text{CT number} = \frac{\mu - \mu_w}{\mu_w} \times 1000 \qquad (9\text{-}3)$$

where μ_w is the attenuation coefficient of water. On the basis of this definition, two points are defined precisely on the CT number scale. The first is water with a CT number of 0 and the second is air with a CT number of −1000. Because water is similar to the soft tissue in terms of attenuation characteristics, it is important to establish its accuracy for CT scanners. Nearly all CT manufacturers provide phantoms filled with water for such testing. When the phantom is scanned, the average CT number in the water portion should be fairly close to 0.

Linearity is another important parameter in CT image quality. *Linearity* refers to the relationship of CT numbers to the linear attenuation coefficients of the object to be imaged. This can be checked by a daily calibration test, during which an appropriate phantom is scanned to ensure that the CT numbers for water and other known materials of which the phantom is made are correct. Such phantom characteristics are given in Table 9-1. For illustration, Figure 9-23 depicts a linearity section of the Catphan with the large cylinders filled with Teflon, Delrin, acrylic, polystyrene, air, polymethylpentene, and low-density polyethylene. The CT numbers of the reconstructed cylinders are used to check the acceptance of the CT system. The average CT numbers can also be plotted as a function of the attenuation coefficients of the phantom materials. The relationship should be a straight line (Fig. 9-24) if the scanner is in good working order (Bushong, 1997).

Uniformity

CT number uniformity dictates that for a uniform phantom, the CT number measurement should not change with the location of the selected regions of interest (ROI) or with the phantom position relative to the isocenter of the scanner. For illustration, Figure 9-25 shows a reconstructed 20-cm water phantom. Theoretically, the average CT numbers in two ROI locations should be identical. Because of the effect of

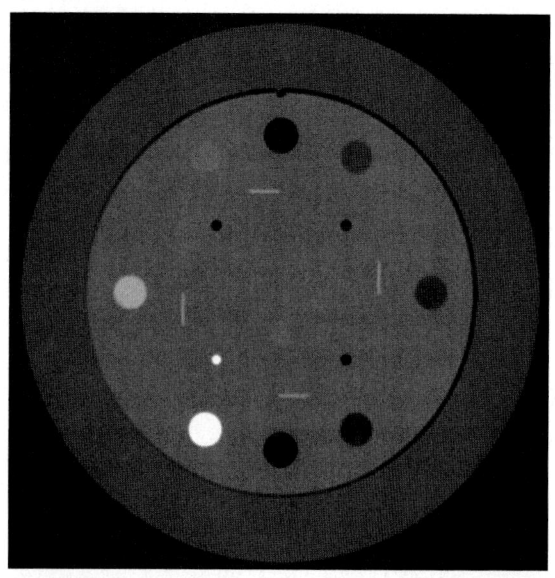

FIGURE 9-23 Linearity insert of the Catphan. The eight larger cylinders are filled with Teflon, Delrin, acrylic, polystyrene, air, PMP, and LDPE.

TABLE 9-1 Characteristics of the American Association of Physicists in Medicine Computed Tomography Phantom

Material	Density (g/ml)	Linear Attenuation Coefficient (cm^{-1}) at 60 keV	Approximate CT Number
Polyethylene, C_2H_4	0.94	0.185	−85
Polystyrene, C_8H_8	1.05	0.196	−10
Nylon, $C_6H_{11}NO$	1.15	0.222	100
Lexan, $C_{16}H_{14}O$	1.20	0.223	115
Plexiglas, $C_5H_8O_2$	1.19	0.229	130
Water, H_2O	1.00	0.206	0

Modified from Bushong S: *Radiologic science for technologists*, ed 9, St Louis, 2009, Mosby.

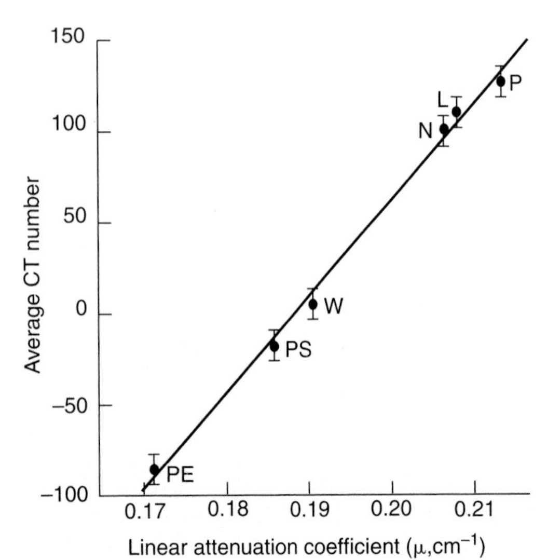

FIGURE 9-24 Plot of average CT numbers as a function of linear attenuation coefficients. This indicates acceptable CT linearity if the relationship is a straight line. (From Bushong S: *Radiologic science for technologists*, ed 9, St Louis, 2009, Mosby.)

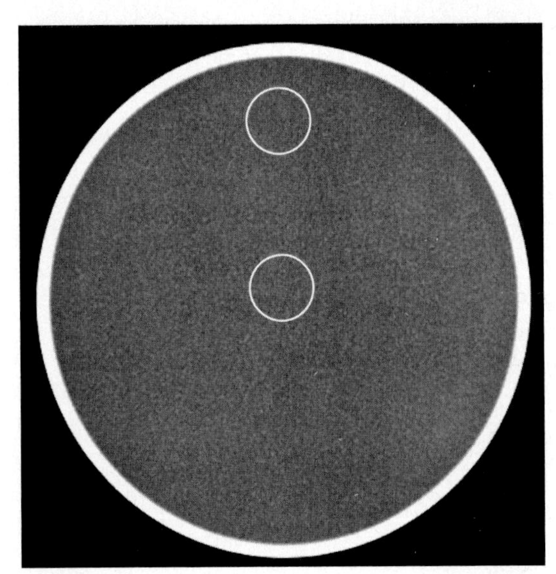

FIGURE 9-25 Water phantom for CT number uniformity measurement.

beam hardening, scatter, stability of the CT system, and many other factors, the CT number uniformity can only be maintained within a reasonable range (typically 2 HU). As long as the operator understands the system limitations and the factors that influence the performance, he or she can avoid potential pitfalls of using absolute CT numbers for diagnosis.

NOISE

Measurements

On the basis of the discussion on LCD, the importance of image noise is obvious. Image noise is measured typically on uniform phantoms. To perform noise measurement, the standard deviation, σ, within an ROI of the reconstructed image, $f(i,j)$, is calculated as follows:

$$\delta = \sqrt{\frac{\sum_{i,j \in \mathrm{ROI}} [f(i,j) - \bar{f}]^2}{N - 1}} \tag{9-4}$$

where i and j are indices of the two-dimensional image, N is the total number of pixels inside the ROI, and f is the average pixel intensity and is calculated by the following equation:

$$\bar{f} = \frac{1}{N} \sum_{i,j \in \mathrm{ROI}} f(i,j) \tag{9-5}$$

In both equations, the summation is two dimensional over the ROI. For robustness, several ROIs are often used and the average value of the measured standard deviations is reported.

Noise Sources

Three major sources contribute to the noise in the image. The first source is the quantum noise determined by the x-ray flux or the number of detected x-ray photons. It is influenced by the scanning techniques (e.g., x-ray tube voltage, tube current, slice thickness, scan speed, and helical pitch), the scanner efficiency (e.g., detector quantum efficiency, detector geometrical efficiency, amber-penumbra ratio), and patient (e.g., patient size, amount of bones and soft tissues in the scanning plane). The scanning technique dictates the number of x-ray photons that reach the patient, and the scanner efficiency determines the percentage of the x-ray photons exiting the patient converted to useful signals. The LCD section briefly discusses the tradeoffs of different acquisition parameters. As long as the tradeoffs are well understood, these options can be used effectively to combat noise. More advanced scanners offer features that allow the operator to select a noise level, and the CT system will determine the x-ray tube current required to achieve a specified noise level. Because the patient anatomy changes with location, the x-ray tube current typically changes as a function of tube angle as well as the location along the patient long axis.

The second source that influences the noise performance is the inherent physical limitations of the system. These include the electronic noise in the detector photodiode, the electronic noise in the data acquisition system (DAS), scattered radiation, and many other factors. Figure 9-26 shows an oval phantom scanned with two different DAS's while all other acquisition parameters were kept constant. Significant reduction in image noise can be observed with the lower-noise DAS.

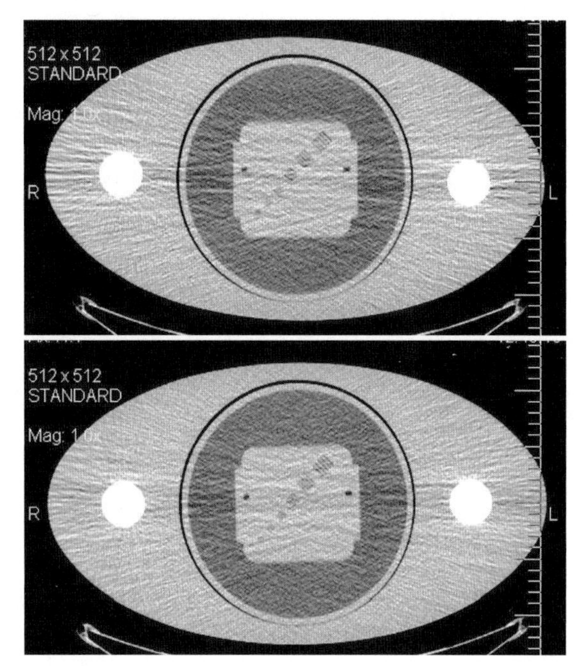

FIGURE 9-26 Illustration of DAS noise impact. *Top*, Old vintage DAS; *bottom*, new low-noise DAS.

The third noise-influencing factor is the reconstruction parameters. In general, a high-resolution reconstruction kernel produces an increased noise level. This is mainly because these kernels preserve or enhance high-frequency contents in the projection. Unfortunately, most noise presents itself as high-frequency signals. An example of the impact of filter kernel selection on noise is shown in Figure 9-8. Note that the noise level of Figure 9-8, *B*, is significantly higher than in Figure 9-8, *A*.

Noise Power Spectrum

It should be pointed out that standard deviation alone is insufficient to fully characterize the noise in the image. This is because noise in the reconstructed images is no longer white. This characteristic can be described by the noise power spectrum, or Wiener spectrum (Riederer et al, 1978). Figure 9-27 shows that the noise power spectrum is obtained with the Fourier transform to break down the image noise into its frequency components. To illustrate the impact of noise spectrum on the image, Figure 9-28 shows a low-contrast phantom scanned with different tube currents and reconstructed with different kernels, one with the standard kernel and the other with the bone kernel. The tube currents were selected such that both images have the same standard deviation. However, the visibility of the low-contrast objects is clearly different. This demonstrates the importance of the fact that, to fully characterize the noise in the image, standard deviation alone is insufficient.

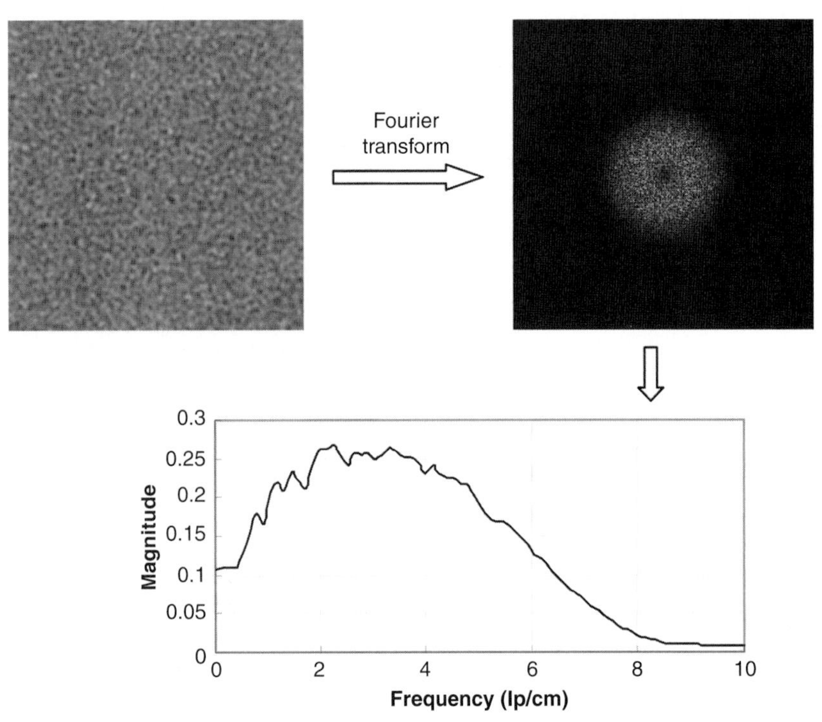

FIGURE 9-27 Generation of noise power spectrum.

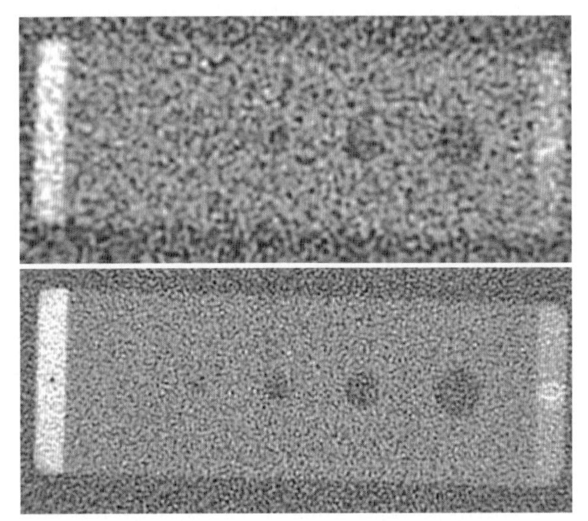

FIGURE 9-28 Illustration of noise power spectrum impact. Both images have identical standard deviations.

IMAGE ARTIFACT

Definition and General Discussion

Artifacts can degrade image quality, affect the perceptibility of detail, or even lead to misdiagnosis. This can cause serious problems for the radiologist who has to provide a diagnosis from images obtained by the technologist. Therefore it is mandatory that the technologist understand the nature of artifacts in CT.

In general, an *artifact* is "a distortion or error in an image that is unrelated to the subject being studied" (Morgan, 1983). Specifically, a *CT image artifact* is defined as "any discrepancy between the reconstructed CT numbers in the image and the true attenuation coefficients of the object" (Hsieh,

1995). This definition is comprehensive and implies that anything that causes an incorrect measurement of transmission readings by the detectors will result in an image artifact. Because CT numbers represent gray shades in the image, incorrect measurements will produce incorrect CT numbers that do not represent the attenuation coefficients of the object. These errors result in various artifacts that affect the appearance of the CT image.

In CT, artifacts arise from a number of sources, including the patient, inappropriate selection of protocols, reconstruction process, problems relating to the equipment such as malfunctions or imperfections, and fundamental limitation of physics. In a typical commercial CT system, an image is reconstructed from 10^6 independent projection samples. The contribution of each projection reading, on the other hand, is not limited to an isolated point in the reconstructed image as a result of the convolution and back-projection process discussed in Chapter 6. This is a radical departure from conventional radiographic imaging, in which each measured sample affects only the value of a single pixel in the resulting image. As a result, the probability of an artifact for CT is significantly higher compared with the conventional radiograph. Given the numerous sources of artifacts and the complexity of the artifact manifestation, it is impossible to cover this topic in a short section. This chapter focuses, instead, on the most important artifacts in routine clinical applications. Interested readers can refer to Hsieh (2003) for more comprehensive coverage on this topic.

Types and Causes

Artifacts in CT can be classified according to cause and appearance. In the classification of artifacts on the basis of their appearance in the image, four major categories can be identified, including streaks, shadings, rings and bands, and "miscellaneous" factors such as the basket weave and moiré patterns (Fig. 9-29) (Table 9-2). Streak artifacts may appear as intense straight lines across an image, which may be caused by improper sampling of the data (aliasing), partial volume averaging, motion, metal, beam hardening, noise, spiral/helical scanning, and mechanical failure or imperfections. Streak artifacts are often caused by errors of isolated projection readings (isolated channels and views). These discrepancies are enhanced by the convolution process and manifested into lines during the back-projection, as shown in Figure 9-29, *A*.

Ring or band artifacts are produced when the projection readings of a single channel or a group of channels consistently deviate from the truth. The can be the result of defective detector cells or DAS channels, deficiencies in system calibration, or a suboptimal image-generation process.

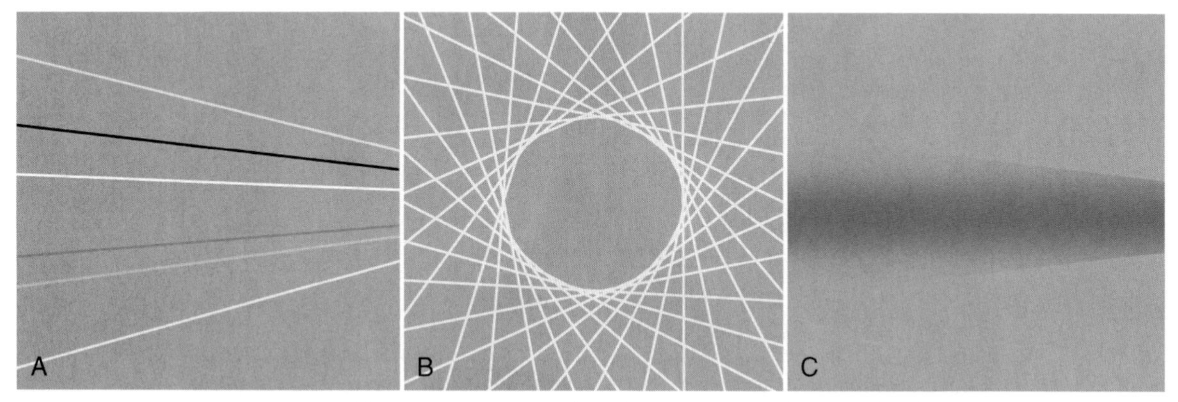

FIGURE 9-29 Different appearances of artifacts. **A**, Streak. **B**, Ring. **C**, shading.

TABLE 9-2 Classification of Artifacts on the Basis of Appearance

Appearance	Cause
Streaks	Improper sampling of data; partial volume averaging; patient motion; metal; beam hardening; noise; spiral/helical scanning; mechanical failure
Shading	Partial volume averaging; beam hardening; spiral/helical scanning; scatter radiation; off-focal radiation; incomplete projections
Rings and bands	Bad detector channels in third-generation CT scanners

This is predominately a third-generation CT scanner phenomenon. Because a detector channel reading is always mapped to a straight line that is at a fixed distance to the isocenter of the system, a defective reading forms a ring pattern during the backprojection process, as illustrated in Figure 9-29, *B*.

Shading artifacts often appear near objects of high densities and can be caused by beam hardening, partial volume averaging, spiral/helical scanning, scatter radiation, off-focal radiation, and incomplete projections. They are formed by the gradual deviation of a group of projection readings over a limited range of views, as shown in Figure 9-29, *C*.

Common Artifacts and Correction Techniques

Patient Motion Artifacts

Patient motion can be voluntary or involuntary. Voluntary motion is directly controlled by the patient, such as swallowing or respiratory motion. Involuntary motion is not under the direct control of the patient, such as head motion with injury, peristalsis, and cardiac motion, as shown in Figures 9-30, *A*, and 9-31, *A*. Both voluntary and involuntary motions appear as streaks that are usually tangential to high-contrast edges of the moving part.

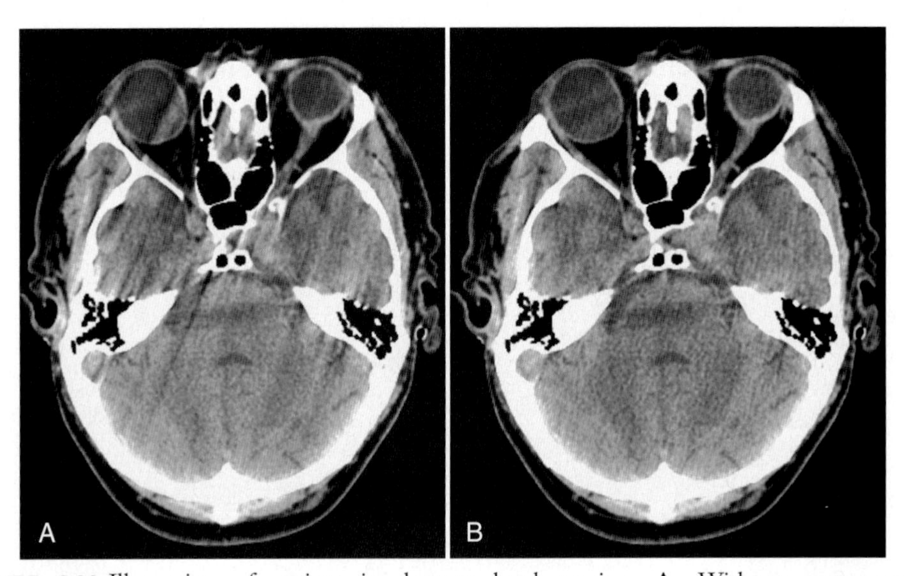

FIGURE 9-30 Illustration of patient involuntary head motion. **A,** Without compensation. **B,** With correction.

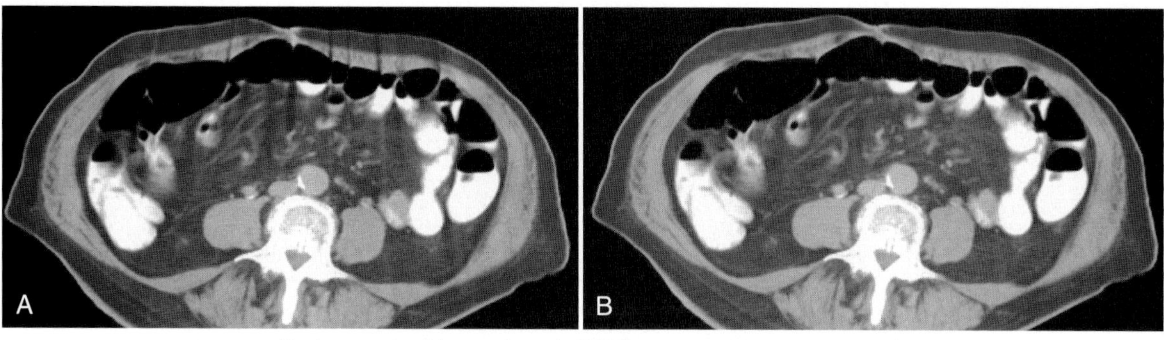

FIGURE 9-31 Patient peristaltic motion. **A,** Without compensation. **B,** With correction.

Additionally, motion artifacts can arise from movement of oral contrast in the gastrointestinal tract.

The appearance of streaks results from the inability of the reconstruction algorithm to deal with data inconsistencies in voxel attenuation arising from the edge of the moving part. There are several methods to reduce CT artifacts from motion. For patient movements such as breathing and swallowing, it is important to immobilize patients and use positioning aids to make them comfortable and to ensure that patients understand the importance of remaining still and following instructions during scanning. Another useful motion artifact reduction technique is to shorten the scan time, as discussed in the temporal resolution section of this chapter. Correction of motion artifacts can also be accomplished with software such as underscan weighting, as shown in Figures 9-30, *B*, and 9-31, *B* (Hsieh, 2003), and physiological gating such as ECG-gated cardiac, as demonstrated in Figure 9-21.

Metal Artifacts

The presence of metal objects in the patient also causes artifacts. Metallic materials such as prosthetic devices, dental fillings, surgical clips, and electrodes give rise to streak artifacts on the image (Fig. 9-32). The creation of these artifacts and a method of correction are illustrated in Figure 9-33. As shown in Figure 9-33, *A*, the metal object is highly attenuating to the radiation, which results in significant error in projection profiles. The error is the combined effects of signal underrange, beam hardening, partial volume, and limited dynamic range of the acquisition and reconstruction systems. The loss of information leads to the appearance of typical star-shaped streaks. It should be pointed out that patient motion is often a major culprit in exacerbating the appearance of artifacts, as illustrated in Figure 9-34 with a pacemaker lead in a patient's heart.

Metal artifacts can be reduced by the removal of all external metal objects from the patient. Software such as the metal artifact reduction (MAR) program can be used to complete the incomplete profile through interpolation (Fig. 9-33, *B*). The procedure is described as follows (Felsenberg et al, 1988):

1. Acquisition and storage of the raw data
2. Reconstruction of a CT image
3. Identification of the implant

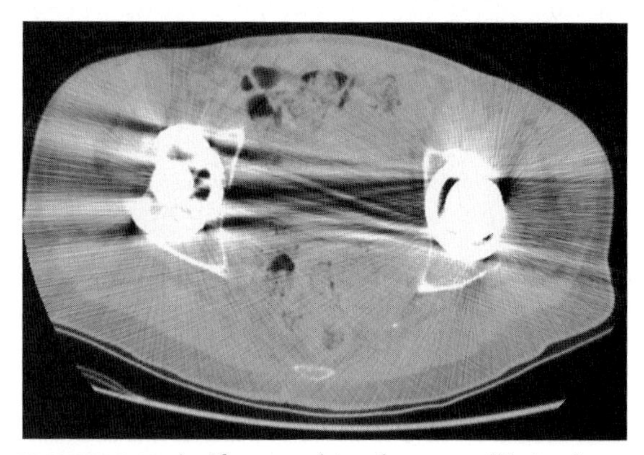

FIGURE 9-32 Artifacts resulting from metallic implants.

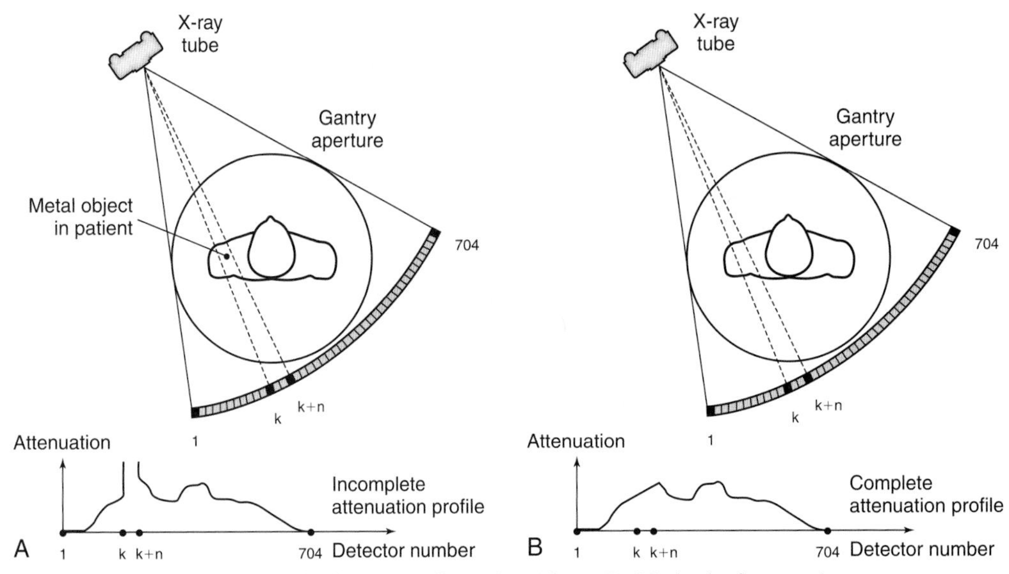

FIGURE 9-33 **A,** Creation of metal artifacts. **B,** Method of correction.

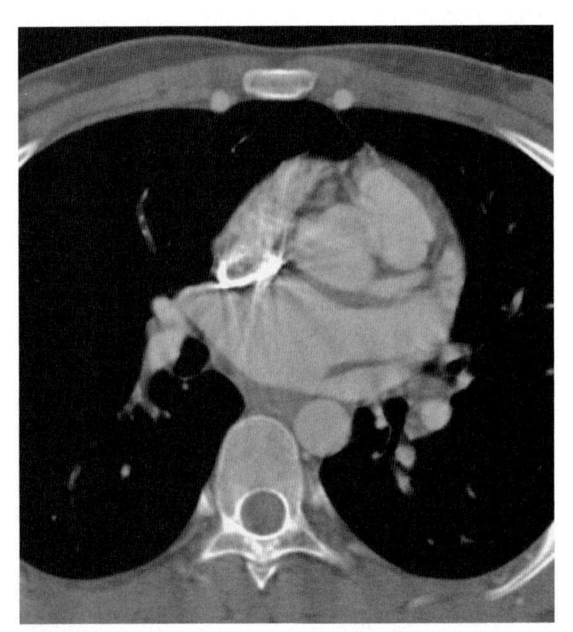

FIGURE 9-34 Illustration of the impact of patient motion on metal artifacts.

4. Automatic definition of the boundaries of the implant within the projection data. For each projection, the implant boundaries are automatically defined within the given ROI by the use of given threshold values.
5. Linear interpolation of the missing projection data
6. Reconstruction of the artifact-reduced image from the newly computed projection data

It should be pointed out that, although metal artifact correction has been the focus of many studies over decades, an effective and robust method is yet to be found. This is due not only to the complexity of the problem (e.g., different type and shape of metals, patient motion, and partial volume), but also to the challenging clinical needs. Radiologists are often interested in the region immediately adjacent to the metal implant to assess the patient condition. Many correction methods, such as the one outlined previously, do not preserve the integrity of such regions.

Beam-Hardening Artifacts

Beam hardening refers to an increase in the mean energy of the x-ray beam as it passes through the patient. As the object size increases, the mean energy shifts to the right because lower energy

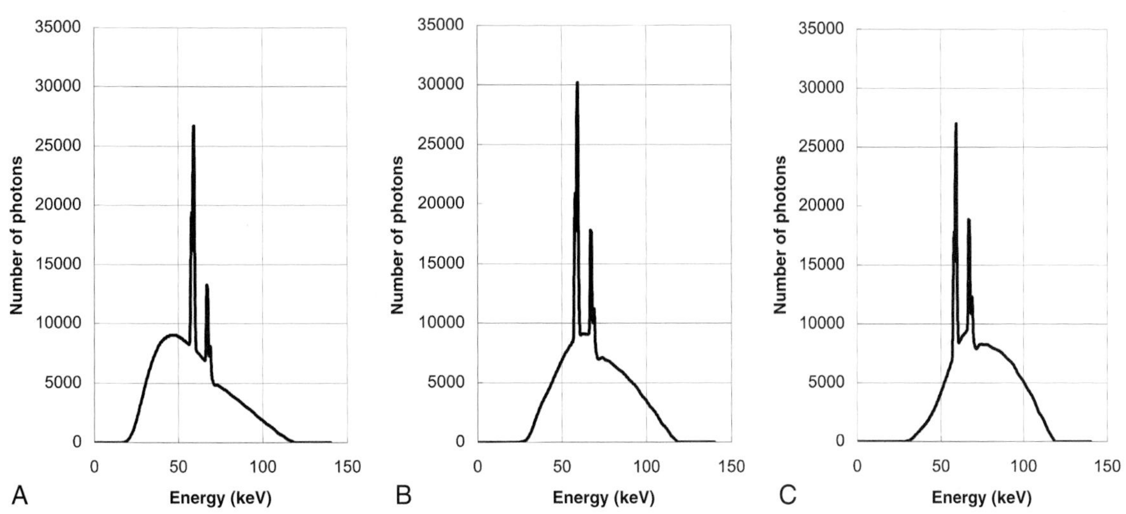

FIGURE 9-35 Effect of beam hardening as the x-ray beam traverses different object sizes. **A,** Original spectrum. **B,** After traversing 15 cm water. **C,** After traversing 30 cm water.

photons are absorbed preferentially as the beam passes through the object. For illustration, we depict the original x-ray tube spectrum, the spectrum after traversing 15 cm water, and the spectrum after traversing 30 cm water (Figure 9-35). For each graph, the number of detected x-ray photons is kept to one million. Note that as the x-ray spectrum is modified, the CT numbers of certain structures change. Additionally, because radiation beams have different path lengths through the object (Fig. 9-36), the x-ray beam spectrum becomes channel dependent. The top portion of Figure 9-36 shows a short and a long path length, which results in different degrees of beam hardening. There is less beam hardening at the periphery of the object, where the radiation path is short, compared with the center of the object, where the radiation path is longer. The bottom portion of Figure 9-36 depicts the intensity profiles of the reconstructed images. Ideally, the intensity should be constant for a uniform object, as shown by the thick solid line. Because of the beam-hardening effect, errors in CT numbers increase gradually from the periphery to the center of the object, as depicted by the dotted line. This artifact can be corrected by performance of a polynomial mapping of the measured projections before the reconstruction (Hsieh, 2003). Figure 9-37 shows two reconstructed images of a 35-cm water phantom with *(B)* and without *(A)* beam-hardening correction.

The beam-hardening effect is material dependent. When dense bones or contrast agents are

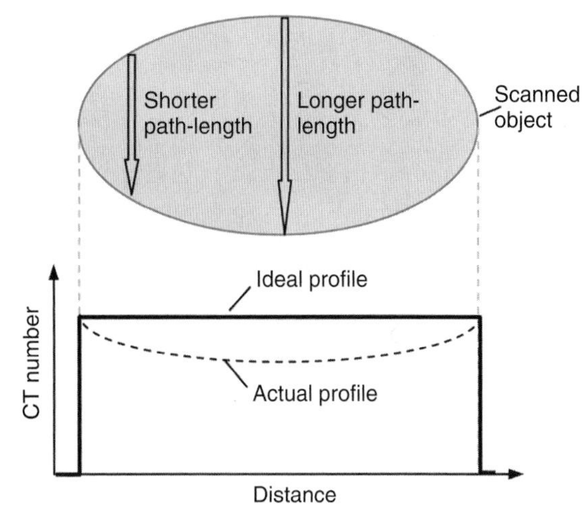

FIGURE 9-36 Illustration of beam-hardening effect.

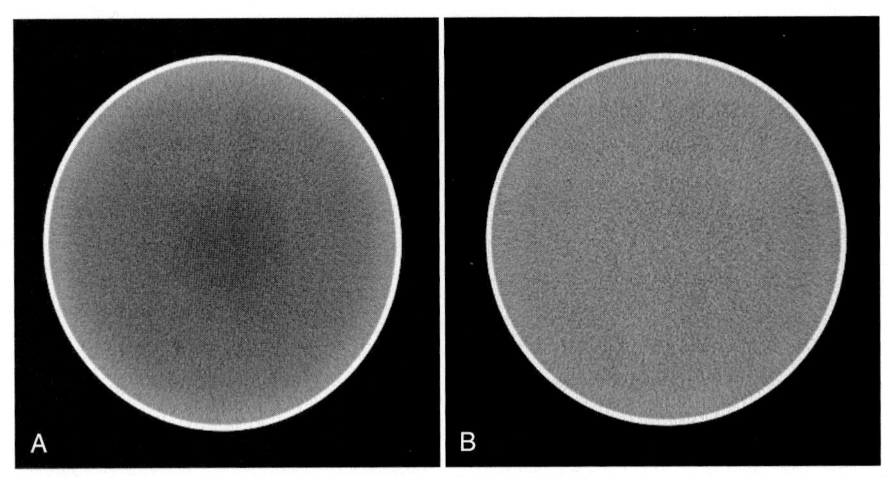

FIGURE 9-37 Reconstructed images of a 35-cm water phantom. **A,** Without beam-hardening correction. **B,** With beam-hardening correction.

present in the beam path, dark shading artifacts can result because the beam-hardening correction applied to soft tissue does not work well for bones. This effect is demonstrated in Figure 9-38, *A*. Note the dark banding connecting the temporal bones. It has been shown that iterative correction is effective in combating such artifacts, as shown by Figure 9-38, *B* (Joseph and Ruth, 1997).

Partial Volume Artifacts

CT numbers are based on the linear attenuation coefficients for a voxel of tissue. If the voxel

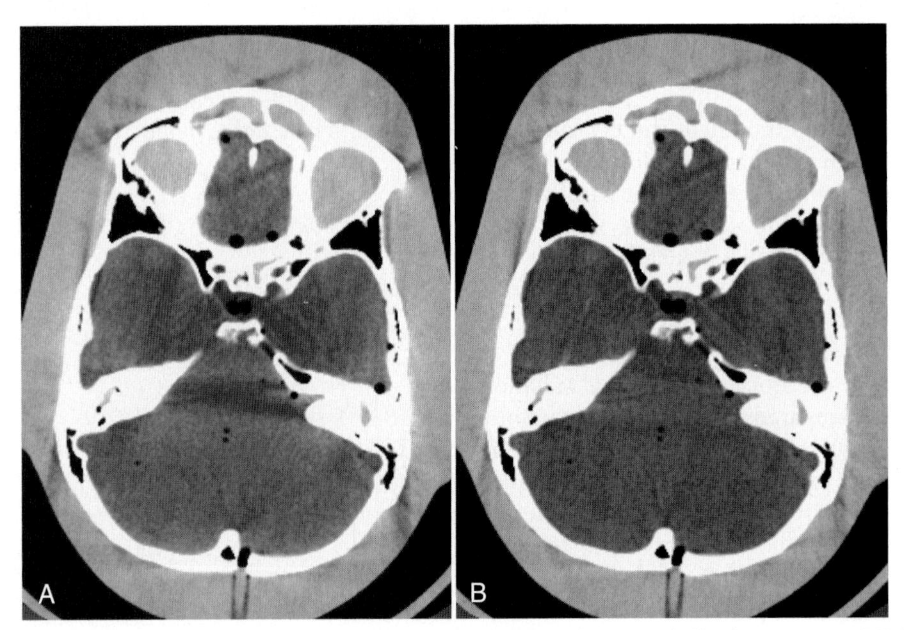

FIGURE 9-38 Illustration of bone beam hardening with a human skull phantom. **A,** Without correction. **B,** With correction.

contains only one tissue type, the calculation will not be problematic. For example, if the tissue in the voxel is gray matter, the CT number is computed at around 43. If the voxel contains three similar tissue types in which the CT numbers are close together—for example, blood (CT number 40), gray matter (43), and white matter (46)—then the CT number for that voxel is based on an average of the three tissues. This is known as *partial volume averaging*.

When the voxel contains multiple materials that are significantly different (e.g., soft tissue and bone), partial volume averaging can lead to partial volume artifacts (Heuscher and Vembar, 1999). In Figure 9-39, *A*, the detector measures x-ray intensity transmitted from the bone, I_1, and soft tissue, I_2, at the same time. Mathematically, the total intensity is measured as $I_1 + I_2$. To convert from intensities to line integrals for reconstruction, it is necessary to perform the logarithmic operation. Because of the nonlinear nature of the operator, it is clear that:

$$\ln(I_1 + I_2) \neq \ln(I_1) + \ln(I_2) \quad (9\text{-}6)$$

These inaccuracies result in partial volume artifacts in the image, which appear as bands and streaks (Fig. 9-40, *A*).

Partial volume artifacts can be reduced with thinner slice acquisitions and computer algorithms (Hsieh, 1995). It is interesting to note that the thin-slice data acquisition comes naturally with the multislice CT. When the two intensities, I_1 and I_2, are measured with two separate detector cells, as shown in Figure 9-39, *B*, the object within each slice width is uniform and logarithm operation is performed on the two intensities individually. Figure 9-40, *B*, shows the same

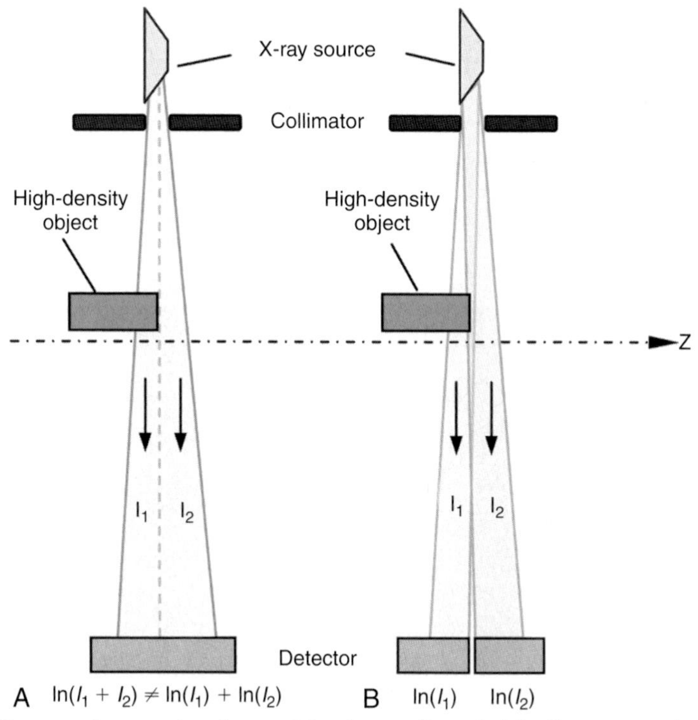

FIGURE 9-39 Cause and correction for partial volume effect. **A,** Nonlinear operation of logarithm. **B,** Thin slice scanning.

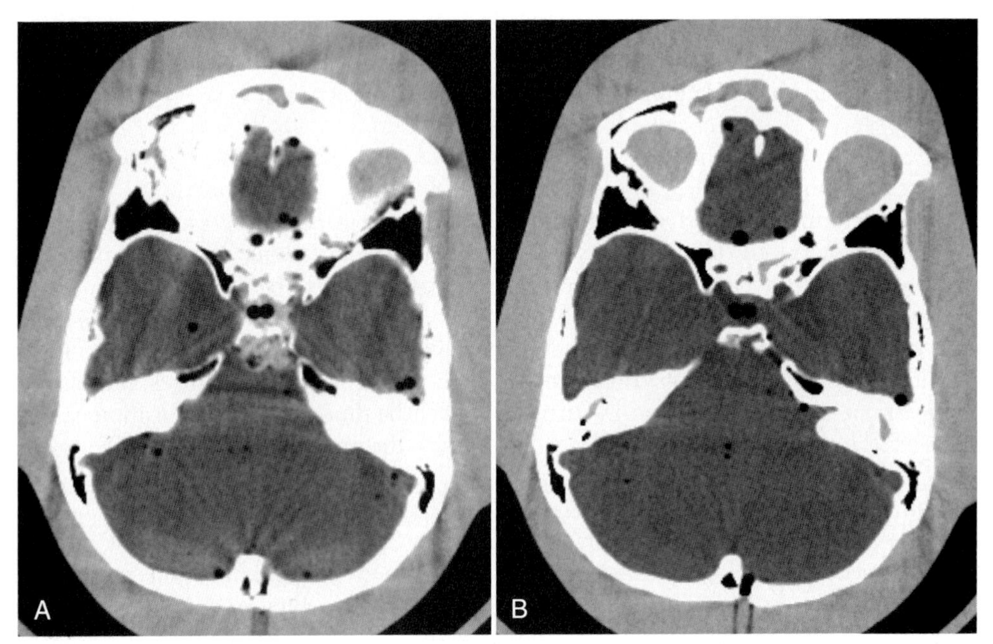

FIGURE 9-40 Partial volume effect. **A,** 7-mm detector aperture. **B,** 1-mm detector aperture.

phantom scanned with a thinner slice; the partial volume artifacts are nearly eliminated.

It is worth pointing out that partial volume artifacts can occur even with thin-slice acquisition if special attention is not paid to other accessories near the patient. As an example, Figure 9-41, *A*, shows a patient head supported by a high-density extension that ends abruptly at the mid brain location. Because of the sharp structure of this particular device, even a 1-mm slice thickness is insufficient to avoid partial volume artifacts, as demonstrated by the severe shading at the lower

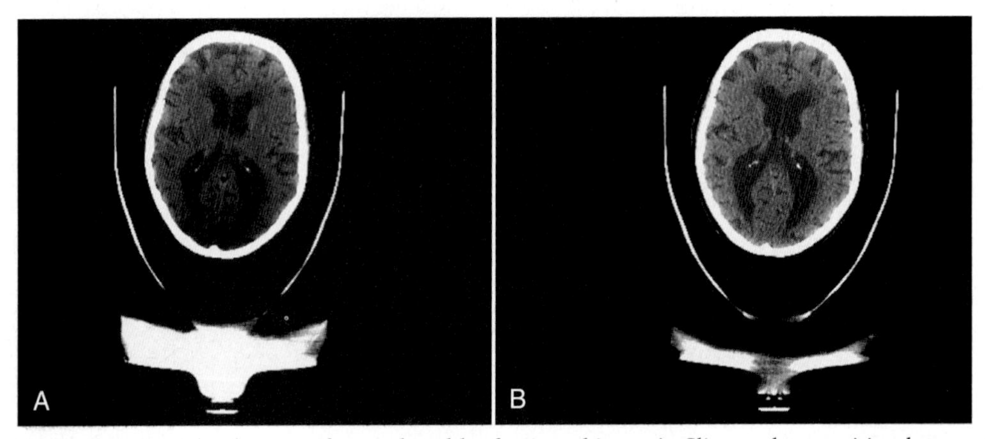

FIGURE 9-41 Partial volume artifacts induced by foreign objects. **A,** Slice at the transition between thicker and thinner part of the holder. **B,** Slice at the thinner part of the holder.

portion of the brain. Note that an adjacent slice *(B)*, which is located 1 mm apart, is free from such artifacts because the supporting structure becomes homogeneous within this slice.

Aliasing Artifacts

The sampling theorem states that to faithfully represent a continuous signal (e.g., intensity profile of a patient), the sampling frequency f_N (the number of rays/cm in the fan beam) must be at least twice the highest frequency content in the signal, f_H. Mathematically, this can be expressed as follows:

$$f_N \geq 2f_H \tag{9-7}$$

If this criterion, the Nyquist criterion, is not met, aliasing artifacts (streaks) can result after the reconstruction process. During CT data acquisition, the original continuous signal is sampled to a discrete form both spatially (each projection is sampled by multiple detector channels) and temporally (each data acquisition is divided into multiple views). Consequently, aliasing artifacts can arise from insufficient projection sampling or from insufficient view sampling. For illustration, Figure 9-42 shows a torso phantom that was scanned with half the normal number of views.

Various methods are available to minimize aliasing artifacts. In some cases the number of views or number of ray samples per view can be increased (Fig. 9-43) to meet the Nyquist requirements. The convolution kernel used in the reconstruction can also be modified so that only frequencies below the Nyquist frequency are allowed into the filtered projection. In this case, a tradeoff is made between the aliasing artifact reduction and spatial resolution of the reconstructed image.

Noise-Induced Artifacts

Noise is influenced partially by the number of photons that strike the detector. Photon starvation can occur as a result of poor patient positioning in the scan SFOV and poor selection of exposure techniques (peak kV, mA), scan speed, and limitations of the CT scanner such as maximum tube power. More photons mean less noise and a stronger detector signal, whereas fewer photons result in more noise and a weaker detector signal. When it is

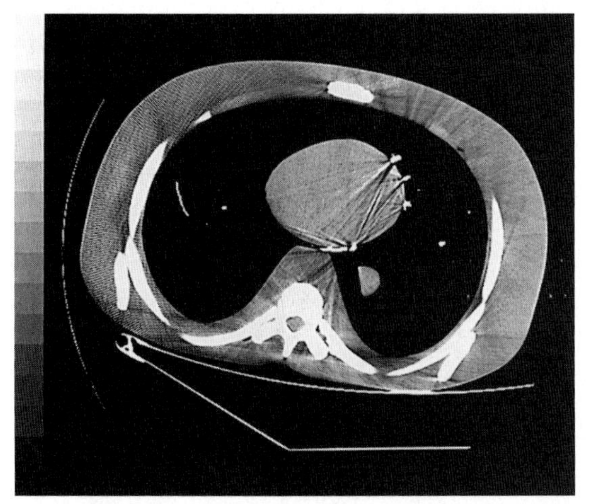

FIGURE 9-42 View aliasing artifacts resulting from 50% of the normal number of views used to scan this torso phantom. The artifacts are apparent at the periphery of the phantom.

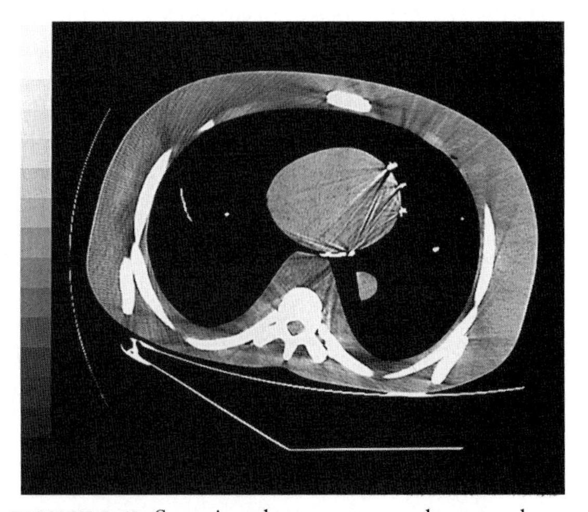

FIGURE 9-43 Scanning the same torso phantom shown in Figure 11-42 at the Nyquist criterion can reduce view aliasing artifacts.

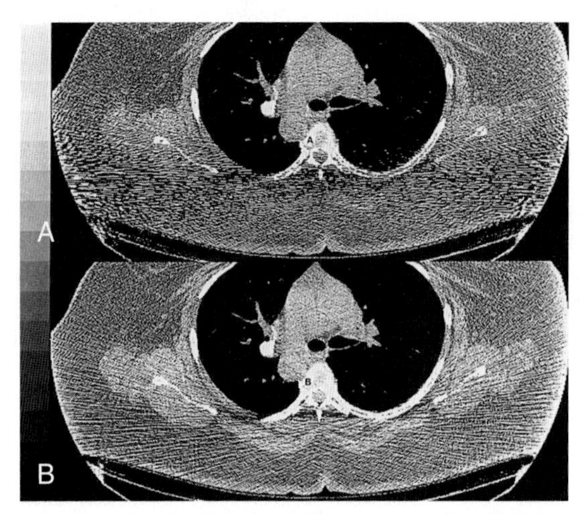

FIGURE 9-44 A, Streak artifacts can arise from an increase in noise resulting from reduced photons at the detector. **B,** Correction of the streaks by adaptive filtering.

combined with the electronic noise and the logarithmic operation, photon starvation often leads to severe streak artifacts, as shown in Figure 9-44, *A*.

The technologist should optimize patient positioning, scan speed, and exposure technique factors to correct streak artifacts. These artifacts can also be reduced with adaptive filtering algorithms (Fig. 9-44, *B*). These algorithms dynamically adjust the amount of smoothing operation on the basis of the x-ray flux level at each projection channel. By selectively smoothing only the channels that contribute to the streaking artifacts and by varying the degree of smoothing on the basis of the noise level of the signal, the technologist can achieve the objectives of simultaneously reducing the streak artifacts in the images and preserving the spatial resolution of the system (Hsieh, 1998).

Another type of the noise-induced artifact is related to the noise nonuniformity. When the noise within the reconstruction FOV is highly heterogeneous, it can produce bright and dark horizontal strips in the MIP or VR images, as shown in Figure 9-45, *A*. This type of artifact can be reduced with either an improved reconstruction algorithm or advanced image processing. Both approaches produce a more uniform noise pattern in the final image (Fig. 9-45, *B*).

Scatter

Scattered radiation is a fundamental phenomenon associated with the interaction between x-ray photons and matter. It reduces the object contrast in conventional radiography and produces artifacts in CT. Scattered radiation has been controlled effectively in the past by placing a postpatient collimator in front of the detector to reject any photons that do not follow the straight-line path between the x-ray source and the detector cell. With the introduction of multislice and volumetric CT, the volume that is exposed to the x-ray radiation increases significantly while the detector aperture reduces. As a result, the scatter-to-primary ratio (ratio of the scattered signal versus true signal) increases. The one-dimensional collimator plates are no longer sufficient, as

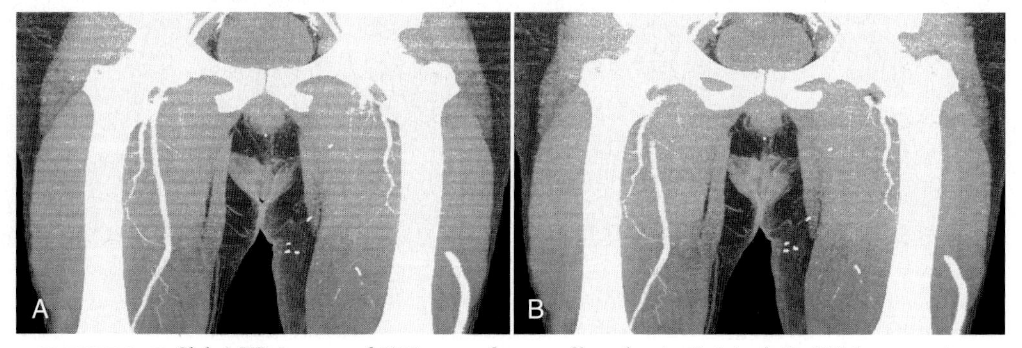

FIGURE 9-45 Slab MIP images of 87.9 mm of a runoff study. **A,** Original. **B,** With correction.

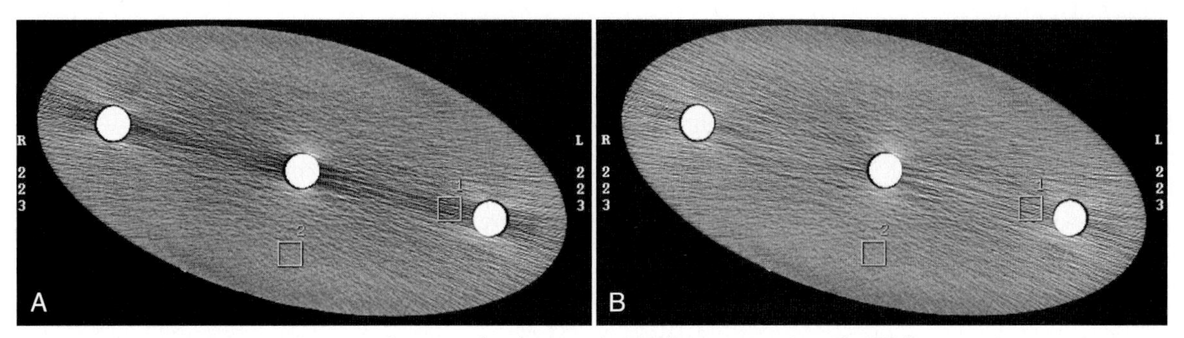

FIGURE 9-46 Impact of scattered radiation. **A,** Without correction. **B,** With correction.

demonstrated by Figure 9-46, *A*. Note the dark shading artifacts connecting the dense rods.

Scatter-induced artifacts can be corrected with algorithms by carefully measuring or estimating the scatter distribution in the projection. The estimated scatter can then be removed from the measured intensities to arrive at the true signals that represent the line integrals of the scanned object. Figure 9-46, *B*, depicts the same scan reconstructed with a software scatter correction. A uniform background is restored.

Cone-Beam Artifacts

The cone-beam artifact is a complicated subject. It is impossible to cover this topic in a subsection. At a very high level, cone-beam artifacts are caused by incomplete or insufficient projection samples as a result of the cone-beam geometry of multislice CT. Understanding the subject involves discussions of the cone-beam reconstruction theory. Given the limited scope of this section, this chapter only provides a specific example of the cone-beam artifact produced with one of the popular reconstruction algorithms: FDK algorithm (Feldkamp et al, 1984). For illustration, a simulation of a helical body phantom is scanned in a step-and-shoot mode with a 64 × 0.625 mm detector configuration (Tang et al, 2005). The comparison of a relatively centered slice (Fig. 9-47, *A*) and an edge slice (Fig. 9-47, *B*) shows both distortions of the dense

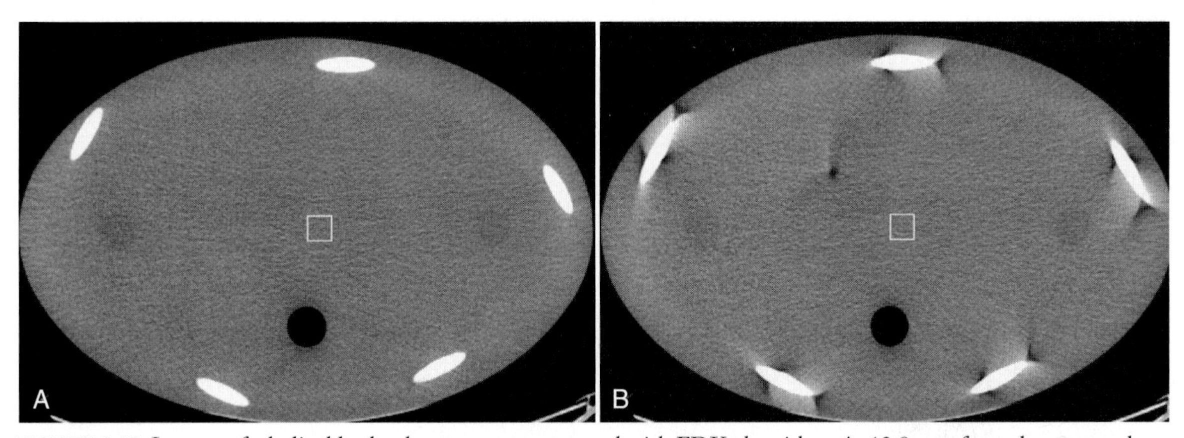

FIGURE 9-47 Images of a helical body phantom reconstructed with FDK algorithm. **A,** 12.8 mm from the center plane. **B,** 17.8 mm from the center plane.

oval objects as well as shading artifacts nearby. The dense oval objects are ellipsoids positioned at a steep angle with respect to the patient's long axis to accentuate the artifacts. Reduction and elimination of cone-beam artifacts have been the focus of intense investigations in recent years, and this research will likely continue for years to come.

QUALITY CONTROL

Quality control is an integral part of equipment testing and maintenance programs in hospitals. Quality control ensures the optimal performance of the CT scanner through a series of daily, monthly, and annual tests for spatial resolution, contrast resolution, noise, slice width, peak kV waveform, average CT number of water, standard deviation of CT numbers in water, and radiation scatter and leakage. These tests constitute a general quality control program for CT scanners and need to be documented.

REFERENCES

Barnes GT, Lakshminarayanan AV: Computed tomography: physical principles and image quality considerations. In Lee JK, et al, editors: *Computed tomography with MRI correction*, ed 2, New York, 1981, Raven Press.

Blumenfeld SM, Glover G: Spatial resolution in computed tomography. In Newton TH, Potts DG, editors: *Radiology of the skull and brain: technical aspects of computed tomography*, vol. 5, St Louis, 1981, Mosby.

Bushong S: *Radiologic science for technologists*, ed 9, St Louis, 2009, Mosby.

Curry TS et al: *Christensen's physics of diagnostic radiology*, ed 4, Philadelphia, 1990, Lea & Febiger.

Feldkamp LA et al: Practical cone-beam algorithm, *J Opt Soc Am* 1:612-619, 1984.

Felsenberg D et al: Reduction of metal artifacts in computed tomography-clinical experience and results, *Electromedica* 56:97-104, 1988.

Goodenough DJ et al: Development of a phantom for evaluation and assurance of image quality in CT scanning, *Opt Eng* 16:52-65, 1977.

Hanson KM: Noise and contrast and discrimination in computed tomography. In Newton TH, Potts DG, editors: *Radiology of the skull and brain: technical aspects of computed tomography*, vol. 5, St Louis, 1981, Mosby.

Heuscher DJ, Vembar M: Reduced partial volume artifacts using spiral computed tomography and integrating spiral interpolator, *Med Phys* 26:276-287, 1999.

Hounsfield GN: Potential uses of more accurate CT absorption values by filtering, *AJR Am J Roentgenol* 131:103-106, 1978.

Hsieh J: Image artifacts, causes and correction. In Goldman LW, Fowlkes JB, editors: *Medical CT and ultrasound: current technology and applications*, College Park, Md, 1995, American Association of Physicists in Medicine.

Hsieh J: Adaptive artifact reduction in computed tomography resulting from x-ray photon noise, *Med Phys* 25:2139-2147, 1998.

Hsieh J: Investigation of the slice sensitivity profile for step-and-shoot mode multi-slice CT, *Med Phys* 28:491-500, 2001.

Hsieh J: *Computed tomography: principles, design, artifacts, and recent advances*, Seattle, 2003, SPIE Press.

Hsieh J et al: Non-uniform phase coded image reconstruction for cardiac CT, *Radiology* 213:401-406, 1999.

Joseph PM, Ruth C: Method for simultaneous correction of spectrum hardening artifacts in CT images containing both bone and iodine, *Med Phys* 24: 1629-1643, 1997.

Kachelriess M et al: ECG-correlated imaging of the heart with subsecond multislice spiral CT, *IEEE Trans Med Imag* 19:888-901, 2000.

Kalender WA, Polacin A: Physical performance characteristics of spiral CT scanning, *Med Phys* 18: 910-915, 1991.

Mayo JR: High-resolution computed tomography: technical aspects, *Radiol Clin North Am* 29: 1043–1048, 1991.

McCollough CH, Zink FE: Performance evaluation of CT systems, In Goldman LW, Fowlkes JB, editors: *Categorical courses in diagnostic radiology physics: CT and US cross-sectional imaging*, pp 189-207, Oak Brook, Ill, 2000, Radiological Society of North America.

Morgan CL: *Basic principles of computed tomography*, Baltimore, 1983, University Park Press.

Parker DL: Optimal short scan convolution reconstruction for fan-beam CT, *Med Phys* 9:254-257, 1982.

Pfeiler M et al: Some guiding ideas on image recording in computerized axial tomography, *Electromedica* 1:19-25, 1976.

Riederer SJ et al: The noise power spectrum in computer x-ray tomography, *Phys Med Biol* 23:446-454, 1978.

Robb RA, Mortin RL: Principle and instrumentation for dynamic x-ray computed tomography. In Marcus ML, et al, editors: *Cardiac imaging: a comparison to Braunwald's heart disease*, Philadelphia, 1991, WB Saunders.

Tang XY et al: A three-dimensional weighted cone beam filtered backprojection (CB-FBP) algorithm for image reconstruction in volumetric CT under a circular source trajectory, *Phys Med Biol* 50:3889–3905, 2005.

Chapter 10

Radiation Dose in Computed Tomography

Chapter Outline

CT USE AND DOSE TRENDS

Since its introduction in the early 1970s, computed tomography (CT) has played a significant role in the detection and management of human diseases in medicine. The technical evolution of CT has been dynamic, ranging from the first-generation single-slice "stop-and-go" technique to multislice volume scanning. The growth of volume CT scanners continues at a rapid rate, from 16- to 64-slice systems to the more recent 320-slice CT scanner. These developments have created a wide variety of clinical applications such as CT colonography, cardiac CT imaging, and CT screening (Brenner, 2006), for example. Furthermore, there has been an increase in CT use worldwide (Amis et al, 2007; Lee et al, 2007; Mukundan et al, 2007). For example, in the United States alone it has been estimated that the number of CT scans increased from 40 million in 2000 to 65 million in 2004 and it is expected to increase to 100 million in 2010 (Baker and Tilak, 2007). In association with the expanding use of CT in medicine, one other major concern that is receiving increasing attention in the literature relates to the potential for high radiation doses delivered by CT scanners (Amis et al, 2007; Baker and Tilak, 2007; Cody and McNitt-Gray, 2006; Colang et al, 2007; ECRI, 2007; Frush, 2006; Goodman and Brink, 2006; Martin and Semelka 2007; Moore et al, 2006; Siegel, 2006), and the potential risks of CT scanning (Brenner and Elliston, 2004; Brenner and Hall, 2007; Brenner et al, 2001; Wise, 2003).

With this in mind, all individuals working in CT, such as radiologists, technologists, medical physicists, physicians and manufacturers alike, should ask themselves three central questions: Why are the doses in CT so high? What is the dose to the patient at my institution? What can be done to reduce the high exposures in CT to protect both patients and personnel?

There are several reasons why these questions are important, as mentioned previously; however, perhaps the most important reason for understanding radiation dose in CT relates to the radiation risks (Brenner, 2006; Huda and Vance, 2007). In this regard, the dose for a CT examination may have to be estimated to make decisions regarding the benefits versus the risks of the procedure. CT manufacturers are now required by law to provide a dose table that shows the doses delivered to patients from their CT scanners.

The purpose of this chapter is to outline the fundamental concepts of radiation dose in CT. In particular, topics such as radiation quantities and their units, factors affecting dose in CT, CT dosimetry including dose descriptors, phantoms and measurement concepts, automatic exposure control (AEC) in CT, dose reduction technology, and radiation protection considerations are described.

RADIATION QUANTITIES AND THEIR UNITS

The literature on radiation dose in CT reports the dose in CT using various radiation quantities (exposure, absorbed dose, and effective dose) and their associated units, Roentgens, rads, and rems (old units), respectively, or coulombs per kilogram, Grays, and Sieverts (International System of units = SI units), respectively (Bushberg et al, 2004; McNitt-Gray, 2002; Seeram, 2001). For this reason, a brief review of these quantities and units is in order. The radiation quantities of relevance to this chapter are exposure, absorbed dose, and effective dose. For a more detailed description, the interested reader may refer to a report by Huda (2006).

Exposure

The radiation quantity exposure refers to the concentration of radiation at a particular point on the patient. Exposure is easy to measure with an ionization chamber positioned at the point of measurement. Radiation falling on the chamber ionizes the air in the chamber to produce ion pairs (charges). The exposure is a measure of the amount of ionization produced in a specific mass of air by x-rays or gamma radiation. The ionization indicates the amount of radiation to which a patient is exposed.

The unit of exposure is the Roentgen (R), the conventional unit, or the coulomb per kilogram (C/kg), the SI unit. One Roentgen produces 2.58×10^{-4} C/kg of air at standard temperature and pressure. Exposure is reported in the literature in milliroentgens (mR), a much smaller unit (1 R = 1000 mR) or in microcoulombs/kilogram (μC/kg) where 1 R = 258 μC/kg.

Absorbed Dose

The absorbed dose, or radiation dose as it is popularly referred to, is the amount of energy absorbed per unit mass of material (patient). Any risk associated with radiation is related to the amount of energy absorbed, and this quantity is particularly important in radiation protection.

The old unit of absorbed dose is the rad (r), which is equal to an energy absorption of 100 ergs per gram of absorber. The SI unit of absorbed dose is the Gray (Gy), so named in honor of Louis Harold Gray, a British radiobiologist who devised ways to measure the absorbed dose. One Gy is equal to 1 joule per kilogram (J/kg) or 1 r is equal to 0.01 Gy or 100 r is equal to 1 Gy. Relevant submultiples of the Gray are 1 centigray (cGy), which equals 1 r and 1 milligray (mGy), which equals 100 millirads (mrads). For the sake of simplicity, 1 r is approximately equal to 0.01 Gy.

Effective Dose

The quantity effective dose, E, previously referred to as the effective dose equivalent, is used to quantify the risk from partial-body exposure to that from an equivalent whole-body dose. The term is used to take into account the type of radiation (because different types of radiation can produce varying degrees of biological damage) and the radiosensitivity of different tissues (because some tissues are more sensitive than others).

As described by McNitt-Gray (2002), E is a "weighted average of organ doses" and can be expressed mathematically as follows:

$$E = \sum_{T} (D_{T,R} \cdot W_T \cdot W_R)$$

where $D_{T,R}$ is the absorbed dose to the tissue (T), W_T is the tissue-weighting factor, W_R is the radiation-weighting factor, and the symbol $\sum$ is the "sum of." These factors can be obtained from previously calculated tables (Bushong, 2009).

Although the old unit of effective dose is the rem, the SI unit is the Sievert (Sv), where 1 Sv = 100 rems. The effective dose relates exposure to risk. As noted by Brenner (2006), "...relevant organ doses for CT examinations are on the order of 15 mSv or less." Brenner also notes that "...there is good epidemiologic evidence of increased cancer risk for children exposed to acute doses of 10 mSv (or more) and for adults exposed to acute doses of 50 mSv (or more)."

To put this in perspective, Huda (2006) emphasizes that "the total amount of radiation that a patient receives in any radiographic examination is best quantified by the effective dose, which is related to the risk of carcinogenesis, and with the induction of genetic effects. Effective doses with radiographic imaging are smaller than natural background (3 mSv/yr). Effective doses from common fluoroscopic and CT examinations are comparable to natural background and may be much higher with interventional radiology procedures."

It is interesting to recall that the dose limits for occupationally exposed individuals (radiologists and technologists, for example) are given in mSv. The International Commission on Radiological Protection (ICRP) dose limit for radiation workers is 20 mSv per year. Although the dose limits for radiation workers in the United States is 50 mSv per year, it is 20 mSv per year for workers in Canada (Bushong, 2009).

RADIATION BIOEFFECTS

One of the reasons why technologists and radiologists should have a clear understanding of the dose in CT relates to radiation bioeffects. These effects are classified as stochastic and deterministic (nonstochastic). It is not within the scope of this chapter to describe the details of these effects; however, for the sake of relating these effects to dose in CT, a brief review is in order.

Stochastic Effects

Stochastic effects are those effects for which the probability (rather than the severity) of the effect occurring depends on the dose. The probability increases with increasing dose, and there is no threshold dose for these effects. The linear no threshold (LNT) dose-response model is a radiation risk model most favored by radiobiologists in estimating the risk of exposure in radiology (Bushong, 2009). Medical radiation protection standards, guidelines, and recommendations are based on this model.

The LNT dose-response model states that the radiation risk increases as the dose increases and that there is no threshold dose. Even a small dose has the potential to cause a biological effect. There is no risk-free dose. Examples of stochastic effects include cancer, leukemia, and hereditary effects. Stochastic effects are considered late effects because they occur years after the exposure. The interested reader should refer to the report by Brenner et al (2001) for a thorough review of the increased risk of certain cancers from CT exposures, most notably in children. Additionally, Brenner (2006) provides the imaging community with a report dealing with the radiation risks in diagnostic radiology.

Deterministic Effects

Deterministic effects (nonstochastic effects) are those effects for which the severity of the effect (rather than the probability of the effect) increases with increasing dose and for which there is a threshold dose. Below the threshold dose, these effects are not observed. Threshold doses are considered to be relatively high doses that can kill cells and cause degenerative changes in tissues that have been exposed to radiation. Examples of deterministic effects include skin erythema, epilation, pericarditis, and cataracts. The threshold dose for cataracts, for example, is about 2 Gy (200 rads). A study by Huda and Vance (2007) on radiation doses from CT in children and adults, showed that "representative organ absorbed doses in CT are substantially lower than threshold doses for the induction of deterministic effects."

As patients undergo several examinations, it may be possible to reach the threshold dose for certain deterministic effects.

PATIENT EXPOSURE PATTERNS IN RADIOGRAPHY AND CT

It is clearly apparent that the geometry of the x-ray beam and the way in which the patient is exposed to the beam is different in radiographic imaging and in CT imaging, as shown in Figure 10-1, *A* and *B*. In radiography, the x-ray tube is typically above the patient in a fixed position as the examination is conducted, and the shape of the beam is a cone. This shape is sometimes referred to as open-beam geometry. Although the entrance exposure is 100%, it is sometimes used to represent risk; however, this is an overestimation because the dose decreases as it passes through the patient. Such decrease is due to attenuation and the inverse square law. The dose distribution for radiographic imaging is illustrated in Figure 10-1, *A*.

In CT, the exposure pattern is somewhat different than that of radiography because of the geometric aspects of the beam and the scanning procedure. In general, the beam is well collimated to describe a fan-shaped beam that rotates around the patient at least for 360 degrees. The x-ray tube

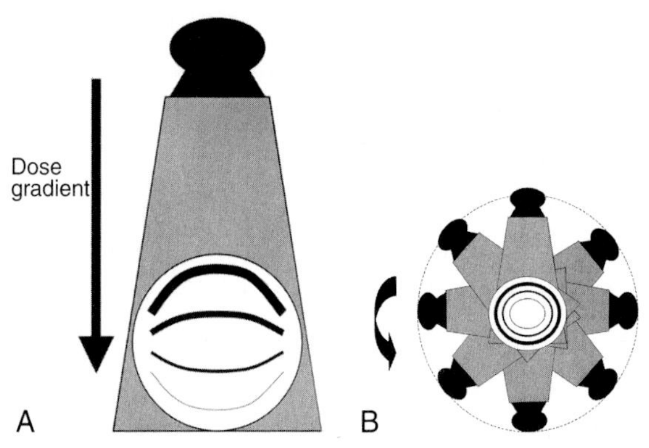

FIGURE 10-1 **A,** The typical dose distribution for radiographic imaging. The entrance skin dose is greater than the exit skin dose, as illustrated by the thickness of the lines, where the thicker lines denote a higher dose. **B,** The typical dose distribution for CT imaging showing that the dose is greater at the entrance surface of the patient (thick lines) and decreases toward the center of the patient (thin lines). (From McNitt-Gray MF: Radiation dose in CT, *Radiographics* 22:1541-1553, 2002. Reproduced by permission of Radiological Society of North American and the author.)

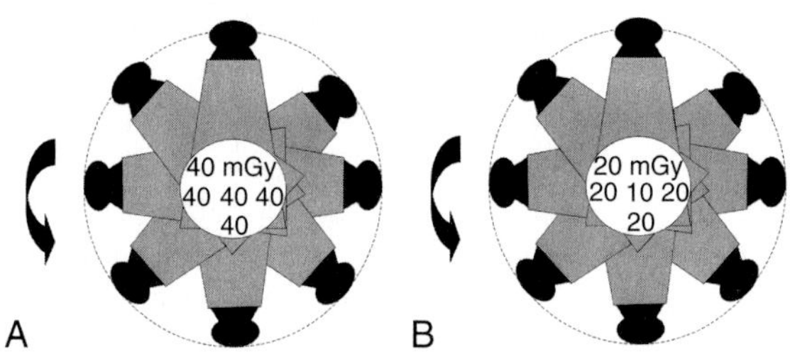

FIGURE 10-2 Typical dose values for a 16-cm diameter head phantom **(A)** and a 32-cm diameter body phantom **(B)**. (From McNitt-Gray MF: Radiation dose in CT, *Radiographics* 22:1541-1553, 2002. Reproduced by permission of Radiological Society of North America and the author.)

is not fixed as in radiography but assumes several positions during one complete revolution around the patient. In modern multislice CT scanners, the fan-shaped beam has now become a cone-shaped beam (see Chapter 12). The dose distribution pattern is more uniform in CT (Fig. 10-1, *B*) compared with radiography because the x-ray beam is rotating 360 degrees around the patient's body. Typical dose values for a 16-centimeter (cm) diameter head phantom and a 32-cm diameter body phantom are given in Figure 10-2, *A* and *B*, respectively.

CT SCANNER X-RAY BEAM GEOMETRY

The term *beam geometry* refers to the size and shape of the x-ray beam emanating from the x-ray tube and passing through the patient to strike a set of detectors that collects radiation attenuation data. The beam geometry and scanning process of CT imaging are shown in Figure 10-3, in which a fan-shaped x-ray beam and an array of detectors rotate 360 degrees around the patient to collect attenuation data. The table moves during the scanning process, and the x-ray tube traces a spiral or helical beam path around the patient.

Figure 10-4, *A*, shows the same fan-shaped x-ray beam viewed from the side with the thickness exaggerated for clarity. If the longitudinal (cranial-caudal) axis of the patient is defined as the *z*-axis, then in theory the intensity of the radiation beam along that axis can be graphed. Ideally the radiation intensity measured along the *z*-axis would have equal intensity everywhere inside the beam and would have no intensity on either side. Figure 10-4, *B*, shows this ideal rectangular intensity profile of the radiation beam. In reality, the radiation intensity measured along the *z*-axis has smoother edges and appears as a bell-shaped curve. The dose distribution is almost always wider than the nominal slice width (SW).

The dose distribution is given by the function $D(z)$, which describes an arbitrarily shaped dose intensity along the patient axis. In general, the shape of $D(z)$ varies among CT scanners. $D(z)$ is extremely important to dose in CT because it is this dose distribution that is being measured. The instrumentation and methods used to measure

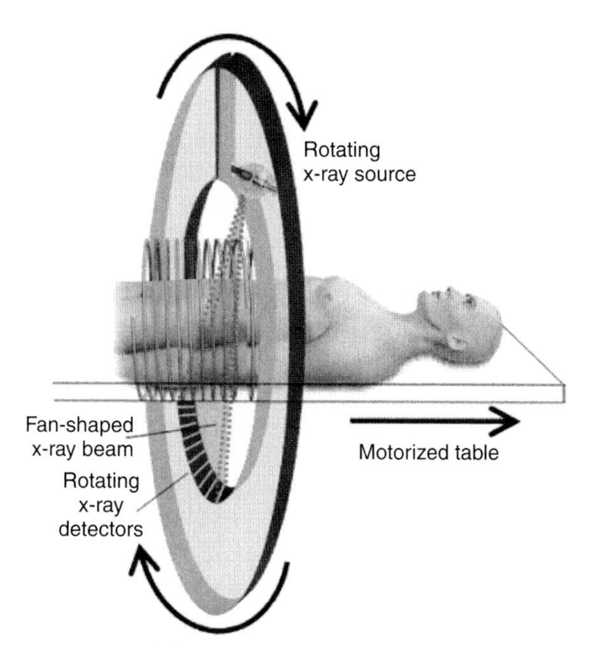

FIGURE 10-3 The scanning principles of CT imaging in which the x-ray beam and detectors rotate 360 degrees around the patient to collect attenuation data used to build up the image. In this diagram, a fan-shaped beam is used and the table moves during data acquisition to trace a spiral or helical beam path around the patient. This process is referred to as spiral or helical CT scanning. (From Brenner D: Radiation risks in diagnostic radiology. In Radiological Society of North America: *Categorical course in diagnostic radiology physics: from invisible to visible—the science and practice of x-ray imaging and radiation dose optimization*, pp 41-50, 2006, Radiological Society of North America. Reproduced by permission of Radiological Society of North America and the author.)

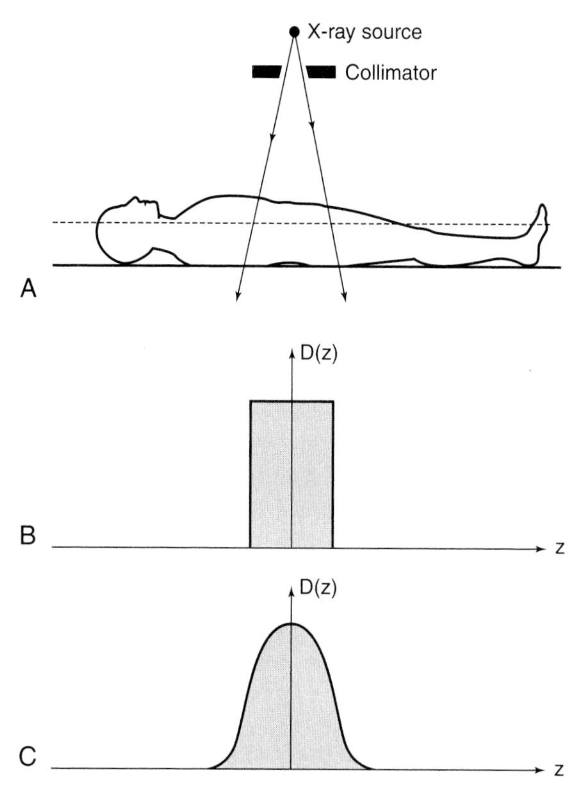

FIGURE 10-4 **A,** The width of the x-ray beam is viewed from the side. The collimator near the x-ray source (the width is exaggerated for clarity) determines the beam width. **B,** An ideal dose distribution along the **z** axis is shown. It has a flat top and steep sides and is the same width as the x-ray beam. **C,** A more realistic bell-shaped dose distribution curve is typical of most CT scanners.

patient dose from a CT scanner is referred to as CT dosimetry, and it is uniquely different compared with the dosimetry of projection radiographic imaging.

CT DOSIMETRY CONCEPTS

CT dosimetry is an important concept for CT technologists for several reasons. First, technologists can compare their hospital CT doses with the national average to find out whether their radiation protection efforts are comparable to those of others. Second, technologists can participate effectively in informing both the public and other hospital personnel (physicians and nurses, for example) about the dose in CT. Third, and perhaps more important, CT technologists can assist the medical physicist with not only performing the actual dose measurements (this has been identified as one of the duties of a certified medical physicist by the

American College of Radiology) but also being a more integral part of CT acceptance testing and continuing quality control procedures. Finally, a knowledge of CT dosimetry will assist the technologist in conducting dose measurements in cases where there is no medical physicist to perform this task.

It is not within the scope of this text to describe how to conduct the actual dose measurements and how to estimate the radiation doses to patients because these are topics within the domain of medical physicists. It is important, however, to highlight several important and essential concepts, including types of dosimeters used to measure CT doses, CT dosimetry phantoms, and dose descriptors specific to CT.

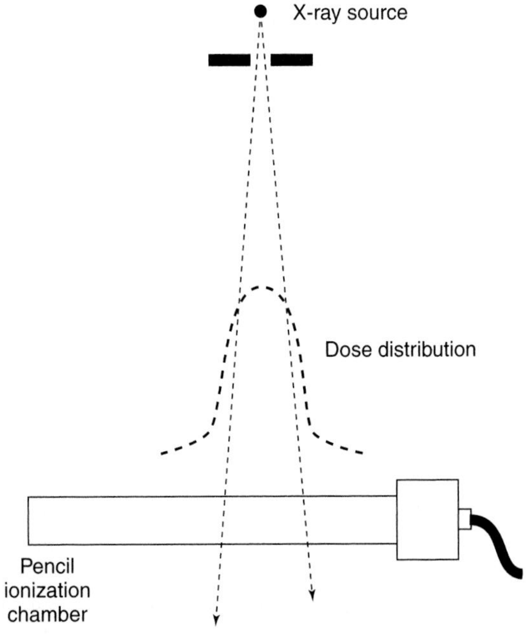

FIGURE 10-5 An ionization chamber effectively performs the integral in equation 10-2 by intercepting the radiation beam and sensing the dose from all parts of the dose distribution curve. The charge emitted from the chamber is proportional to the area-under-the-dose-distribution curve.

Types of Dosimeters

In the past, several types of dosimeters were used to measure the dose in CT. These include film dosimeters, thermoluminescent dosimeters (TLDs), and specially designed ionization chambers. In 1981, the Bureau of Radiological Health (BRH), now the Center for Devices and Radiological Health (CDRH), introduced what could be noted as a significant step toward CT dose measurement. The method suggested by the CDRH uses a pencil ionization chamber. Recently, solid-state metal oxide semiconductor field effect transistors (MOSFET) are being used in CT dosimetry studies because they are more sensitive than TLDs and they provide an instant read out and can be reused immediately. For further details, the interested reader may refer to one such study by Mukundan et al (2007) that used MOSFET dosimetry to assess the dose to the orbits in pediatric CT imaging, for further details. In addition, those interested in the use of the TLD in CT dosimetry may refer to a report by Moore et al (2006).

Although many dose measurement methods are available, only the pencil ionization chamber method, or what the CDRH referred to as the CT dose index (CTDI) method, is described in this chapter. The ionization chamber method is the easiest and probably the most accurate, and it is used almost exclusively to report dose.

Ionization Chamber

An ionization chamber is an instrument used to accurately quantify radiation exposure. The ionization chamber shown in Figure 10-5 consists of a small air-filled container with thin walls that allow radiation to pass through easily. As the high-energy photons (x-rays) collide with air molecules enclosed within the ionization chamber, some of the molecules are "ionized" (i.e., one or more electrons are knocked from some molecules). These free electrons can be collected on a conducting wire or plate and measured as electric charge. The amount of collected charge is proportional to the amount of ionization, which is proportional to the amount of radiation that passes through the chamber. The charge is removed from the ionization chamber and measured with a very sensitive instrument known as an *electrometer*. The total electric charge generated by an x-ray beam is represented by Q and measured in coulombs (one coulomb = 1.6×10^{19} electrons).

Phantoms for CT Dose Measurement

To standardize the measurement of the dose and provide a clinically realistic geometry, the BRH researchers suggested that the ionization chamber be placed in one of two cylindrical phantoms during the radiation measurement. The smaller phantom simulates a patient's head and the larger phantom simulates a "body" or torso (Fig. 10-6). Both phantoms are 15 cm in length. The diameter of the "head" phantom is 16 cm, and the diameter of the "body" phantom is 32 cm. Both phantoms are solid acrylic with holes drilled through the phantom at specified locations to accommodate the pencil ionization chamber (Fig. 10-7). Acrylic plugs are placed in the holes unoccupied by the ionization chamber. Figure 10-8 shows a pencil ionization chamber about to be inserted into a CT scanner dosimetry phantom. The holes that are not being used for the ionization chamber are filled with acrylic plugs. Careful examination of the plug reveals a small hole that can be seen through its diameter. This hole is centered end to end in the plug and is visible in the CT image of the dosimetry phantom if the x-ray beam is centered on the phantom and passes through the hole. The appearance of the hole in the image verifies that the x-ray beam is striking the center of the phantom.

The procedure for measurement is to place the ionization chamber in one of the phantom holes, take a scan, and record the amount of charge emitted from the chamber. Then the chamber is moved to the next hole, the plug is placed in the original chamber hole, and the procedure is repeated. Moving the chamber to another hole (e.g., from the anterior to the posterior) allows the dose to be determined at a variety of locations within the phantom. Generally, the dose varies among locations, even when the same technique is used. For example, the dose at the anterior location of the phantom differs from the dose at the posterior location, which differs from the dose on the patient's right side, and so on. It is usually prudent to measure the dose at several locations for a given technique.

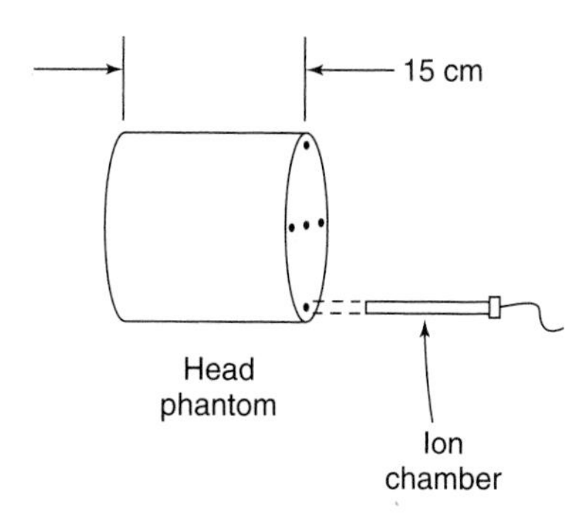

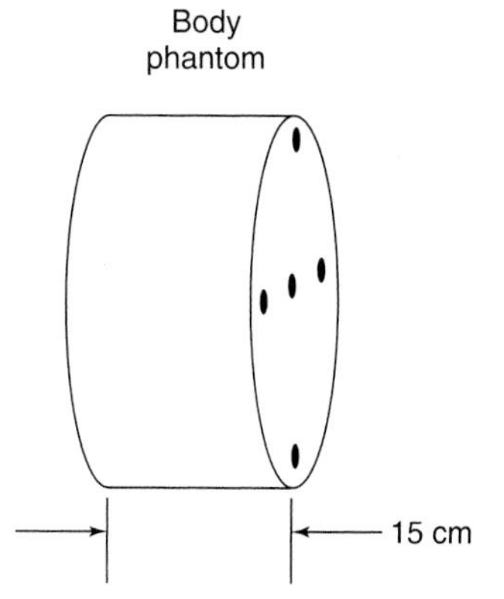

FIGURE 10-6 The "head" and "body" CT scanner dosimetry phantoms are solid acrylic with holes placed strategically to receive a pencil ionization chamber. Although the phantoms differ in diameter, they are both 15 cm long.

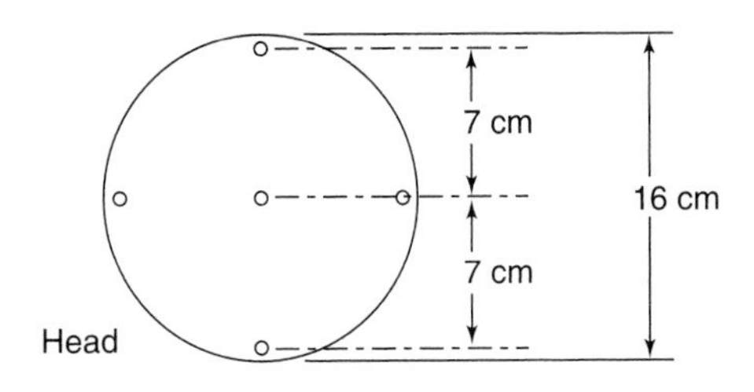

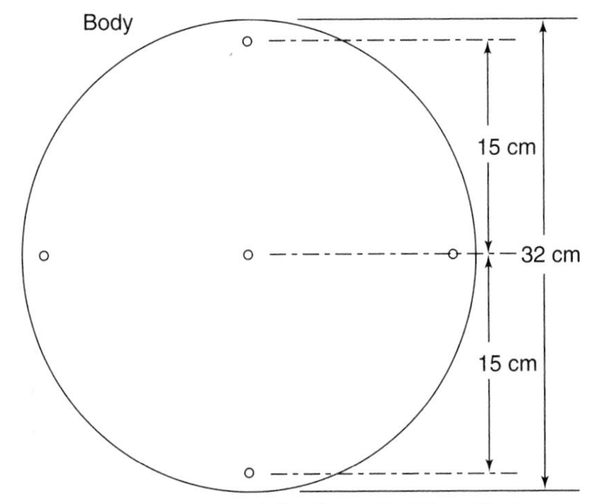

FIGURE 10-7 A view of the face of a "head" phantom *(top)* and a "body" phantom *(bottom)*. Dimensions and location of the ionization chamber holes are shown. Diameters of the holes are typically 1 cm and should be drilled to match the outer diameter of the ionization chamber.

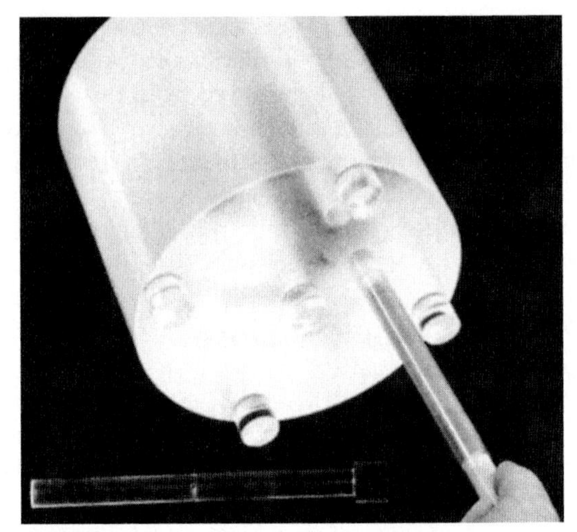

FIGURE 10-8 A pencil ionization chamber about to be inserted in a "head" CT scanner dosimetry phantom. The holes that are not being used for the ionization chamber are filled with acrylic plugs *(bottom)*. The appearance of the hole in the image verifies that the x-ray beam is striking the center of the phantom.

CT Dose Descriptors

The earlier dose studies reported CT doses by using various terms to describe the absorbed dose in a CT examination. These included single-scan peak dose, multiple-scan peak dose, dose profile, and others such as multiple-scan average dose (MSAD). These results led the CDRH to introduce and recommend the use of CTDI and MSAD in the Federal Performance Standard as the dose descriptors specific to CT. For example, because the early CT examinations consist of a series of "stop-and-go" scans (slices), the MSAD was the dose descriptor for use in a clinical situation at that time. The MSAD concept will be highlighted for historical reasons only.

Additionally, another dose descriptor, the dose length product (DLP) has been identified and used in some studies; it is available for CT scanners and is linked to the CTDI (McNitt-Gray, 2002).

Multiple-Scan Average Dose

The MSAD was the first CT dose descriptor to be identified (McNitt-Gray, 2002). To use the MSAD, a series of CT scans is performed on a patient (Fig. 10-9). Between each scan, the patient is moved a bed index (BI) distance. Each slice delivers the characteristic bell-shaped dose represented by the curves at the top of Figure 10-9. If the doses from all scans are summed, the resulting total patient dose resembles the oscillating curve at the bottom of Figure 10-9. In the regions where the bell curves overlap, the resultant dose is higher than that from just one scan. If the total dose distribution curve is known (bottom curve), the

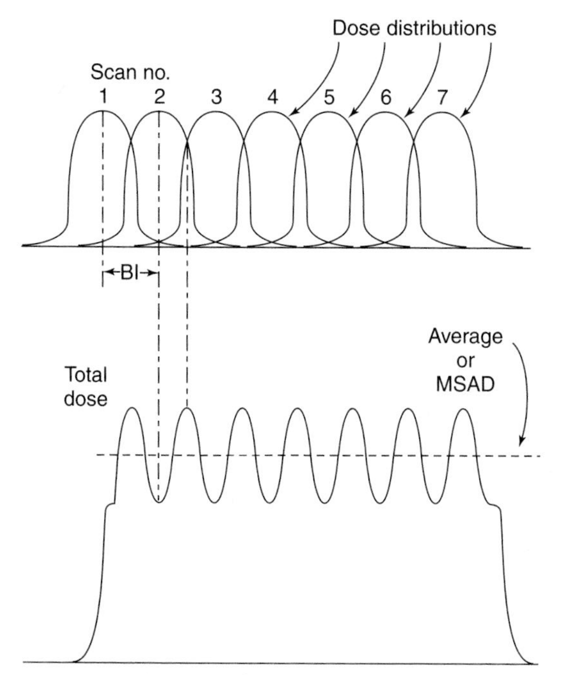

FIGURE 10-9 A series of seven scans spaced (bed indexing) apart along the z-axis disburses seven bell-shaped dose distribution curves *(top)*. When the doses from this series are summed, the resultant total dose appears as the bottom curve. The total dose curve has peaks where the bell-shaped curves overlap. The dotted line through the total dose curve is the multiple scan average dose.

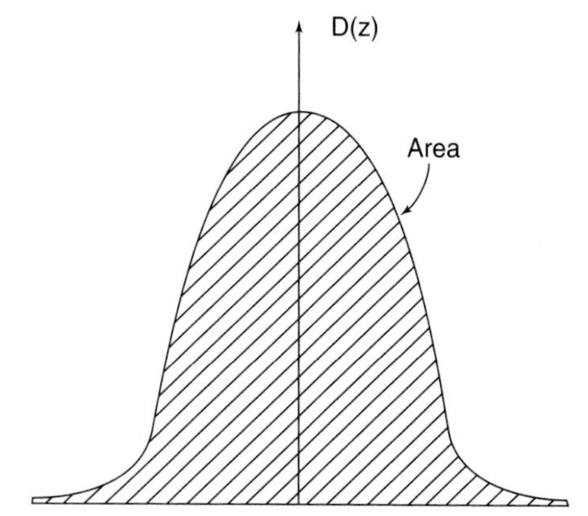

FIGURE 10-10 The integral in equation 10-2 is numerically equal to the area (shaded region) of the dose distribution curve.

MSAD (dotted straight line) can be calculated by mathematically sampling the peaks and valleys of the multiple scan dose curve. This can be written as follows:

$$\text{MSAD} = \text{CTDI} \times \text{SW/BI} \qquad (10\text{-}1)$$

where SW is slice width in millimeters and BI is bed index or slice spacing.

CT Dose Index

The CTDI was the next CT dose descriptor after the MSAD. It was developed by the U.S. Food and Drug Administration (FDA) and was therefore labeled CTDI_{FDA} (Boone, 2007). CTDI_{FDA} has evolved to its present form with several notable changes. These are highlighted in this subsection of the chapter.

The CTDI_{FDA} is defined as follows:

$$\text{CTDI}_{\text{FDA}} = \frac{1}{n \cdot \text{SW}} \int_{-7}^{+7} D(z)dz \qquad (10\text{-}2)$$

where n is the number of distinct planes of data collected during one revolution, *SW* is the nominal slice width in millimeters), *D*(z) is the dose distribution, and z is the dimension along the patient's axis. For axial (nonspiral/helical) CT scanners and spiral/helical CT scanners with a single row of detectors, $n = 1$. For multislice CT scanners, n is the number of active detector rows (n = 16) during the scan.

The CTDI_{FDA} represents the mean absorbed dose in the scanned object volume and therefore the unit of the CTDI is the Gy with relevant submultiples such as the centigray (cGy) and the mGy.

This equation is not as complicated as it appears. The integral sign ($\int$) merely instructs the user to determine the area under a single curve *D*(z). Figure 10-10 demonstrates the value of this integral by shading the area under a typical dose distribution curve. If this area is divided by the number of slices times the slice width $\{(n)(SW)\}$, the result is the CTDI_{FDA}.

This definition, which was accepted by the International Electrotechnical Commission (IEC) (IEC, 2001), is good for essentially all shapes of dose distribution curves *D*(z) that are emitted by CT scanners. Note that increasing the area under the curve can increase the $CTDI_{FDA}$. The area can be increased by either increasing the intensity of radiation, which raises the height of the curve, or by widening the curve, usually by opening the x-ray collimators near the x-ray tube. Either case increases the $CTDI_{FDA}$ and ultimately increases the radiation dose to the patient.

For axial CT scanners, as the slice spacing increases, there is a greater likelihood that relevant tissue will be "missed" (it falls between the slices) in the scan sequence, thus limiting the amount that the BI can be increased. Conversely, when the BI is made smaller, the slices become closer together, more overlap of adjacent dose distributions occurs, and the average dose increases. When the SW equals the BI, the MSAD is numerically equal to the $CTDI_{FDA}$.

The $CTDI_{FDA}$ has evolved from its initial stage of measurement for 14 contiguous slices where the integration would be from −7 to +7. The fixed length of the pencil ionization chamber "meant that only 14 sections of 7-mm thickness could be measured with that chamber alone. To measure $CTDI_{FDA}$ for thinner sections, sometimes lead sleeves were used to cover the part of the chamber that exceeded 14 section widths" (McNitt-Gray, 2002).

This shortcoming was solved by introducing another dose index, the $CTDI_{100}$, which "relaxed the constraint on 14 sections and allowed calculation of the index for 100 mm along the length of the entire pencil ionization chamber, regardless of the nominal slice width being used" (McNitt-Gray, 2002). The index is given by the equation

$$CTDI_{100} = (1/nT)\int_{-50}^{50} D(z)dz \tag{10-3}$$

where nT is the nominal collimated slice thickness.

The next major change in the CT dose descriptor is the introduction of the weighted CTDI ($CTDI_W$) to account for the average dose in the x-y axis of the patient instead of the z-axis. This can be done using a phantom where the pencil ionization chamber is positioned in the center ($CTDI_{center}$) and at the periphery ($CTDI_{periphery}$) of the phantom (see Fig. 10-7). In this case the following algebraic expression can be used to calculate the $CTDI_W$ as provided by McNitt-Gray (2002):

$$CTDI_W = (1/3)(CTDI_{100})_{center} + (2/3)(CTDI_{100})_{periphery} \tag{10-4}$$

Several examples of the $CTDI_W$ for head and body dose phantoms at 120 kilovolts (kV) for five CT scanners are given in a report by Huda and Vance (2007). They state that for the following scanners; LightSpeed Plus (GE Healthcare), Mx8000 IDT (Philips Medical Systems), Sensation 16 (Siemens Medical Solutions), 7000 TS (Shimadzu Corporation), and the Aquilion Multi (Toshiba Medical Systems), the $CTDI_W$ (mGy/milliampere [mA]) for the head were 0.180, 0.130, 0.190, 0.180, and 0.190 respectively. For the body, the $CTDI_W$ were 0.094, 0.066, 0.069, 0.103, and 0.105, respectively.

To consider the dose in the z-axis, yet another dose descriptor was developed. This is the $CTDI_{volume}$, which can be calculated with the following relationship for spiral//helical CT imaging:

$$CTDI_{volume} = CTDI_W/Pitch \tag{10-5}$$

It is important to note that the term *pitch* has been defined by the IEC as a ratio of the distance the table travels per revolution (in millimeters) to the total nominal beam collimation (in millimeters). For a pitch of 1, the $CTDI_{volume}$ is equal to the $CTDI_W$; for a pitch of 1.5, the $CTDI_{volume}$ is equal to $CTDI_W/1.5$.

Dose Length Product

As mentioned earlier, the DLP is yet another dose descriptor used in CT dose studies and reported in the literature and on CT scanners. Although the $CTDI_{volume}$ provides a measurement of the exposure per slice of tissue, the DLP provides a measurement of the total amount of exposure for a series of scans. The DLP can be calculated if the length of the irradiated volume (scan length) and the $CTDI_{volume}$ are known by using the following relationship:

$$DLP = CTDI_{volume} \times \text{Scan length} \quad (10\text{-}6)$$

It is important to note that, although the $CTDI_{volume}$ is not dependent on the scan length, the DLP is directionally proportional to the scan length.

In summary, McNitt-Gray (2002) informs the radiologic community that "these CTDI descriptors are obviously meant to serve as an index of radiation dose due to CT scanning and are not meant to serve as an accurate estimate of the radiation dose incurred by an individual patient. Although the phantom measurements are meant to be reflective of an attenuation environment somewhat similar to a patient, the homogeneous polymethyl methacrylate phantom does not simulate the different tissue types and heterogeneities of a real patient."

Measuring the CT Dose Index

It is not within the scope of this book to describe the details of how to measure the CTDI because this is a task for the medical physicist. However, the following steps are noteworthy, using the phantoms and pencil ionization chamber described earlier:

1. The pencil ionization chamber is placed into one of the holes in the phantom, perpendicular to the fan of the radiation beam (i.e., the chamber is placed parallel to the longitudinal axis of the patient) (see Fig. 10-5), and the other holes are plugged with acrylic plugs.
2. An exposure is made for a single scan, and the chamber measures the exposure (not dose). The chamber intercepts the entire narrow width of the x-ray beam. The x-ray beam must be positioned in the center of the chamber.
3. The chamber converts the x-rays into charge. This charge represents the integral in Equation 10-2.
4. The ionization chamber receives radiation from all parts of the dose distribution $D(z)$ because of its length. The total charge from the ionization chamber is proportional to the integral in the CTDI definition. Mathematically, this is expressed as follows:

$$Q = \frac{1}{C_f} \int_{-\infty}^{+\infty} D(z)dz \quad (10\text{-}7)$$

where Q is the total charge collected during a single scan and C_f is the calibration factor of the ionization chamber. Because the ionization chamber measures exposure and not the dose, a conversion factor (the f factor) must be included in C_f, which converts exposure (in Roentgens) to dose (cGy; recall that 1 cGy = 1 rad). The value of the f factor at CT scanner x-ray energies is approximately 0.94 cGy/Roentgen.

An interesting point to note about the CTDI is that the integration range is restricted to single-slice CT scanners collimated to beam widths of 10 mm and less (Boone, 2007) and to 100 mm for the $CTDI_{100}$. As pointed out by Cody and McNitt-Gray (2006), "with the advent of multidetectors scanners with beam widths from 25 to 40 mm (and a prototype that has a nominal collimated beam width of 128 mm (Mori et al, 2006), the 100 mm pencil chamber will not be able to capture all of the primary and scatter radiation in the CTDI phantoms. In addition, CTDI is measured in a single transverse scan so that the pencil chamber can integrate the radiation dose profile, assuming a contiguous transverse scanning protocol; approximations are made to calculate dose when helical scanning is performed....therefore, methods are being developed to measure radiation dose better for multidetector CT (and also for cone beam CT) as well as to measure estimated actual radiation does to patients." For example, the nominal beam width for the 256-slice CT scanner is 128 mm; therefore, the integration range has increased to 300 mm for an accurate measurement of the dose from this CT scanner (Mori et al, 2006). These investigators have developed what they call the dose profile integral (DPI). In addition, in a letter to the editor of *Medical Physics*, Dixon (2006) proposes that a Farmer ion chamber be used to measure the dose with a phantom "using the exact protocol that would be used for patients, instead of a single transverse scan, removing the need to make approximations or corrections for helical scanning" (Cody and McNitt, 2006). Other investigators have used MOSFET technology as well to assess dose in CT (Dixon, 2003; Muhundan et al, 2007.

These measurement and dose estimation methods are not described further in this text; however, the interested reader should refer to the reports by Dixon (2003, 2006).

FACTORS AFFECTING DOSE IN CT

Several factors affect the dose in CT. These fall into two categories, namely, those that have a direct effect on the dose and those that have an indirect effect on the dose (Cody and McNitt-Gray, 2006; Kalra et al, 2004a; McNitt-Gray, 2002). Although the direct factors are those factors that increase or decrease the dose to the patient and are under the direct control of the technologist, the indirect factors are those that "have a direct influence on image quality, but no direct effect on radiation dose; for example, the reconstruction filter" (McNitt, 2002). It is beyond the scope of this chapter to describe all of these factors; however, only the factors that have a direct effect on the dose to the patient, and which the technologist has some degree of control, are reviewed. These include the exposure technique factors, x-ray beam collimation, pitch, patient centering, number of detectors, and overranging, also referred to as z-overscanning.

Exposure Technique Factors

Exposure technique factors are characterized by the tube potential defined by the kilovoltage; tube current, defined by the milliamperage; and the exposure time in seconds. The product of the milliamperage and the exposure time is the milliamperage-seconds (mAs). The technologist can select these factors manually or they can be selected by using AEC. AEC uses a technique known as automatic tube current modulation, which is described later in the chapter.

Constant Milliamperage-Seconds

The term *constant mAs* refers to the selection of milliamperage and time (in seconds) separately or mAs on some scanners before the scan begins, keeping all other technical factors constant. The mAs determines the quantity of photons (dose) incident on the patient for the duration of the exposure. The dose is directly proportional to the mAs, and therefore if the mAs is doubled, the dose will be doubled. The results of different amounts of mAs on the dose (mGy and mGy/mAs) using a phantom and a 64-slice CT scanner are provided in Table 10-1. It is clearly apparent that as the mAs increases, the dose increases proportionally. For example, the $CTDI_w$ (mGy) for a 32-cm diameter body phantom using 110 mAs and 220 mAs is 7.4 and 15 mGy, respectively, when all other technical scanning factors remain constant (Cody and McNitt-Gray, 2006).

Effective Milliamperage-Seconds

The *effective mAs* is a term used for multislice CT scanners that denotes the mAs per slice. This is given by the following relationship:

$$\text{Effective mAs} = \text{True mAs/pitch} \qquad (10\text{-}8)$$

This expression simply implies that, to keep the effective mAs constant, as the pitch increases, the

TABLE 10-1 Changes in $CTDI_w$ in a 32-cm Diameter Body Phantom as a Function of Tube Current-Time Product for Both Constant Rotation Time Settings and Constant Current Settings

Tube Current (mA)	Rotation Times (s)	Tube Current-Time Product (mAs)	$CTDI_W$ (mGy)	$CTDI_W$/mAs (mGy/mAs)	% $CTDI_W$/mAs Difference 220 mAs
220	0.5	110	7.4	0.068	0.0
440	0.5	220	15	0.068	—
580	0.5	290	19.8	0.069	+1.5
440	0.33	145	9.94	0.068	0.0
440	0.375	165	11.3	0.068	0.0
440	1.0	440	30.2	0.069	+1.5

Note: All other factors were held constant at 120 kVp with 20 channels and 1.2-mm channel width (20 × 1.2 mm).
From Cody, McNitt-Gray: CT image quality and patient radiation dose: definitions, methods, and trade-offs. In Radiological Society of North America: *Categorical course in diagnostic radiology physics: from invisible to visible—the science and practice of x-ray imaging and radiation dose optimization*, Chicago, 2006, Radiological Society of North Ameria. Reproduced by permission of Radiological Society of North America and the authors.

true mAs must be increased as well (Cody and McNitt-Gray, 2006). For example, increasing the pitch from, say, 1 to 2, increases the mAs per rotation from 100 to 200 while the relative $CTDI_{vol}$ remains the same (Lewis, 2005).

Peak Kilovoltage

The peak kilovoltage (kVp) determines the penetrating power of the photons coming from the x-ray tube. Higher kVp means that the photons have higher energies and can penetrate thicker objects compared with lower kVp x-ray beams. In CT generally, for adult imaging, high kVp techniques are used, such as 120 kVp, for example. The radiation dose is proportional to the square of the kVp (Bushberg et al, 2004). This means that the quantity of photons increases by the square of the kVp. A 72-kVp technique will have fewer photons than a kVp of 82, all factors held constant.

The results of different amounts of kVp on the dose (mGy and mGy/mAs) with a 64-slice spiral/helical CT scanner are provided in Table 10-2. It is clearly apparent that as the kVp increases, the dose increases. For example, the $CTDI_w$ (mGy) for a 32-cm diameter body phantom using an 80 kV and a 140 kVp beam is 5.2 and 24.9 mGy, respectively, when all other technical scanning factors remain constant (Cody and McNitt-Gray, 2006).

Collimation (Z-Axis Geometric Efficiency)

In CT, the collimation is used to define the beam width for the examination. Collimation schemes are different between single-slice (single detector row along the z-axis) and multislice (multidetector rows along the z-axis) CT scanners. The collimation reflects the efficient use of the x-ray beam at the detector, as shown in Figure 10-11. The shaded portion represents the penumbra that is caused by the finite size of the x-ray tube focal spot. It is clearly apparent that on a single-slice CT scanner the entire beam width plus the penumbra fall on the detectors. The penumbra, however, is not used to produce the image, but it does affect the patient dose.

On multislice CT scanners, the beam width, including the penumbra, would fall on a finite set of detectors depending on the scanner, but

TABLE 10-2 Changes in $CTDI_w$ in a 32-cm Diameter Body Phantom as a Function of Tube Potential (kV)

Peak Voltage (kVp)	$CTDI_W$ (mGy)	$CTDI_W$/mAs (mGy/mAs)	% Difference from 120-kVp Setting
80	18.0	0.073	−63.6
100	32.3	0.131	−34.6
120	49.4	0.200	—
140	68.2	0.276	+38.2

Note: All other factors were held constant at a 0.75-second rotation time, 330 mA, collimation of 12 channels with 1.5-mm channel width (12 × 1.5 mm), and head bowtie filtration.
From Cody, McNitt-Gray: CT image quality and patient radiation dose: definitions, methods, and trade-offs. In Radiological Society of North America: *Categorical course in diagnostic radiology physics: from invisible to visible—the science and practice of x-ray imaging and radiation dose optimization*, Chicago, 2006, Radiological Society of North America. Reproduced by permission of Radiological Society of North America and the authors.

the penumbra would not be used to produce the image (because the intensity of the beam at the penumbra regions is less than the intensity at the center of the beam). To address this problem, the beam width (collimation) is increased so that the penumbra extends beyond the active detectors that will receive the central beam intensity (Lewis, 2005). The ratio of the area under the z-axis dose profile falling on the active detectors to the area under the total z-axis dose profile is referred to as the z-axis geometric efficiency (IEC, 2001).

Cody and McNitt-Gray (2006) have shown that for a 32-cm diameter phantom, as beam widths increase from 18.0 mm, 19.2 mm, 24.0 mm, and 28.8 mm, the $CTDI_w$ (mGy) changes from 15.7 mGy, 16.8 mGy, 15.0 mGy, and 13.9 mGy, respectively (all other technical factors held constant). Additionally, Lewis (2005) indicates that "scanners that acquire a greater number of simultaneous slices have an advantage in terms of z-axis geometric efficiency. This is because for narrow slice widths a wider total collimation can be used....On multislice scanners z-axis geometric efficiencies are generally in the range of 80-98% for collimators of 10mm and above, and about 55-75% for collimators of around 5mm. For collimators around 1-2mm z-axis geometric efficiencies are as low as 25% on some systems, although in dual slice mode, they can be much higher. Therefore the reduced geometric efficiency of multislice scanners, for wider collimators most commonly used, leads to dose increases around 10% when compared to single slice systems. However very narrow collimations can result in a tripling, or more, in dose."

Pitch

The term *pitch* is one common to spiral/helical CT scanners, sometimes called *spiral pitch* or *helical pitch* depending on the manufacturer of the scanner. As defined by the IEC, pitch is a ratio of the distance the table travels per rotation to the total collimated x-ray beam width. The relationship between the absorbed dose and pitch is as follows:

$$\text{Dose} \propto 1/\text{Pitch} \quad (10\text{-}9)$$

Therefore if the pitch increases by 2, the dose will be reduced to one half. It is important, however, to note that this relationship only holds true when the pitch changes and all other factors remain constant. For constant mAs (100 mAs per rotation), if the pitch changes from 1 to 2, the relative $CTDI_{vol}$ decreases from 1.0 to 0.5mGy (Lewis, 2005).

Number of Detectors

In a study comparing the dose from multislice CT scanners, Moore et al (2006) demonstrated that the measured radiation dose is inversely proportional to the number of detector rows. They showed that there is a trend that as the number of detector rows increases from 4, 8, to 16 detector rows, the dose decreases with both standard and near identical technique (Moore et al, 2006).

Overranging (Z-Overscanning)

In spiral/helical CT scanning, it is important to realize that to image the planned length of tissue required for the examination and that is of interest to the radiologist, additional rotations before and after the planned length are essential for the image reconstruction process. This is referred to as overranging or z-overscanning (Van der Molen and Gelijns, 2007; Tzedakis et al, 2007), of which the components and definitions developed by Van der Molen and Gelijns (2007) are clearly illustrated in Figure 10-12. It is clear that there are two definitions of overranging:

1. Definition 1: This refers to the difference between the planned and exposed scan length.
2. Definition 2: This refers to the difference between the imaged and the exposed scan length.

Overranging increases the dose to the patient, which is validated in studies conducted by Tzedakis et al (2007) on pediatric patients and by Van der Molen and Gelijns (2007). For example, Tzedakis et al (2007) concluded that "in all cases normalized effective dose values were found to increase with increasing z-overscanning. The percentage differences in normalized data between axial and helical scans may reach 43%, 70%, 36%, and 26% for head-neck, chest, abdomen-pelvis, and trunk studies, respectively." Van der Molen and Gelijns (2007), for example, concluded that "overranging is reconstruction algorithm specific, and its length generally increases with collimation and pitch, while the effect of section width is variable. Overranging may lead to substantial but unnoticed exposure to radiosensitive organs."

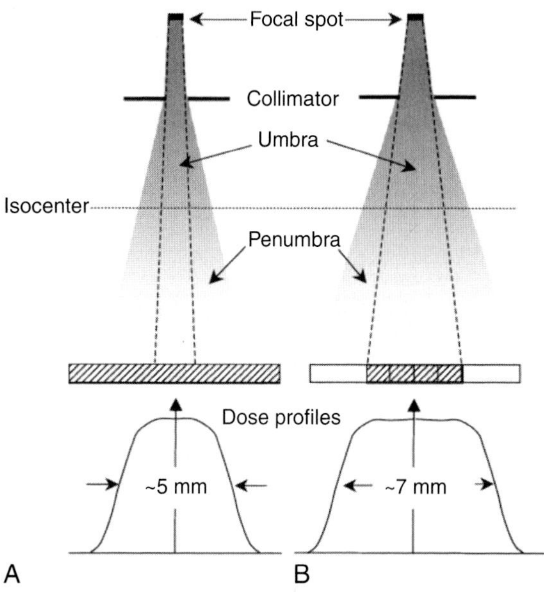

FIGURE 10-11 The implications of focal spot penumbra on dose. In **A** the geometry of a single-slice scanner collimated to a nominal slice width of 4 mm is illustrated. The umbra and all the penumbra contribute to image formation, resulting in a dose profile of 5 mm that, when corrected to the isocenter, closely corresponds to the nominal slice width of 4 mm. In **B** the geometry for a multislice scanner collimated to a nominal 4 × 1 mm beam width may be compared. The collimators must be opened to ensure that each of the four 1-mm wide detector rows receives similar umbral radiation. The penumbral radiation is not used in the image reconstruction, and the resulting dose profile is approximately 7 mm in width. (From Heggie JCP et al: Importance of optimization of multi-slice computed tomography scan protocols, *Aust Radiol* 50:278-285, 2006. Reproduced by permission of Blackwell Publications, Oxford, England.)

Patient Centering

Another factor affecting the dose to the patient that is under the control of the technologist is that of patient centering. The patient must be

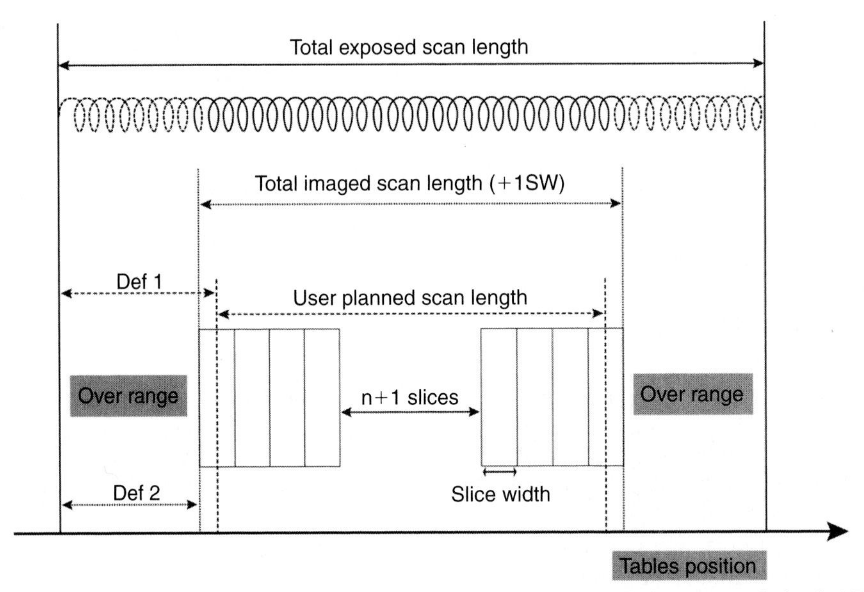

FIGURE 10-12 Simplified depiction of overranging components and definitions at helical CT scanning. To the planned scan length, one section width *(SW)* is automatically added so imaged scan length is slightly longer. Extra rotations needed for image reconstruction are added to imaged length, resulting in longer exposed scan length. Definitions of overranging vary; either the difference between planned and exposed scan length *(Def 1)* or the difference between imaged and exposed scan length *(Def 2)* is used. (From Van der Molen AJ, Geleijns J: Overranging in multisection CT: quantification and relative contribution to dose—comparison of four 16-section CT scanners, *Radiology* 242:208-216, 2007. Reproduced by permission of Radiological Society of North America and the authors.)

centered in the gantry isocenter for accurate imaging of the anatomy. Inaccurate patient centering (miscentering) as shown in Figure 10-13 degrades the image quality and increases the dose to the patient, especially with the use of AEC in CT (Li et al, 2007; Toth et al, 2007). Additionally, the use of bowtie filters in CT scanners is intended to serve basically two purposes: to shape the beam intensity within the scan field-of-view (SFOV) and to produce a more uniform beam at the detectors (Chapter 5). The x-ray beam is filtered; therefore, the bowtie filter actually plays a small role in reducing the dose to the patient because the low energy photons are removed and thus the beam becomes harder, that is, the mean energy of the beam increases. Improper centering of the patient in the gantry isocenter as shown in Figure 10-13 can lead to an increase in surface dose as well as the peripheral dose to the patient (Li et al, 2007; Toth et al, 2007).

In a study on the effect of patient centering on CT dose and image noise, Toth et al (2007) showed that, for a 32-cm CTDI body phantom, a miscentering of about 3 cm and 6 cm can result in an increase in doses by 18% and 41%, respectively. Similar results were obtained by Li et al (2007). Furthermore, a miscentering in elevation by 20 to 60 mm with a mean position 23 millimeters below the isocenter can result in a dose increase of up to 140% "with a mean dose penalty of 33% assuming that the tube current is increased

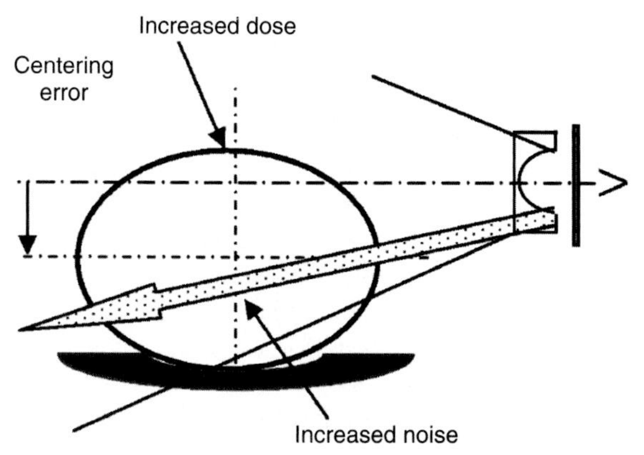

FIGURE 10-13 A patient who is miscentered in the scan field of view can be expected to have degraded bowtie filter performance with an undesired increase in both dose and noise. (From Toth et al: How patient centering affects CT dose and noise, *Med Phys* 34:3093-3101, 2007. Reproduced by the American Association of Physicists in Medicine.)

to compensate for the increased noise due to miscentering" (Toth et al, 2007).

These findings are positive proof that technologists should always center the patient accurately in the gantry isocenter to avoid image noise problems and reduce the dose to the patient.

Automatic Tube Current Modulation

AEC is now commonplace on CT scanners. AEC uses a technique referred to as automatic tube current modulation (ATCM) to optimize the dose to the patient while maintaining constant image quality regardless of the size of the patient in the z-axis and the attenuation changes in the x-y axis (Brisse et al, 2007; Toth et al, 2007). ATCM has been hailed as "the most important technique for maintaining constant image quality while optimizing radiation dose" (Li et al, 2007). For this reason, ATCM is described in detail in the next section of the chapter.

AUTOMATIC TUBE CURRENT MODULATION

ATCM is a technical development in CT based on the fundamental principles of AEC. AEC is not a new concept for radiologic technologists, for it is used extensively in radiography and fluoroscopy. The purpose of AEC in radiography, for example, is to provide a level of image quality (expressed as optical density for film-based radiography) in which there is consistent optical density for any examination (e.g., chest x-ray) regardless of the thickness (small, medium, and large) of the patient. This level of image quality (optical density) is controlled by varying the duration of the exposure on the basis of the size of patient being imaged. For example, although the duration of the exposure will be shorter for smaller patients, it will be longer for larger patients, and therefore images of the same body parts on these patients will all have a consistent level of optical density.

Problem with Setting Manual Milliamperage Techniques

In CT, the exposure technique factors (mAs and kVp) do not have a direct effect on the image density and contrast, respectively (as they do in film-based radiography), because CT is a digital imaging modality. The dose to the patient is directly proportional to the mA, and in the past, CT technologists selected the mA values for patients manually. Lewis (2005) explains one of the problems with setting the mA values manually. She notes "the attenuation of the x-ray beam increases with the thickness of material in its path, and for approximately every 4 cm of soft tissue, the x-ray beam intensity halves. In order to achieve the same transmitted x-ray intensity, and thereby the same level of image noise, changing from a 16 cm to a 20 cm diameter phantom requires a doubling of the mA. Changing from a 32 cm to a 48 cm phantom, the mA should in theory, be increased by a factor of 16. Systems which automatically adapt the overall tube current based on actual patient attenuation remove the guesswork from selecting the appropriate mA setting" (Lewis, 2005).

Definition of Automatic Tube Current Modulation

In CT, ATCM refers to the automatic control of the mA in two directions of the patient (the x-y axis and the z-axis) during data acquisition (scanning process) by use of specific technical procedures that take into consideration not only the patient size but also the attenuation differences of the various tissues. The overall goal of ATCM is to provide consistent image quality despite the size of the patient and the tissue attenuation differences and to control the dose to the patient (Brisse et al, 2007; Kalra et al, 2004b; Li et al, 2007; McCollough et al, 2006; Toth et al, 2007) compared with manual mA selection techniques. Although the automatic control of the tube current (mA) in the x-y axis (in-plane) is referred to as angular modulation, changing the tube current automatically in the z-axis (through-plane) is referred to as z-axis modulation or longitudinal modulation. When used together, that is, angular-longitudinal tube current modulation, AEC is the result (Goodman and Brink, 2006).

The use of angular-longitudinal modulation can reduce the dose by as much as 52% compared with use of only the angular modulation technique (Goodman and Brink, 2006).

Historical Background

ATCM techniques can be traced back to 1981, when Haaga et al (1981) suggested its use as a dose reduction strategy in CT while not compromising the needed image quality to make a diagnosis. This was followed by efforts of several others, such as General Electric (GE) Medical Systems in 1994 and researchers such as Kalender, who in 1999 published two reports describing dose reductions as much as 40% with ATCM techniques (McCollough et al, 2006). Later in 2001, a number of CT manufacturers such as GE Healthcare, Philips, Siemens, and Toshiba introduced ATCM techniques referred to by several names. For example, angular modulation systems are referred to as Smart Scan (GE Healthcare), DOM-Dose Modulation (Philips), and Care Dose (Siemens). In addition, different names are used for both angular-longitudinal modulation systems, such as for example; Smart mA (GE Healthcare), Z-DOM (Philips), CareDose 4D (Siemens), and Sure Exposure (Toshiba).

Basic Principles of Operation

In CT AEC, the tube current (mA) is adjusted in real time during the scanning of a patient on the basis of differences in radiation attenuation in the transverse or x-y direction (in-plane) and the z-axis or longitudinal direction (through-plane) during the rotation of the tube and detectors. In addition, these tube current modulation techniques require some knowledge of the attenuation characteristics of the patient, and second, the operator must first set up the defined level of image quality (image noise target value) needed for the examination (Cody and McNitt-Gray, 2006; Lewis, 2005; McCollough et al, 2006). Each of these will be described briefly.

Longitudinal (Z-Axis) Tube Current Modulation

Longitudinal (z-axis) tube current modulation (z-axis TCM) is based on differences in attenuation among body parts. For example, thicker body parts such as the abdomen and pelvis will attenuate the radiation more than thinner body parts, such as the head, neck, and chest regions. The technique of z-axis TCM is designed (using a specific computer algorithm) to change the mA automatically as the patient is scanned from, say, head to toe (along the z-axis) while maintaining a constant (uniform) noise level (image noise target values) for different thicknesses of body parts examined. This is clearly shown in Figure 10-14.

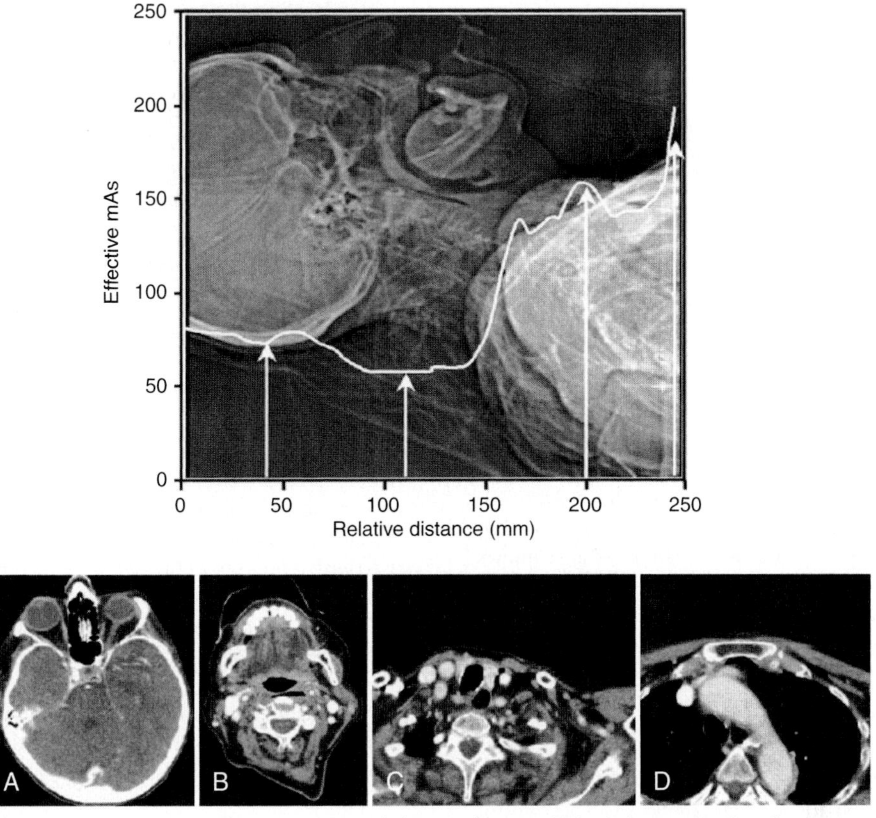

FIGURE 10-14 The z-axis tube current modulation during CT of the neck. On the basis of the attenuation measurements made during the acquisition of the scan projection radiograph, the scanner software adjusts the effective mAs on the fly during the acquisition of the axial images. Axial images shown through orbits (**A**), midcervical vertebrae (**B**), the apex of the lung (**C**), and the aortic arch (**D**) require 75, 58, 160, and 200 mAs respectively, at 120 kVp. (From Heggie JCP et al: Importance of optimization of multi-slice computed tomography scan protocols, *Aust Radiol* 50:278-285, 2006. Reproduced by permission of Blackwell Publications, Oxford, England.)

Angular (X-Y Axis) Tube Current Modulation

Angular (x-y axis) tube current modulation (x-y axis TCM) is based on the fact that the radiation attenuation varies from the anteroposterior (AP) projection (low attenuation) to the lateral projection (high attenuation) as the tube rotates around (gantry rotation) the patient. Although the high attenuation projections will require higher mA values, the low attenuation projections will require lower mA values, as illustrated in Figure 10-15. The x-y axis TCM algorithm ensures that a constant (uniform) noise level is maintained during the scanning process.

Angular-Longitudinal Tube Current Modulation

Figure 10-16 illustrates a method where both x-y axis and z-axis modulation can be used

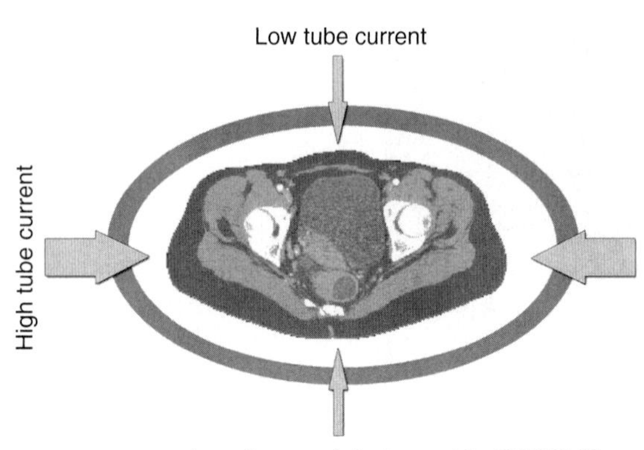

FIGURE 10-15 Angular modulation with CARE Dose (Siemens Medical Solutions) ATCM technique. On-line modulation of tube current is performed at different projections in the x-y plane within each 360-degree x-ray tube rotation. Thin arrows indicate reduction of tube current relative to higher tube current *(thick arrows)*. (From Kalra M et al: Techniques and applications of automatic tube current modulation for CT, *Radiology* 233:649-657, 2004. Reproduced by permission of the Radiological Society of North America and the authors.)

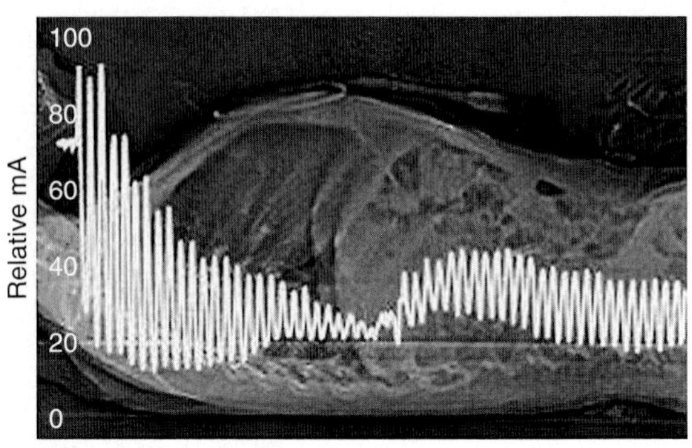

FIGURE 10-16 Graph of tube current *(mA)* superimposed on a CT projection radiograph shows the variation in tube current as a function of time (and, hence, table position along the z-axis) at spiral CT in a 6-year-old child. An adult scanning protocol and an AEC system (CareDose 4D, Siemens Medical Solutions) were used with a reference effective tube current-time product of 165 mAs. The mean effective tube current-time product for actual scanning was 38 mAs (effective tube current-time product = tube current-time product/pitch). (From McCollough C et al: CT dose reduction and dose management tools: overview of available options, *Radiographics* 26:503-512, 2006. Reproduced by permission of the Radiological Society of North America and the authors.)

together to therefore provide the "most comprehensive approach to CT dose reduction because the x-ray dose is adjusted according to the patient-specific attenuation in all three planes" (McCollough et al, 2006).

Approaches to Obtaining Attenuation Characteristics of the Patient

The attenuation characteristics of the patient are one of the first pieces of information that is required to use of AEC systems in CT imaging (that is, vary the mA during the scanning process and keep the image noise constant regardless of the gantry rotation and the z-axis position). Such information is currently obtained by two different schemes. Although the first approach uses a CT scanned projection radiograph (SPR), the typical "scout view" (also referred to as ScoutView, Topogram, or the Scanogram depending on the CT vendor), the second approach makes use of "on-line" data "from the preceding 180° of rotation to modulate the mA" (Lewis, 2005).

Defined Level of Image Quality in CT Automatic Exposure Control

The second requirement when AEC is used in CT imaging is that operators must set up the defined level of image quality on their respective CT scanners. The approaches from four CT vendors include a noise index (GE Healthcare), a reference image (Philips), a quality reference mAs (Siemens), and the standard deviation of CT numbers or an image quality level (Toshiba). Each of these is briefly described in Table 10-3. Essentially, the fundamental basis for these methods, as outlined in Table 10-1, rests on several important points:

1. A CT projection radiograph is required from which attenuation data are obtained.
2. An image quality index is prescribed (prescription of the mA). This index related to the noise

TABLE 10-3 Image Quality Paradigms to Help the Computed Tomography Operator Select the Desired Level of Image Quality in Automatic Exposure Control in Computed Tomography

CT Vendor	Image Quality Paradigm	Description*
GE Healthcare	Noise Index	The noise index is referenced to the standard deviation of CT numbers within the region of interest in a water phantom of a specific size. A look-up table is then used to map the patient-specific attenuation values measured on the CT projection radiograph ("scout" image) to tube current values for each gantry rotation according to a proprietary algorithm. The algorithm is designed to maintain the same noise level as the attenuation values change from one rotation to the next. Different noise indices may be required for patients of different sizes.
Philips	Reference Image	In a process that the manufacturer calls automatic current setting, the user selects an acceptable patient examination, and the system saves the image (including the raw CT projection data and the CT projection radiograph, or "surview") as the reference data for comparison with the CT projection radiograph and data obtained from other patients in examinations for the same diagnostic task. The comparison is performed with the use of a proprietary algorithm and on a protocol-by-protocol basis (i.e., for a given examination type) to enable the automated selection of the appropriate tube current values by the scanner.
Siemens	Quality Reference mAs	For each examination type (i.e., protocol) the user selects the effective tube current-time product (tube current-time product/pitch) typically used for a CT in a patient with a weight of approximately 80 kg. (For pediatric protocols the effective tube current-time product that should be selected is that typically used for a CT in a 20-kg patient.) The noise target (standard deviation of the CT numbers) is varied on the basis of patient size by using an empirical algorithm; thus, image noise is not kept constant for all patients but is adjusted according to an empirical impression on image quality. CT projection radiography ("topograms") for each patient is used to predict the tube current curve (with variations along the x-y and z-axes) that will yield the desired image quality, given the patient's size and anatomy. An on-line feedback system fine-tunes the actual tube current values during scanning to precisely match the patient-specific attenuation values at all angles (as opposed to the attenuation values estimated on the basis of one angle of the CT projection radiograph).

*McCollough et al: CT dose reduction and dose management tools: overview of available options, *Radiographics* 26:503-512, 2006.

Continued

TABLE 10-3 Image Quality Paradigms to Help the Computed Tomography Operator Select the Desired Level of Image Quality in Automatic Exposure Control in Computed Tomography—cont'd

CT Vendor	Image Quality Paradigm	Description*
Toshiba	1. Standard deviation of CT numbers 2. Image quality level	Both methods are referenced to the standard deviation of CT numbers measured in a patient-equivalent water phantom. Data from the patient's CT projection radiograph (scanogram) are used to map the selected image quality to tube current values.

*McCollough et al: CT dose reduction and dose management tools: overview of available options, *Radiographics* 26:503-512, 2006.

level (standard deviation of the CT numbers in a water phantom) (Lewis, 2005), or
3. A referenced image is selected (from previous examinations) that has the image quality required and the mA is adjusted to produce the same level of image quality as the referenced image when scanning other patients.
4. These methods are based on the use of proprietary algorithms.

IMAGE QUALITY AND DOSE: OPERATOR CONSIDERATIONS

It is clearly apparent from the foregoing discussion that image quality and dose are closely related. Image quality includes spatial resolution, contrast resolution, and noise. Although spatial resolution depends on geometric factors (such as focal spot size, slice thickness, and pixel size, for example), contrast resolution and noise depend on both the quality (beam energy) and quantity (number of x-ray photons) of the radiation beam. Several mathematical equations have been derived to express the relationship between dose and image quality (Bushong, 2009). For CT operators, the following mathematical expression is important:

$$\text{Dose} = \text{Intensity} \times \text{Beam energy}/\text{Noise}^2 \times \text{Pixel size}^3 \times \text{Slice thickness}$$

where intensity and beam energy depend on mA and kVp, respectively, and noise depends on the number of photons detected. This expression is read as follows: dose is directly proportional to the product of mA and kVp and inversely proportional to the product of noise squared, pixel size cubed, and slice thickness.

The expression also implies the following about dose and image quality:

1. To reduce the noise in an image by a factor of 2 requires an increase in the dose by a factor of 4.
2. To improve the spatial resolution (pixel size) by a factor of 2 (keeping the noise constant) requires an increase in the dose by a factor of 8.
3. To decrease the slice thickness by a factor of 2 requires an increase in the dose by a factor of 2 (keeping the noise constant).
4. To decrease both the slice thickness and the pixel size by a factor of 2 requires an increase in the dose by a factor of 16 ($2^3 \times 2 = 2 \times 2 \times 2 \times 2$).

5. Increasing mA and kVp increases the dose proportionally. For example, a twofold increase in mA increases the dose by a factor of 2. Additionally, doubling the dose will require an increase by the square of the kVp.

CT DOSE OPTIMIZATION

In this chapter, two points have been made clear so far. First, CT is rapidly expanding in its use in medicine. Second, a major concern that is receiving increasing attention in the literature relates to the potential for high radiation doses delivered by CT scanners and the potential biologic risks of CT scanning (Brenner and Elliston, 2004; Brenner et al, 2001). With these notions in mind, there have been increasing efforts to reduce the dose to the patient without compromising the image quality needed to make a diagnosis. One such significant approach is that of dose optimization, and to date various strategies have been devised to help CT users reduce the dose to the patient while maintaining optimal image quality (Heggie et al, 2006; Kalra et al, 2004a; Lewis, 2005; McCollough et al, 2006).

What Is Dose Optimization?

Optimization is a radiation protection principle that is intended to ensure that doses delivered to patients are kept as low as is reasonably achievable (ALARA). Essentially, the principle of optimization refers to reducing radiation dose while maintaining the required image quality needed for making a diagnosis. Dose optimization is especially important for digital imaging modalities such as computed radiography and CT, for example, where the potential for high doses exists (Brenner and Hall, 2007).

Dose Optimization Strategies

As described in this chapter, a number of factors affect the dose to the patient in CT. These include the scan parameters such as exposure technique factors (constant and effective mAs and kVp), collimation (z-axis geometric efficiency), pitch, number of detectors, overranging (z-overscanning), patient centering, and ATCM. To effectively reduce the dose and maintain the needed image quality, users must have systematic approaches or strategies to CT dose optimization.

Several authors have described various dose optimization strategies in CT, especially in multislice CT (Frush, 2004; Heggie et al, 2006; Kalra et al, 2004a; Kanal et al, 2007; Lai and Frush, 2006; Lewis, 2005; McCollough et al, 2006; Winkler, 2003; Winkler and Mather, 2005). It is not within the scope of this chapter to describe details of these strategies; however, it is noteworthy to highlight the essential guiding principles. Several strategies that emerge as common themes relate to the mAs, kVp, collimation, slice thickness, scanned volume, pitch, and the use of ATCM techniques. In CT dose optimization, Heggie et al (2006) present a summary of the main items to consider, as listed in Box 10-1.

Dose optimization has received increasing attention in pediatric CT. Lai and Frush (2006) and Goodman and Brink (2006), for example, present excellent overviews on this topic, examining not only trends and patterns of CT use, radiation risks from CT, and how radiologists can manage CT dose but also focus on the technical factors for dose management such as controlling tube current and voltage, the influence of gantry cycle time, choice of pitch and detector width, and finally the use of tube current modulation techniques. For example, Lai and Frush (2006) emphasize the importance of the radiologist to ensure that all examinations ordered should be justified and that the need for communications between ordering physicians and radiologists is vital as a first step to CT dose reduction. Additionally, they point out that the CT protocols used must include various technical parameters that optimize the dose to the patient without compromising the needed image quality. In this regard, they state that increasing the detector width from

BOX 10-1 *Optimization Technique*

Use sequential as opposed to helical techniques for head scans
Avoid transferring scan protocols applicable to one scanner to another without due consideration to differences in scanner filtration and geometry
Keep scanned volume to minimum and scan in one large block rather than multiple smaller blocks. However, see text for possible exceptions
Use widest x-ray beam collimation consistent with clinical requirements
Consider using a lower tube potential for CT angiography
Keep the effective mAs, which is defined as the mAs/pitch, as low as clinically indicated
Use tube current modulation technology with an appropriately selected reference effective mAs or noise index. For optimum performance of modulation technology, the SPR that is of clinical relevance must be acquired over the full length of the patient by using the same kVp that will be subsequently used for the axial image acquisition
Minimize use of multiphasic examinations

The primary parameters that have an impact of CT dose optimization.
From Heggie et al: Importance in optimization of multi-slice computed tomography scan protocols, *Aust Radiol* 50:278-285, 2006. Reproduced by permission Blackwell Publishing Limited, Oxford, England.

0.625 to 1.25 for a 16-slice CT scanner while holding all other factors constant will result in a reduced dose to the patient. Finally, they also advocate the use of age- or weight-adjusted CT protocols and the use of ATCM techniques. In addition, interesting study on optimizing image quality and radiation dose in CT pulmonary angiography showed that by decreasing the peak kilovoltage from 120 to 100 kVp, the dose to the patient is reduced significantly without loss of objective or subjective image quality (Heyer et al, 2007).

RADIATION PROTECTION CONSIDERATIONS

The dose optimization strategies described so far focus on methods to reduce the dose to the patient. What about the protection of personnel in CT scanning? Radiation protection of both patients and personnel in medicine is guided by two triads that are intended to ensure that medical radiation workers work within the ALARA (as low as reasonable achievable) philosophy of the ICRP. One triad deals with radiation protection actions, and the other triad addresses the radiation protection principles (Seeram, 2001).

Radiation Protection Actions

Radiation protection actions include the use of time, shielding, and distance, which are intended to protect both patients and personnel in radiology. For example, because dose is proportional to the time of exposure, to protect personnel in CT, it is essential to minimize the time spent in the CT scan room during the exposure.

Distance, on the other hand, is a major dose reduction action because the dose is inversely proportional to the square of the distance. This means that the further one is away from the radiation source, the less the dose received. In CT, because the patient is the main source of scatter, technologists should stand back as far away from the patient as possible if there is a need to be present in the scan room during scanning. This implies that the use of a power injector that can be controlled from outside the scan room is recommended. If a hand injector is used, then a long tubing should be used.

Shielding is intended to protect not only patients (gonadal, breast, eyes, and thyroid shielding) but also personnel and members of the public. Patients are often concerned about the exposure of their gonads during a CT examination. Because most of the gonadal exposure will come from internal scatter and not from the primary beam (unless the gonadal region was being examined), there is no need for this concern. Technologists, however, could place gonadal shielding on the patient because it may alleviate any fears about the risks of being exposed to radiation. Shields can also be used to protect the eyes, breast, and thyroid of patients undergoing CT examinations (Fricke et al, 2003; Kennedy et al, 2007). Although some of the shields are made of flexible, nonlead (bismuth) composition, lead may also be used (Kennedy et al, 2007) to provide significant dose reduction to these critical organs.

When personnel are expected to be present in the CT scan room during the exposure, lead aprons should be worn (for the same reason that gonadal shields are placed on patients) because of the presence of scatter (Bushong, 2009).

Because scatter radiation is present during a CT examination and strikes the walls of the CT room, should these walls be shielded to protect members of the public or other radiation workers who are present outside the room. The use of minimum shielding in the form of thick plate-glass control room viewing windows and gypsum wall board with no lead content can sometimes provide the minimum required shielding.

Radiation Protection Principles

Radiation protection principles deal with justification, optimization, and dose limitation, principles that are vital to radiation protection regulation.

Justification involves the concept of net benefit, that is, there must be a benefit associated with every exposure. This requirement is intended for referring physicians and is one effort to reduce doses to patients undergoing x-ray examinations.

Optimization is a principle that is intended to ensure that doses delivered to patients are kept as low as is reasonably achievable (ALARA), economic and social factors being taken into account. In implementing ALARA, technologists should always apply all relevant technical radiation protection practices to ensure that the dose is optimized and that image quality is not compromised, as discussed earlier in the chapter.

The concept of dose limitation is a major integral component of regulatory guidance on radiation protection. This concept addresses the dose that an individual receives annually or accumulates over a working lifetime. These doses should be within the limits established by international organizations such as the ICRP and other national bodies such as the National Council on Radiation Protection. These recommended limits are intended to reduce the probability of stochastic effects and to prevent detrimental deterministic effects. These dose limits are beyond the scope of this chapter.

REFERENCES

Amis ES et al: American College of Radiology white paper on radiation dose in medicine, *J Am Coll Radiol* 4:272-284, 2007.

Baker SR, Tilak GS: CT spurs concern over thyroid cancer, *Diagn Imag* 25-27, 51, 2006.

Barr HJ et al: Focusing in on dose reduction, *AJR Am J Roentgenol* 186:1716-1717, 2006.

Boone JM: The trouble with the $CTDI_{100}$, *Med Phys* 34:1364-1371, 2007.

Boone JM et al: Dose reduction in pediatric CT: a rational approach, *Radiology* 228:352-360, 2003.

Brenner DJ: It is time to retire the computed tomography dose index (CTDI) for CT quality assurance and dose optimization, *Med Phys* 33:1189-1191, 2006.

Brenner DJ, Elliston CD: Estimated radiation risks potentially associated with full body CT screening, *Radiology* 232:735-738, 2004.

Brenner DJ, Hall EJ: CT–an increasing source of radiation exposure, *N Engl J Med* 22:2277-2284, 2007.

Brenner DJ et al: Estimated risks of radiation-induced fatal cancer from pediatric CT, *AJR Am J Roentgenol* 176:289-296, 2001.

Brisse HJ et al: Automatic exposure control in multichannel CT with tube current modulation to achieve a constant level of image noise: experimental assessment on pediatric phantoms, *Med Phys* 34:3018-3032, 2007.

Bushberg AT et al: *The essential physics of medical imaging*, ed. 2, Philadelphia, 2004, Lippincott-Williams.

Bushong S: *Radiologic science for technologists*, ed 9, St Louis, 2009, Mosby-Year Book.

Cody D, McNitt-Gray: CT image quality and patient dose. Definitions, methods and trade-offs. *RSNA Categorical course in diagnostic radiology physics: from invisible to visible-the science and practice of x-ray imaging and radiation dose optimization*, 2006.

Coolang JE et al: Patient dose from CT: a literature review, *Radiol Technol* 79:17-26, 2007.

Dixon RL: A new look at CT dose measurement: beyond CTDI, *Med Phys* 30:1272-1280, 2003.

Dixon RL: Restructuring CT dosimetry–a realistic strategy for the future Requiem for the pencil chamber, *Med Phys* 33:3973-3976, 2006.

ECRI: Radiation dose in CT, *Health Devices* 36:41-63, 2007.

Fricke BL et al: In-plane bismuth breast shields for pediatric CT: effects on radiation dose and image quality using experimental and clinical data, *AJR Am J Roentgenol* 180:407-411, 2003.

Frush DP: Review of radiation issues for computed tomography, *Semin Untrasound CT MRI* 25:17-24, 2004.

Frush DP: Pediatric CT quality and radiation dose: clinical perspective. In *Radiological Society of North America: Categorical course in diagnostic radiology physics: from invisible to visible—the science and practice of x-ray imaging and radiation dose optimization*, pp 167-182, 2006, Radiological Society of North America.

Goodman TR, Brink JA: adult CT: controlling dose and image quality. In *Radiological Society of North America: Categorical course in diagnostic radiology physics: from invisible to visible—the science and practice of x-ray imaging and radiation dose optimization*, pp 157-165, 2006, Radiological Society of North America.

Haaga JR et al: The effect of mAs variation upon computed tomography image quality as evaluated by in vivo and in vitro studies, *Radiology* 138:449-454, 1981.

Heggie JCP et al: Importance of optimization of multislice computed tomography scan protocols, *Aust Radiol* 50:278-285, 2006.

Heyer CM et al: Image quality and radiation exposure at pulmonary CT angiography with 100- or 120-kVp protocol, *Radiology* 245:577-583, 2007.

Huda W: Medical radiation dosimetry. In *Radiological Society of North America Categorical course in diagnostic radiology physics: from invisible to visible—the science and practice of x-ray imaging and radiation dose optimization*, pp 29-39, Chicago, 2006, Radiological Society of North America.

Huda W, Vance A: Patient radiation dsoes from adult and pediatric CT, *AJR Am J Roentgenol* 188:540-546, 2007.

Huda W et al: How do radiographic techniques affect image quality and patient doses in CT? *Semin Ultrasound CT MRI* 23:411-422, 2003.

International Electrotechnical Commission (IEC): Particular requirements for the safety of x-ray equipment for CT, *Ed 2 60601-2-44*, 2001.

Kalender W et al: Dose reduction in CT by anatomically adapted tube current modulation. II. Phantom measurements, *Med Phys* 26:2248-2253, 1999.

Kalra MK et al: Strategies for CT radiation dose optimization, *Radiology* 230:619-628, 2004a.

Kalra MK et al: Techniques and applications of automatic tube current modulation for CT, *Radiology* 233:649-657, 2004b.

Kanal KM et al: Impact of operator-selected image noise index and reconstruction slice thickness on patient radiation dose in 64-MDCT, *AJR Am J Roentgenol* 189:219-225, 2007.

Kennedy EV et al: Investigation into the effects of lead shielding for fetal dose reduction in CT pulmonary angiography, *Br J Radiol* 80:631-638, 2007.

Lai KC, Frush DP: Managing the radiation dose from pediatric CT, *Appl Radiol* April 13-20, 2006.

Larson DB et al: Informing parents about CT exposure in children: it's OK to tell them, *AJR Am J Roentgenol* 189:271-275, 2007.

Lee C et al: Organ and effective doses in pediatric patients undergoing helical multislice computed tomography examination, *Med Phys* 34:1858-1873, 2007.

Lewis M: *Radiation dose issues in multi-slice CT scanning*, London, 2005, St. George's Hospital.

Lewis M: *Principles and implementation of automatic exposure control systems in CT*, London, 2007, St. George's Hospital.

Li J et al: Automatic patient centering for MDCT: effect on radiation dose, *AJR Am J Roentgenol* 188:547-552, 2007.

Martin DR, Semelka RC: Health effects of ionizing radiation from diagnostic CT imaging: consideration of alternative imaging strategies, *Appl Radiol* March 20-29, 2007.

McCollough CH et al: CT dose reduction and dose management tools: overview of available options, *Radiographics* 26:503-512, 2006.
McCollough CH et al: Dose performance of a 64-channel dual source CT scanner, *Radiology* 243:775-784, 2007.
McNitt-Gray MF: Radiation dose in CT, *Radiographics* 22:1541-1553, 2002.
Moore WH et al: Comparison of MDCT radiation dose: a phantom study, *AJR Am J Roentgenol* 187:W498-W502, 2006.
Mori S et al: Comparison of patient doses in 256-slice CT and 16-slice CT scanners, *Br J Radiol* 79:56-61, 2006a.
Mori S et al: Conversion factor for CT dosimetry to assess patient dose using a 256-slice CT scanner, *Br J Radiol* 79:888-892, 2006b.
Mori S et al: Physical performance evaluation of a 256-slice CT scanner for 4-dimensional imaging, *Med Phys* 31:1348-1356, 2004.
Mukundan S et al: MOSFET dosimetry for radiation dose assessment of bismuth shielding of the eye in children, *AJR Am J Roentgenol* 188:16-48, 2007.
Seeram E: *Tech guide to radiation protection*, Boston, 2001, Blackwell Science.
Siegel E: Primum non nocere: a call for a re-evaluation of radiation doses used in CT, *Appl Radiol* April 6, 8, 2006.
Toth et al: The influence of patient centering on CT dose and image noise, *Med Phys* 34:3093-3101, 2007.
Tzedakis A et al: Influence of z overscanning on normalized effective doses calculated for pediatric patients undergoing multidetector CT examinations, *Med Phys* 34:1163-1172, 2007.
Van der Molen AJ: Geleijns J: Overranging in multisection CT: quantification and relative contribution to dose—comparison of four 16-section CT scanners, *Radiology* 242:208-216, 2007.
Winkler ML: Knowledgeable use of MDCT minimizes dose, *Diagn Imag* 2003.
Winkler M, Mather R: CT risk minimized by optimal system design, *Toshiba Med Syst* July 18-23, 2005.

Chapter 11

Single-Slice Spiral/Helical Computed Tomography: Physical Principles and Instrumentation

Chapter Outline

In 1990 the first computed tomography (CT) scanner to perform volume data acquisition was introduced (Kalender, 1995). This scanner was invented to overcome the problems imposed by conventional (slice-by-slice scanning) CT scanners. In addition, the scanners provide shorter scan times to subsecond levels and improvement in three-dimensional (3D) imaging. These scanners are referred to as single-slice *spiral/helical CT scanners* (SSCT) or volume CT scanners on the basis of the beam geometry used during data acquisition.

The purpose of the chapter is to introduce the language of SSCT scanning and describe the fundamental concepts of spiral/helical data acquisition, image reconstruction, major system components, basic scan parameters, and the advantages and limitations of SSCT scanners.

It is important to note that, more recently, multislice CT (MSCT) scanners have become available (see Chapter 1) and are rapidly replacing SSCT scanners. The physical principles and technology of MSCT scanners are described in detail in Chapter 12.

The technical principles and concepts of SSCT scanners described in this chapter serve to lay the foundations necessary for a good understanding of MSCT scanners.

HISTORICAL BACKGROUND

In the Beginning

An early pioneer in the development of the technique of volume scanning in CT was Dr. Willi A. Kalender (see Chapter 1) of the Institute of Medical Physics at the University of Erlangen, Germany. Kalender started work on spiral CT in 1988 with Peter Vock from Switzerland, and in 1989 he described the technical details and clinical applications of spiral CT to the Radiological Society of North America (RSNA) meeting in Chicago. Other early investigators included Mori (1987), various Japanese researchers, and Bresler and Skrabecz (1993).

Terminology Controversy

Kalender and Vock's presentation at the RSNA in 1989 resulted in a flurry of activities related to volume scanning. An interesting debate that surfaced in the early literature was related to the terminology to best describe the method of volume data acquisition. Should volume scanning be called spiral CT or helical CT? In a letter to the editors of the *American Journal of Roentgenology (AJR)*, Towers (1993) used an illustration (Fig. 11-1) to describe the fundamental differences between spiral CT and helical CT. Towers noted that the term *helical* describes a cylindrical configuration, whereas *spiral* refers to both cylindrical and conic configurations. He therefore recommended the use of the term *spiral CT*.

In another letter to the editors of *AJR*, Silverman et al (1994) argued that the term *helical CT* "best describes this new CT technology."

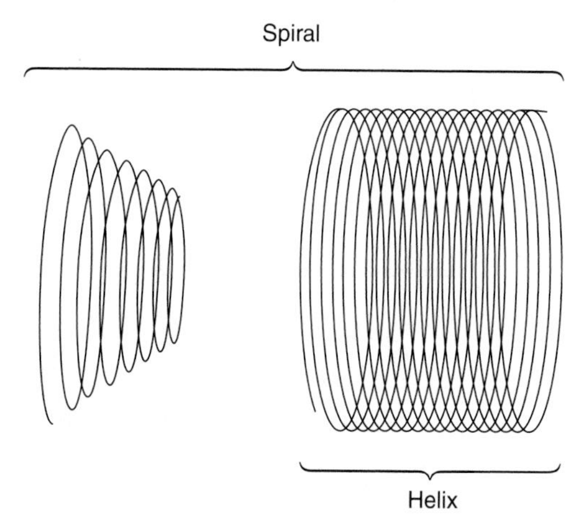

FIGURE 11-1 Spiral geometries. The helix is one type of spiral. (From Towers MJ: Spiral or helical CT? [letter], *AJR Am J Roentgenol* 161:901, 1993.)

Dr. Mark Bahn of the Mallinckrodt Institute of Radiology offered mathematical definitions to support this view. He pointed out that mathematical dictionaries (Baker, 1961; James and James, 1976) provide more technical definitions of these two terms: a spiral describes a curve on a plane surface; a helix describes a curve in 3D space.

In response, Kalender (1994a) submitted a letter (Appendix A) to the editors of *Radiology* to support use of the term *spiral CT*, which convinced the editors to accept either term for CT papers published in *Radiology*. This book uses both terms as synonyms, as suggested by Kalender (1994a).

CONVENTIONAL SLICE-BY-SLICE CT SCANNING

Scanning Sequence

In conventional CT scanning, the x-ray tube rotates around the patient to collect data from a single slice of tissue, followed by table indexing so that the next contiguous slice can be scanned. This process is repeated until data from several contiguous slices have been collected. The scanning sequence for this type of data acquisition consists of four distinct steps (Fig. 11-2).

In the first step, the x-ray tube must be accelerated to a constant speed of rotation. This means that the cables that supply power to the x-ray tube must be long enough to allow for the full 360-degree rotation. During this rotation (step 2), the x-ray tube produces x-rays that are transmitted through the patient to fall on the detectors, which measure the relative transmission values (data). At this particular point, the patient holds a breath, and data are collected from a specific axial slice. In step 3, the patient resumes breathing while the x-ray tube slows to a stop. In step 4, it is necessary to unwind the cable because of the 360-degree rotation and to move the patient and table so that the next contiguous slice can be scanned.

This four-step process is repeated until all the required contiguous axial slices have been scanned. The time it takes to accomplish steps 1, 3, and 4 is referred to as the *interscan delay time* (ISD).

Slices are usually collected in groups while the patient holds a breath, with the ISD after each pair of slices. Between two groups of slices is an

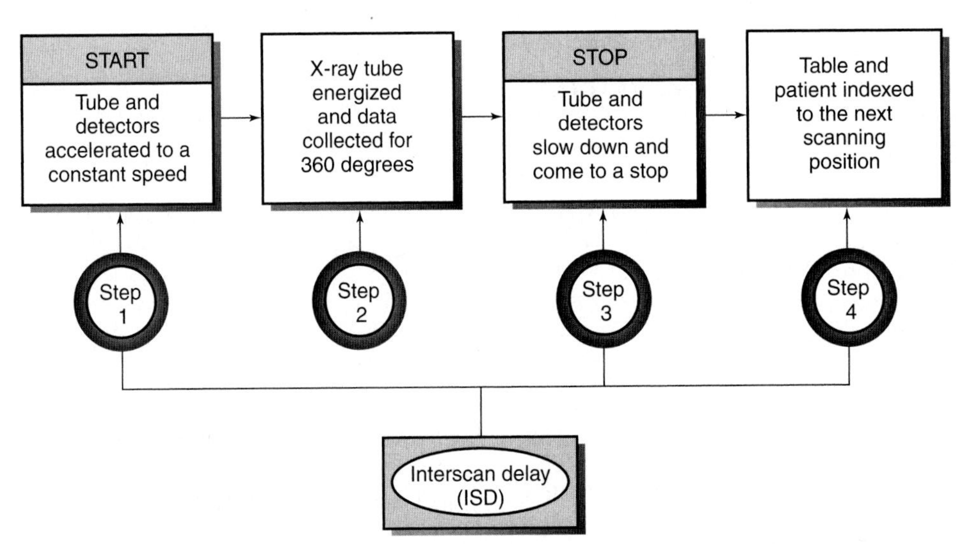

FIGURE 11-2 Characteristic four-step process of slice-by-slice sequential CT scanning.

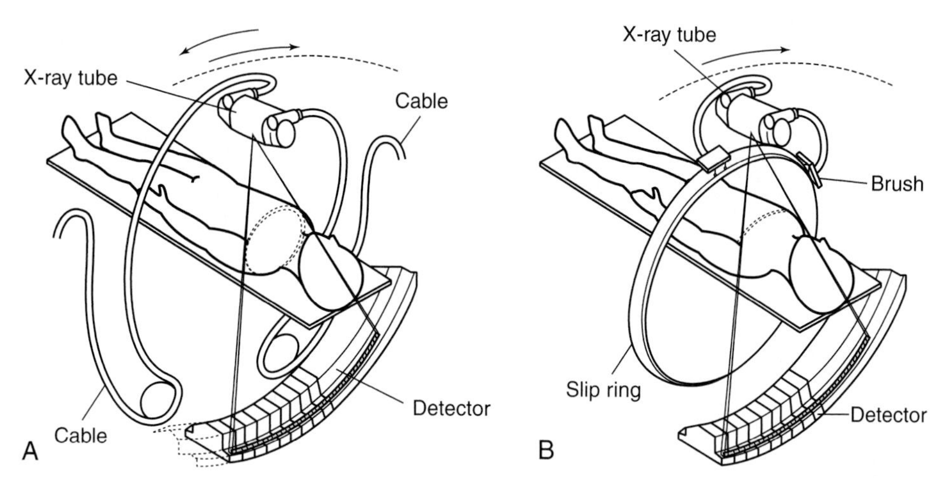

FIGURE 11-3 One advance in CT technology that facilitates CT fluoroscopy is continuous scanning by using slip-ring technology. The cable wraparound typical of conventional slice-by-slice CT results in a delay that prevents real-time image reconstruction and display. **A,** Reciprocating rotation. **B,** Fast continuous rotation. (From Ozaki M: Development of a real-time reconstruction system for CT fluorography, *Toshiba Med Rev* 53:12-17, 1995.)

intergroup delay, and it is at this point that the patient breathes. Additionally, the scan rate is expressed as the following ratio:

$$\text{Scan rate} = \frac{\text{No. of scans per group}}{\text{sum of time to collect slices} + \text{IGD}}$$

If the study requires more slices, its duration would have to be increased. This requirement places an additional burden on the patient to remain still to ensure that images obtained are free of motion artifacts.

Limitations

The limitations imposed by slice-by-slice sequential CT scanning include the following:

1. Longer examination times because of the stop-start action necessary for patient breathing, table indexing, and cable unwinding. This gives rise to the ISD. The cable wraparound and unwinding is shown in Figure 11-3, *A*. This wraparound results from the fixed length of the high-voltage cable, which follows the x-ray tube as it rotates through 360 degrees around the patient. The cable is unwound during the imaging of the next slice. In Figure 11-3, *B*, the cable wraparound process is eliminated through the use of slip-ring technology, which allows the x-ray tube to rotate continuously as the patient moves continuously through the gantry. This is spiral/helical CT scanning.
2. Certain portions of the anatomy are omitted because the patient respiration phase may not always be consistent between scans (Fig. 11-4). For example, it has been reported that lesions in the liver smaller than 1 centimeter (cm) may be missed because of inconsistent levels of inspiration. This omission of anatomy is often referred to as *slice-to-slice misregistration.*
3. Inaccurate generation of 3D images and multiplanar reformatted images, attributed to the inconsistent levels of inspiration from scan to scan. The result is the appearance of "steplike" contours in 3D images. Figure 11-5 illustrates production of the stairstep artifact and its elimination with spiral/helical CT.
4. Only a few slices are scanned during maximum contrast enhancement when the contrast

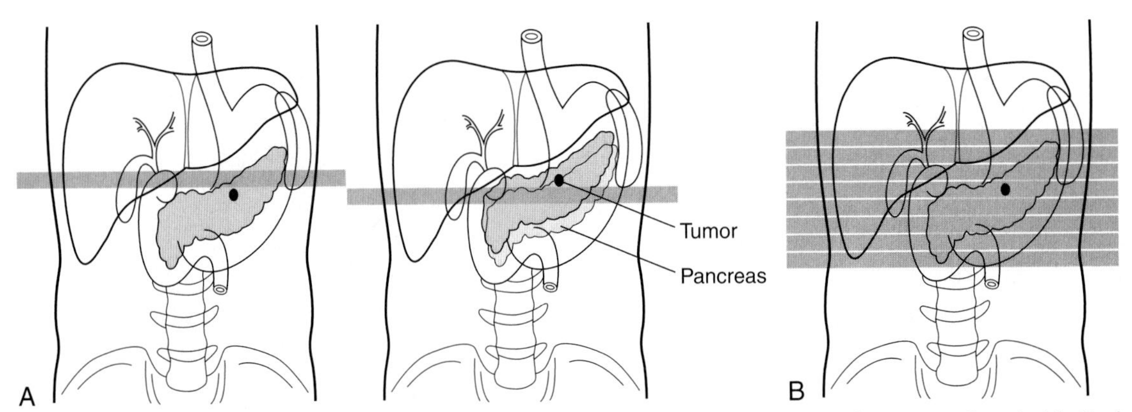

FIGURE 11-4 Removal of the effects of different levels of respiration. **A,** Conventional scanning. In spiral/helical CT scanning **(B)** there is no shifting of lesions because of different levels of respiration. (Courtesy Toshiba America Medical Systems, Tustin, Calif.)

enhancement technique is used. These problems may be overcome if the scan rate is increased and the ISD is eliminated, both of which are technologically feasible. The scan time can be increased by decreasing the time to accomplish the four steps shown in Figure 11-2. The ISD can be eliminated by having the tube (and detector) rotate continuously around the patient (instead of the start-stop action characteristic of slice-by-slice sequential CT scanning) while simultaneously translating the patient through the gantry aperture at a faster speed. Data are acquired during the patient translation.

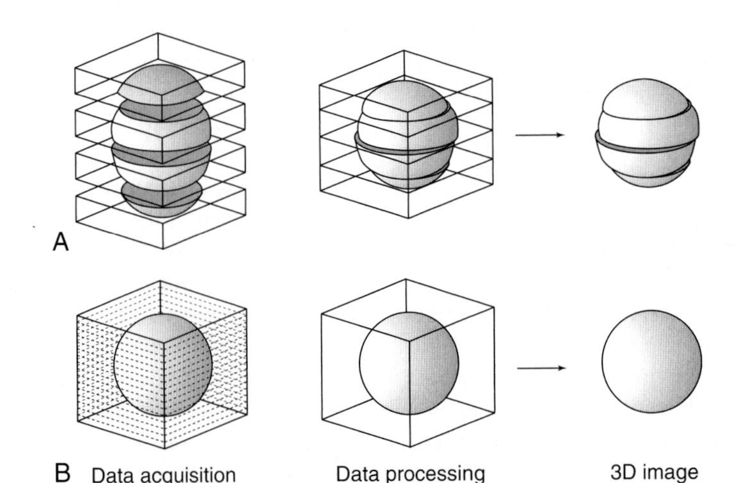

FIGURE 11-5 Comparison of the accuracy of 3D reconstruction for conventional **(A)** and spiral/helical **(B)** CT scanning. (Courtesy Toshiba America Medical Systems, Tustin, Calif.)

This chapter concentrates on methods to remove the ISD with the goal of acquiring the data continuously rather than in slices. This technique is only possible with continuous rotation scanners based on slip-ring technology.

PRINCIPLES OF SSCT SCANNERS

The introduction of CT scanners that can scan rapidly with scan times shorter than 1 second has led to the development of the SSCT scanner. The overall goal of this scanner is to increase the volume coverage speed compared with that of the conventional CT scanner.

To do this efficiently requires that the x-ray tube rotate continuously around the patient while the patient moves through the gantry aperture during the scanning to cover an entire volume of tissue (compared with a single slice characteristic of conventional CT scanners). Rotation of the x-ray tube coupled with patient translation through the gantry aperture traces an x-ray beam path with respect to the patient (Fig. 11-6). The path geometry describes a spiral or helical winding and therefore has been referred to as *spiral/helical* CT. Other terms considered synonymous are *spiral volume* CT and *helical volumetric CT*.

Because a one-dimensional (1D) detector array is used, only a single slice is acquired during one rotation of the tube. Because there are several rotations per required length of anatomy imaged (volume of tissue scanned), several slices of tissue and corresponding images can be computer generated for the volume of the anatomy scanned during a single breath-hold.

Requirements for Volume Scanning

Because the data in spiral/helical CT are collected in volumes rather than slices, the following requirements must be met:

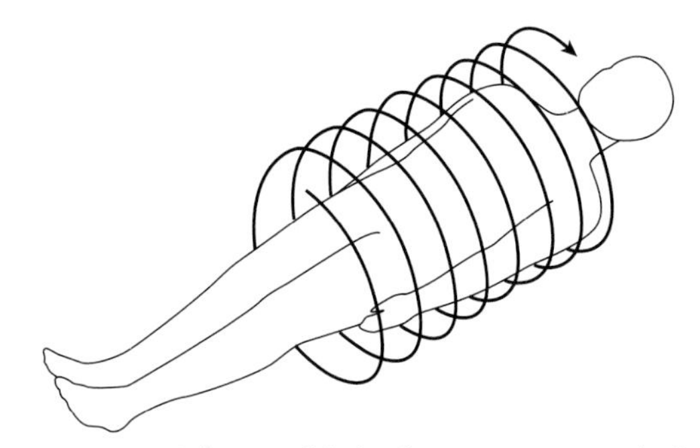

FIGURE 11-6 The spiral/helical geometry created when the x-ray tube rotates continuously around the patient with simultaneous patient translation.

1. Continuously rotating scanner based on slip-ring technology
2. Continuous couch movement
3. Increase in loadability of the x-ray tube, capable of delivering at least 200 milliamperes per revolution continuously throughout the time it takes to scan the volume of tissue
4. Increased cooling capacity of the x-ray tube
5. Spiral/helical weighting algorithm
6. Mass memory buffer to store the vast amount of data collected

Data Acquisition

The first step in volume scanning is data acquisition (Fig. 11-7). The x-ray tube traces a spiral/helical path with a radius equal to the distance from the focal spot to the center of rotation. This results in an entire volume of tissue being scanned during a single breath-hold compared with slice-by-slice imaging (Fig. 11-8).

Transporting the patient too quickly leads to image degradation caused by motion artifacts or may cause the patient to feel motion sickness. It is therefore important that the patient moves at a constant speed. In general, patients are moved at a table speed of about 10 millimeters (mm) per second during a continuous 1-second scanning. If a 24-second scan is taken, then the anatomic volume scanned is 240 mm (24 cm). Scanning times differ

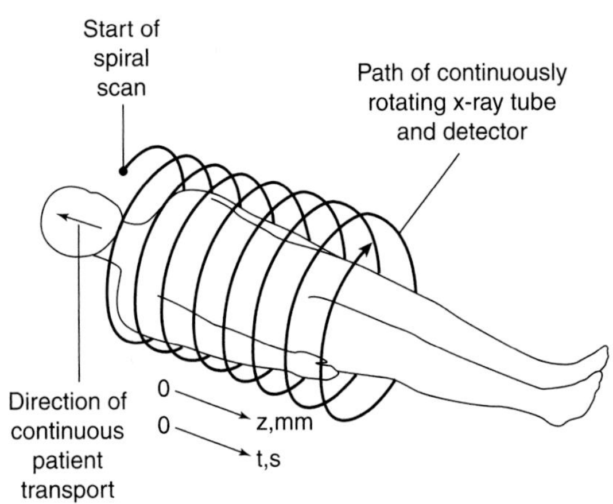

FIGURE 11-7 First step in spiral/helical CT: data acquisition. As the patient is transported through the gantry aperture, the x-ray tube traces a spiral path around the patient, collecting data as it rotates.

by manufacturer but average about 32 seconds. In addition the slice thickness may range from 1 to 10 cm.

Several problems can result from data acquisition with spiral geometry:

1. There is no defined slice, and thus localization of a particular slice is difficult.

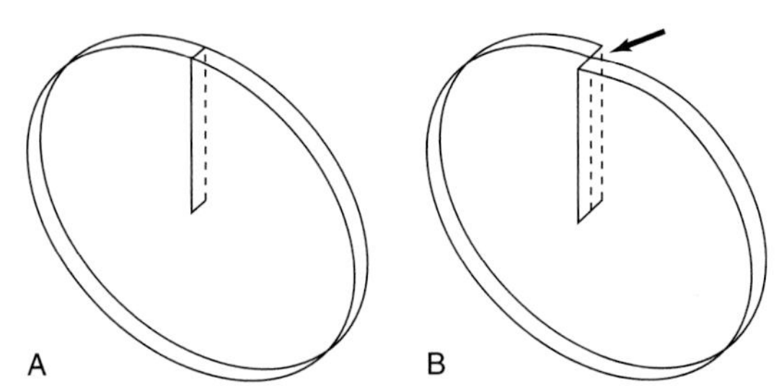

FIGURE 11-9 Geometry of the slice volume characteristic of conventional CT scanning **(A)** and spiral/helical CT scanning **(B)**.

2. The geometry of the slice volume is different for spiral/helical scans compared with conventional CT scans (Fig. 11-9). Figure 11-10 explains the origin of the slice volume shown in Figure 11-9, *B*. In conventional slice-by-slice CT, the tube rotates around the patient for 360 degrees to collect a complete set of data in planar geometry for each individual slice shown in Figure 11-9, *A*. This data set is said to be consistent; that is, it is collected from one slice or plane. In spiral/helical volume CT scanning, the x-ray tube rotates continuously as the patient moves through the gantry continuously as well. In this situation, data are

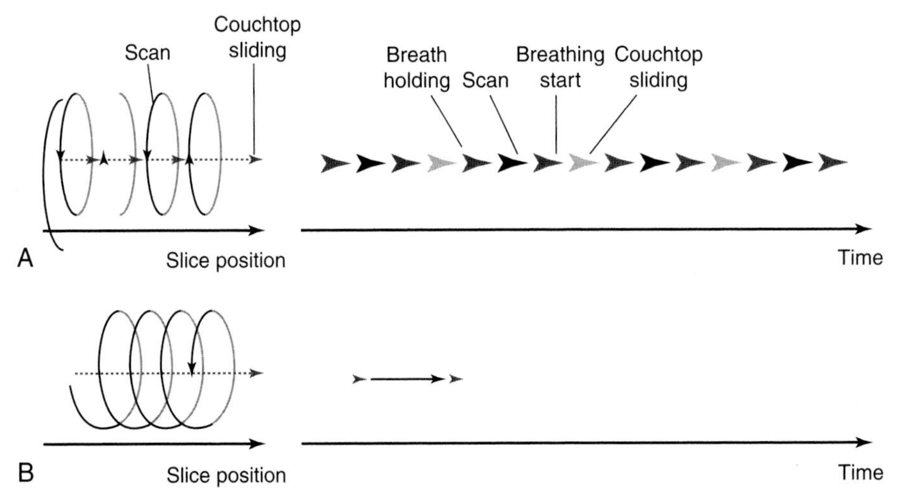

FIGURE 11-8 Comparison of conventional **(A)** and spiral/helical **(B)** CT scanning sequences. (From Tohki Y: The helical scanning technique, *Toshiba Med Rev* 38:1-5, 1991.)

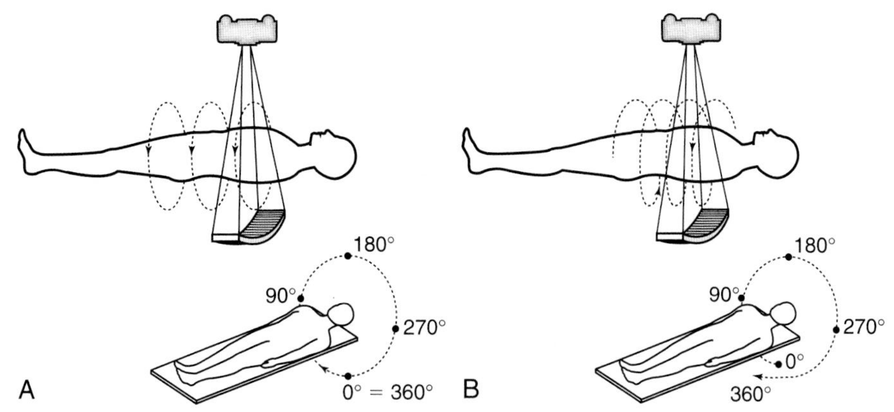

FIGURE 11-10 Data acquisition geometries for conventional slice-by-slice CT **(A)** and spiral/helical CT **(B)**.

now collected in nonplanar geometry, resulting in the diagram shown in Figure 11-9, *B*. The data are collected from different regions of the volume and not through a particular plane.

3. The effective slice thickness increases because it is influenced by the width of the fan beam and the speed of the table.
4. Because of the absence of a defined slice, the projection data are inconsistent (consistent projection data are needed to satisfy the standard reconstruction process).
5. When inconsistent projection data are used with the standard reconstruction process, streak artifacts akin to motion artifacts are clearly apparent on the image.

These problems can be solved through the use of special postprocessing techniques. One such method involves a "dedicated reconstruction algorithm that synthesizes raw data representing a perfectly planar slice from the original spiral data by interpolation" (Kalender, 1995). Interpolation is a mathematical technique whereby an unknown value can be estimated given two known values on either side (see Chapter 6). Interpolation and extrapolation are illustrated in Figure 11-11.

Image Reconstruction

Inconsistent data that are obtained from 360-degree spiral/helical scan rotation are used directly in the image reconstruction process. Motion artifacts are apparent as shown in Figure 11-12, *A*, for phantom images and in Figure 11-13, *A*, for patient images.

To eliminate these motion artifacts arising from the continuous movement of the patient during scanning, two steps are needed:

1. Calculation (using interpolation) of a planar data set from the tissue volume data set for every image (Fig. 11-14). The planar data set (the image plane in Fig. 11-14) approximates the transverse axial section as with conventional CT. Within the volume scanned, a slice can be selected anywhere between the start and end

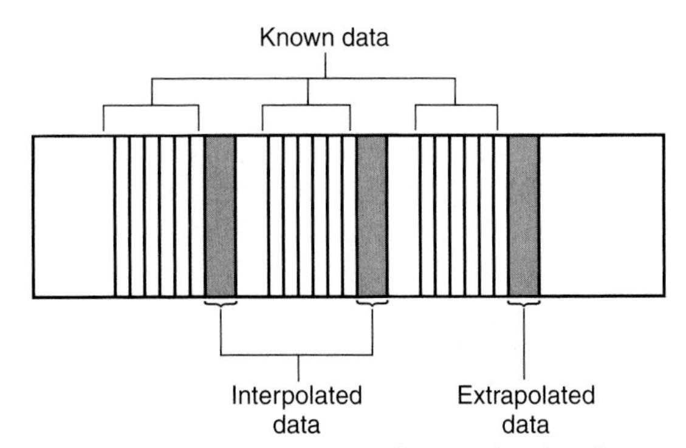

FIGURE 11-11 A comparison of interpolated and extrapolated data.

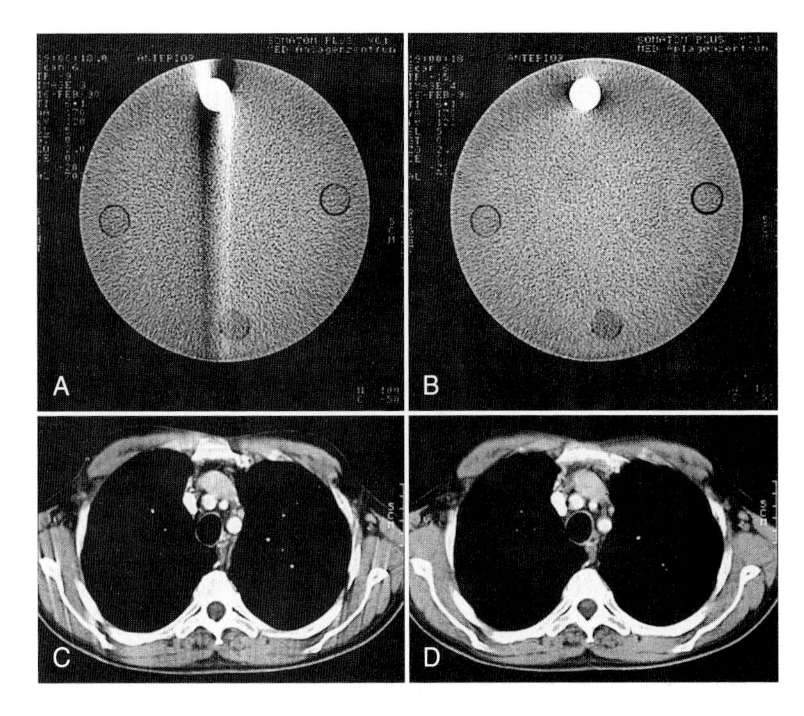

FIGURE 11-12 Comparison of image quality using direct reconstruction of the spiral data **(A, C)** as opposed to reconstruction using the interpolation algorithm **(B, D)** for phantom **(A, B)** and mediastinal **(C, D)** studies. The streak artifacts are removed when the interpolation algorithm is used. (From Kalender WA et al: Spiral CT scanning for fast and continuous volume data acquisition. In Fuchs WA, editor: *Advances in CT*, New York, 1990, Springer-Verlag.)

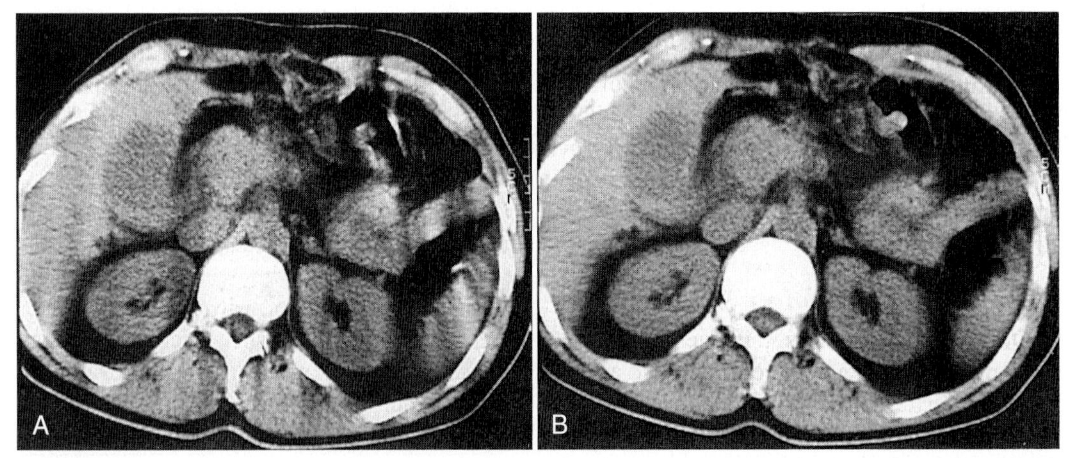

FIGURE 11-13 Image reconstruction principles in spiral/helical CT. **A,** Direct reconstruction of an image from a 360-degree spiral segment results in motion artifacts. **B,** Image reconstruction from a planar data set calculated by slice interpolation from the spiral data set results in images free of artifacts. (From Kalender W: Principles and performance of spiral CT. In Goldman LW, Fowlkes JB, editors: *Medical CT and ultrasound: current technology and applications*, College Park, Maryland, 1995, American Association of Physics in Medicine.)

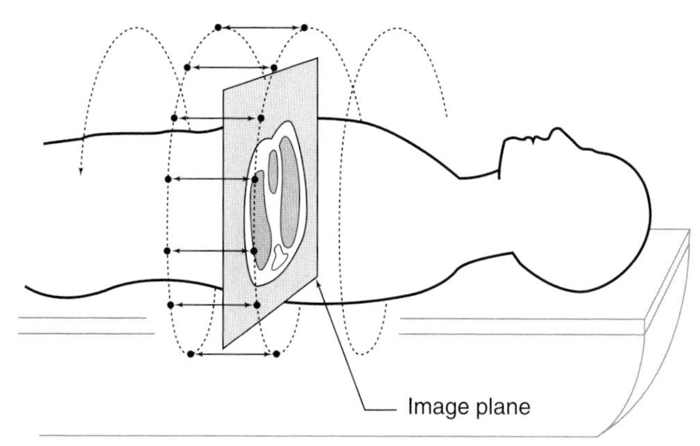

FIGURE 11-14 The first step to produce an image in spiral/helical CT scanning is to calculate a planar data set (image plane) from the volume data set (measured data). This is accomplished by using linear interpolation.

positions in addition to the spacing and the number of slices (Fig. 11-15).

2. Reconstruction of images similar to conventional CT by use of the filtered back-projection algorithm. The results of these two processes are free of blurring as shown in Figure 11-13, *B*.

A number of interpolation algorithms are used to produce the planar data set, and linear interpolation (LI) represents the "simplest approach" (Kalender, 1995). Two interpolation algorithms for single-slice spiral/helical CT are the 360-degree LI algorithm and the 180-degree LI algorithm.

360-Degree Linear Interpolation Algorithm

The 360-degree LI algorithm was the interpolation algorithm used during the initial development of spiral/helical CT scanners (Fig. 11-16). The basis

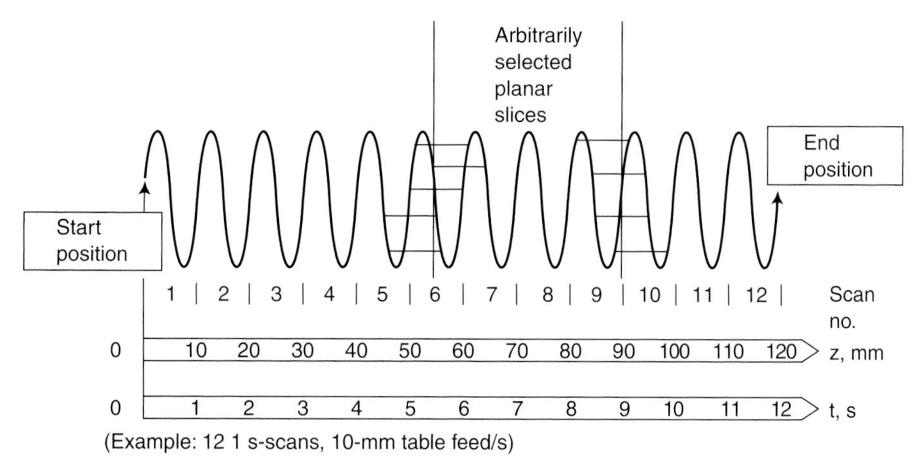

FIGURE 11-15 The second major step in spiral/helical CT is interpolation. Images of arbitrarily selected slices can be reconstructed with an interpolation algorithm. (Courtesy Siemens Medical Systems, Iselin, NJ.)

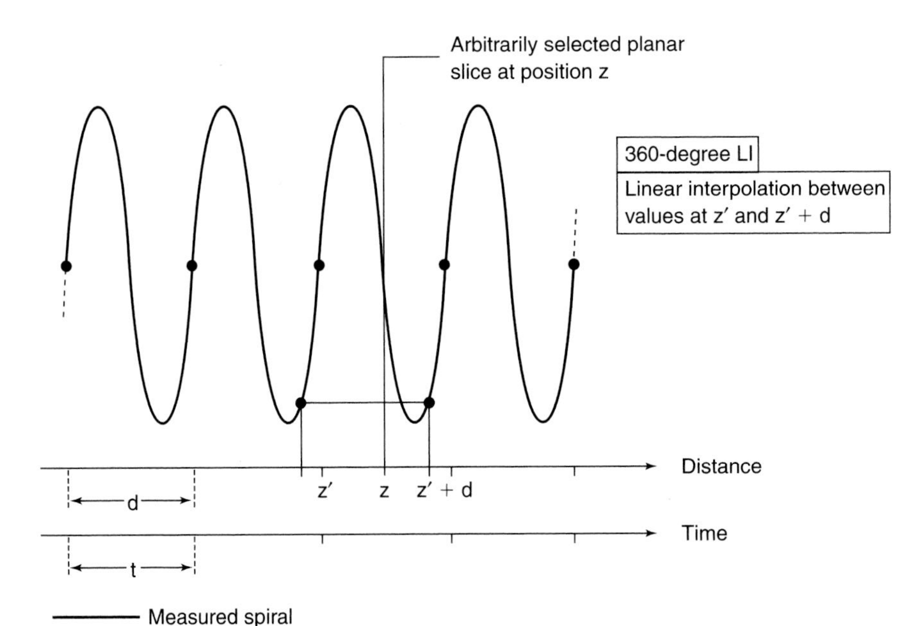

FIGURE 11-16 The 360-degree LI algorithm. LI between points Z' and $Z' + d$ was most commonly used in the early days of spiral/helical scanning to estimate data that would have been obtained in planar geometry for an arbitrarily selected image position Z.

for this algorithm is illustrated in Figure 11-16. The planar slice is interpolated by use of data points measured 360 degrees apart. The fundamental problem with the 360-degree LI algorithm is related to the image quality of the planar slice. This algorithm broadens the slice sensitivity profile (SSP) and hence degrades image quality. To overcome this problem, the 180-degree LI algorithm was introduced.

180-Degree Linear Interpolation Algorithm

The 180-degree LI algorithm improves the image quality of the 360-degree LI algorithm by using points that are closer to the planar slice to be interpolated (Fig. 11-17). The basic difference between the 360-degree and the 180-degree LI algorithms is that a second spiral (the dotted line in Fig. 11-17) is calculated from the measured spiral/helical data set and is offset by 180 degrees. In this situation, the planar slice can then be interpolated with use of data points that are closer to it compared with the 360-degree LI algorithm. This process improves on the SSP and therefore enhances image quality.

In addition to the algorithms, Kalender (1995) states that "higher-order nonlinear interpolation algorithms can be implemented. While they preserve the shape of the sensitivity profiles even better, their influence on noise and image quality is not easy to predict and control. On a given scanner, the exact algorithm and above all its implementation, which may have significant influence on image quality and artifact behavior, are not documented as they are considered confidential by the manufacturers in most cases." These algorithms are not within the scope of this book. The reader should refer to Kalender (2005) for a further description of nonlinear interpolation algorithms.

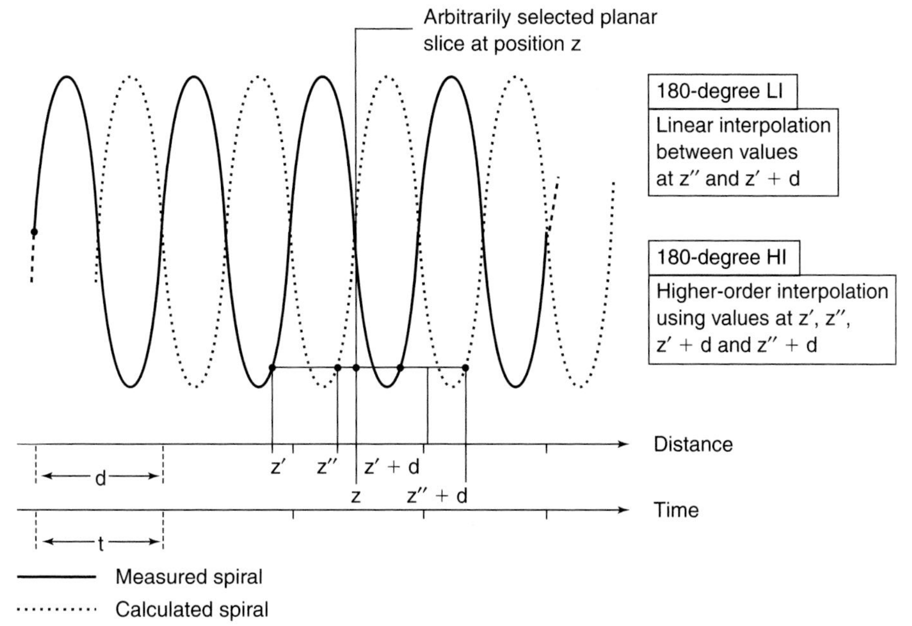

FIGURE 11-17 The 180-degree LI algorithm. Interpolation between measured data points derived from 180-degree opposite views allows to limit the scan range used per image. Higher-order interpolation schemes can also be implemented.

INSTRUMENTATION

Spiral/helical CT scanners (Fig. 11-18) are not different in external appearance from conventional CT scanners. However, there are significant differences in several major equipment components.

Equipment Components

A block diagram of the major equipment components of a spiral/helical CT scanner is shown in Figure 11-19. The most noteworthy feature is the use of slip rings to connect the stationary and rotating parts of the scanner.

The rotating part of the system consists of the x-ray tube, high-voltage generator, detectors, and detector electronics (DAS). The stationary part consists of the front-end memory and computer and the first-stage high-voltage component.

The x-ray tube and detectors rotate continuously during data collection because the cable wraparound problem has been eliminated by slip-ring technology. Because large amounts of projection data are collected very quickly, increased storage is needed. This is accommodated by the front-end memory, fast solid state, and magnetic disk storage.

In spiral/helical CT scanners, the x-ray tube is energized for longer periods of time compared with conventional CT tubes. This characteristic requires x-ray tubes that are physically larger than conventional x-ray tubes and have heat storage capacities greater than 3 million heat units (MHU) and anode cooling rates of 1 MHU per minute (Bushong, 2004).

X-ray detectors for single-slice spiral/helical CT scanning are 1D arrays and should be solid state because their overall efficiency is greater than gas ionization detectors.

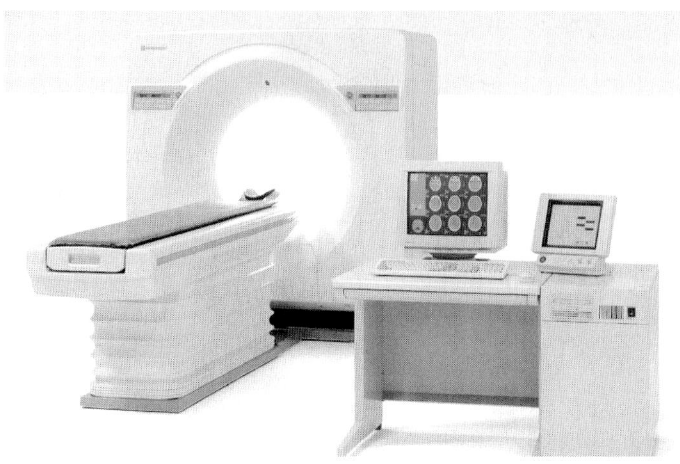

FIGURE 11-18 A spiral/helical CT scanner is similar in external appearance to conventional CT scanners. (Courtesy Shimadzu Medical Systems, Seattle, Wash.)

The high-voltage generator for spiral/helical CT scanners is a high-frequency generator with a high power output. The high-voltage generator is mounted on the rotating frame of the CT gantry and positioned close to the x-ray tube (see Fig. 11-19). X-ray tubes operate at high voltages (about 80 to 140 peak kilovolts) to produce x-rays with the intensity needed for CT scanning. At such high voltages, arcing between the brushes and rings of the gantry may occur during scanning. To solve this problem, one approach is to divide the power supply into a first stage on the stationary part of the scanner, where the voltage is increased to an intermediate level, and a second stage on the rotating part of the scanner, where the voltage is increased to the required high voltages needed for x-ray production and finally rectified to direct current potential (see Fig. 11-19) (Napel, 1995). Another approach passes a low voltage across the brushes to the slip rings, the high-voltage generator, and then the x-ray tube. In both designs, only a low to intermediate voltage is applied to the brush/slip-ring interface, thus decreasing the chances of arcing.

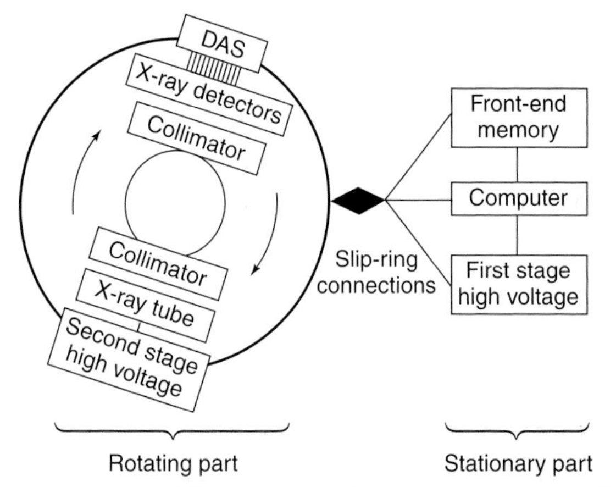

FIGURE 11-19 The major equipment components of a spiral/helical CT scanner. Connection between the stationary and rotating parts of the scanner is made possible by slip-ring technology.

Slip-Ring Technology

One of the major technical factors that contribute to the success of spiral/helical CT scanning is slip-ring technology (see Fig. 11-19). The purpose of the slip ring is to allow the x-ray tube and detectors (in third-generation CT systems, see Fig. 11-19) to rotate continuously so that a volume of the patient, rather than one slice, can be scanned very quickly in a single breath hold. The slip rings also eliminate the long, high-tension cables to the x-ray tube used in conventional start-stop CT scanners. As the x-ray tube rotates continuously, the patient also moves continuously through the gantry aperture so that data can be acquired from a volume of tissue.

The technical aspects of using slip rings for data acquisition are described in Chapter 5. These include the design and power supply to the rings and a comparison of low-voltage and high-voltage slip-ring CT scanners in terms of the high voltage supplied to the x-ray tube.

BASIC SCAN PARAMETERS

Several scan parameters for spiral/helical CT are the same as for conventional CT; however, there are a few parameters and a set of terms associated only with spiral/helical CT. Typical parameters include spiral scan time, table feed per 360-degree rotation, table speed, number of revolutions, scan range or volume coverage, z-axis (the axis of rotation of the scanner or the longitudinal axis of the patient), collimation, and the reconstruction increment and z-interpolation ("calculation of planar attenuation data for desired table position interpolation between data points measured for the same projection angle at neighboring z-axis positions [synonyms: slice interpolation, section interpolation, z-axis interpolation]") algorithms (Kalender, 1995). It is not within the scope of this chapter to describe all these parameters; however, the pitch, volume coverage, collimation, table speed, and reconstruction increment are highlighted here.

Pitch

The *pitch* is a term associated with a fastener, and it is actually the distance between the turns on the fastener. In spiral/helical CT, the pitch is defined as the distance (in mm) that the CT table moves during one revolution of the x-ray tube (Fig. 11-20). The pitch is used to calculate the pitch ratio, which is a ratio of the pitch to the slice thickness or beam collimation. The pitch ratio is as follows:

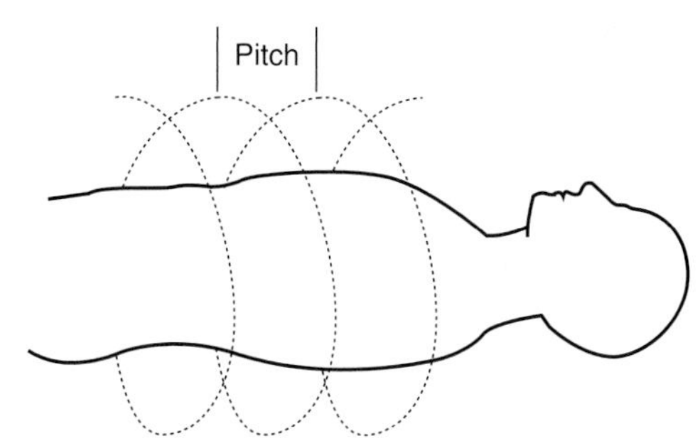

FIGURE 11-20 The pitch is the distance the CT table moves during one complete revolution of the x-ray tube.

$$\text{Pitch} = \frac{\text{distance the table travels during 360-degree revolution}}{\text{Slice thickness or beam collimation}}$$

When the distance the table travels during one complete revolution of the x-ray tube equals the slice thickness or beam collimation, the pitch ratio (pitch) is 1:1, or simply 1. A pitch of 1 results in the best image quality in spiral/helical CT scanning. The pitch can be increased to increase volume coverage and speed up the scanning process (Fig. 11-21). Pitch is of particular significance because it affects image quality and patient dose and also plays a role in the overall outcome of the clinical examination.

Volume Coverage

The volume coverage is given by the following relationship:

$$\text{Volume coverage} = \text{Pitch} \times \text{Slice thickness or Beam collimation} \times \text{Scan time}$$

for fixed scan time and fixed slice thickness (Bushong, 2004).

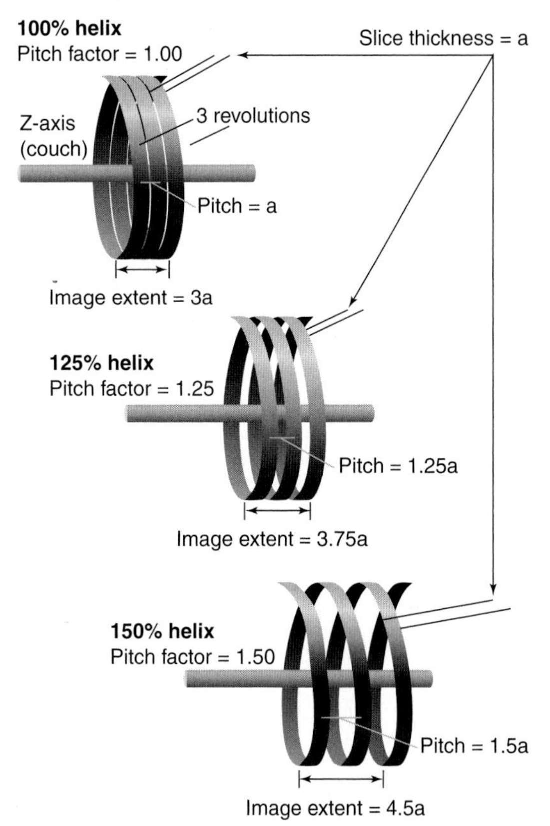

FIGURE 11-21 The pitch can be increased to increase volume coverage quickly, although image quality degrades.

Another factor that influences the volume coverage is gantry rotation time. The volume coverage in this case becomes:

$$\text{Volume coverage} = \frac{\text{pitch} \times \text{collimation} \times \text{scan time}}{\text{gantry rotation time}}$$

Collimation and Table Speed

Collimation determines the slice thickness and in most cases is equal to the table increment (a pitch of 1). Collimation selection also depends on the type of tissue to be examined. Smaller structures usually require narrow collimation, whereas larger structures are imaged with wider collimation.

Another parameter of importance is the table increment (mm per second), also referred to as the *table feed* or *table speed.* As the table increment increases with respect to the collimation, pitch increases, resulting in a loss of image quality. To cover a certain volume, it is important to keep in mind two parameters that influence image quality: collimation and table incrementation. The goal is to use the smallest possible collimation at a pitch of 2 (with 180-degree interpolation algorithm). Hence, for a volume length of 30 cm, either a 5-mm or 8-mm collimation can be used with a table speed of 10 mm.

Scan Time

Another operator-defined parameter in spiral/helical CT that affects the outcome of the examination is the scan time, which refers to the duration of the scan. The choice of scan time depends on the patient's respiratory condition. Most current scanners feature various spiral/helical scan modes (Fig. 11-22) for patients who have difficulty holding the breath. For example, in a multistep spiral/helical scan mode, multiple scans are obtained with a pause between scans to enable patients to breathe so that the required length of tissue can be imaged successfully.

Reconstruction Increment

Another parameter unique to spiral/helical CT is the reconstruction increment (RI), also referred to as the *reconstruction interval* or *reconstruction spacing*. The RI determines the degree of sectional overlap to improve image quality. As RI decreases, image quality generally improves. Urban et al (1993) found that for the detection of small lesions in the liver, a 50% overlap (Fig. 11-23) resulted in better visualization of these lesions by 10%. In a set of simulations conducted by Brink et al (1994) to find whether an increased degree of overlap would provide better results, the researchers

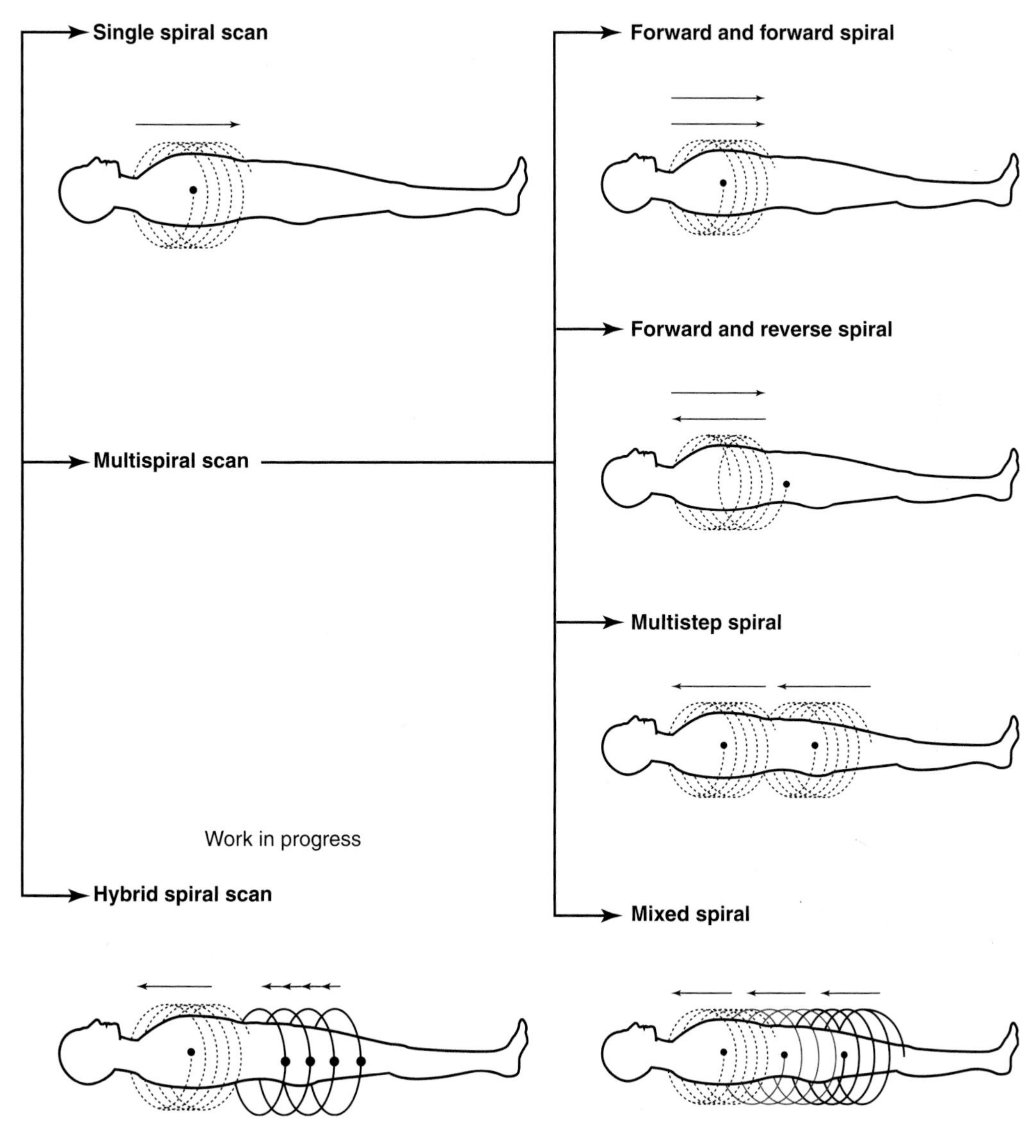

FIGURE 11-22 Various spiral/helical scan modes can be used to accommodate the needs of the examination. For example, the multistep spiral scan mode can accommodate patients who have difficulty holding the breath for prolonged scan times.

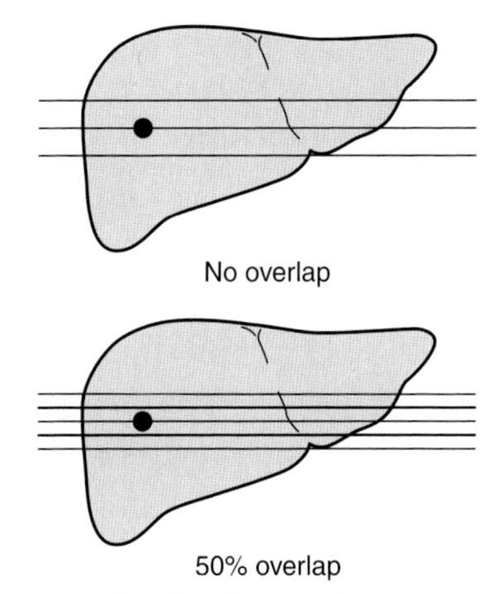

FIGURE 11-23 Overlapping sections may result in better visualization of lesions.

recommended "reconstructing one or two sections per table increment for routine diagnosis and at least three sections per table increment for multidimensional imaging."

SSCT/CONVENTIONAL CT: IMAGE QUALITY/DOSE COMPARISON

In this section, a comparison is made of SSCT scanners and conventional CT scanners on several image quality parameters. These are discussed here to provide the reader with some historical notes relating to the performance of the SSCT scanners introduced and used in the past.

A number of workers have investigated the physical performance characteristics of spiral/helical CT (Kalender et al, 1994b). These characteristics include image quality parameters such as spatial resolution, image uniformity, and contrast; image noise and slice sensitivity profiles; radiation dose; and artifacts.

In general, most characteristics appear to be affected only slightly. As noted by Kalender (1995), image quality in spiral/helical CT is equivalent to that of conventional CT "in every respect" because the basic imaging parameters are the same.

Spatial and Contrast Resolution

For the same image reconstruction parameters, contrast and spatial resolution should be about the same for both spiral/helical CT and conventional CT. For example, measurements of the scan plane (image plane) spatial resolution conducted by Kalender (1995) with a standard poly(methyl methacrylate (Perspex) hole pattern phantom demonstrate this similarity between spatial resolution for conventional CT and spiral/helical CT. The visual evidence is shown in Figure 11-24. However, as noted by Kalender (1995), the contrast for small objects and the spatial resolution along the z-axis (longitudinal direction) may be somewhat different. For example, in simulations, phantom experiments, and specimen studies that compared contrast and spatial resolution along the z-axis for both conventional and spiral/helical CT, Kalender et al (1994) found that spiral/helical CT provides "significantly better" contrast and spatial separation of 5-mm spheres imaged with a 5-mm slice thickness.

Noise

Noise in spiral/helical CT is affected by a range of parameters, including beam intensity, beam quality (energy), slice thickness, and matrix size (pixel size). Additionally, noise in spiral/helical CT is also affected by the interpolation algorithm. Compared with conventional CT (all other factors held constant), the 360-degree LI algorithm produces less noise; however, when the 360-degree LI and the 180-degree LI algorithms were compared, it was found that the 180-degree LI algorithm produced more noise and thus degraded image quality (Kalender, 1994b). However, this problem has little effect on the image quality of bony structures because the subject contrast of bone is greater than its surrounding soft tissues (Fig. 11-25).

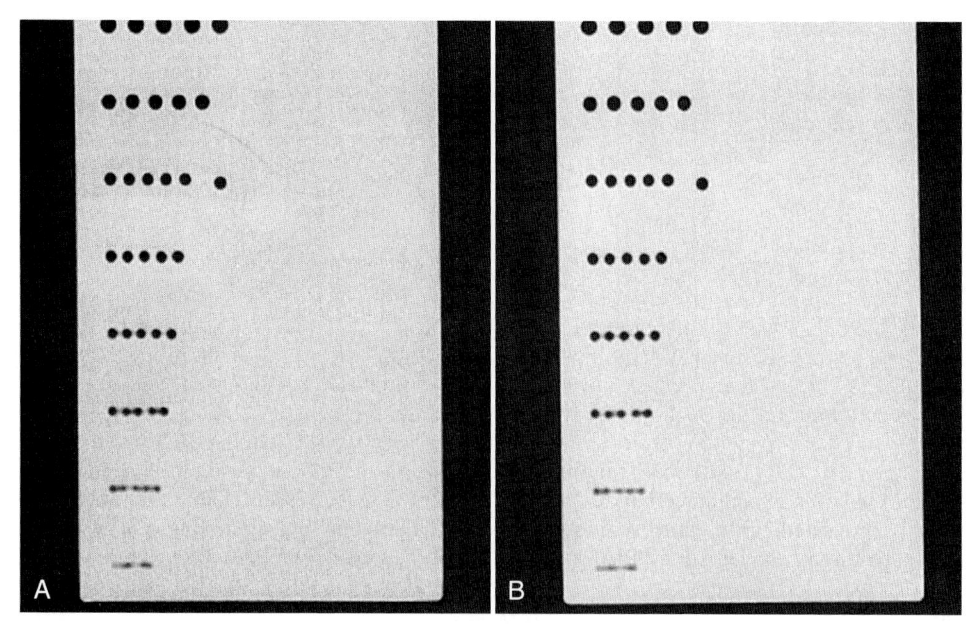

FIGURE 11-24 The spatial resolution as measured by a Perspex hole pattern phantom is the same for conventional CT **(A)** and spiral/helical CT **(B)** for the same reconstruction parameters. (From Kalender WA: Technical foundations of spiral CT, *Semin Ultrasound CT MRI* 15:81-89, 1994.)

Slice Sensitivity Profile

The SSP "describes how thick a section is imaged and to what extent details within the section contribute to the signal" (Kalender, 1994b). For conventional CT, the shape of the SSP is rectangular (Fig. 11-26, *A*). The section thickness is measured in the middle of the rectangle. This point is referred to as the full width at half maximum (FWHM). For spiral/helical CT, the SSP also depends on the pitch and the interpolation algorithm. Figure 11-26, *B*, shows the SSPs for a pitch of 1 and 2. Figure 11-26, *C*, shows SSPs for a 180-degree LI algorithm and a 360-degree algorithm. The SSP degrades with a pitch of 2 and a 360-degree LI algorithm. (The FWHM does not approximate closely the actual slice thickness selected.) As the SSP widens, image quality degrades.

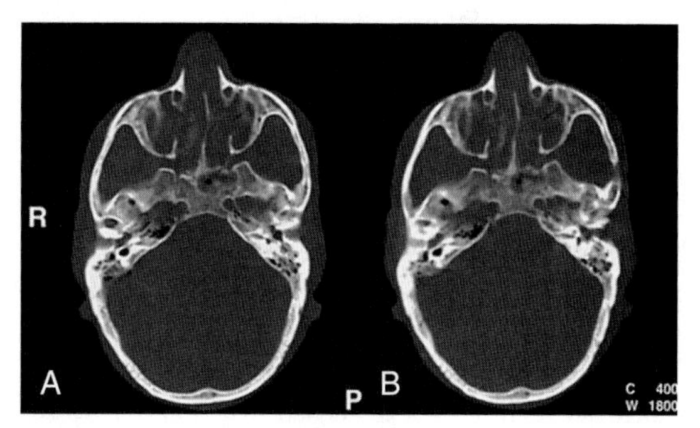

FIGURE 11-25 The difference in image quality and noise in studies carried out using a pitch of 1 (360-degree interpolation algorithm) and a pitch of 2 (180-degree interpolation algorithm) may be inconsequential in bone studies because of the high inherent subject contrast, especially when other imaging parameters are optimized, as evidenced by these phantom studies. **A,** Pitch 1, 360 degrees. **B,** Pitch 2, 180 degrees. (From Cinnamon J: *Multislice volumetric spiral CT: principles and applications*, Liege, Belgium, 1998, Massoz.)

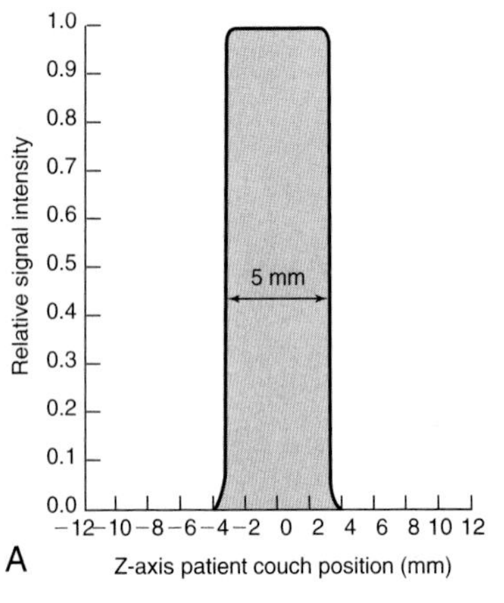

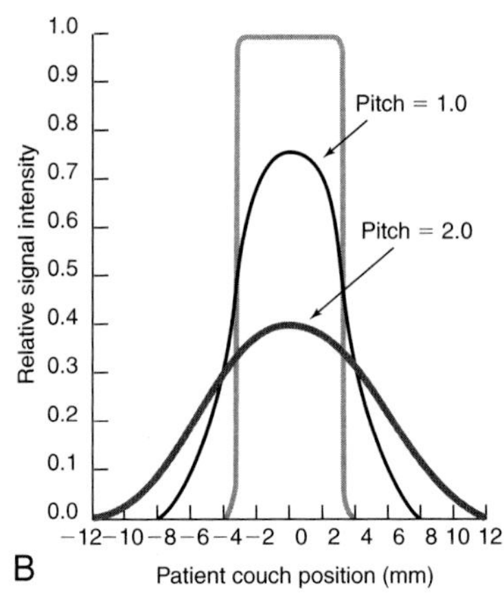

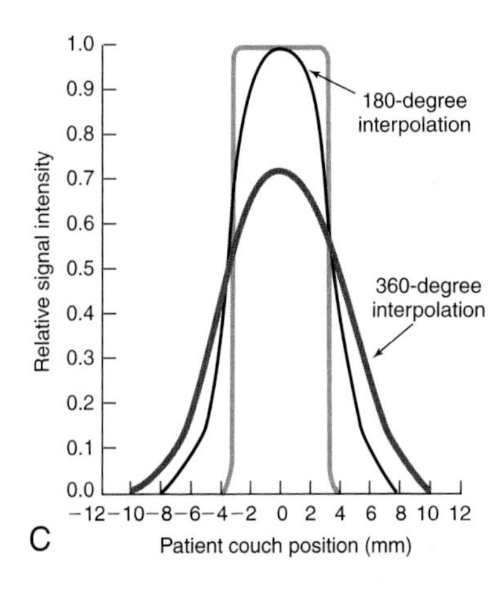

FIGURE 11-26 The SSP for conventional CT and spiral/helical CT. **A,** The SSP is almost a rectangle and closely approximates the slice thickness. **B,** The SSPs for spiral/helical CT are shown for a pitch of 1 and a pitch of 2. **C,** The influence of two linear interpolation algorithms on SSP. SSP is wider for the 360-degree LI, resulting in a loss of image quality.

Dose Comparison

During the early development and use of spiral/helical CT, it was thought that the dose would be higher simply from volume data acquisition. Comparison studies show that the dose in conventional CT is about equal to that of spiral/helical CT.

There are several reasons why patient dose is less in SSCT than in conventional CT, as follows:

1. Tube currents in spiral/helical CT are set to lower values than in conventional CT.
2. Spiral/helical CT largely eliminates the need to retake single scans.
3. Spiral/helical CT arbitrarily calculates overlapping images from one spiral scan without renewed exposure, whereas conventional CT must take many overlapping images to obtain high display quality.
4. Unlike contiguous scanning, spiral/helical CT can reduce patient dose by using pitch values >1 (Kalender, 1994b).

The effective doses from spiral/helical CT for the head, chest, abdomen and pelvis are 1.1, 6.7, 4.3, and 2.7 millisieverts (mSv), respectively (Kalender, 1994b). The effective dose allows the quantification of the risk from partial-body exposure on the basis of that received from an equal whole-body dose.

Huda et al (1997), for example, reported effective dose range from 1.5 to 5.3 mSv for abdominal examinations in pediatric and adult patients.

To place all this in perspective, the effective dose from natural background radiation is about 2.4 mSv per year (Kalender, 1994b).

TECHNICAL APPLICATIONS OF SSCT

In addition to the routine imaging modes that generate transverse axial images, the volume scanning capability of spiral/helical CT opens new dimensions in CT imaging. The vast amount of data collected from the patient volumes, when subjected to appropriate computer processing, have created techniques such as real-time CT fluoroscopy (continuous imaging), 3D imaging, CT angiography, and virtual reality imaging or CT endoscopy.

Today these applications have become more refined and efficient, and they provide additional clinical information for the medical management of the patient. Each of these technical applications of volume CT scanning are described further in later chapters.

REFERENCES

Baker CCT: *Dictionary of mathematics*, New York, 1961, Hart.

Bresler Y, Skrabacz C: Optimal interpolation in helical scan 3D computerized tomography, *Natl Sci Found* MIP88-10412:1472-1475, 1993.

Brink JA et al: Helical CT: principles and technical considerations, *Radiographics* 14:887-893, 1994.

Bushong S: *Radiologic science for technologists*, ed 8, Philadelphia, 2004, Mosby.

Gay SB, Matthews AB: Ten reasons why spiral CT is worth a million bucks, *Diagn Imag* Nov 111-113, 1998.

Huda W et al: An approach for the estimation of effective radiation dose in CT for pediatric patients, *Radiology* 203:417-422, 1997.

James G, James R, editors: *Mathematics dictionary*, ed 4, New York, 1976, Van Nostrand Reinhold.

Kalender WA: Spiral or helical CT: right or wrong? *Radiology* 193:583, 1994a.

Kalender WA: Technical foundations of spiral CT, *Semin Ultrasound CT MRI* 15:81-89, 1994b.

Kalender WA: Principles and performance of spiral CT. In Goldman LW, Fowlkes JB, editors: *Medical CT and ultrasound: current technology and applications*, College Park, Maryland, 1995, American Association of Physics in Medicine.

Kalender WA: *Computed tomography-fundamentals, system technology, image quality, applications*, Erlangen, 2005, Publicis.

Kalender WA et al: A comparison of conventional and spiral CT: an experimental study on the detection of spherical lesions, *CAT* 18:167-176, 1994.

McGhee PI, Humphreys S: Radiation dose associated with spiral computed tomography, *J Can Assoc Radiol* 45:124-129, 1944.

Mori I: Computerized tomographic apparatus utilizing a radiation source, U.S. Patent No. 4630202, 1987.

Napel SA: Basic principles of spiral CT. In Fishman ED, Jeffrey RBJr, editors: *Spiral CT: principles, techniques, and clinical applications*, New York, 1995, Raven Press.

Silverman PM et al: Helical vs spiral, *AJR Am J Roentgenol* 162:1247, 1994.

Towers MJ: Spiral geometries: the helix is one type of spiral. From spiral or helical CT? [letter], *AJR Am J Roentgenol* 161:901, 1993.

Urban BA et al: Detection of focal hepatic lesions with spiral CT: comparison of 4-mm and 8-mm interscan spacing, *AJR Am J Roentgenol* 160: 783-787, 1993.

Multislice Spiral/Helical Computed Tomography: Physical Principles and Instrumentation

Chapter Outline

LIMITATIONS OF SINGLE-SLICE VOLUME CT SCANNERS

Ever since its introduction in 1990, single-slice volume computed tomography (CT) has been used successfully in many body CT imaging applications in which speed and volume coverage are important. Volume coverage and speed can be increased by using higher pitch ratios; however, higher pitch ratios in single-slice volume CT scanning degrade image quality (z-axis resolution) and produce image artifacts. In single-slice volume CT, the volume coverage speed is limited, especially in clinical applications that demand large-volume scanning with critical timing requirements and optimum image quality (z-axis resolution and low image artifacts), such as CT angiography with three-dimensional (3D), multiplanar reformatting or reconstruction (MPR), and maximum intensity projection (MIP) techniques (Hu, 1999a). Single-slice volume CT is based on the use of a single row of detectors (one-dimensional [1D] detector array). Because the x-ray beam is highly collimated to the size of the detector array, only a small percentage of x-rays emitted by the tube is used in the imaging process. This situation is described as poor geometric efficiency. Also, single-slice volume CT uses the 360-degree linear interpolation algorithm (LIA) and the 180-degree LIA to improve the problems imposed by the 360-degree LIA, such as poor image quality and artifact production. However, the 180-degree LIA produces more noise while preserving the detail (slice sensitivity and spatial resolution). Additionally, the time duration for covering defined volumes in single-slice volume CT (several seconds) is limited by several factors, such as the ability of some patients, particularly those who are critically ill, to maintain a single breath-hold during volume scanning and the heat loading of the x-ray tube.

Single-slice volume CT is also limited in its ability to meet the needs of time-critical clinical examinations such as multiphase organ dynamic studies and CT angiography, in which both arterial and venous phases are extremely important, with smaller amounts of contrast media. The use of higher pitch ratios to solve these problems degrades the slice sensitivity profile (detail). Therefore, other methods are needed to overcome these limitations to improve the performance of single-slice volume CT in terms of better use of the x-ray output (improved geometric efficiency) and scan parameters affecting image quality and volume coverage.

Multislice CT offers "substantial improvement of the volume coverage speed performance" (Hu, 1999a). This means that multislice CT provides faster scanning and higher resolution for a number of clinical applications (Taguchi and Aradate, 1998). One of the most conspicuous differences between multislice CT and single-slice volume CT is that the former uses a multiple row of detectors (two-dimensional [2D] detector array), whereas the latter uses a single row of detectors (1D detector array), as is clearly illustrated in Figure 12-1.

EVOLUTION OF MULTISLICE CT SCANNERS

Terminology

Several terms are used in the literature to refer to multislice CT. These include multisection CT, multidetector CT, multidetector row CT, and multichannel CT (Cody and Mahesh, 2007; Douglas-Akinwande et al, 2006). Each of these terms appears to focus on a particular outcome characteristic. For example, although the terms *multislice* and *multisection* focus on images, the terms *multidetector* and *multidetector row* focus on the detectors used during the scanning. Finally, the term *multichannel* refers to the

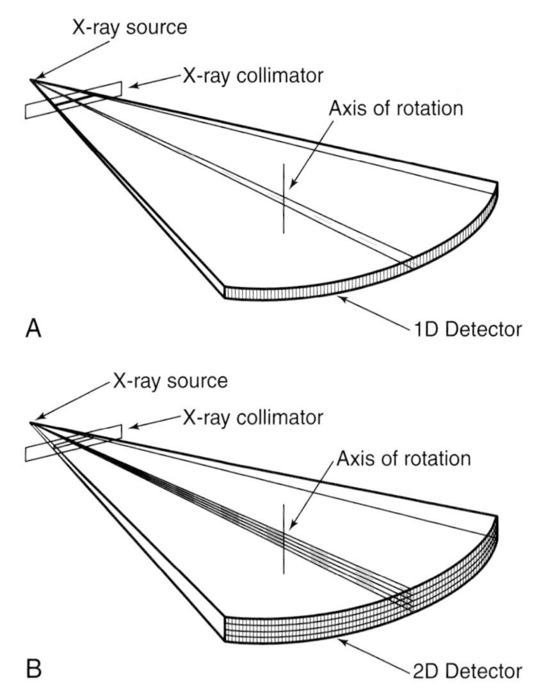

FIGURE 12-1 One of the most conspicuous differences between a single-slice volume CT scanner and a multislice CT scanner is the detector design. **A,** A 1D detector is used in single-slice systems. **B,** A 2D detector array is characteristic of multislice CT systems.

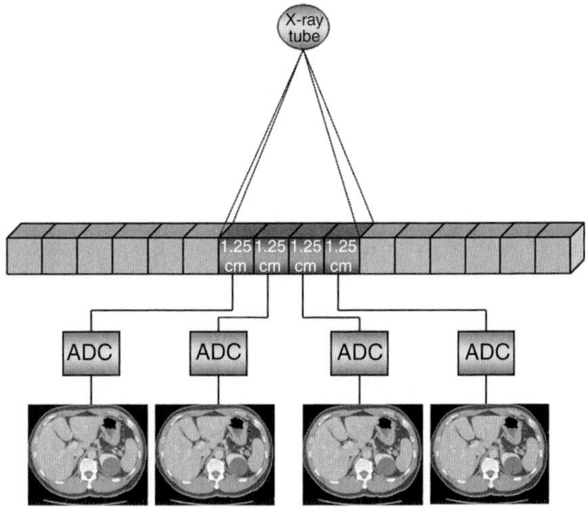

FIGURE 12-2 A diagrammatic illustration of how the detector elements from a multislice CT detector can be electronically combined to create slices of different thicknesses.

function of the data acquisition system (DAS). In this textbook, the term *multislice CT* will be used because it has become commonplace not only in the literature but also in clinical practice (Dowsett et al, 2006; Kachelriess, 2006; Kalender, 2005).

A CT detector consists of basically two major components: a radiation sensor coupled to suitable electronics such as photodiodes and analog-to-digital converters (ADCs) (see Chapter 5). Although the radiation sensors convert x-ray photons to light, the photodiodes convert the light into electrical current (signal) that must be digitized before it is sent to a digital computer for processing. The electronics are carefully configured to the sensor elements (cells) of the CT detector and in this regard represent the data acquisition channels. As seen in Figure 12-2, the detector consists of 16 elements or cells, each 1.25 millimeters (mm) in size, and the x-ray beam is collimated to fall on four of these cells. Therefore four signals are collected per gantry rotation from each of the four cells and sent to the four ADCs to produce four slices, each 1.25 mm thick. For eight 1.25-mm thick slices, the x-ray beam would fall on eight detector elements. For four 2.5-mm thick slices, the beam would be collimated to fall on eight detector elements, where two 1.25-mm elements would be combined to produce a 2.5-mm thick slice, and so on. This electronic combination (or binning) of detector elements is described in more detail later in the chapter.

The evolution of multislice CT technology is outlined in Figure 12-3. Its overall goal is to improve volume coverage speed performance; therefore, scanning is at higher speeds with higher pitch ratios to cover large volumes with equivalent image quality compared with single-slice volume CT scanners introduced in the 1990s. The 256 CT scanner was introduced by the Toshiba Corporation Medical Systems Division as a prototype high-speed 3D CT scanner for imaging the entire heart in one complete rotation. The high-speed 3D scanner will use larger area detectors to scan larger volumes at high speeds and subsequently display all images in 3D. Finally, in 2008, Toshiba Medical Systems introduced a new 320 CT scanner. These two scanners will be described briefly later in the chapter.

Subsecond Scanners

Scanning time continues to decrease from the 5 minutes needed by the original EMI scanner to as low as one half second at present. The engineering barriers to be overcome in reaching this gantry speed are formidable. The acceleration on gantry components such as the tube and generator can reach 13 gravities (G), considerably more than experienced by the space shuttle at lift off. Some interesting technologic developments have accompanied the design of these high-speed CT systems.

To prevent anode movement under the stress of subsecond acceleration, new x-ray tubes have the anode mounted on a shaft that extends along the tube, providing support on both sides of the anode. This design has distinct advantages over the traditional method of supporting a massive anode from the rear only. Other innovative developments in tube design for CT include grounded anodes and a technique to reduce off-focal x-rays. Virtually all medical x-ray tubes have applied the potential difference equally between cathode and anode so that the cathode can be at 75 kilovolts (kV) while the anode is at 75 kV. This requires a substantial gap between the anode and the tube housing to reduce the possibility of arcs. With all the voltage placed on the cathode and the anode at ground potential, the tube housing can be brought into close proximity to the anode, which facilitates heat transfer and markedly improves anode cooling rate. Recoil electrons, which normally are reattracted to the anode

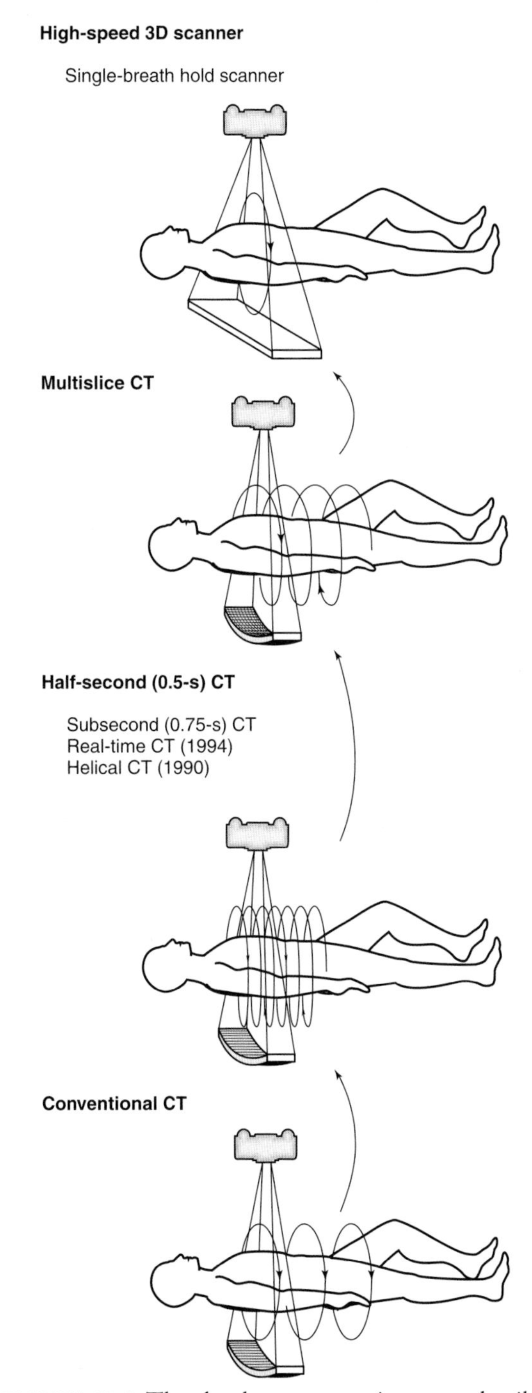

FIGURE 12-3 The development continuum and milestones for Toshiba's CT scanners.

and generate off-focal x-rays, can now be collected on a special collimator located near the anode. This eliminates off-focal x-rays that can reduce image quality and reduces the anode heat loading by about 30%, thereby reducing tube cooling delays during routine scanning.

The clinical benefits of subsecond scanning include reduced motion artifact and greater scan coverage. Patient movement during CT scanning, whether by cardiac motion, breathing, or peristalsis, may cause artifacts because filtered back-projection reconstruction combines all the views acquired during the scan rotation to cancel artifacts. Movement of any object in the field of view (FOV) during gantry rotation prevents accurate elimination of artifacts with consequent loss of image quality. If the moving object has notably high or low contrast, such as bone, calculi, or air, the artifacts are particularly noticeable. Unfortunately, the left ventricle and pulmonary vessels near the heart move so quickly that scans would have to be completed in less than 20 to 25 milliseconds to completely eliminate all blurring. This is a far shorter time than is possible with conventional CT scanners and is even difficult for electron-beam CTs, which are extremely fast. Even so, the half-second scanners, which can acquire "partial" (i.e., less than 360-degree rotation) images in 250 to 320 milliseconds have made it feasible to obtain considerably better images of the heart and chest than is possible with a 1-second system. An example is the ability of these scanners to use gated reconstruction, in which the raw scan data for image reconstruction can be selected on the basis of the patient's electrocardiogram (ECG). Reconstruction of a gated "partial" image during cardiac diastole, when the heart is relatively quiescent, can show fairly sharp ventricular borders and calcium in the coronary arteries.

Prospective gating can also be used in which the patient's ECG triggers the actual scan acquisition. This is a relatively simple technique, although it is not applicable to spiral/helical scanning.

A less dramatic but very practical benefit of subsecond scan times is the increased spiral/helical coverage that can become available. For the same pitch and scan duration, a half-second scanner will cover twice the anatomy that can be acquired with a 1-second scanner.

Alternatively, the half-second scanner could cover the same area by using 50% of the slice thickness, which improves z-axis resolution and leads to better image quality in 3D and multiplanar reconstructions. Clinical applications, such as CT angiography (CTA), can benefit from increased patient coverage without increasing pitch. This assumes that the system generator is able to produce enough power to accommodate the faster scans. For example, a 250-milliampere (mA) image of the abdomen requires a tube current of 500 mA in a half-second scanner.

Dual-Slice CT Scanners

The history of scanning more than one slice at a time (actually two-slice scanners) dates back to one of the early EMI (London, United Kingdom) CT scanners, which became available in 1972, and the Siemens SIRETOM (Siemens Medical Solutions, Germany) CT scanner, which appeared in 1974. These scanners used two detectors and they are based on the translate/rotate method of data collection over 180 degrees. The next major step to multislice CT scanning appeared in 1993, with the introduction of the first dual-slice volume CT scanner, the Elscint CT-TWIN (Elscint, Hackensack, NJ). The most significant difference between the dual-slice volume CT scanner and its single-slice counterpart is shown in Figure 12-4. As can be seen, the dual scanner slice geometry is based on a fan-beam of x-rays falling on two rows of detectors (Fig. 12-4, *A*) instead of one row of detectors, characteristic of the single-slice CT scanner beam geometry (Fig. 12-4, *B*).

The dual-slice whole-body fan-beam CT scanner offers improved volume coverage speed performance compared with the single-slice volume CT scanner, reducing the scan time by 50% while maintaining image quality for the same scanned volume.

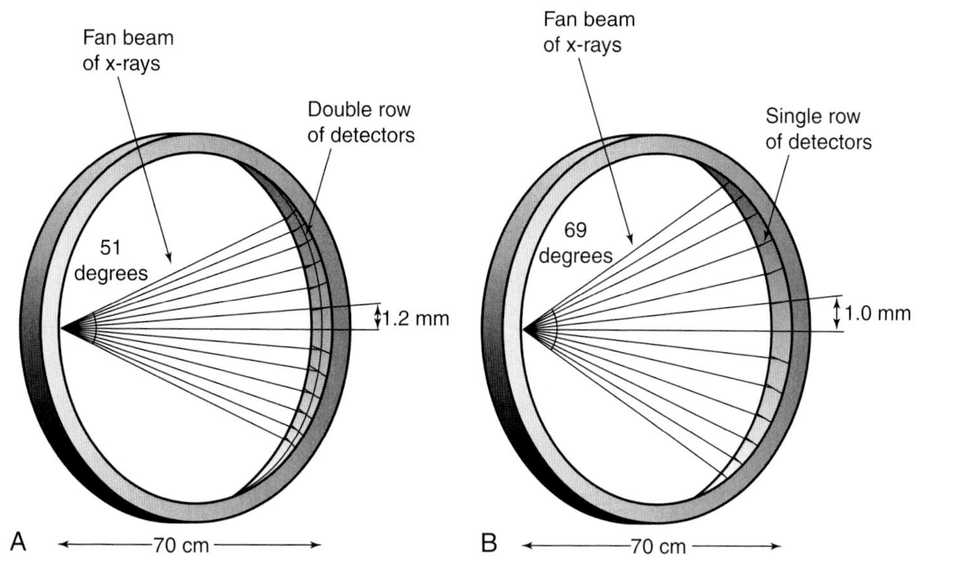

FIGURE 12-4 **A,** Dual scanner slice geometry based on far beam of x-rays falling on two rows of detectors. **B,** Single-slice CT scanner based on far beam of x-rays falling on one row of detectors.

Multislice CT Scanners

The dual-slice whole-body fan-beam CT technology paved the way for the development of other multislice CT scanners. These scanners were introduced at the 1998 meeting of the Radiological Society of North America in Chicago. They are based on spiral/helical scanning using multiple detector rows ranging between 8, 16, 32, 40, 64, (Kohl, 2006a), 256 (Mori et. al, 2006a), and more recently 320 (Toshiba Medical Systems, 2008) depending on the manufacturer. The 256-slice prototype scanner paved the way to the most recent commercially available multislice CT scanner, the 320 dynamic volume CT scanner. This scanner is highlighted later in the chapter.

The overall goal of the multislice CT scanner is to improve the volume coverage speed performance of both single-slice and dual-slice CT scanners. For example, a multislice CT scanner with *N*-detector rows (*N* slices) will be *N* times faster than its single-row (one slice) counterpart. Thus, multislice CT opens new avenues and opportunities to improve the quality of care afforded to patients because it now offers a wide range of new clinical applications afforded by recent technological developments.

PHYSICAL PRINCIPLES

Although the fundamental physics and flow of data are the same as conventional and spiral/helical CT scanners, multislice CT scanners introduce several new concepts relating to detector technology, the geometry of data acquisition, slice selection, and multislice image reconstruction algorithms.

Data Acquisition

Data acquisition is one of two mechanisms that affect image quality in CT (the other is image reconstruction). This section examines data

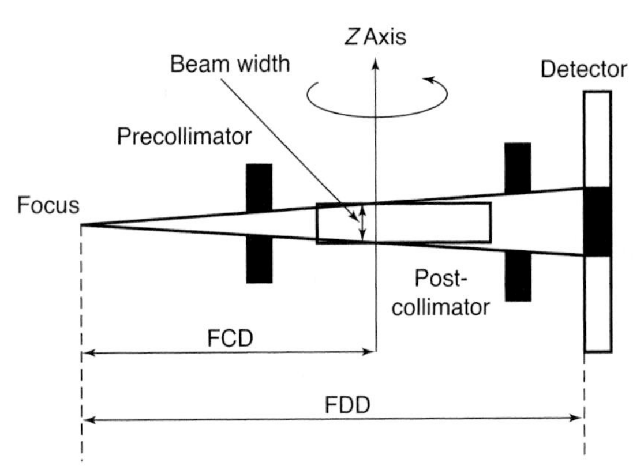

FIGURE 12-5 A side view of the basic data acquisition geometry for single-slice volume CT scanners. *FCD*, Focus isocenter distance; *FDD*, focus detector distance.

acquisition in multislice CT with respect to beam geometry and basic parameters such as collimation, slice thickness, and pitch; but first a brief review of data acquisition in single-slice CT is in order.

Single-Slice CT

The basic data acquisition geometry for single-slice volume CT is shown in Figure 12-5. This is a third-generation scheme in which the x-ray tube is coupled to a single-row detector array positioned in the z axis.

Collimation

The x-ray beam collimation system is designed to ensure a constant beam width because the precollimator and postcollimator widths are equal. The beam may or may not be collimated at the detector array. The width of the precollimator defines the slice thickness (z-axis resolution or spatial resolution) and affects the volume coverage speed performance. Although thin collimation results in better resolution and takes longer to scan a specified volume, wide collimation results in less resolution but provides better volume coverage speed. The beam width (BW) is measured in the z-axis at the center of rotation for a single-row detector array, and it is defined by the precollimator width, which determines the thickness for a single slice. A collimator width of 8 mm falling on a 1D detector array will provide a slice thickness of 8 mm.

Beam Geometry

The x-ray beam geometry for single-slice CT describes a small fan (see Fig. 12-5) and is referred to as a *parallel fan-beam geometry*.

Pitch

The pitch for single-slice volume CT is defined as the ratio of the distance the table translates per gantry rotation to the BW or precollimator width. As noted by Hu (1999a), "the table advancement per rotation of twice the x-ray beam collimation appears to be the limit of the volume coverage speed performance of a single-slice CT, and further increase in the table translation would result in clinically unusable images."

Slice Thickness

In single-slice volume CT, the thickness of the slice is determined by the pitch and the width of the precollimator (which also defines the BW) at the center of rotation (see Fig. 12-5).

Multislice CT

The data acquisition geometry for multislice CT is shown in Figure 12-6 (see also Fig. 12-1, *B*). Perhaps the most conspicuous difference between the data acquisition geometry in Figure 12-1 and Figure 12-6 is the multirow detector array (specifically 4) coupled to the x-ray tube to describe a third-generation geometry (see Fig. 12-6, *A*). This 2D detector array is what Hu (1999a) refers to as the "enabling component" of a multislice CT scanner. Other important and unique features of multislice data acquisition relate to collimation, beam geometry, and pitch.

Collimation

The fundamental collimation scheme is shown in Figure 12-1, *B*. The beam is collimated by a precollimator to fall on the entire multirow detector array. The BW is still defined in the z-axis at the center of rotation but now is for a four-row

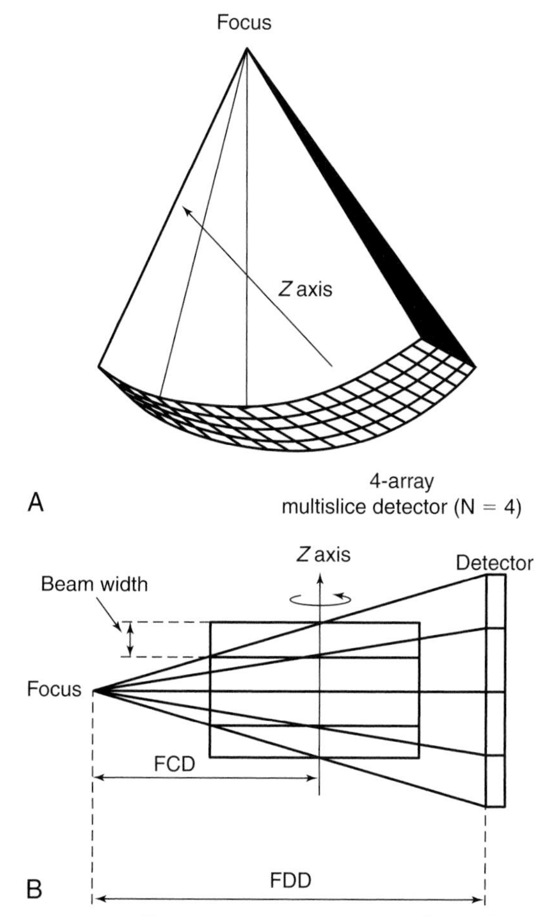

FIGURE 12-6 Data acquisition geometry for multislice CT. **A,** The coordinate system. **B,** A cross-section (side view).

multislice detector array, as shown in Figure 12-6, *B*. This width will be for four slices and is prescribed by the precollimator. A precollimator width of 8 mm that falls on a four-row multislice detector array will produce four slices, each with a thickness of 2 mm (i.e., 8 mm—the total beam width in the z-axis at the center of rotation divided by 4). This is unlike the single-slice counterpart, which provides a slice thickness of 8 mm with its 8 mm wide precollimator. In addition, the four slices are a result of the division of the total x-ray beam into multiple beams, depending on the number of arrays in the 2D detector system.

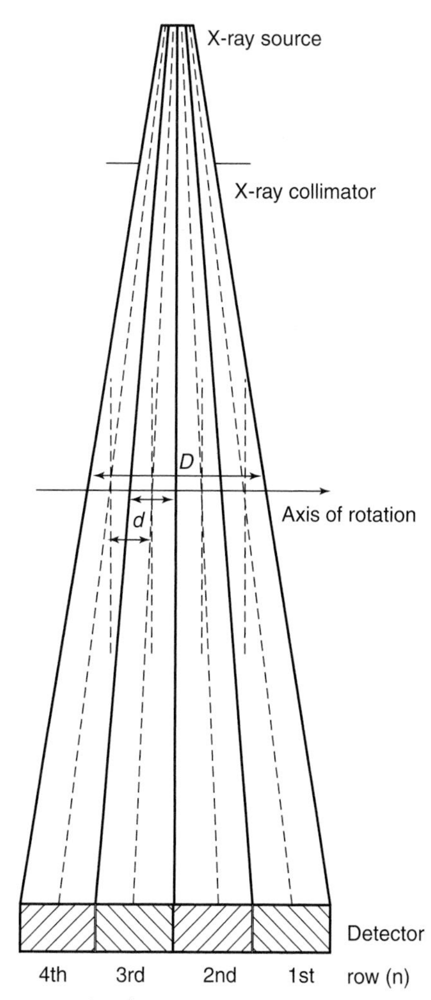

FIGURE 12-7 A side view or cross-section of a multislice CT beam geometry from the x-ray tube to a four-row multislice detector array system.

These multiple beams are the result of the detector row collimation or the detector row aperture (Hu, 1999a).

Figure 12-7 is a side view of a multislice CT scanner beam from the x-ray tube to the detectors. D is the width of the x-ray beam collimator and is measured at the axis of rotation; N is the number of detector rows; and d represents the detector row collimation. Hu (1999a) explains that, if the gaps between the adjacent detector rows are small and can be ignored, the detector row spacing is equal

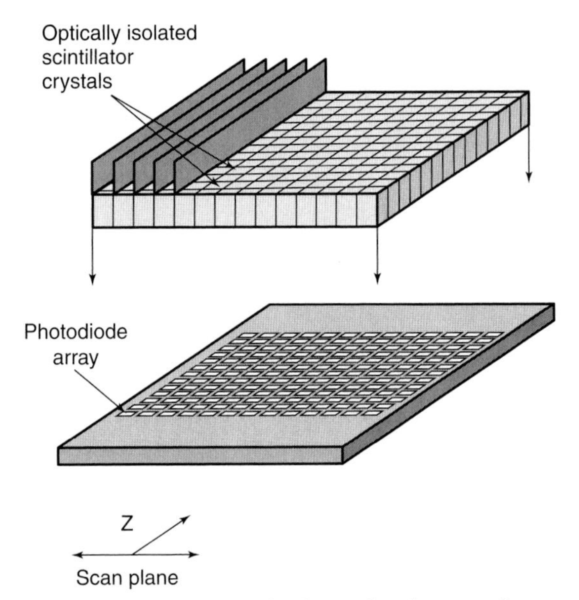

FIGURE 12-8 A proposed scheme for the use of postcollimation in multislice CT to reduce scattered radiation falling on a 2D detector array. The collimators are positioned between detector columns similar to conventional CT single-row detector arrays.

to the detector row collimation (*d*). The detector row collimation *d* and the x-ray beam collimation *D* has the following relationship:

$$d\ (mm) = D\ (mm)/N$$

where *N* is the number of detector rows. In single-slice CT, the detector row collimation equals and is interchangeable with the x-ray beam collimation. "In multislice CT, the detector row collimation is only 1/*N* of the x-ray beam collimation." This makes it possible "to simultaneously achieve high volume coverage speed and high z axis resolution. In general, the larger the number of detector rows N, the better the volume coverage speed performance."

For example, if the x-ray prepatient collimation width (x-ray beam collimation) is 20 mm and the scanner has a four-row detector array, the detector row collimation is as follows:

$$d\ (mm) = D\ (mm)/N$$

in which *d* is the detector row collimation, *N* is the number of detector rows, and *D* is the x-ray beam collimator width (20/4 = 5 mm).

Alternatively,

$$d = 1/N \times \text{X-ray beam collimator width}$$
$$d = 1/4 \times 20$$
$$= 5\ mm$$

As the beam width increases in the z direction to cover the number of rows in the 2D detector system, the amount of scattered radiation increases because a wide area of the patient is scanned. To minimize scattered radiation, antiscatter collimation may be used at the detector array (postcollimation). One such scheme is shown in Figure 12-8. Another scheme is illustrated later.

Beam Geometry

As the number of detector rows in a multirow detector array increases, the beam becomes wider to cover the 2D detector array (Fig. 12-9; see also Fig. 12-7). The beam must cover the length of the detector array. This coverage is influenced by the fan angle of the beam, in which a wider fan angle will cover a longer detector array. The beam must also cover the width of the detector array, which is defined by the number of rows in the detector array. A larger number of rows will result in a wider beam (large cone beam) in the z-axis direction.

A cone beam geometry produces more beam divergence along the z-axis compared with fan-beam geometry. For this reason, increasing the number of detector rows in multislice CT creates a need for a different approach to the interpolation process (compared with single-slice spiral/helical interpolation) because the rays that contribute to the imaging process are more oblique. In addition, the number of detector rows plays an important role in slice thickness selection and volume coverage.

Pitch

The pitch, *P*, for single-slice CT is defined as the ratio of the distance, *L*, the tabletop travels for one

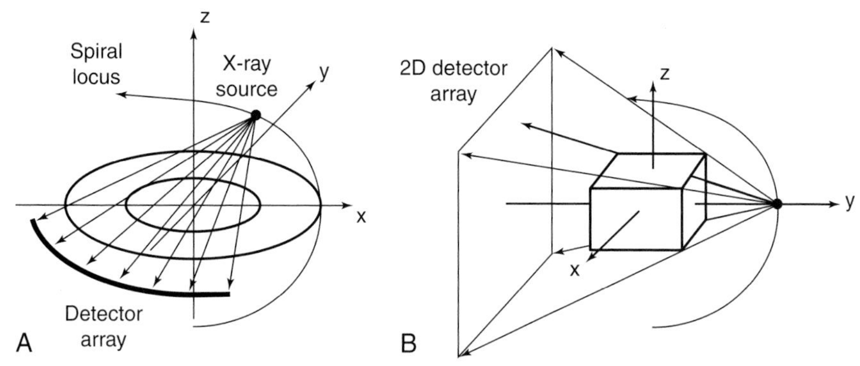

FIGURE 12-9 **A,** The fan-beam geometry of single-row 1D detectors, in which the rays at the detector array are almost parallel and close together. **B,** The concept of cone-beam geometry typical of multirow 2D detectors. The cone beam results in a wider divergence of rays at the detector array than the fan-beam geometry of single-row 1D detectors.

complete rotation of the x-ray tube to the x-ray beam collimation. This collimation defines the BW for a single-row detector array at the center of rotation (see Fig. 12-5). The thickness of the slice is determined by the BW at the center of rotation.

In the past, the definition of pitch was somewhat varied and controversial. For example, Hu (1999a) extends the single-slice pitch definition (Equation 12-1).

$$\text{Multislice CT pitch} = \text{Table movement per rotation} / \text{detector row collimation (or spacing)} \quad (12\text{-}1)$$

As noted by He (1999), "the key difference here is that multislice CT beam collimation is much wider than the smallest detector row used for data acquisition. In the 4-slice scanner case, for example, one scan mode is 4 × 2.5 mm, table speed is 7.5 mm/rotation, beam width is 10 mm. So if we used our definition, the pitch value would be 7.5 mm/2.5 mm = 3. However, one could also argue that the pitch should be 7.5 mm/10 mm = 0.75. There are good arguments for either definition here."

Taguchi and Aradate (1998) define the pitch, *P*, in a 4-slice scanner (four-row detector array) as:

$$P = L/BW \quad (12\text{-}2)$$

where *L* is table speed per rotation and BW is the beam width in the z-axis for a 1-row detector array, at the center of rotation (see Fig. 12-5). For a four-slice scanner, each slice is defined by BW (see Fig. 12-6). In this case, four slices are acquired at the same time, and the helical pitch is increased by a factor of four compared with single-slice volume CT (Fig. 12-10).

In addition, Kalender (2005) defines pitch for a multislice CT scanner with a four-row detector array as "the table feed, *d*, per full rotation relative to the slice width, *S*, of a single detector row (rather than relative to the total detector width)." Mathematically, this can be expressed as shown in Equation 12-3:

$$\text{Pitch} = d/s \quad (12\text{-}3)$$

Although pitch for single-slice volume CT is defined in terms of the table speed per rotation, the definition of pitch for multislice CT is varied

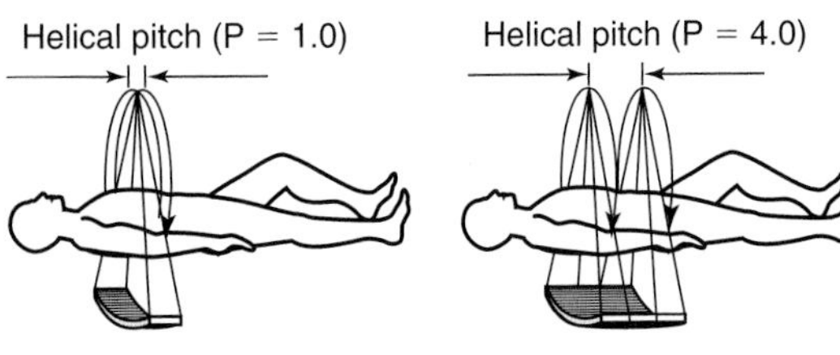

FIGURE 12-10 A comparison of the pitch between single-slice and multislice CT data acquisition. In the multislice case, the pitch is increased by a factor of 4, which allows for increased volume coverage in less time without a loss of image quality.

and is based on the table speed per rotation and either the slice thickness, the detector row collimation, or the BW at the center of rotation, depending on the manufacturer.

International Electrotechnical Commission Definition of Pitch

In 1999, the International Electrotechnical Commission (IEC) introduced a definition of pitch, which is stated in the IEC document 60601 regulation for CT, as a means of addressing the variations in definitions offered by different manufacturers (IEC, 1999). The IEC recommends the following:

$$\text{Pitch (P)} = \text{Distance the table travels per rotation (d)} / \text{Total collimation (W)} \quad (12\text{-}4)$$

The total collimation, on the other hand, is equal to the number of slices (M) times the collimated slice thickness (S). Algebraically, the pitch can now be expressed as follows:

$$P = d/W \text{ or } P = d/M \bullet S \quad (12\text{-}5)$$

Pitch is an important and familiar parameter in spiral/helical scanning that combines the table distance traveled per 360-degree rotation with the slice thickness. Pitch relates to the volume covered and also to patient dose. A pitch of less than 1 is effectively the same as overlapping slices and imparts a high dose. Conversely, pitches of greater than 1 result in reduced patient dose. The introduction of multislice detectors requires a reevaluation of the definition of pitch.

For a patient dose comparable to current single-slice scanners at a pitch of 1, a four-slice scanner would require a beam pitch of 1 or a slice pitch of 4. As an example, selection of 4 × 5-mm slices with a table speed of 20 mm per rotation should result in approximately the same patient dose as from a single-slice scanner operated with a 5-mm slice at 5 mm per rotation table speed. Whether this is true in practice depends on the collimator design of the specific scanner.

Slice Thickness

In multislice CT, the slice thickness is determined by the BW (see Fig. 12-6), the pitch, and other factors such as the shape and width of the reconstruction filter in the z-axis. The details of slice thickness selection for multislice CT scanners are described later in the chapter under the subsection "Slice Thickness Selection."

Image Reconstruction

In conventional step-and-shoot CT (conventional CT), a fan-beam geometry and a single-row detector array are used in the data acquisition process, and all rays pass through the image plane (planar section), the slice of interest. With this condition, a fan-beam reconstruction algorithm, specifically, the filtered back-projection algorithm is used for image reconstruction.

Single-Slice Spiral/Helical Reconstruction

In single-slice spiral/helical CT (single-slice CT), the fan-beam geometry is maintained and a single-row detector array is used in the data acquisition process. In conventional CT, the patient is stationary during scanning, whereas in single-slice CT the patient is moving continuously through the gantry aperture during a 360-degree rotation of the x-ray tube and detectors. In this case, all rays do not pass through the image plane.

A fan-beam geometry is used, so the fan-beam reconstruction algorithm used in conventional CT is used for image reconstruction. During data acquisition, the fan-beam traces a spiral/helical path around the patient, as shown in Figure 12-11. Because all rays do not pass through the image plane (planar section), single-slice spiral/helical CT requires an additional step of first calculating a planar section. This is done by interpolation, using data points on either side of the section.

The first interpolation algorithm used was 360-degree linear interpolation (360 degrees LI), in which the distance between the two data points used in the interpolation was represented by *s* in Figure 12-11. In an effort to improve the image quality resulting from the 360-degree LI, a different algorithm was developed on the basis of the mathematical fact that a CT view from a specific angle contains the same information as a view in the opposite direction (at 180 degrees). The 180-degree view, when flipped and used for interpolated reconstruction, is referred to as *complementary data*, as opposed to the direct, measured data. With a 180-degree LI, data points are now closer to the image plane. The distance between the two points used for interpolation is now *s*/2. This equation involves calculation of a complementary data set *(dashed lines)* using the direct fan-beam data set or measurements *(solid lines)*. The distance between the two points used for interpolation is referred to as the *z-gap* (Hu, 1999a). The z-gap affects image quality so that, the smaller the z-gap, the better the image quality. In single-slice spiral/helical CT, increased volume coverage can be achieved with increased pitch; however, as the pitch increases, image quality decreases because the z-gap becomes larger. This is one motivating factor for the development of multislice CT.

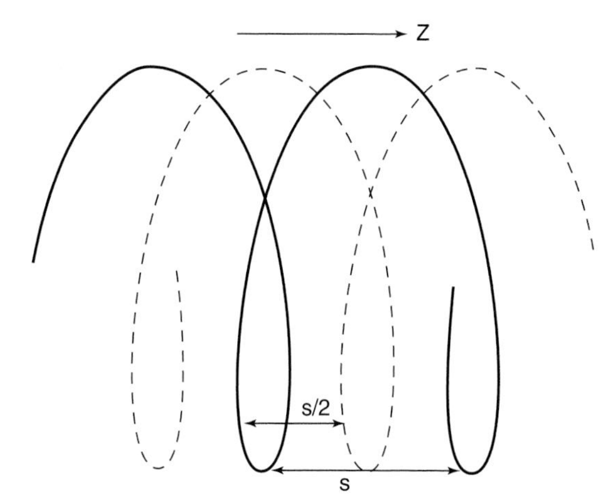

FIGURE 12-11 The spiral/helical trace of a single-row detector array in single-slice volume CT. The distance of the data points used for 360-degree LI and 180-degree LI are *s* and *s/2*, respectively.

Multislice Reconstruction

One of the most conspicuous differences between single-slice CT and multislice CT is that the latter uses a new detector technology in which the number of detector rows can vary from four to 320 (at the time of writing this chapter). These multiple detector rows result in a large 2D detector array. Because of this, a cone-beam geometry results instead of the fan-beam geometry characteristic of single-slice CT systems. Cone-beam geometry produces an increase in the beam divergence, which now poses a fundamental problem because all the rays do not pass through the image plane. Rays at the periphery of the beam lie outside the image plane. Approximate cone-beam reconstruction algorithms have been developed for solving this problem (Kudo and Saito, 1991); however, these particular algorithms demand extensive calculations (compared with fan-beam algorithms) and are not suitable for use in medical imaging.

Special fan-beam reconstructions (Hu, 1999a; Taguchi and Aradate, 1998) have been developed for multislice CT in its present state. In deriving an algorithm for image reconstruction in multislice CT, a logical first step is to extend the principles of 360-degree LI and 180-degree LI used in single-slice CT to multislice CT. To examine this extension, consider Figure 12-12, which shows the spiral/helical path of a four-row detector array

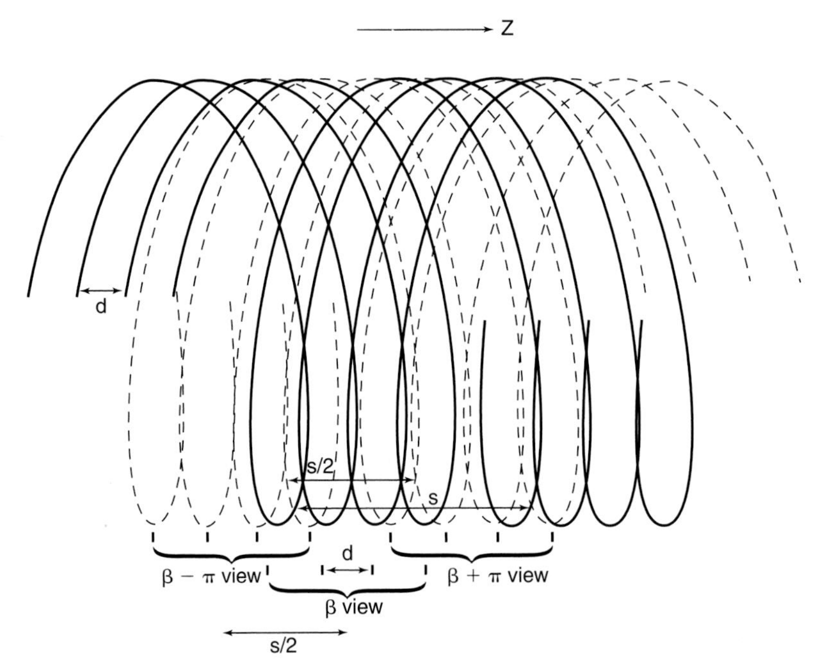

FIGURE 12-12 The spiral/helical trace of a four-row detector array in multislice CT. See text for further explanation.

used in multislice CT. For a 360-degree LI, the distance between the two points used for interpolation of a planar section is *s*, the same distance as in Figure 12-11 for single-slice CT. With a 180-degree LI, the distance of the data points is *s/2* (distance between the solid and dashed lines of the same detector row). The z-gap is the same as in single-slice CT.

Multislice CT for up to Four Detector Rows

In multislice CT, the z-gap is determined by the pitch (as in single-slice CT) and by the detector row spacing, *d*. "As the helical pitch varies, distinctively different z sampling patterns and therefore interlacing helix patterns may result in multislice helical CT" (Hu, 1999a). This is illustrated in Figure 12-13 for a four-row detector array for two different pitches. At a pitch of 2:1 (Fig. 12-13, *A*) the distance between the points used for interpolation, the z-gap, is *d*, "which is the same as the displacement from one solid helix to the next. This causes a high degree of overlap between different helices, generating highly redundant projection measurements at certain z-positions. Because of this high degree of redundancy (or inefficiency) in z-sampling, the overall z-sampling spacing (i.e., the z-gap of the interlacing helix pattern) is still *d*, not any better than its single-slice counterpart" (Hu, 1999a).

Increased pitch in multislice CT from 2:1 to 3:1 (Fig. 12-13, *B*) results in a z-gap of *d/2*, a much shorter distance. In this case the volume coverage speed can be increased. In addition, because the z-gap is less as the pitch increases, better image quality results. Hu (1999a) points out that "the volume coverage speed performance of the multislice scanner is substantially better than its single-slice counterpart, and so the selection of helical pitches is very critical to its performance. The pitch selection is determined by the consideration of the z-sampling efficiency and conventional factors such as volume coverage speed (which disfavors very low helical pitch); slice profile; and image artifacts, which disfavor very high helical pitch." The preferred helical pitches are those that represent the preferred tradeoffs for various applications.

Alternatively, Figures 12-14, 12-15, 12-16, and 12-17 can be used to explain the problem and solution described previously. The unwound helical path for single-slice CT is shown in Figure 12-14 for both direct and complementary data. The image plane is interpolated using two points from the direct data and the complementary data on either side of it (image plane). Extending the single-slice concept to the multislice case as shown in Figure 12-15 results in a superimposition of the complementary and direct data for each of the detector rows in the four-row array. Note also that the z-gap is larger, and this results in image degradation. Additionally, the superimposition does not allow for efficient z-sampling. A pitch of 4 is not as preferable as a pitch of 2 because of the redundancy in the data sampling.

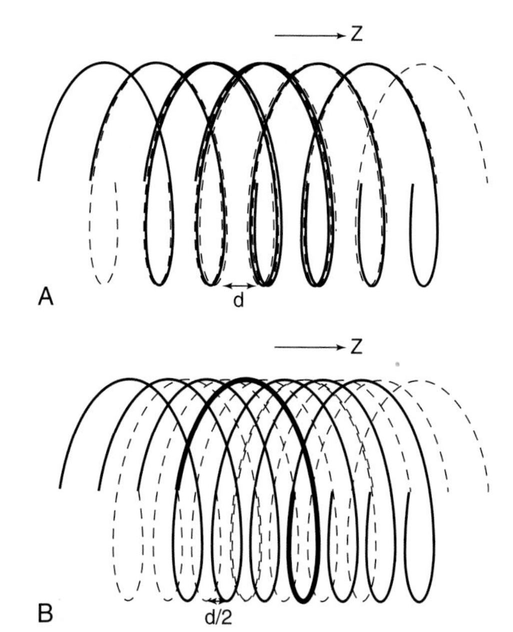

FIGURE 12-13 Spiral/helical traces for a four-row detector array in multislice CT at a pitch of 2:1 **(A)** and a pitch of 3:1 **(B)**.

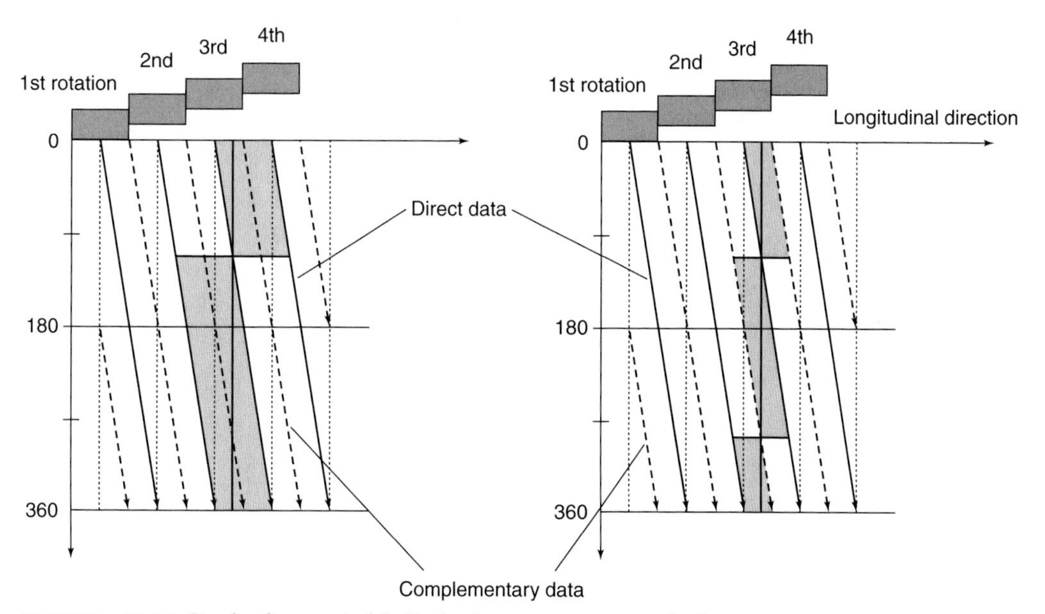

FIGURE 12-14 Single-slice spiral/helical data are generated from many gantry rotations. Reconstruction of an image in a single plane on the patient axis involves the interpolation of views in front of and behind the image plane. The use of complementary data reduces effective slice thickness but increases noise.

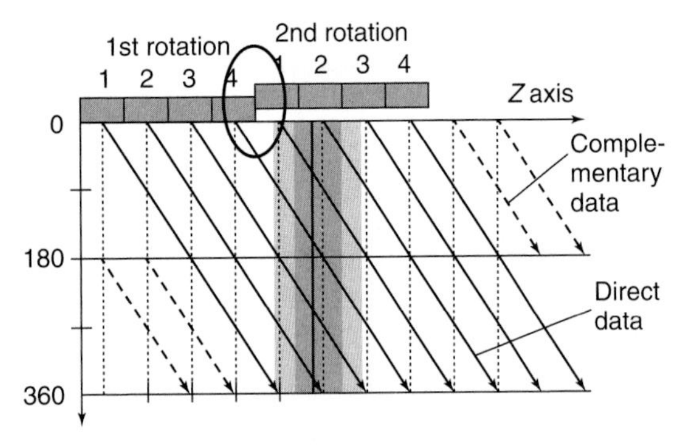

FIGURE 12-15 Rotation of a multislice detector with an even integer pitch causes the overlap of direct and complementary data from different slices. This duplication reduces the amount of information available for image reconstruction and affects image quality.

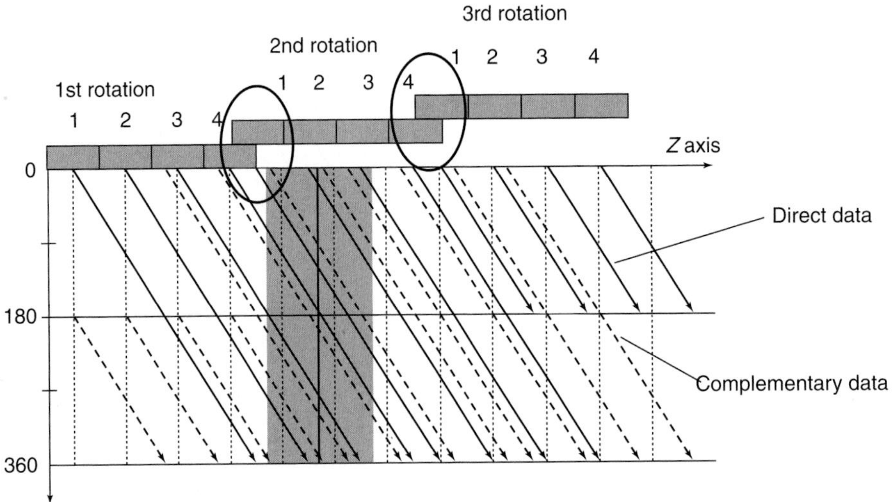

FIGURE 12-16 Careful choice of multislice pitch avoids the duplication of direct and complementary data so that image quality is not compromised.

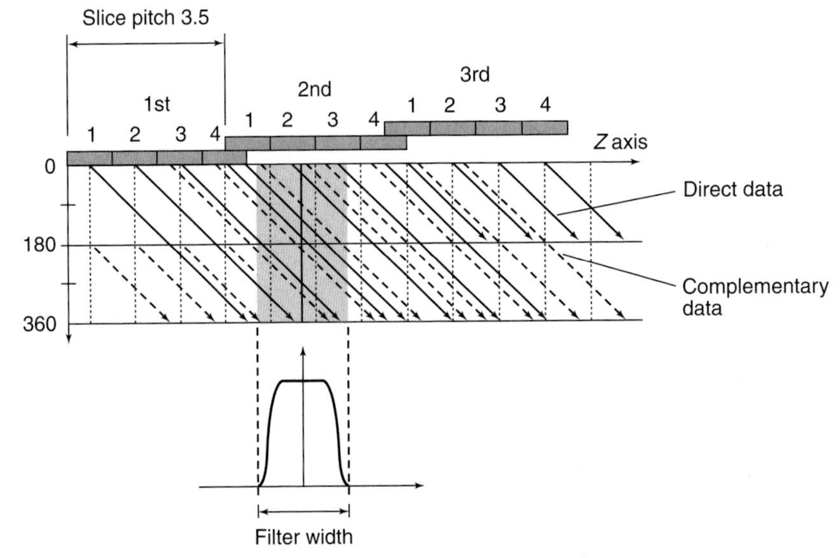

FIGURE 12-17 Filters may be used to average data along the z-axis and provide more tradeoff options between effective slice thickness and image noise to the operator.

Figure 12-16 provides a solution to the problem imposed by Figure 12-15. By separating the direct and complementary data trails, efficient z-sampling can be achieved (Saito, 1998). Taguchi and Aradate (1998) referred to this as *optimized sampling scan.* Figure 12-16 is with a pitch of 3.5 less than that of Figure 12-15 (pitch of 4). These figures indicate that a slight compromise in helical pitch (just 0.5) produces amazing improvement in the data sampling pattern.

The detector design for multislice CT allows the operator to select variable slice thicknesses on the basis of the requirements of the examination. The new algorithms for multislice CT also allow for the reconstruction of these variable slice thicknesses. These new algorithms address problems (image quality degradation) arising from the increase in speed (hence volume coverage) of the patient moving through the gantry aperture when the pitch is increased. Additionally, these algorithms provide for the selection of the slice thicknesses that meet the needs of the examination.

Two such algorithms were developed by Taguchi and Aradate (1998) and by Hu (1999a). These algorithms are almost identical (including the algorithm developed by Siemens Medical Systems) and are based on the same philosophy (Hu, 1999b; Taguchi, 1999).

In general, these algorithms are based on the following steps:

1. *Spiral/helical scanning by interlaced sampling* In this step, smaller z-gaps are obtained by adjusting or selecting the pitch to separate the complementary data from the direct data.
2. *Longitudinal interpolation by z-filtering* Another unique aspect of multislice data reconstruction involves averaging data in the z-axis direction. Interpolation of spiral/helical data is still needed, but the fact that the density of data points in this dimension is greater than with single-slice scanners is advantageous. One approach to image reconstruction uses a filter in the z-axis to select and weight the data points to be used in the averaging (Taguchi and Aradate, 1998) (Fig. 12-17). This is a method of a filtering process in the longitudinal *(z)* direction. Assuming some range with a width called the *filter width* (FW) in the longitudinal *(z)* direction (see Fig. 12-17), all data sampled within that range are processed by weighted summation. The filter parameters (e.g., FW and shape) can control the spatial resolution in the longitudinal direction, the image noise, and the image quality. Again, pitch selection is flexible and should be carefully selected. A practical advantage of this technique is that the size and shape of the filter can be selected by the operator for more control over the effective slice thickness versus noise tradeoff. As can be seen in Figure 12-17, the selection of different FWs provides considerably more control over effective slice thickness than has generally been available with single-slice spiral/helical reconstruction. FW can also substantially affect image noise compared with conventional 180- or 360-degree linear interpolation.
3. *Fan-beam reconstruction* This algorithm can be used if the number of detector rows is small. Hu (1999a) uses multiple parallel fan beams to approximate the cone-beam geometry characteristic of multislice CT. The algorithm used by Taguchi and Aradate (1998) is also based on a fan-beam method. Additionally, Saito (1998) labels the algorithm multislice cone-beam tomography reconstruction method (MUSCOT). The effect of MUSCOT on image quality is shown in Figure 12-18. Compared with single-slice CT (180-degree LI), MUSCOT provides good image quality "at a scanning speed that is about three times faster than that for single-slice CT" (Taguchi and Aradate, 1998).

Multislice CT for 16 or More Detector Rows

The previous description lends itself to multislice CT scanners with up to four detector rows. These scanners use a 2D detector array in which the x-ray beam is now opened in two dimensions to cover the entire detector array. The divergence of the beam describes a cone beam rather than a fan

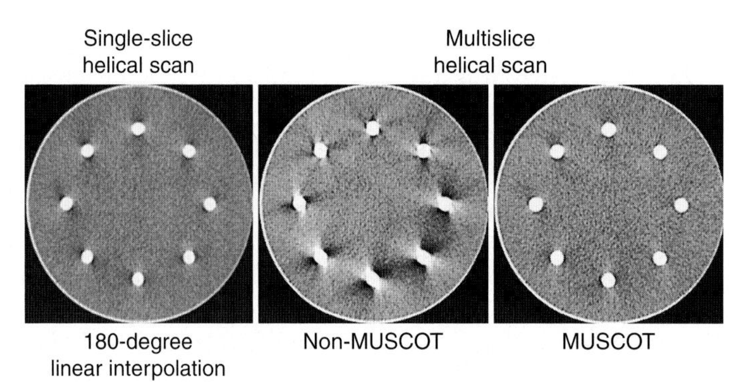

FIGURE 12-18 The difference in image quality of a ball phantom obtained with a 180-degree LI algorithm (single-slice CT) and with and without the MUSCOT algorithm used for multislice CT imaging. (From Saito Y: Multislice x-ray CT scanner, *Med Rev* 66:1-8, 1998.)

beam, and therefore the scanning geometry is now referred to as a cone beam. The nature and problems of using a cone beam with algorithms designed for fan-beam CT scanning geometries are outlined in Chapter 6 on image reconstruction in CT. One of the problems, for example, is related to cone-beam artifacts (streaks, for example) that degrade image quality.

The algorithms for four-slice scanners described earlier ignore the cone-beam geometry in four-slice multislice CT scanners because these algorithms assume that the measurement rays are parallel and perpendicular to the z-axis (longitudinal axis), a

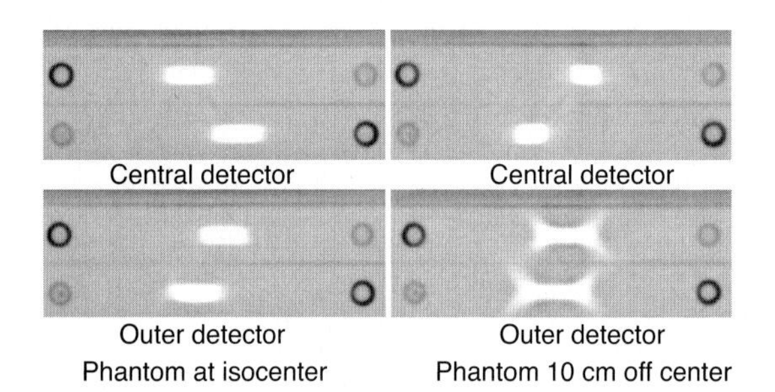

FIGURE 12-19 The appearance of streaking artifacts that occur with imaging of nonuniform objects in the z-axis with a 16-slice (cone beam) CT scanner. The artifacts are more pronounced for those created by the outer detectors and worsen if the object is not positioned accurately in the isocenter. (Courtesy ImPACT Scan, London, United Kingdom.)

condition that satisfies the filtered back-projection (FBP) algorithm. Basically, the measurement rays for a planar data set are obtained by interpolation with 360-degree LI or 180-degree LI algorithms similar to those for single-slice spiral/helical CT scanners (Chapter 11), followed by the well-established and proven FBP algorithm.

As the number of detector rows increase from four to 16 to 64 and beyond, the cone beam becomes larger and cone-beam artifacts become more pronounced, especially if the object imaged is not perfectly centered in the isocenter of the CT gantry (Figure 12-19). The outer detectors receive more oblique rays compared with the central set of detectors. The effects of cone-beam geometries on image quality for these 16-slice and beyond multislice CT scanners cannot be ignored. The cone-beam angle, for example, increases by up to 16, and previous interpolation algorithms are not useful for these large cone angles (Mather, 2005a). Therefore, cone-beam algorithms are needed to address these increasing cone-beam geometries and minimize cone-beam artifacts.

Cone-Beam Algorithms: An Overview

Cone-beam algorithms fall into two classes, namely, (1) exact algorithms and (2) approximate algorithms. Although exact algorithms for cone-beam data have not been successful in recent times (Kalender, 2005), they are also "computationally complex and difficult to implement" (Mather, 2005a). For these reasons, they are not described in this book. On the other hand, approximate cone-beam algorithms fall into two categories: 3D algorithms and 2D algorithms (Chen et al, 2003). Two such algorithms that have become commonplace in multislice CT scanners are as follows:

1. Feldkamp-Davis-Kress (FDK), also simply referred to as the Feldkamp-type 3D algorithm
2. Advanced single-slice rebinning (ASSR) 2D approximate algorithm

Feldkamp-Davis-Kress Algorithm

The fundamental basis of the FDK algorithm is illustrated in Figure 12-20. As can be seen, the FDK algorithm simply is an extension of the 2D FBP for fan-beam geometry into a 3D FBP for cone-beam geometry (Chen et al, 2003; Kachelriess et al, 2006).

This algorithm is more extensive than the 2D FBP algorithm, and it is more commonplace for use with cone-beam CT scanners (Feldkamp et al, 1984). Although the 2D FBP algorithm filters the acquired data from one-dimensional detectors, followed by a 2D fan-beam back-projection, the FDK algorithm filters the data acquired from 2D detectors (3D data set) followed by a 3D cone-beam back projection (Kalender, 2005).

There are several modifications of the FDK algorithm (referred to as Feldkamp-type algorithms) for use in multislice CT scanners; however, the principles of these algorithms are beyond the scope of this book. Two examples of these algorithms in use on some multislice CT scanners are the true cone-beam tomography (TCOT) Feldkamp-based algorithm developed by Toshiba Medical Systems, which can handle data from large cone angles, and the extended parallel back-projection (EPBP) algorithm developed by Siemens for scanners with more than 64 slices per/rotation.

A basic problem with the Feldkamp-type algorithms is that they "cannot incorporate 2D back projection hardware already available in conventional medical CT systems" (Chen et al, 2003; Kachelriess, 2006). This problem however can be solved by 2D approximate algorithms.

Two-Dimensional Approximate Algorithm

The main goal of the 2D approximate algorithms "is to provide an image quality close to that of a three-dimensional reconstruction algorithm using two-dimensional and back projection methods" (Chen et al, 2003). The principle is based on the notion of *rebinning*, a term used to describe the resorting of the 3D data collected from the cone-beam acquisition (geometry) to a set of 2D fan-beam projection data and subsequently use the conventional 2D FBP algorithm to reconstruct transaxial images, as illustrated in Figure 12-21.

One early rebinning method was the single-slice rebinning (SSR) algorithm; however, it did not produce acceptable image quality for multislice CT scanners with large cone angles. Therefore, other methods were developed to solve this problem by use of a technique called tilted plane reconstruction (TPR) (Chen et al, 2003). The TPR method requires that the plane to be reconstructed is tilted (oblique) to fit the spiral/helical path of the x-ray beam to reduce cone-beam artifacts. One popular TPR algorithm is the ASSR algorithm used by General Electric (GE) Healthcare and by Siemens Medical Solutions.

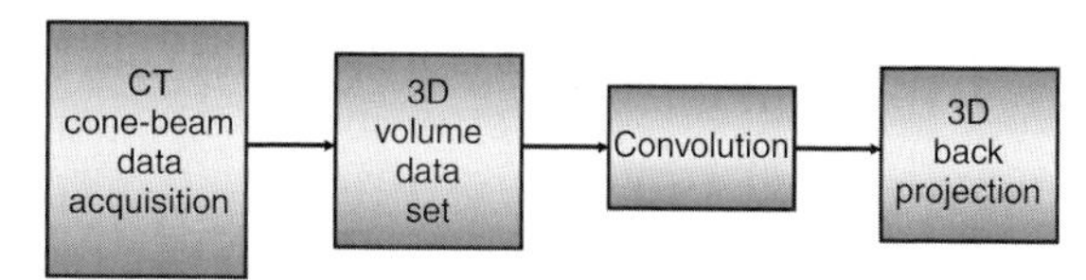

FIGURE 12-20 The most fundamental representation of the FDK algorithm for conebeam reconstruction. First, cone-beam projections of the 3D object are obtained, followed by preweighting and filtering (convolution). Finally, 3D back-projection is performed along the identical beam geometry (rays) as used for the initial cone-beam data acquisition.

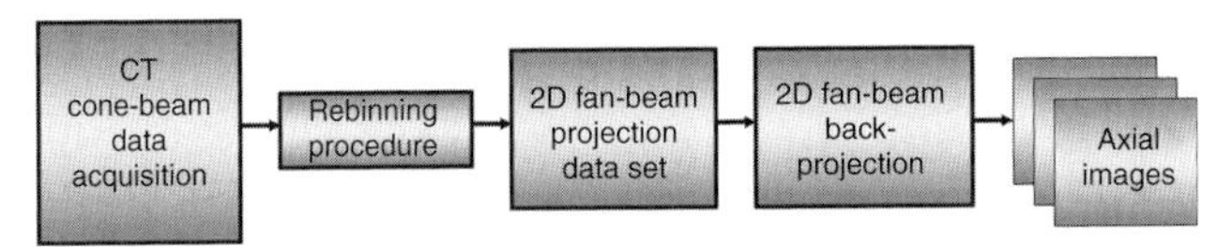

FIGURE 12-21 The basic steps of the 2D approximate reconstruction algorithm for wide cone-beam CT scanners. The acquired cone-beam data are rebinned into a 2D fan-beam projection data set that is finally back-projected by use of the 2D fan-beam reconstruction algorithm to create a set of axial images.

The fundamental steps of the ASSR algorithm, clearly illustrated in Figure 12-22, are as follows:

1. The image planes to be reconstructed make use of 180-degree segments of the spiral/helical path of the x-ray beam to obtain optimized oblique images (semicircles) because they are tilted to fit the spiral path along the z-axis of the patient.
2. The measured cone beam data are then rebinned (resorted) to produce a large number of overlapping tilted reconstruction planes that can cover the entire volume of tissue imaged.
3. In the third step, z-axis reformation (z-axis filtering) is performed to produce axial images by using the conventional 2D reconstruction algorithm on the tilted planes.
4. Finally, step 3 produces an axial image data set.

One of the fundamental problems with the ASSR algorithm is related to smaller pitch values. To solve this problem, the adaptive multiplane reconstruction (AMPR) algorithm was introduced. The AMPR algorithm is an extension of the ASSR algorithm and determines the z-axis resolution by allowing the free selection of pitch values and slice thickness (Flohr et al, 2005).

Another multislice cone-beam reconstruction algorithm that is somewhat related to the AMPR algorithm is the weighted hyperplane reconstruction (WHR) algorithm. A hyperplane is a concept in geometry. In a 2D (x, y) space, a hyperplane is a line, whereas in a 3D (x, y, z) space, a hyperplane is an ordinary plane that separates the space into two halves (OED, 2008). How this algorithm works is summarized by Flohr et al (2005) as follows:

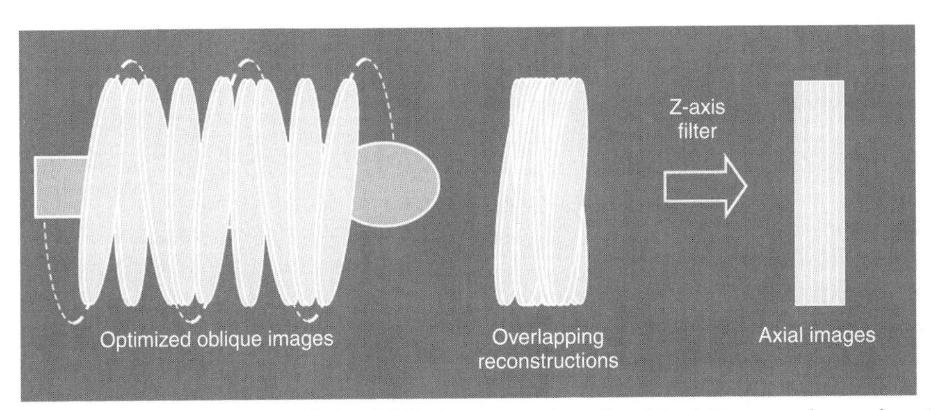

FIGURE 12-22 The basic steps of the ASSR reconstruction algorithm. See text for explanation. (Courtesy ImPACT Scan, London, United Kingdom.)

"Similar to the AMPR, 3D reconstruction is split into a series of two-dimensional reconstructions. Instead of reconstruction of traditional transverse sections, convex hyperplanes are proposed as the region of reconstruction. The increasing spiral overlap with decreasing pitch is handled by introducing subsets of detector rows, which are sufficient to reconstruct an image at a given pitch value. At a pitch of 0.5625 with a 16-slice scanner the data collected by detector rows one to nine form a complete projection data set. Similarly, projections from detector rows two to 10 can be used to reconstruct another image at the same z-axis position. Projections from detector rows three to 11 yield a third image and so on....The final image is based on a weighted average of the sub-images."

For a more detailed treatment of cone-beam algorithms, the interested reader should refer to the works of Kalender (2005) and Flohr et al (2005).

INSTRUMENTATION

In describing the instrumentation for multislice CT systems, it is essential to focus on the major components responsible for data acquisition, image reconstruction, image display and manipulation, image processing, image storage, recording, and image transmission.

The flow of data in multislice CT parallels that of conventional step-and-shoot CT and includes x-ray production and transmission through the patient and conversion of x-rays into electrical signals, which are subsequently converted into digital data for processing by a digital computer. Digital data in the computer are then converted into image data through image reconstruction, to be displayed on a monitor for viewing by an observer. However, the detector technology in multislice CT is one of the most significant developments in the evolution of CT. Other components of significance are the DAS and the image reconstruction system for multislice CT scanning.

The major equipment components for multislice CT are the data acquisition components, patient couch or table, the computer system, and the operator console, as shown in Figure 12-23.

Data Acquisition Components

The multislice CT gantry houses the x-ray generator, the x-ray tube, and detectors, as well as the detector electronics (DAS). Almost all multislice CT scanners are based on the third-generation system design, in which the x-ray tube and detectors are coupled and rotate continuously during continuous patient translation through the gantry aperture. Such data collection strategy is possible by the use of slip-ring technology (see Chapter 5).

X-Ray Generator

The x-ray generator is a compact, lightweight, high-frequency generator that provides a stable high voltage to the x-ray tube to ensure efficient production of x-rays. The power output of these generators varies depending on the manufacturer. Typical values can range from around 60 kilowatts (kW) to 90 kW.

X-Ray Tube

The x-ray tube is a rotating-anode tube capable of high heat storage capacity with high anode and tube housing cooling rates. The x-ray beam is

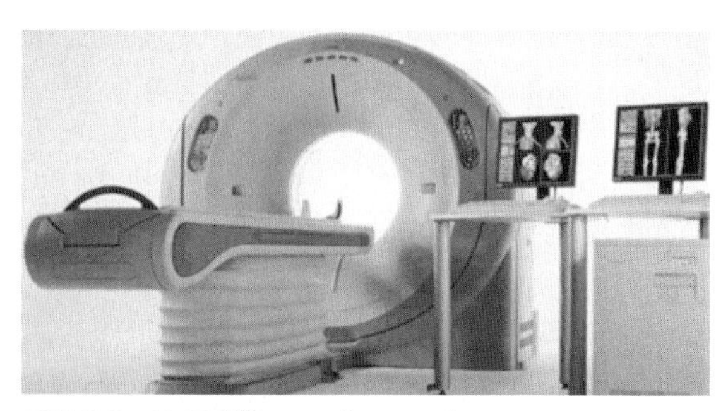

FIGURE 12-23 The major equipment components (gantry, patient couch, computer, and operator's console) of a multislice CT scanner. (Courtesy Toshiba Medical Systems.)

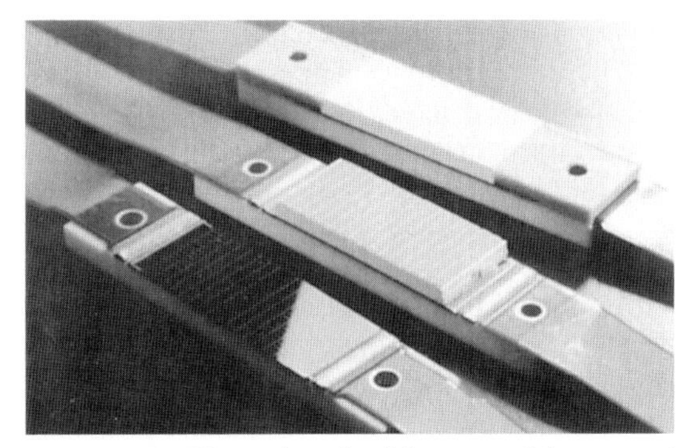

FIGURE 12-24 Examples of solid-state multirow matrix detector arrays for multislice CT scanning. These detectors are used in the GE LightSpeed QX/I CT scanner, and consist of 16 rows with 912 channels and 14,592 individual elements. (Courtesy General Electric Healthcare; Milwaukee, Wis.)

usually fan shaped and emanates from either a small or large focal spot. X-ray tubes for multislice CT provide for a range of selectable peak kilovolts (kVp) and mAs, such as 80, 100, 120, and 140 kVp and 10 to 500 mA in increments of 10 mA. See Chapter 5 for a more detailed description of x-ray tubes, including the most recent design for use with multislice CT scanners

Multislice Detectors

Multislice detectors have evolved over time and therefore they are described in the next subsection of this chapter.

Multislice CT Detectors

The first clinical scanner, the EMI Mark 1, and several of its successors recorded two image slices simultaneously in an effort to offset their agonizingly slow scan speeds. In 1992, Elscint introduced the first modern multislice scanner, which used dual detector banks. A major difference between the EMI Mark 1 and Elscint scanners was that a particular image from the Elscint system could take advantage of data acquired by both detector banks, whereas the old EMI scanner, which predated spiral/helical acquisition, simply generated two independent images.

Detectors capable of providing more than two slices for CT scanners were introduced in 1998. At present, they allow acquisition of up to 320 slices simultaneously, and their design suggests that this number may increase in the future. This dramatic technical advance promises to have a major impact on the way CT is used in clinical practice. The tremendous increase in the rate of data collection will influence routine CT applications and create new areas for CT imaging.

Types of Detectors

As noted earlier in this chapter, the most significant difference between single-slice CT and multislice CT is the detector technology. These detectors are solid-state scintillation detectors (Fig. 12-24).

There are three types of detectors for use in multislice CT scanning (Cody and Mahesh, 2007; Dowsett et al, 2006; Kachelriess, 2006; Kohl, 2005). These are as follows:

1. Uniform or matrix detectors (also referred to as *fixed-array detectors* or *linear array detectors*)
2. Nonuniform or variable detectors (also referred to as adaptive-array detectors)
3. Hybrid detectors

Several different approaches to the construction of these detectors are available (Fig.12-25). As can be seen in Figure 12-25, detector arrays in the z-axis can be uniform, with all elements of the same dimensions or nonuniform to reduce the number of elements needed for thicker slices. An advantage of the nonuniform elements is the reduction of dead space (the gap between detector elements to ensure optical isolation). On the other hand, this arrangement offers less flexibility for the future, when slice numbers greater than 320 will be practical. Element dimensions shown are "effective" detector sizes, calculated at the center of gantry rotation where slice thickness is measured. The size and distribution of detector elements in the x-y plane are similar to those in current single-slice systems. Consequently, spatial

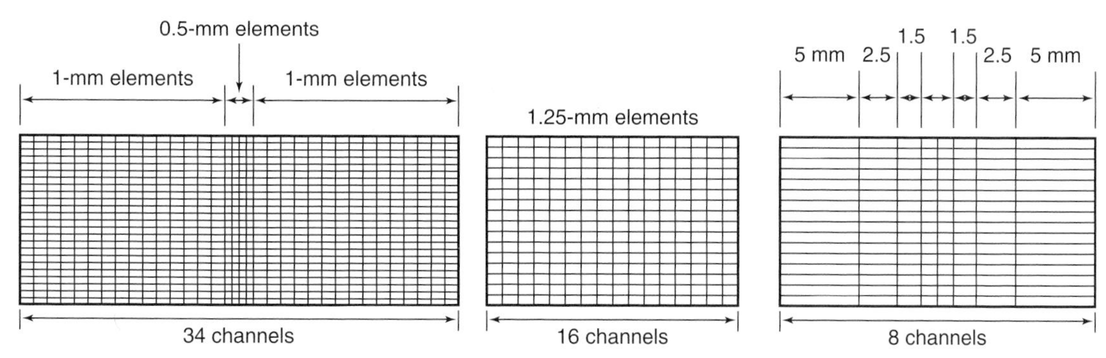

FIGURE 12-25 Multirow CT detector designs. Detector elements may be uniform or nonuniform. See text for further explanation.

or high-contrast resolution is unlikely to change significantly. Such arrays can involve more than 30,000 individual detector elements.

Detector Materials

As described in Chapter 5, detectors in CT fall into two categories; gas ionization detectors and solid-state detectors. It is important to note, however, that multislice CT scanners do not use gas ionization detectors such as xenon detectors (used in the earlier single-slice CT scanners) because they have low quantum detection efficiency (<50%) and low x-ray absorption (Dowsett et al, 2006; Kachelriess, 2006; Kohl, 2005).

The detector elements of multislice CT scanners use solid-state materials (scintillation crystals or ceramics) such as cadmium tungstate and, more recently, rare earth materials such as gadolinium oxysulfide or yttrium-gadolinium oxide, gadolinium oxide, or ceramics (Dowsett et al, 2006; Kohl, 2005). The detectors are doped with suitable dopants (europium, for example) to decrease afterglow below 0.1% at 100 milliseconds (Dowsett et al, 2006).

These materials convert x-ray photons to visible light that is subsequently detected by photodiodes (see Chapter 5).

Properties of Detectors

It is beyond the scope of this text to discuss the physical properties of CT detectors; however, Dowsett et al (2006) emphasize that detectors for multislice CT scanners should have several properties. These include a large dynamic range, high quantum absorption efficiency, high luminescence efficiency, good geometric efficiency, small afterglow, and high precision machineability. In addition, they note that all detector elements must have a uniform response. Readers interested in these properties should refer to the work of Dowsett et al (2006).

Detector Configuration

The term *detector configuration* is a term that "describes the number of data collection channels and the effective section thickness determined by the data acquisition system settings" (Dalrymple et al, 2007). Multislice CT detectors can be configured in several ways by combining various detector elements electronically (or binning) to produce the desired slice thickness required for the examination, at the isocenter. Typical slice thicknesses that can be obtained are as follows:

- 2 × 0.5 mm, 4 × 1.0 mm, 4 × 5.0 mm, 2 × 8.0 mm, 2 × 10 mm for four-slice adaptive array detector
- 16 × 0.5 mm, 16 × 1.0 mm, 16 × 2.0 mm for a 16-slice fixed array detector
- 40 × 0.625 mm and 32 × 1.25mm for a 40-slice fixed array detector
- 64 × 0.5 mm and 32 × 1.0 mm for a 64-slice fixed array detector

The reader should consult the manufacturer data sheets for specific slice thicknesses offered by their scanners.

Slice Thickness Selection

As mentioned earlier, individual slice widths (Fig. 12-26) are generally defined by the number of detector elements grouped (or binned) into each data channel (Dalrymple et al, 2007). The smallest slice width available is determined by the smallest single detector element. An exception to this generalization occurs in the nonuniform array shown in Figure 12-26, in which two 0.5-mm slices can be acquired by moving the collimator leaves inward so that only the inner half of the two central 1-mm elements are exposed to the x-ray beam. Similarly, four 1-mm slices are acquired by irradiating the two central elements and two thirds of the adjacent 1.5-mm elements. Slice width is defined at the center of rotation (center of the gantry aperture), so the actual detector dimensions for that slice will be greater because of the magnification produced by beam divergence. The x-ray beam width, as defined by the prepatient collimators, will be approximately four times the slice width.

The slice, as defined by the tissue irradiated during the rotation of a multislice detector, is significantly different from that of a single-detector scanner (Fig. 12-27). This is an extension of the problem with the earlier dual-detector scanners. In this case, however, the outer two slices are considerably more affected by beam divergence than are the inner two slices.

The significance of this geometric nonuniformity may be most severe in the case of conventional scanning. Reconstruction of the CT image involves all views acquired throughout the 360 degrees of data collection. When views from different angles are actually measuring quite different tissue pathways,

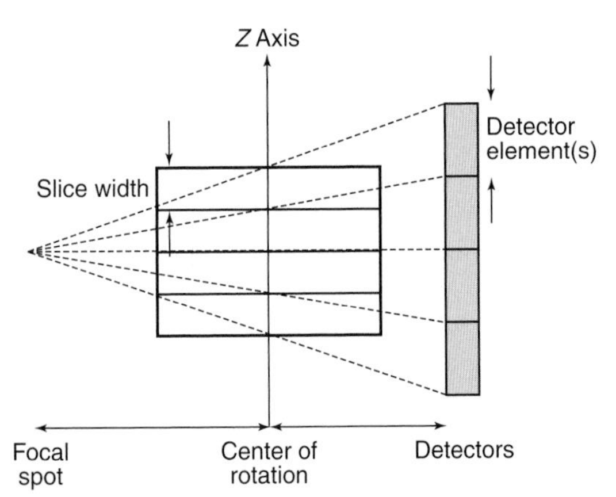

FIGURE 12-26 Slice geometry in multislice scanners. The number of detector elements grouped together determines the size of the slice. Slice width is defined at the center of gantry rotation.

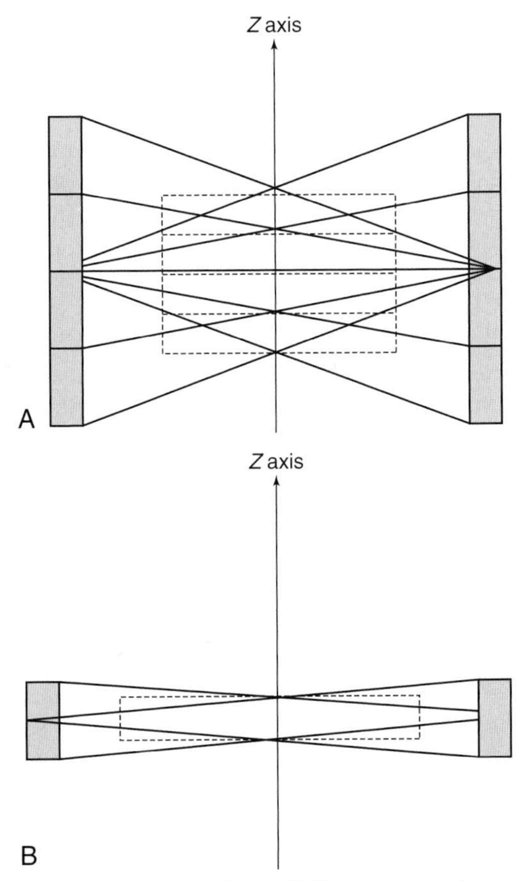

FIGURE 12-27 Comparison of slice geometry between multislice **(A)** and single-slice **(B)** scanners. The x-ray beams are shown at opposite sides of gantry rotation. Although the diagram is exaggerated, there is more beam divergence with the multislice system.

there will be varying degrees of volume averaging with an increased likelihood of artifact and inaccurate reconstruction. If detector size is increased in future scanners to add more slices, this geometric situation will be further exaggerated. With the x-ray beam fan extended in the z-axis, as well as the x-y plane, a reconstruction algorithm that is different from those used for single-slice scanners is needed to process the raw data (Hu, 1999a; Taguchi and Aradate, 1998).

The signals from the individual detector elements are fed to four DASs through a bank of switches that combines the signals from the appropriate number of elements into the slice width selected by the operator (Fig. 12-28).

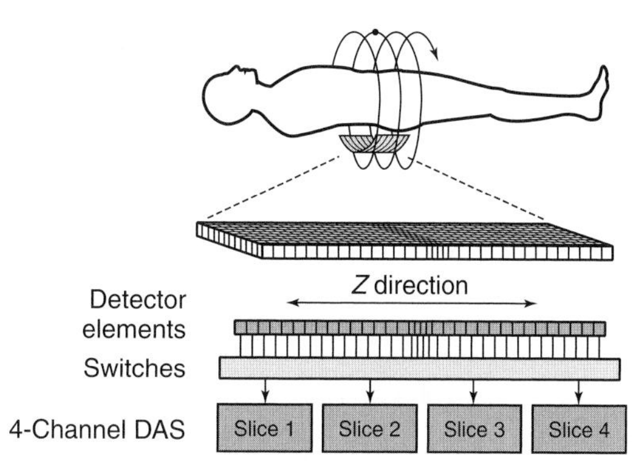

FIGURE 12-28 Switches group the signal from individual detector elements. The signals are then transferred to one of four DASs that generate the four simultaneous slices. Additional DAS channels can be added in the future.

Detector elements outside the selected slices are switched off and do not contribute any signal to the DAS. Patient dose is controlled by prepatient collimators that restrict the x-ray beam to only those detector elements needed for the four data slices. At present, the slice thickness must be selected before scanning, and it is not possible to narrow the slice width after data collection. Summing slices after scanning to create fewer, thicker images is certainly feasible and can have clinical value. In this case, it would be possible to return to the thinner slices if clinically indicated and if the raw data were still available.

Figure 12-29 provides examples of various combinations of detector elements for both fixed array and adaptive array detectors for multislice CT imaging. In addition, the detector module of a 64-slice multislice CT scanner (SOMOTOM Sensation 64, Siemens Medical Solutions, Germany) together with its antiscatter collimators (diagonally cut) is shown in Figure 12-30.

The design of the multirow detector influences the speed of acquisition of the slices and the resolution of the slices, as shown in Figure 12-31.

Data Acquisition System

Another major component of the gantry is the DAS, the detector electronics responsible mainly for digitizing the signals from the detectors before they are sent to the computer for processing. Figure 12-31 shows an example of a DAS coupled to the multirow detector array by switches. In this case, four slices are acquired at the same time because of the presence of four DAS systems (four times the electrical circuits compared with single-slice CT systems) (Saito, 1998). Regardless of which four slices are required for the examination, the switches can be turned on and off to ensure that the appropriate detector segments are exposed to x-rays.

Patient Table

The patient table, or couch, features are essentially similar to those associated with single-slice CT and conventional step-and-shoot CT scanners. The purpose of the table is to support the patient and to facilitate multislice CT scanning through the variable speed of travel of the tabletop and its wide range of movement. The table can be raised and lowered to accommodate positioning of the patient in the gantry aperture and to facilitate easy transfer of the patient from the scanner to a

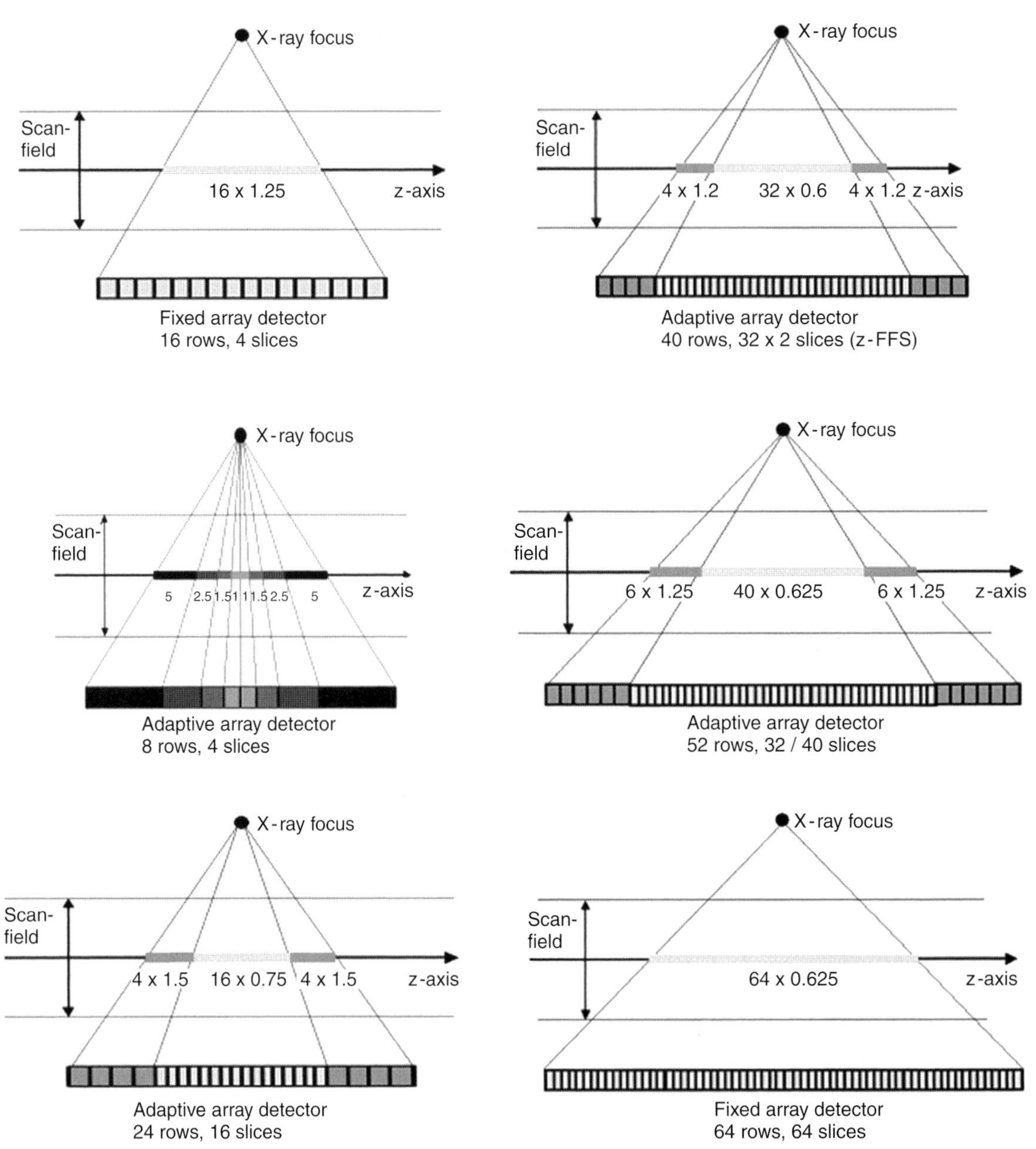

FIGURE 12-29 Examples of the use of fixed-array and adaptive-array detectors in multislice CT scanners in determining the slice thicknesses to be obtained. (From Kohl G: The evolution and state-of-the-art principles of multi-slice computed tomography, *Proc Am Thorac Soc* 2:470-476, 2005. Reproduced by kind permission.)

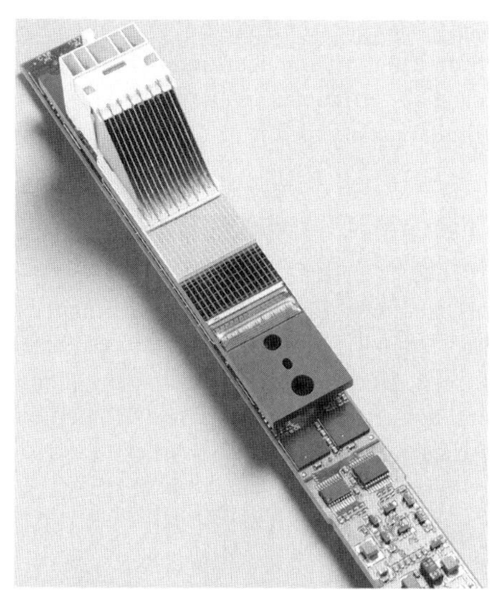

FIGURE 12-30 Photo of a detector module for the Siemens 64-slice SOMATOM Sensation multislice CT scanner showing the electronics and the antiscatter collimators that are cut diagonally (left side of the detector module). (From Kohl G: The evolution and state-of-the-art principles of multi-slice computed tomography, *Proc Am Thorac Soc* 2:470-476, 2005. Reproduced by kind permission.)

bed or gurney and vice versa. Movement of the tabletop in the longitudinal direction also facilitates patient position in the gantry aperture, with variable scannable ranges.

Patient tables for CT are equipped with a head holder or headrest to ensure patient comfort during the examination. In an emergency during the examination, the movement of the table can be controlled manually to ensure patient safety.

Computer System

The computer system for multislice CT receives data from the data acquisition system and the operator, who inputs patient data and various examination protocols. These systems must be capable of handling vast amounts of data collected by the 2D multirow detector array. These computers have hardware architectures that provide

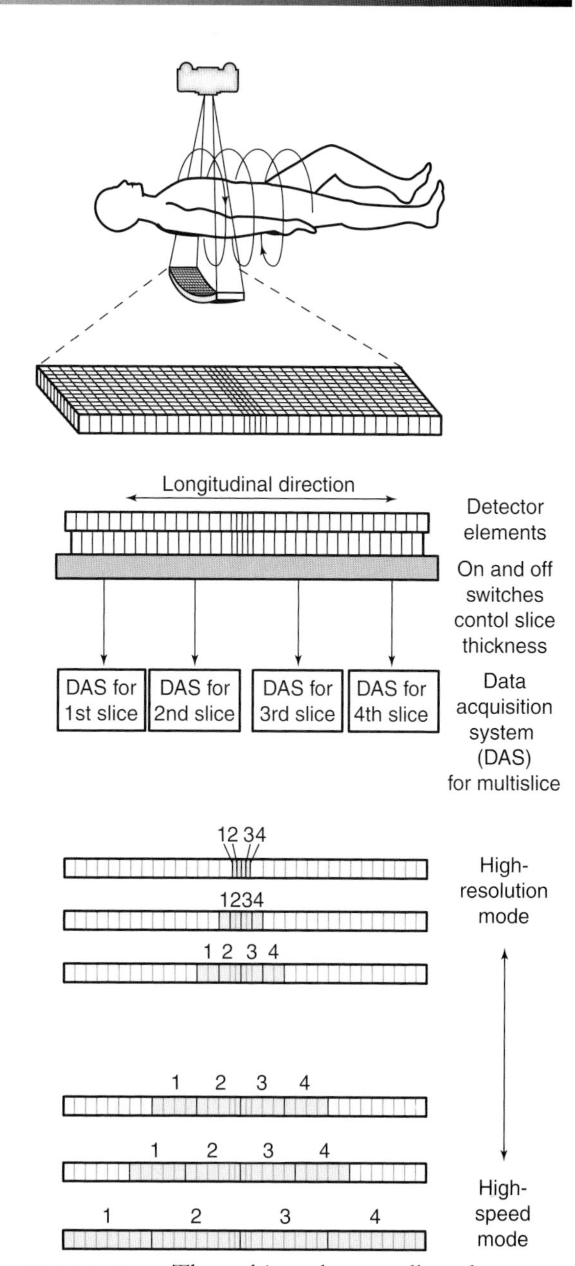

FIGURE 12-31 The multirow detector allows for various selections of slice thicknesses to meet the needs of the examination. Thinner slice thicknesses are selected in the high-resolution mode, whereas thicker slices are selected in the high-speed mode. The slice thickness is varied by turning the switches "on" or "off."

high-speed preprocessing, image reconstruction, and postprocessing operations. Although preprocessing includes various corrections to the raw data, *image reconstruction* refers to the use of multislice reconstruction algorithms for image buildup. On the other hand, postprocessing involves the use of a wide range of image processing and advanced visualization software, such as the generation of 3D and MPR, as well as virtual endoscopic images from the axial data set stored in the computer.

The results of computer processing are displayed for viewing by an observer on a monitor. Several characteristics of the monitor are important to the observer, such as the display matrix, bandwidth, display memory, and the gray level and color resolution.

Data storage devices for holding the raw data and image data include hard disks, usually of the Winchester type with high storage capacities, and erasable optical disks of the magneto-optical type.

Operator Console

The operator console allows the operator to interact with the scanner before, during, and after the examination. Essentially the major components include the keyboard, mouse, monitor, and other controls for the execution of specialized functions.

The operator console controls the entire CT scanner system and facilitates the selection of scan parameters and scan control (automatic or manual), image storage, communication, image reconstruction, image processing, windowing, and control of the gantry, and x-ray tube rotation. The console allows for communication of images to other parts of the department and hospital and other remote sites through the use of local and wide area networks. The multislice CT console also supports full digital imaging and communication in medicine (DICOM) connectivity to other equipment, such as network printers, for example. Multislice CT consoles also provide for the use of a wide range of software options for image processing, such as 3D imaging, virtual endoscopy, maximum intensity projection, MPR reconstruction, cardiac applications, and dental CT and bone mineral analysis.

ISOTROPIC IMAGING

One of the major goals of developing scanners with an increasing number of slices (4, 8, 16, 32, 40, 64, 320 slices) per rotation of the x-ray tube and detectors around the patient is to achieve isotropic imaging.

Definition

Several technical developments in multislice CT scanners have made it possible to perform isotropic imaging. The term *isotropic* is used to refer to the size of the voxels used in a volume data set. When the slice thickness is equal to the pixel size, all dimensions of the voxel (x, y, z) are equal. In other words, the voxel is a perfect cube, and the data set acquired is said to be isotropic. If, however, all voxels dimensions are not equal, that is, the slice thickness is not equal to the pixel size, for example, the data set acquired is said to be anisotropic. The geometry of both isotropic and anisotropic data is clearly illustrated in Figure 12-32.

Goals

One of the major goals of isotropic imaging in CT is to achieve excellent spatial resolution (detail) in all imaging planes, especially in MPR and 3D imaging. In addition, there are other benefits as well (Dalrymple et al, 2007; Paulson et al, 2004, 2005), but at the expense of more dose to the patient. Furthermore, the use of narrow collimation increases the scanning time. As noted by Dalrymple et al (2007), "the parameters that affect the radiation dose and exposure time vary considerably according to scanner design and these variations determine the proportions of the

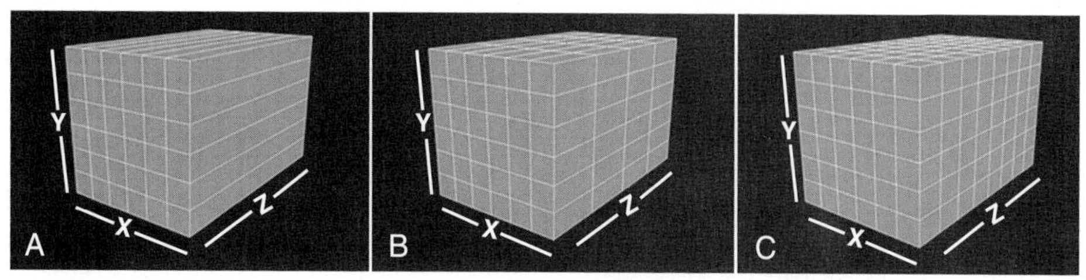

FIGURE 12-32 Geometry of isotropic and anisotropic acquisitions. Anisotropic data consist of voxels that have a section thickness greater than the x- and y-axis dimensions of the facing pixels. Section thickness along the z-axis is four times the size of each pixel in **A** but only twice the size of each pixel in **B.** Although both data sets are anisotropic, there is a significant difference in image quality for 3D applications, with improved longitudinal spatial resolution in **B** compared with that in **A.** When the section thickness is equal to the pixel size, as in **C,** the data are isotropic. (From Dalrymple NC et al: Price of isotropy in multidetector CT, *Radiographics* 27:49-62, 2007. Figure and legend reproduced by permission of the Radiological Society of North America and the authors.)

trade-off in increased radiation dose and scanning time relative to the voxel size." Therefore, in MSCT scanning, personnel should have a working knowledge of how voxel size affects not only the spatial resolution but also the radiation dose. Such understanding ensures that personnel work within the ALARA (as low as reasonably achievable) philosophy to optimize the image quality and radiation dose.

Data Acquisition

Isotropic imaging with 4-, 16-, 40-, and 64-channel multislice CT scanners has been described in some detail by Dalrymple et al (2007). One of the major technical parameters that have an effect on isotropy is the detector configuration, that is, how the detector elements are used together with the effective slice thickness. Although the four-channel multislice CT scanner can achieve near isotropic imaging, the 16-, 32-, 40-, and 64-channel multislice CT scanners can produce isotropic voxels, hence achieve isotropy. As demonstrated by Dalrymple et al (2007), the scanners (beyond four-slice) can also produce voxels that are anisotropic.

The detector configurations and voxel dimensions for isotropic and anisotropic imaging are illustrated in Figure 12-33, *A*, for a 16-channel CT scanner and in Figure 12-34, *A*, for a 64-channel CT scanner. The fundamental principles for isotropic reconstructed voxels are shown in Figures 12-33, *A*, and 12-34, *A*, and anisotropic reconstructed voxels are illustrated in Figures 12-33, *B*, and 12-34, *B*. The effects of isotropic data acquisition and anisotropic data acquisition on 3D volume-rendered images are shown in Figure 12-35 and Figure 12-36 for 16- and 64-channel CT scanners, respectively.

IMAGE QUALITY CONSIDERATIONS

Image quality in CT is described in detail in Chapter 9. Essentially there are three main parameters: spatial resolution, contrast resolution, and noise. Spatial resolution, the ability of the scanner to image fine detail, is measured in line pairs per centimeter. Contrast resolution or low-contrast resolution or tissue resolution is the ability of the scanner to discriminate small differences in tissue contrast. Noise, on the other hand, is a fluctuation of CT numbers from point to point in the image for a scan of uniform material such as water. Noise degrades image quality and affects the

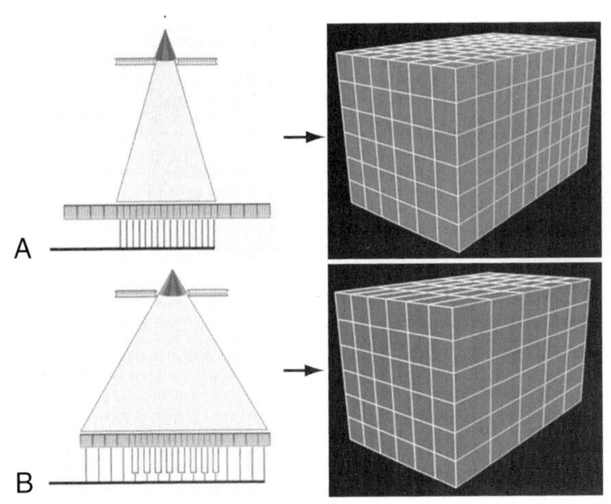

FIGURE 12-33 Detector configurations and voxel dimensions at 16-channel multidetector CT. **A,** *Left,* Diagram shows narrow collimation, with exposure of only the central 16 detector elements. Each element functions as a separate unit, and 16 sections with a thickness of 0.625 mm each are acquired per gantry rotation. *Right,* Diagram shows that the reconstructed voxels are isotropic, with about equal length in each dimension. **B,** *Left,* Diagram shows wide collimation, with exposure not only of the central small elements but also of larger elements at the periphery. Central elements function in pairs, and peripheral elements are used individually. As a result, 16 sections with a thickness of 1.25 mm each are acquired per rotation. *Right,* Diagram shows that reconstructed voxels are anisotropic, about twice as long in the longitudinal plane as in the transverse plane. (From Dalrymple NC et al: Price of isotropy in multidetector CT, *Radiographics* 27:49-62, 2007. Figure and legend reproduced by permission of the Radiological Society of North America and the authors.)

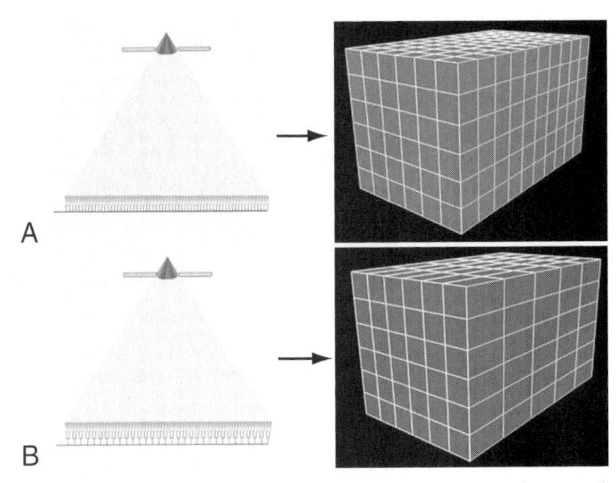

FIGURE 12-34 Detector configurations and voxel dimensions at 64-channel multidetector CT. Because the width of the incident beam does not change between detector configurations, the concepts of narrow and wide collimation do not apply. **A,** *Left:* Diagram shows the detector configuration for thin-section acquisitions. With each detector element used individually, 64 sections with a thickness of 0.625 mm each are acquired per gantry rotation, resulting in long-axis coverage of 40 mm. *Right:* Diagram shows that reconstructed voxels in this mode are isotropic, with approximately equal length in each dimension. **B,** *Left:* Diagram shows the detector configuration for acquisition of thicker sections. Although the beam collimation does not change, the data acquisition system pairs the elements for the receipt of data. As a result, 32 sections with a thickness of 1.25 mm each are acquired per gantry rotation, while long-axis coverage remains constant. *Right:* Diagram shows that reconstructed voxels in this mode are anisotropic, approximately twice as large in the longitudinal plane as in the transverse plane. (From Dalrymple NC et al: Price of isotropy in multidetector CT, *Radiographics* 27:49-62, 2007. Figure and legend reproduced by permission of the Radiological Society of North America and the authors.)

perceptibility of detail. Artifacts can also degrade image quality and cause problems in image interpretation.

In multislice CT, these parameters are the same in terms of definition. Recall that the purpose of multislice CT is to improve on the performance of single-slice CT in terms of speed and coverage. The volume coverage speed performance in multislice CT is better than its counterpart single-slice CT without compromising image quality.

In addition, image quality depends on radiation dose. Although the dose in CT has received increasing attention in the literature and has been identified as an increasing source of radiation exposure and may be viewed as "a public health issue in the future" (Brenner and Hall, 2007),

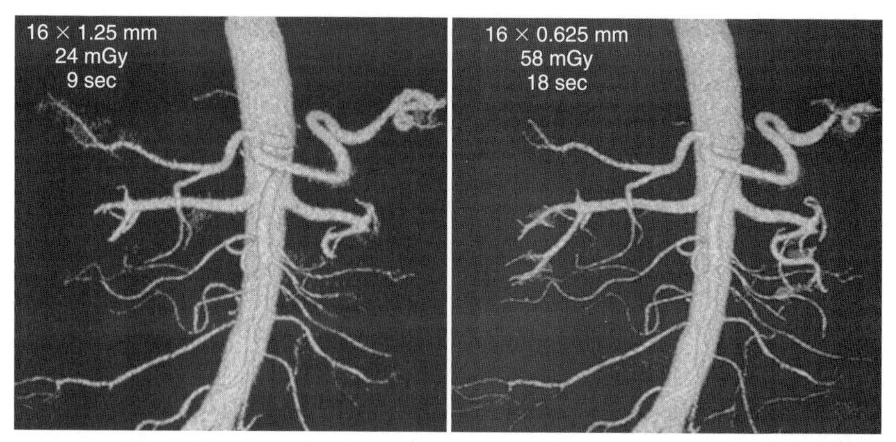

FIGURE 12-35 Three-dimensional volume-rendered images from renal CT angiography with a 16-channel scanner. The first row of data on the images is the detector configuration, the middle row is the volume CT dose index, and the bottom row is the scanning time. **A,** Image reconstructed from anisotropic data provides satisfactory depiction of the aorta and central vessels. **B,** Image reconstructed from isotropic data provides slightly improved definition of smaller vessels. The automated "seed and grow" software program used to create these images provided better depiction of peripheral branches of the renal vessels with the use of isotropic data. (From Dalrymple NC et al: Price of isotropy in multidetector CT, *Radiographics* 27:49-62, 2007. Figure and legend reproduced by permission of the Radiological Society of North America and the authors.)

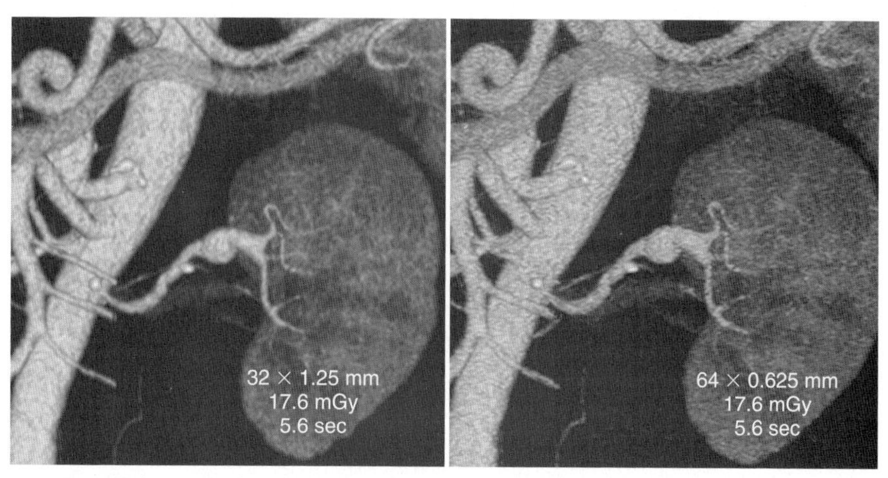

FIGURE 12-36 Volume-rendered images from 64-channel multidetector CT. The first row of data on the images is the detector configuration, the middle row is the volume CT dose index, and the bottom row is the scanning time. **A,** Image reconstructed from anisotropic data (section thickness, 1.25 mm; increment, 0.625 mm) clearly depicts a peripheral aneurysm of the left renal artery. **B,** Image reconstructed from isotropic data (section thickness, 0.625 mm; increment, 0.3 mm) provides sharper definition of vessel margins and allows visualization of small lumbar and mesenteric vessel branches. (From Dalrymple NC et al: Price of isotropy in multidetector CT, *Radiographics* 27:49-62, 2007. Figure and legend reproduced by permission of the Radiological Society of North America and the authors.)

there have been increasing technical efforts to reduce this dose not only to adults but to children in particular. One such dose reduction technology is the tube current modulation techniques introduced by manufacturers. Dose in CT is described in detail in Chapter 10.

Acceptance testing and research studies will provide verification on image quality parameters and more information on the performance of multislice CT scanners in the image quality and radiation dose arenas.

BEYOND 64-SLICE MULTISLICE CT SCANNERS: FOUR-DIMENSIONAL IMAGING

Limitations of Previous Multislice CT Scanners

The technical evolution of multislice CT scanners from 16-slice, 32-slice, 40-slice, and 64-slice CT scanners has resulted in numerous clinical benefits not only to enhance diagnosis but also for use in radiation therapy and surgical simulation, for example. One such benefit of multislice CT imaging is improved 3D imaging of anatomical structures. It is still a problem, however, to obtain dynamic 3D images of the beating heart in cardiac imaging, for example. Dynamic 3D is referred to as four-dimensional imaging (Mori et al, 2004). In addition, these multislice CT scanners can increase the dose to patients (Brenner and Hall, 2007), create image artifacts especially in cardiac CT imaging as a result of the beating heart, and have limited organ coverage because of the size of the detector (20-40 mm). The latter implies that two or more rotations are needed to cover the entire organ, such as the heart or lungs. To solve these problems, two other multislice scanners have been developed and are being implemented into clinical practice. These two scanners are the 256-slice and 320-slice CT scanners.

The 256-Slice Beta Four-Dimensional CT Scanner

The first model of the 256-slice 4D CT scanner was developed at the National Institute of Radiological Sciences in Japan in 2003. The major goal of this scanner is to produce four-dimensional CT images with a wide-area detector capable of covering the entire organ (heart or lung) in a single rotation rather than multiple rotations.

The second model of the 256-slice four-dimensional CT scanner (Fig. 12-37, *A*) is based on the

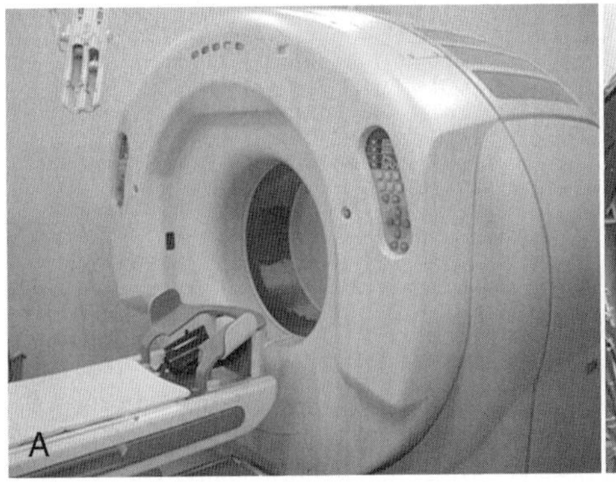

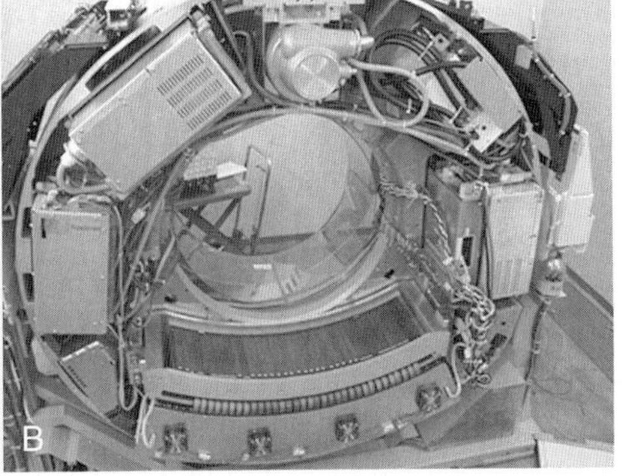

FIGURE 12-37 The second model of the 256-slice beta four-dimensional CT scanner showing the external gantry and table in **A** and the x-ray tube, wide area detector, and associated electronics mounted on the rotating frame of the gantry. (**A,** Courtesy Shinichiro Mori, Radiological Protection Section, National Institute of Radiological Sciences, Japan. **B,** Courtesy Toshiba Medical Systems.)

design of the first model, and in 2006 and 2007 this model prototype scanner was installed in three centers for clinical beta trials. These centers include the Fujita Health University in Nagoya, Japan; the National Cancer Center in Tokyo, Japan; and Johns Hopkins University in Baltimore, Maryland.

The most conspicuous difference is the use of a wide-area 2D detector mounted on the gantry frame of a 16-slice CT scanner (Aquilion, Toshiba Medical Systems, Tokyo Japan), as shown in Figure 12-37, *B*. The scanner uses a cone beam with a larger cone angle (about 13 degrees) compared with the previous multislice CT scanners to cover a wider FOV. The total beam width is 128 mm, four times the size of the Aquilion 16-slice CT scanner (Toshiba Medical Systems). This wide beam ensures complete coverage of the entire organ (heart) in one complete rotation (Fig. 12-38).

The 256-slice four-dimensional CT scanner has 912 (transverse) × 256 (craniocaudal) detector elements, each approximately 0.5 mm × 0.5 mm at the center of rotation. The 128-mm total BW allows for the continuous use of several collimation sets. The detector element is made of a gadolinium oxysulfide (Gd_2O_2S) and a single crystal silicon photodiode as used in the current multislice CT scanners.

The rotation time is 0.5 seconds per rotation and the dynamic range is 18 bits. The reconstruction algorithm used in this scanner is the Feldkamp cone-beam algorithm. Real-time reconstruction processing is done by 32 field programmable gate arrays (FPGSs-Virtex II Pro, Xilinx, San Jose, Calif.) with a clock speed of 125 megahertz. Volumes of 256 × 256 × 128 can be produced.

The clinical beta testing program of the 256-slice CT scanner laid the foundations for the design of a new multislice CT scanner designed to image the entire heart, for example, in a single rotation. This scanner is Toshiba's 320-slice Aquilion ONE Dynamic Volume CT scanner (Toshiba Medical Systems), which is described briefly in the next section.

The 320-Slice Dynamic Volume CT Scanner

In 2007, the 320-slice CT scanner referred to as the AquilionONE MSCT scanner (Fig. 12-39)

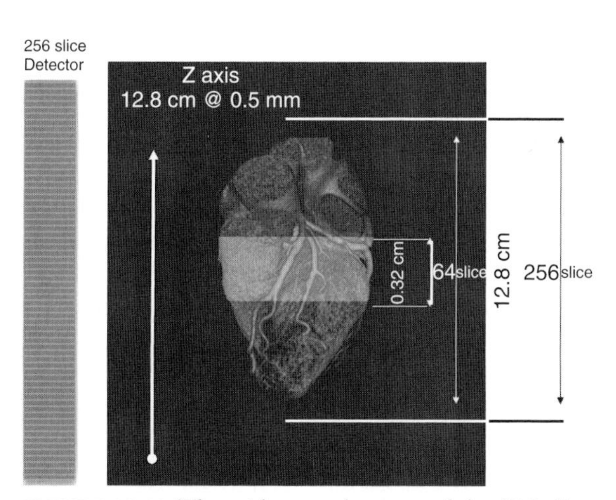

FIGURE 12-38 The wide area detector of the 256-slice beta four-dimensional CT scanner ensures coverage of the entire heart with one complete rotation. (Courtesy Toshiba Medical Systems.)

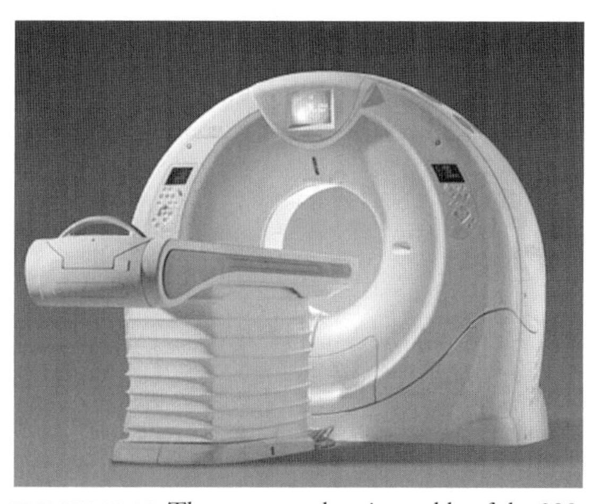

FIGURE 12-39 The gantry and patient table of the 320-slice dynamic volume CT scanner. (Courtesy Toshiba Medical Systems.)

was introduced at the Radiological Society of North America meeting in Chicago. One of the characteristic technical features of this scanner is its wide-area 2D detector that ensures a field coverage of 160 mm (compared with 128 mm of the 256-slice prototype CT scanner). The detector design is such that the number of detector rows is 320 ultrahigh resolution detector elements. This feature allows for scanning the entire anatomical structures such as the heart, lungs, and brain, in a single rotation and therefore not requiring the spiral/helical scanning principle.

This high-speed volume scanner features a rotation time of 350 milliseconds, which is needed to provide a temporal resolution for imaging the entire heart in one heartbeat with excellent spatial and contrast resolution at lower doses (Mather, 2007). In addition, the reconstruction time is fast (less than 10 seconds) and is made possible through the use of specially designed reconstruction processors.

A major challenge in the development of this wide area detector CT volume scanner is the large cone angle because the beam divergence is much greater than that of the 256-slice scanner. To address this problem, Toshiba developed an FDK-based algorithm called the coneXact reconstruction algorithm to eliminate any cone-beam image artifacts.

The 320-slice volume scanner can be used in neurological imaging, cardiac imaging, and other body applications where entire organs (chest, for example) can be scanned very quickly. Such scanning results in large data sets that will provide more information for the radiologist to use in diagnostic management of the patient.

BEYOND SINGLE-SOURCE MULTISLICE CT SCANNERS: DUAL-SOURCE CT SCANNER

In 2006, a CT scanner primarily for cardiac imaging (and other applications as well) was introduced at the Radiological Society of North America meeting. This scanner, the dual-source CT scanner introduced by Siemens Medical Solutions (Forchheim, Germany), featured a unique design incorporating two x-ray tubes coupled to two detector systems that in this manner provided a scanner with two DASs.

CT imaging of the heart with multislice CT scanners dates back to 1999 and, because the heart is in constant motion (beating heart), temporal resolution is essential to avoid motion artifacts. Additionally, for cardiac imaging with CT, it is important to cover the entire heart in a single breath-hold. Although four-slice CT scanners provided acceptable results, problems with respect to motion artifacts, greater heart rates, long breath-hold times, and limited spatial resolution still persist (Flohr et al, 2006).

The introduction of 16-slice scanners provided improved gains in spatial and temporal resolution compared with four-slice systems. The subsequent arrival and use of 64-slice CT scanners provided further improvements in the technical requirements for cardiac imaging. For example, these scanners provided spatial resolution (by isotropic imaging) and temporal resolution because of the reduction of gantry rotation times to 0.33 milliseconds (necessary to deal with high rates) compared with about 0.375 seconds for 16-slice scanners (Flohr et al, 2006). One of the problems in CT cardiac imaging is to remove the need for heart rate control, and therefore efforts are needed to improve temporal resolution below 100 milliseconds at any heart rate.

To solve these problems, other scanners are needed. One such scanner that was developed was the electron beam CT scanner (see Chapter 5). Although this scanner provided some benefits in imaging (for example, the scanner does not have any moving parts), it did not provide a sufficient signal-to-noise ratio when imaging large patients. Therefore, this scanner "is currently not considered adequate for state-of-the-art cardiac CT imaging or for general radiology applications" (Flohr et al, 2006).

In an effort to further improve the temporal resolution needed for cardiac CT imaging by a factor of 2 (Cody and Mahesh, 2007, and see reference 3 in Cody and Mahesh), another CT scanner, the dual-source CT scanner, dedicated to cardiac imaging, developed by Siemens Medical Solutions, was called the Definition (Forchheim, Germany). The design concept of the scanner is based on the use of two x-ray tubes coupled to two separate detector systems, as mentioned earlier.

Major Technical Components

The major system components of the dual-source CT scanner are illustrated in Figure 12-40. The most noticeable difference between this scanner and other multislice CT scanners is that there are two data acquisitions systems offset by 90 degrees (Engel et al, 2008). Although an acquisition system labeled "Det A" has a scan (FOV coverage of 50 centimeters in diameter, an acquisition system labeled "Det B" is smaller in size compared with "Det A" and has a smaller scan FOV diameter of 26 centimeters. This reduction in size of one acquisition system is due to the restricted space in the gantry.

Each x-ray tube is of the STRATON type (Siemens Medical Solutions, Forchheim, Germany) that uses the z-flying focal spot technique (see Chapter 5) and cone-beam geometry to image two 32-slices (0.6 mm) combined to produce 64 slices per revolution. The detectors are multislice detectors with 40 detector rows of the hybrid design where the central 32 rows would produce a 0.6-mm slice width and the two outer rows provide slice widths of 1.2 mm. In addition, each x-ray tube can be operated separately with regard to the exposure technique (kVp and mA). This feature allows the scanner to perform dual-energy imaging, where one tube can operate at say 80 kVp and the other at say 140 kVp (Flohr, 2006).

Cardiac Imaging with the Dual-Source CT Scanner

The dual-source CT scanner is primarily "well-suited" for cardiac imaging for several reasons

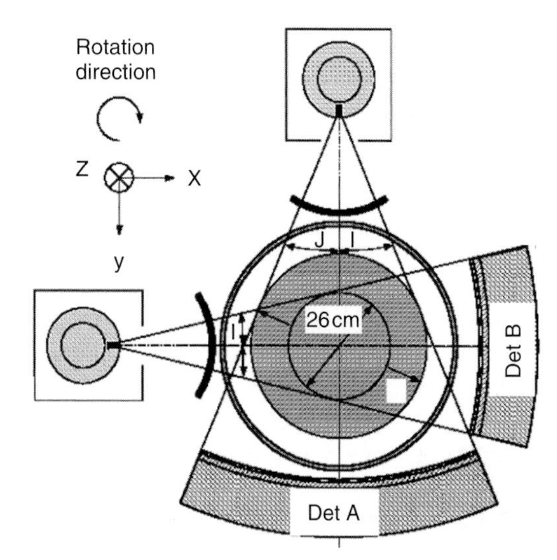

FIGURE 12-40 The major components of the dual-source CT scanner, which consists of two DASs, that is, two x-ray tubes coupled to two separate detector systems, Det A, which covers the entire scan field-of-view (scan FOV = 50 cm in diameter); and Det B, which covers a smaller central scan FOV (26 cm in diameter). See text for further explanation. (From Flohr TG et al: First performance of a dual-source CT (DSCT) system, *Eur Radiol* 16:256-268, 2006. Reproduced by kind permission.)

(Cody and Mahesh, 2007), an important reason being that the design of the system offers excellent temporal resolution compared with other multislice CT scanners. Such resolution is needed to reduce motion artifacts created by the beating heart. Although it is not within the scope of this text to describe the details of cardiac CT imaging, the following points (from several experts) about the DSCT scanner are noteworthy:

1. "Because the minimum rotation speed required for a cardiac CT image is equal to just over one-half of a rotation for a conventional multislice CT scanner, it is also equal to just over one-fourth of a rotation for a dual-source MSCT scanner" (Cody and Mahesh, 2007).

2. The dual-source CT scanner improves the temporal resolution for cardiac CT imaging by a factor of 2 (Cody and Mahesh, 2007).
3. "In a single detector row spiral CT, noise is independent of pitch. Conversely in non-cardiac multi-detector row CT, noise depends on pitch because the spiral interpolation algorithm makes use of redundant data from different detector rows to decrease noise for pitch values less than 1 (and increase noise for pitch values >1. However, in cardiac CT, redundant data cannot be used because such data averaging would degrade the temporal resolution" (Primak et al, 2006).
4. "In addition, linking the heart rate to the pitch (by which a higher rate can be examined by using a higher pitch), effectively reduces the dose to radiation delivered during the examination and can also eliminate the need for additional drugs (e.g., β-blockers) before the cardiac CT examination to reduce the heart rate" (Cody and Mahesh, 2007).
5. "The minimum amount of data required to reconstruct a CT image is 180° plus the angle (in degrees) of the x-ray beam in the plane of the image (known as the fan angle). Hence cardiac algorithms use partial reconstruction technique (180° + the fan angle) to reconstruct an image. These data are collected either during a single cardiac cycle (single segment reconstruction) or during two or more consecutive heartbeats (multi-segment reconstruction). In both cases the number of photons N contributing to the cardiac reconstruction depends only on the tube current and time it takes the gantry to rotate through $180^{\circ 0}$ plus the fan angle, and not the pitch" (Primak et al, 2006). Because faster rotation times require lower pitch values in cardiac multidetector row CT, dose is increased without a commensurate decrease in noise (Primak et al, 2006).
6. "Several steps can be taken to reduce the dose, including lowering the tube current as the x-ray beam crosses over certain areas of the body; decreasing the tube current during certain phases of the cardiac cycle, and using a higher pitch" (Primak et al, 2006).

Other Imaging Applications

Other applications of the dual-source CT scanner include the following:

1. Imaging obese patients. Because the dual-source CT scanner can operate at a higher power rating (higher kW) compared with the lower kW power rating of a single-source CT scanner by using the power of two x-ray tubes, better image quality for obese patients can be obtained.
2. Dual-energy imaging. The dual-source CT scanner overcomes the problems of dual-energy imaging afforded by the earlier CT scanners. The two x-ray tubes can be operated at two different kVp values, producing images with different tissue characterization, because the absorption of x-rays in tissues depends on the kVp of the beam used. For example, scanning at 80 kVp, the CT number for bone and iodine are 670 Hounsfield units (HU) and 296 HU, respectively. At 140 kVp, the CT numbers for bone and iodine are 450 HU and 144 HU, respectively (Siemens Medical Solutions, 2006). This difference is useful in CTA, where it is necessary to separate bone from vessels filled with iodine.
3. Finally, the dual-source CT scanner can perform in a similar manner as a single-source 64-slice CT scanner by using only one acquisition system (one x-ray tube coupled to a detector array) (Siemens Medical Solutions, 2007).

ADVANTAGES OF MULTISLICE CT

The advantages of multislice CT have been outlined by Saito (1998) and Cinnamon (1998), as well as by Kohl (2005), Kalender (2005b), Mather (2005b), Douglas-Akinwande (2006), Kachelriess,

(2006), and Cody and Mahesh (2007). There are several factors in multislice CT scanning that combine to improve not only the spatial and contrast resolution of images but also the temporal resolution (fewer motion artifacts) as well. Furthermore, multislice CT opens up improved gains in other clinical applications such as improved MPR images and 3D rendered images, retrospective creation of thinner or thicker sections from the same raw data, and delivery of intravenously administered iodinated contrast material at faster rates, and so on.

Essentially, these advantages include the following:

1. Increase in speed and volume coverage. In multislice CT, the increase in pitch and the increase in rotation speed of the x-ray tube and detectors allow for a larger volume of the patient to be scanned in less time. Hu (1999a), for example, showed that a four-slice helical/spiral CT scanner is about two times faster than a single-slice CT scanner for comparable image quality.
2. Improved spatial resolution. Multislice CT images thin slices with better isotropic resolution. This is sometimes referred to as *isotropic imaging*, in which case all the sides (axial, vertical, and horizontal) of the voxels in the slice have equal dimensions compared with single-slice CT. This advantage provides improved MPR and 3D images with reduced image artifacts.
3. Efficient use of the x-ray beam. In multislice CT, the x-ray beam width has to be opened to fall on the 2D detector array compared with a single-row detector array characteristic of single-slice CT scanners. The entire beam is thus used to acquire four slices (images) per 360-degree rotation without wasting any portion of the x-ray beam, as opposed to one slice per 360-degree rotation in the single-slice CT case, in which a portion of the x-ray beam is wasted during data acquisition. Such use of the beam increases the life of the x-ray tube. The tube can now be used to produce a large number of thin slices without having to wait for it (x-ray tube) to cool, a problem with single-slice CT systems. In 1999, Kopecky et al (1999) noted that with an x-ray tube with a lifespan of 200,000 seconds, a single-slice CT scanner will provide about 200,000 image (one image/second) compared with 800,000 images for a four-slice multislice CT scanner (same conditions are maintained), "or 1.6 million images if the gantry spins at two revolutions per second, or 3.2 million images if two images are created for each full rotation of 0.5 secs."
4. Reduction of radiation exposure. The development of new dose reduction technology, such as for example, tube current modulation techniques, will play a significant role in CT dose reduction.
5. Improved accuracy in needle placement in CT fluoroscopy. One of the problems with needle placement under CT fluoroscopic control with a single-slice CT scanner is illustrated in Figure 12-41. The image shows that the needle has hit the target, which is simply not the case. This problem is solved with multislice CT scanners that offer CT fluoroscopy because multiple images are obtained. It is apparent in Figure 12-41 that the target has been hit.
6. Cardiac CT imaging. Multislice CT technology has been developed to such a level that "dedicated" CT scanners for imaging the heart such as the dual-source CT scanner and the 320-slice four-dimensional CT scanner are now available commercially. These scanners can image the heart (and other organ systems) with exceptional spatial, contrast, and temporal resolution, as well as with reduced doses compared with 64-slice CT scanners. Additionally, the use of special cardiac reconstruction algorithms can have an impact on artifact reduction when the beating heart is imaged (Cody and Mahesh, 2007; Dowe, 2006; Flohr, 2006; Flohr et al, 2006; Kachelriess, 2006; Mather, 2005b; Mather, 2007; Primak et al, 2006).

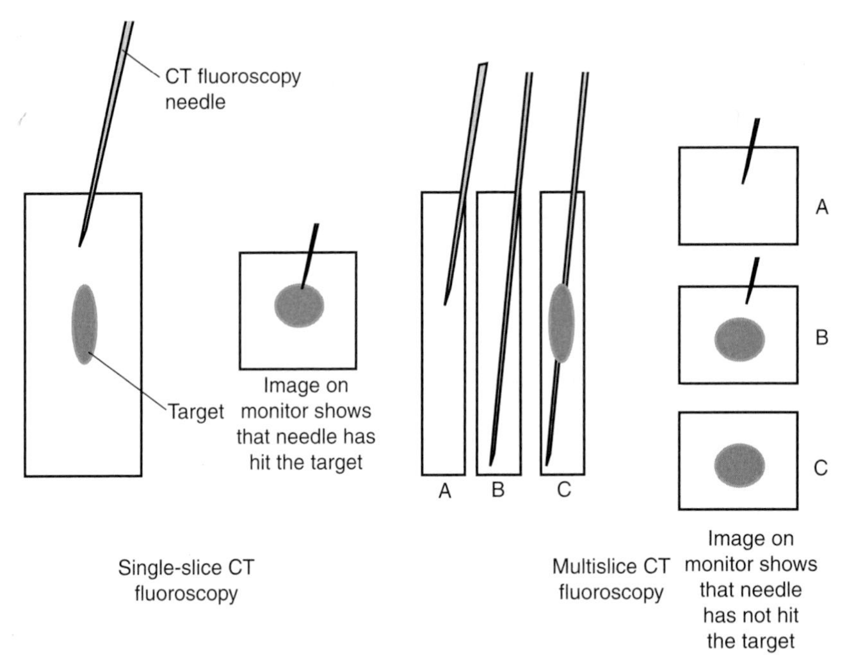

FIGURE. 12-41 A comparison of the accuracy of needle placement in CT fluoroscopy from single-slice CT and multislice CT systems.

CLINICAL APPLICATIONS

The immediate advantages of multislice CT are the speed of volume acquisition and the reduced loading on the x-ray tube. The same anatomic coverage may be obtained in one fourth the time and at one fourth the anode heating with all other parameters remaining the same. The implications for the x-ray tube are enormous. Not only is it possible to perform many more acquisitions before the necessary pause for tube cooling, but the wear and tear on the tube is also greatly reduced for the same scan volume. For example, a full-body scan from head through the pelvis, which would require more than 95 seconds of data collection in a 1-second, single-slice scanner (excluding interscan delays), could be performed in less than 12 seconds of data collection for a half-second multislice system.

Such amazing speed should have immediate value in examinations of trauma and pediatric patients. Better phase differentiation in contrasted studies is now possible, which hopefully will lead to improved diagnostic information. However, just as the introduction of spiral/helical CT emphasized the need for accurate contrast timing, the speed of multislice scanning will make this accuracy even more critical. Accurate contrast tracking techniques such as those available from continuous imaging technology will play an even greater role in the optimization of contrast opacity in both routine and special examinations.

As with spiral/helical scanning, speed may be exchanged for improved image quality. With the single-slice scanner, technique selection must balance the volume to be covered against slice thickness and pitch. Multislice systems offer the possibility of extended coverage with thin slices, which improves z-axis resolution and reduces partial volume averaging. These effects should be particularly noticeable in 3D and MPRs of scan data in CT angiography, for example.

It has been demonstrated that, for example, 0.5-mm slices can be achieved in reasonable scan times, which brings isotropic resolution in 3D reconstructions within reach. This is particularly valuable in cerebral CT angiography for the more accurate visualization of small vessels. Aneurysms and stenoses may be characterized quantitatively to yield better diagnostic information and allow the presurgical preparation of customized stents and other devices for more effective therapy. Similar improvements in CTA of the neck, aorta, and renal vessels are available with these scanners because of the combination of speed and thin slices for high axial resolution. Indeed, examples of peripheral runoff studies are appearing in which superb CT angiograms of the aorta and lower extremities can be completed in 75 seconds with substantially less contrast volume. In addition to more accurate CT angiography, the ability to cover large volumes with excellent spatial resolution should also provide more accurate data sets for the performance of CT endoscopy and the diagnosis of pulmonary embolism.

Another exciting prospect with multislice detectors is the continued development of functional CT imaging. Examples of the usefulness of CT in the evaluation of perfusion and other functions in various parts of the body have been reported. Now that a larger volume of data can be continuously acquired, the potential of CT in functional studies has been fully realized. An application of this technique is the evaluation of brain perfusion through the observation of first-pass contrast flow in patients suspected of acute infarction.

Clinical applications are discussed further in Chapters 17, 18, and 19.

POTENTIAL PROBLEMS

Although multislice scanners offer dramatic advantages compared with their single-slice counterparts, they also have some potential problems. Cases that are currently scanned with thin slices, overlapped reconstruction, and possibly two or more reconstruction algorithms can generate huge numbers of images. Routine studies consisting of hundreds of images are common, and special examinations might involve thousands of images. Obviously, such large data sets present problems for interpretation, recording, distribution, and archiving. Radiologists are now making the diagnosis from "soft" reading of images on workstations, and are reading MPR and 3D reconstructions instead of individual axial images. Reliance on remote locations for diagnosis may strain existing transmission capabilities and necessitate considerably faster systems for the future.

It will no longer be practical to record all CT images on film, and even archiving to digital media may require new strategies such as "stacking" slices or selective archival. Some departmental PACS (picture archiving and communication systems) have already been stretched beyond their capabilities by the flood of new data, and great care is needed in future facility design. The handling of image data may be the next big problem area for CT.

REFERENCES

Brenner DJ, Hall EJ: Computed tomography—an increasing source of radiation exposure, *New Engl J Med* 357:22, 2007.

Chen L et al: General surface reconstruction for cone-beam multislice spiral computed tomography, *Med Phys* 30:2804-2812, 2003.

Cody DD, Mahesh M: Technologic advances in multi-slice CT with a focus on cardiac imaging, *Radiographics* 27:1829-1837, 2007.

Dalrymple NC et al: Price of isotropy in multidetector CT, *Radiographics* 27:49-62, 2007.

Daly B, Templeton PA: Real-time CT fluoroscopy: evolution of a clinical tool, *Radiology* 211:309, 1999.

Douglas-Akinwande AC et al: Multichannel CT: evaluating the spine in postoperative patients with orthopedic hardware, *Radiographics* 26:S97-S110, 2006.
Dowe DA: Prospectively gated CTA dramatically reduces dose, *Diagn Imaging*, 28:S1-S5, 2006.
Dowsett D et al: *The physics of diagnostic imaging*, London, 2006, Hodder Arnold.
Engel KJ et al: X-ray scattering in single- and dual-source CT, *Med Phys* 35:318-332, 2008.
Feldkamp LA et al: Practical cone-beam algorithm, *J Opt Soc Am* 1:612-619, 1984.
Flohr TG et al: Multi-detector row CT systems and image reconstruction techniques, *Radiology* 235:756-773, 2005.
Flohr TG: Radiation dose with dual source CT, *Siemens Med Solutions* June 94-97, 2006.
Flohr TG et al: First performance of a dual-source CT (DSCT) system, *Eur Radiol* 16:256-268, 2006.
He HD: Personal communication, General Electric Medical Systems, 1999.
Hu H: Multislice helical CT: scan and reconstruction, *Med Phys* 26:5, 1999a.
Hu H: Personal communications, 1999b.
IEC (International Electrotechnical Commission): Medical Electrical Equipment-60601 Part 2-44: Particular requirements for the safety of x-ray equipment for computed tomography, Geneva, Switzerland, 1999.
Kachelriess M et al: Extended parallel backprojection for standard three-dimensional and phase-correlated four dimensional axial and spiral cone-beam CT with arbitrary pitch, arbitrary cone angle, and 100% dose usage, *Med Phys* 31:1623-1641, 2004.
Kachelriess M: Clinical x-ray computed tomography. In Schlegel W et al, editors: *New technologies in radiation oncology*, New York, 2006, Springer.
Kalender WA: *Computed tomography: fundamentals, system technology, image quality, applications*, Erlangen, Germany, 2005, Publicis Corporate Publishing.
Kalender WA, Kyriakou Y: Flat-detector computed tomography (FD-CT), *Eur Radiol* 17:2767-2779, 2007.
Kohl G: The evolution and state-of-the-art principles of multi-slice computed tomography, *Proc Am Thorac Soc* 2:470-476, 2005.
Kopecky K et al: Multislice CT spirals past single-slice in diagnostic efficacy, *Diagn Imaging* April: 36-42, 1999.
Kudo H, Saito T: Helical-scan computed tomography using cone-beam projections. In *IEEE Conf. Record 1991 Nuclear Science Symposium and Medical Imaging Conference*, Santa Fe NM, 1958-1962, 1991.
Liang Y, Kruger RA: Dual-slice spiral versus single-slice spiral scanning: comparison of the physical performance of two computed tomography scanners, *Med Phys* 23:205-217, 1996.
Mather R: Meeting the cone-beam challenge—Aquilion's sureCardio™ and TCOT, *Toshiba Med Rev* October 15:16-21, 2005a.
Mather R: Patient focused imaging—Aquilion's low dose vision, *Toshiba Med Rev* July 17:4-8, 2005b.
Mather R: *Aquilion ONE—dynamic volume computed tomography*, 2007, Toshiba Medical Systems.
Meyer CA et al: Real-time CT fluoroscopy: utility in thoracic drainage procedures, *AJR Am J Roentgenol* 171:1097, 1998.
Mori S: Personal communications, 2008.
Mori S et al: Physical performance evaluation of a 256-slice CT-scanner for four-dimensional imaging, *Med Phys* 31:1348-1356, 2004.
Mori S et al: A combination-weighted Feldkamp-based reconstruction algorithm for cone-beam CT, *Phys Med Biol* 51:3953-3965, 2006a.
Mori S et al: Comparison of patient doses in 256-slice CT and 16-slice CT scanners, *Br J Radiol* 79:56-61, 2006b.
Noo F et al: The dual-ellipse cross vertex path for exact reconstruction of long objects in cone-beam tomography, *Phys Med Biol* 42:797-810, 1998.
Oxford English Dictionary: http://oed.com. Accessed September 19, 2008.
Paulson EK et al: MDCT of patients with acute abdominal pain: a new perspective using coronal reformations from submiillimeter isotropic voxels, *AJR Am J Roentgenol* 183:899-906, 2004.
Paulson EK et al: Acute appendicitis: added diagnostic value of coronal reformations from isotropic voxels at multi-detector row CT, *Radiology* 235:879-885, 2005.
Primak AN et al: Relationship between noise, dose, and pitch in cardiac multi-detector row CT, *Radiographics* 26:1785-1794, 2006.
Saito Y: Multislice x-ray CT scanner, *Med Rev* 66:1-8, 1998.
Siemens Medical Solutions: Personal communication, 2006.
Siemens Medical Solutions: Personal communications, 2007.
Taguchi K: Personal communication, 1999.
Taguchi K, Aradate H: Algorithm for image reconstruction in multislice helical CT, *Med Phys* 25:550, 1998.
Toshiba Medical Systems: Personal communications, 2008.

Other Technical Applications of Computed Tomography Imaging: Basic Principles

Chapter Outline

There are several other technical applications of computed tomography (CT) imaging that have been used to image the patient to provide more information to enhance diagnostic interpretation of CT images and also play a role in the medical management of the patient. These applications range from those that have been used successfully in the past, such as subsecond CT scanning (see Chapter 12), CT angiography (CTA), CT fluoroscopy, quantitative CT, and applications of CT in radiation treatment planning, such as CT simulation and image fusion, to other developments. These include CT screening, breast CT, and more recently improved methods for CT imaging of the heart and portable CT scanners.

This chapter presents a description of these technical applications with the goal of setting the stage for a further exploration of these topics. Therefore only the essential technical elements will be introduced, and the interested reader should refer to the literature (journal articles and textbooks) dedicated to a more detailed explanation of the various techniques presented later. The chapter begins with a description of cardiac CT imaging and concludes with a brief introduction to portable CT scanners.

CARDIAC CT IMAGING

The technical advances in CT within the past 10 years have provided the motivation for the development of artifact-free cardiac CT imaging. Two of these advances include faster rotation times and multislice data acquisition methods at submillimeter slice thickness (Blobel et al, 2008; Hsieh et al, 2006). Although the faster rotation times relate to the temporal resolution needed to image the beating heart without motion artifacts, multislice data acquisition addresses the need to cover the organ in its entirety in a single rotation at high spatial resolution. This is necessary to demonstrate the tiny vasculature associated with the anatomy of the heart. The temporal resolution is a measure of the data acquisition time for one image. In addition, multisegment image reconstruction can be used to improve the temporal resolution, which is accomplished by using a set of raw data from a number of cardiac cycles (Blobel et al, 2008). As introduced in Chapter 1, cardiac CT applications include quantitative assessment of coronary artery calcifications, ventricular function assessment, coronary angiography assessment of pulmonary veins, cardiac masses and pericardial disease, and coronary artery bypass grafts and so forth (Prat-Gonzalez et al, 2008).

Although the rotation time for the 64-slice multislice CT (MSCT) scanners is about 330 milliseconds, the temporal resolution is about 165 milliseconds, which is not fast enough to image a fast-beating heart without motion artifacts (Gupta et al, 2006). In an effort to reduce the temporal resolution, two dedicated cardiac CT scanners were introduced: the dual-source CT (DSCT) scanner (Siemens Medical Solutions) and the more recent AquilionONE (Toshiba Medical Systems), a dynamic volume CT scanner.

The AquilionONE scanner features high temporal resolution and covers the entire heart in a single rotation with its wide area detector that offers a 16-centimeter (cm) organ coverage by use of its 320×0.5 millimeter (mm) detector rows. The DSCT scanner, on the other hand, uses two data acquisition systems (two x-ray tubes coupled to two sets of detector arrays) offset by 90 degrees to improve the temporal resolution and scan speed. The characteristic features of these two scanners are described in Chapter 12.

Physics of Cardiac Imaging with Multiple-Row Detector CT

Cardiac CT imaging is now being used almost routinely in large centers throughout the world, and therefore it is essential that users and operators alike (technologists and radiologists) have a firm understanding of the fundamental physics of cardiac CT. Mahesh and Cody (2007) describe such physics comprehensively in a seminal article entitled "Physics of Cardiac Imaging with Multiple-Row Detector CT." This article is reproduced in its entirety in Appendix C. Their coverage includes the following topics:

- Key issues in cardiac imaging with multiple-row detector CT
- Understanding the physics of cardiac imaging
- Temporal resolution
- Spatial resolution
- Pitch
- Radiation risk
- Geometric efficiency
- Artifacts
- Future directions in cardiac imaging

The reader should review this article for details of the physics of cardiac CT imaging.

CT ANGIOGRAPHY: A TECHNICAL OVERVIEW

Definition

A significant advantage of spiral/helical CT data acquisition is its application to three-dimensional (3D) imaging of vascular structures with an intravenous injection of contrast medium. Such an application is referred to as *CT angiography* (Kalender, 2005; Lell et al, 2006).

During spiral/helical data acquisition, the entire area of interest can be scanned during the injection of contrast. Images can be captured when vessels are fully opacified to demonstrate either arterial or venous phase enhancement through the acquisition of both data sets (arterial and venous). CTA has been applied successfully to a number of examinations investigating vascular anatomy problems and diseases. In particular, CTA techniques have proved useful in imaging the neurovasculature, and in particular stroke, coronary artery disease, the abdominal and thoracic aorta, and renal vasculature and in evaluating the vasculature of the abdominal viscera (Gupta et al, 2006; Pomerantz et al, 2006; Schoepf et al, 2007; Tanenbaum, 2006). Specifically, CTA can provide information regarding carotid artery stenosis, intracranial stenosis, venous thrombosis, vascular malformations, and aneurysms (Lell et al, 2006).

CTA is based on 3D imaging techniques to display images of the vasculature through intravenous administration of contrast, differing from conventional intra-arterial angiography. In 1995, the advantages of CTA over conventional angiography were several; they are highlighted in Table 13-1. At the time, one of the major disadvantages of CTA was its poor spatial resolution (Rawlings, 1995); however, MSCT scanners were developed that feature isotropic imaging, where the voxels are perfect cubes (equal dimensions in all three axes, x, y, and z). The 16- to 64-slice scanners can provide isotropic imaging with thin slice images that show a dramatic improvement in the spatial resolution of CTA images (Tanenbaum, 2006). Furthermore, spiral/helical scanning provides increased volume coverage (Fig. 13-1) without the loss of image quality.

Technical Requirements

Several authors, such as Lell et al (2006), Tanenbaum (2006), Jacobs (2006), and Schoepf et al (2007) have described the techniques for CTA with MSCT scanners, and in general they identify at least four major steps that are crucial to carrying out a CTA examination. Careful execution of these steps will serve to optimize the examination and produce high-quality images that will aid the radiologist in making an accurate diagnosis. Essentially these steps include the following:

1. Patient preparation
2. Acquisition parameters
3. Contrast medium administration
4. Image postprocessing techniques

Patient Preparation

A successful CTA examination depends on careful preparation of the patient before the examination. Such preparation requires that both the technologist and radiologist work together to obtain the

TABLE 13-1 Comparison of the Advantages of Computed Tomographic Angiography and Conventional Angiography

Conventional Angiography	CT Angiography
Biplane systems can acquire at most two view angles of a given vascular structure per contrast injection. When required, alternate views and examination of additional structures require added x-ray exposure and contrast media.	CTA acquires an entire volume of 3D data with a single injection of contrast agent. Thus, arbitrary views can be retrospectively targeted and reconstructed without the need for additional iodine or x-ray exposure.
Because an arterial puncture is made, patients must recover from the procedure with close nursing observation and strict bed rest for a minimum of 6 to 8 hours. An overnight hospital stay may also be required. Thus, recovery time adds significantly to the cost of the examination.	Peripheral intravenous injections permit a true outpatient examination with minimal postprocedure observation.
Serious complications from angiography can include reactions to contrast media and thromboembolic complications from catheterization of arteries that can lead to infarctions, strokes, arterial dissections, pseudoaneurysms, and arterial bleeding. Using cerebral angiography as an example, the risk of a neurological complication such as a transient ischemic attack or stroke is about 4% and the risk for development of a permanent neurological deficit from a disabling stroke is about 1%.	Although the contrast agent is the same, peripheral intravenous injections significantly reduce the risk of thromboembolic complications.
Conventional angiography is a projection imaging technique that produces two-dimensional images of 3D structures. Therefore, blood vessels and other structures that overlap in the direction of the projection may obscure the site of interest.	CTA is a 3D examination. Overlying structures may be eliminated by postprocessing.
Conventional angiography is an intraluminal technique and as such does not display mural abnormalities or true mural dimensions, making percent stenosis and aneurysm size measurements difficult.	CT is a cross-sectional imaging modality that exhibits excellent soft tissue discrimination. As such, it has utility for depicting mural thrombus, calcifications, and true mural dimensions.

From Napel SA: Principles and techniques of 3D spiral CT angiography. In Fishman EK, Jeffrey RB Jr, editors: *Spiral CT: principles, techniques and clinical applications*, New York, 1995, Raven Press.

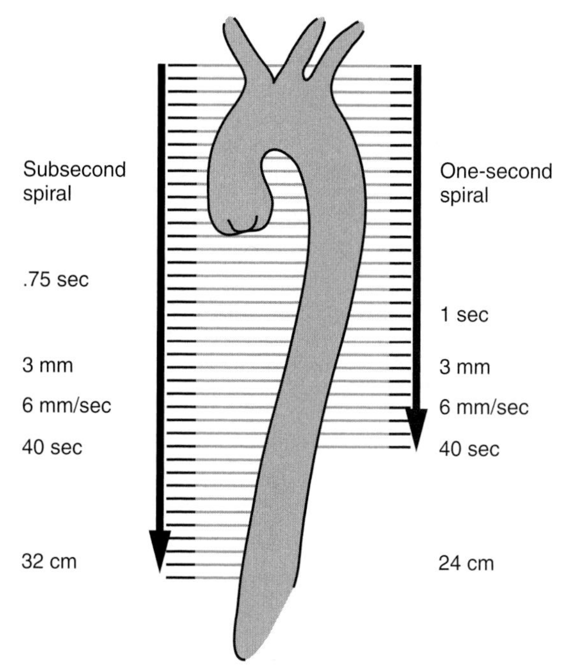

FIGURE 13-1 In CTA, a subsecond spiral/helical scanner increases volume coverage without a loss of image quality compared with its counterpart 1 second spiral/helical scanner. (From Kuszyk BS, Fishman EK: Technical aspects of CT angiography, *Semin Ultrasound CT MRI* 19:394-404, 1998.)

appropriate and correct information from the patient and to ensure that the patient understands the procedure, particularly breath-holding techniques. It is not within the scope of this chapter to describe the specifics of patient preparation because this will differ somewhat from department to department.

Acquisition Parameters

The acquisition parameters include the scan speed, the pitch, the spatial resolution needed, contrast material administration, and the image reconstruction algorithm.

In general, a routine CT examination precedes a CTA examination. The routine examination provides some evidence of the range of anatomy to be scanned. Once the scan distance or scan range, R (mm), has been determined, a number of parameters must be carefully chosen to optimize both the quality of the 3D images and the accuracy of the CTA examination. These parameters include the total spiral/helical scan time, T (seconds); the slice thickness, S (mm); and the speed of the patient through the gantry, that is, the table speed, d (mm/second) (Kalender, 2005).

The table speed (or scan speed), can be calculated by using Equation 13-1 or 13-2 (Kalender, 2005):

$$d = R/T \quad (13\text{-}1)$$

$$d = S \times P/t \quad (13\text{-}2)$$

where s is slice collimation, p is pitch, and t is scan time (seconds) per 360-degree rotation.

The spatial resolution (z-axis or longitudinal resolution) of the CTA images is influenced by the collimation. To image the basal intracranial arteries, for example, a 100-mm length of tissue coverage is necessary. With a four-slice MSCT scanner with a collimated 1-mm section width, a pitch of 1.5, and a gantry rotation time of 0.5 second, the 100-mm volume of tissue can be scanned in 9 seconds. With a 16-slice MSCT scanner with the same pitch and rotation time of the 4-slice MSCT scanner and at a slice width of 0.75 mm, the 100-mm volume can be scanned in 3 seconds (Lell et al, 2006).

In addition, the in-plane spatial resolution is important and is affected by not only the detector design (with thin slices such as 0.5 and 0.75 mm on 16- to 64-slice scanners). As noted by Lell et al (2006), the typical in-plane resolution for a 64-slice scanner with a 0.6-mm detector element is 0.6 to 0.7 mm.

Also influencing the quality of the CTA examination is careful selection of peak kilovolt (kVp) and milliampere (mA) values and the image reconstruction intervals. The selection of kVp and mA used in CTA examinations is usually determined by the size of the patient and the level of noise in the images. To maintain a good signal-to-noise ratio, mA and kVp must be adjusted accordingly. In this respect, Lell et al (2006) and Tanenbaum (2006) point out that 120 kVp is commonly used, mA values selected are based on the size of the patient's body section to be examined, and 140 mAs (effective) is not uncommon. Finally, the role of isotropic imaging (voxels are perfect cubes) has made a significant impact on the quality of CTA images, especially 3D images and reformatted images (Tanenbaum, 2006).

The image reconstruction interval, or increment, refers to the spacing between the center of the slices. Reconstruction intervals are important because they play a role in the quality of the 3D CTA images. Overlapping reconstructions improve the 3D image quality, and a reconstruction increment of 50% to 75% of the slice width can serve as a "reasonable rule of thumb" (Lell et al, 2006). Spatial resolution is also influenced by the reconstruction algorithm used. Lell et al point out that "the ideal kernel would combine low image noise and sharp edge definition, maintaining good low-contrast resolution." Additionally, although soft kernels decrease noise and smooth images, edge enhancement kernels improve sharpness but create increased image noise.

Contrast Medium Administration

Imaging the contrast while it is in the vascular area of interest during the CTA examination is a critical step in the acquisition of images. Contrast injection techniques take into consideration the volume of contrast needed to opacify vascular regions, the contrast injection rate, and the timing between the start of contrast medium injection and the start of the spiral/helical scan. Measuring the contrast circulation times for different patients is important in CTA to ensure that images are recorded when flow-in of contrast is optimum in the vessels. To help with this task, various automated systems such as SmartPrep (General Electric Medical Systems), Siemens Combined Applications to Reduce Exposure (CARE Bolus), and Toshiba's SureStart are available commercially. These products ensure optimized contrast monitoring in CTA. Figure 13-2 demonstrates such optimization with Toshiba's SureStart package. The change in CT number on the image, which is displayed in real time, is monitored by the monitoring scan. When the contrast reaches a set value (threshold), the monitoring scan ends, and the main scan (helical scan) starts automatically to provide images when contrast flow in the vessels is optimum. Figure 13-3 details the essential steps for operating SureStart.

Consideration must be given to the size of the needle and the site of the injection. Various-size intravenous angiocatheters, such as 18- or 20-gauge or 20- or 22-gauge, are commonly inserted into a medial antecubital vein, using injections at rates that vary from 3 to 4 ml per second to 5 ml per second (Lell et al, 2006).

Image Postprocessing Techniques: Visualization Tools

The algorithms used to display 3D images from the axial data set are described in detail in Chapter 14. These algorithms are digital postprocessing techniques or visualization tools, which are used quite extensively in CTA. Currently, the following techniques are commonplace in CTA:

1. Multiplanar reconstruction (MPR), including curved MPR
2. Shaded surface display (SSD)
3. Maximum intensity projection (MIP)
4. Volume rendering (VR)
5. Interactive cine

Furthermore, the student should refer to Lell et al (2006) for an excellent review of the use of these image postprocessing operations in CTA.

Multiplanar Reconstruction

MPR is the first visualization tool for use in CTA. It is simple and faster to reconstruct than any other 3D technique and enables visualization of the volume data set in any plane, including curved planes. However, MPR is less useful in a number of applications, such as visualization of

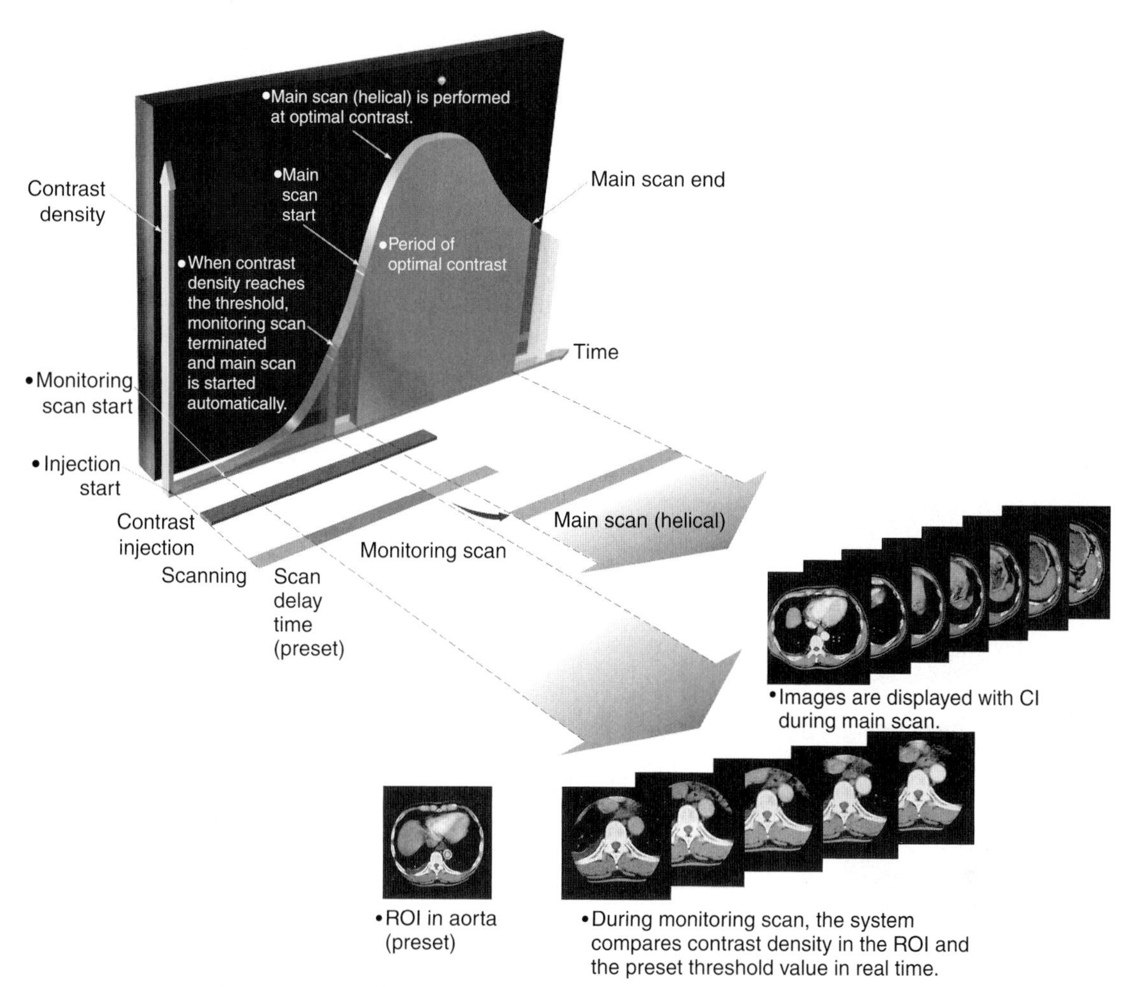

FIGURE 13-2 Optimization of contrast monitoring for CTA examinations using SureStart, an automated package for optimal scan control for contrast studies. *ROI*, Region of interest. (Courtesy Toshiba America Medical Systems, Tustin, Calif.)

complex vessels (circle of Willis) and intracranial arteriovenous malformations. In addition, no editing is required when using MPR in CTA examinations.

The use of isotropic imaging possible with multislice CT scanners offering slices from 16 to 320 per revolution provides excellent spatial resolution because the voxels are perfect cubes under certain imaging conditions. Additionally, a variation of the MPR technique called curved MPR can be used to demonstrate tortuous structures (Lell et al, 2006).

Shaded Surface Display

The SSD visualization tool requires little editing to remove overlapping structures obscuring the vessels. It is faster than VR because it uses only a small fraction of the total axial data set.

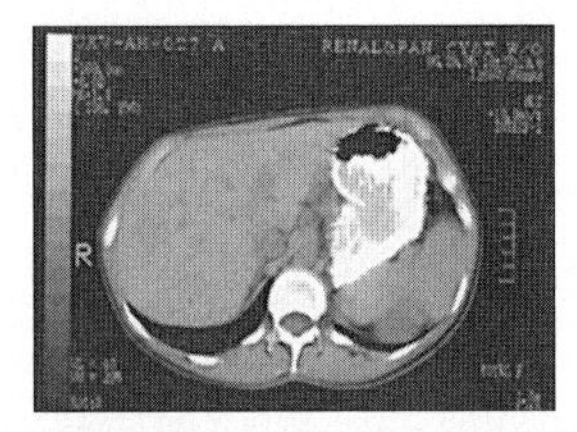

1 Observe the target vessel
The operator views an axial image which includes the structure to be monitored for contrast arrival.

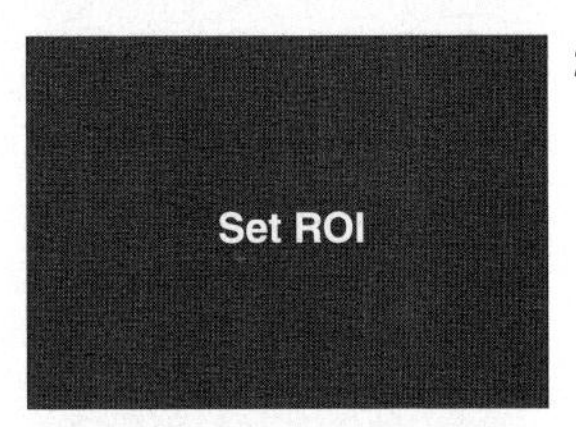

2 Define an ROI and set target threshold
A threshold CT value is assigned to the ROI for automatic initiation of the scan. SureStart operating techniques and preset delay times may be selected at this time.

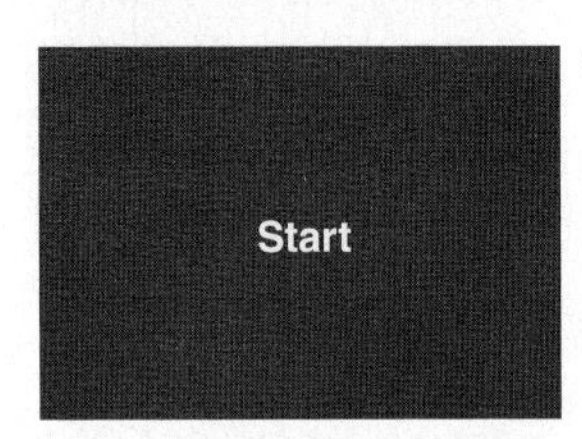

3 Begin SureStart
SureStart preparation is selected from the touch panel of the console. The contrast injection is begun, and the START key is pressed. SureStart imaging commences at the end of a pre-set delay.

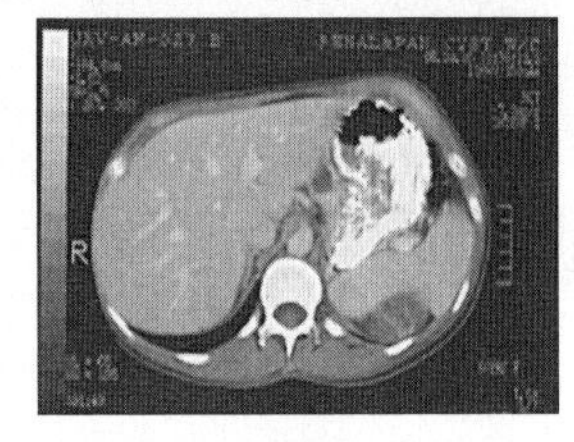

4 Begin scanning
When the ROI CT number matches or exceeds the threshold value, or when the NEXT SCAN key is hit, the next scan in the exam plan sequence is initiated.

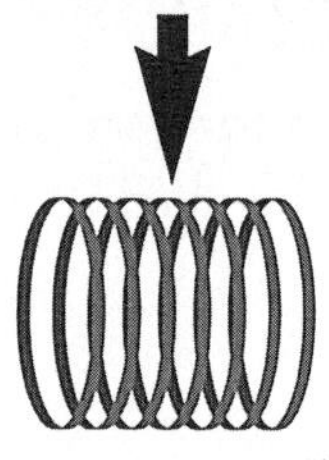

NOTE: SureStart is a selectable element which can be included in any exam plan, and can be followed by helical or dynamic acquisition. SureStart may be interrupted at any time using the ABORT KEY.

FIGURE 13-3 The four essential steps to operating SureStart, Toshiba's automated system for optimized contrast monitoring in CTA. *ROI*, Region of interest. (Courtesy Toshiba America Medical Systems, Tustin, Calif.)

This characteristic can result in artifact generation and images that are not very accurate. SSD images are useful in the display of vascular relationships, vessel origins, and the surface contours of vessels.

Maximum Intensity Projection

The MIP visualization tool is the most frequently used in CTA examinations to display the structure of vessels. It is popular in CT and magnetic resonance imaging (MRI) and is more accurate than

SSD (Kuszyk and Fishman, 1998). Although MIP has proved useful in CTA, it requires editing to remove unwanted structures, such as bone and calcified plaques that prevent the observer from viewing intravascular detail. The MIP can be used successfully to separate out vascular calcifications, lumen thrombus, and intravascular thrombus (Oldendorf and Weber, 1997).

Volume Rendering

Another postprocessing 3D visualization tool that is popular for use in CTA is VR. VR uses all the information in the axial data set to display internal structures (soft tissues, vascular and bony anatomy) and to provide accurate vessel diameters and 3D vascular relationships. In the past, VR was performed only on powerful workstations, and not only was it expensive but also time consuming.

SSD and MIP processing techniques use data from surface and voxel intensities, respectively. However, VR uses all the data in the axial volume data set. Therefore, all voxel information is used in the processing. Developments in computer graphics hardware now make it possible to process VR images at higher speeds and higher frame rates (5 to 20 frames/seconds), thus resulting in real-time rendering.

Kuszyk and Fishman (1998) describe four VR parameters intended to enhance the "accuracy and the practicality of CT angiography." These parameters include windowing (window width and window level), opacity, brightness, and accuracy. Although windowing allows observers to alter the image contrast and density to suit their viewing needs, opacity refers to the degree that structures that are close to the user obscure structures that are further away. Opacity can be varied from 0% to 100%. Higher opacity values produce an appearance similar to surface rendering, which helps to display complex 3D relationships. Lower opacity values allow the user to "see through" structures and can be very useful for such applications as seeing a free-floating thrombus within the lumen of a vein or evaluating bony abnormalities such as tumors that are located below the cortical surface (Kuszyk and Fishman, 1998).

Brightness, on the other hand, provides the observer with the ability to alter the image appearance from 0% to 100%. Kuszyk and Fishman (1998) report that a brightness setting of 100% is useful for a wide range of examinations. Finally, VR provides more accurate results for a number of vascular problems (stenosis, for example) than do SSD and MIP 3D visualization tools (Johnson et al, 1998; Kuszyk et al, 1998). However, Ebert et al (1998) have shown that VR is not without problems. One such problem is that of *interobserver variability*.

These 3D visualization tools are described in detail in Chapter 14.

Interactive Cine

The developments in image processing and display of 3D images have led to interactive cine viewing and display. *Interactive cine* refers to the viewing and evaluation of the images in the axial data set by panning through the set of images. Because each of these images is separated only slightly in time, the rapid display of the set of axial images provides the effect of motion (much like a cine film). Although axial images can be used to provide a diagnosis, 3D images help to demonstrate anatomical relationships and show vessels that run along the z-axis.

CT FLUOROSCOPY

The basis for continuous CT imaging or real-time CT fluoroscopy depends on slip-ring technology, high-speed processing of the data collected from the patient, and a fast processing algorithm for image reconstruction. CT fluoroscopy has been used as a guidance tool in interventional radiology procedures (Carlson et al, 2001; Carlson et al, 2005; Hohl et al, 2008; Kalender, 2005; Kataoka et al, 2006; Paulson et al, 2001).

This section of the chapter focuses on a basic description of the imaging principles, equipment components, image quality, and radiation dose considerations.

Conventional CT as an Interventional Guidance Tool

Conventional slice-by-slice CT has been used as a clinical tool for guidance in nonvascular interventional radiologic procedures, such as percutaneous interventions as biopsies and drainage, together with other techniques (e.g., ultrasonography, conventional fluoroscopy, and MRI). A problem with conventional CT-guided interventional procedure, compared with ultrasonography and fluoroscopy, is the lack of real-time display of images, resulting from a time lag between data collection and image reconstruction. Such image display is especially important during needle puncture of the patient. Conventional CT-guided intervention is also limited in imaging body regions where movement is present, such as the respiratory system and the upper abdominal region. The movement associated with these body regions is responsible for shifting and disappearance of lesions of interest, making localization almost impossible (Daly and Templeton, 1999; Froelich et al, 1997). This results in an unsuccessful examination that must often be repeated.

This limitation of conventional CT-guided interventional technique has been overcome by CT hardware and software that allow current CT scanners to reconstruct and display images in real time with frame rates that can vary from two to eight frames per second, depending on the scanner. Such improvements facilitated the development of CT fluoroscopy (Katada, 1996).

CT Fluoroscopy Fundamentals

Historical Background

In 1993 Dr. K. Katada of the Fujita Health University, School of Health Sciences, in Japan initiated the idea for real-time imaging with use of a CT scanner. Dr. Katada subsequently approached Toshiba CT Systems Design Group with a proposal for decreasing the image reconstruction time, the image matrix size, the number of views, and the field-of-view (Katada, 1996). This resulted in a modification of one of Toshiba's CT scanners to provide images at a rate of three per second with a time delay of 0.83 second. Having conducted preliminary experiments and clinical trials, Katada and colleagues reported their early clinical experience with real-time CT fluoroscopy at the Radiological Society of North America (RSNA) meeting in 1994. The first CT scanner capable of real-time imaging was introduced in North America in 1994.

In 1996 the U.S. Food and Drug Administration approved real-time CT fluoroscopy as a useful clinical tool (Daly and Templeton, 1999). Today, several CT scanner manufacturers offer scanners capable of performing real-time CT fluoroscopy, including Toshiba Medical Systems, Siemens Medical Solutions, Philips Medical Systems, and General Electric Healthcare. These scanners feature multiple-image multidetector row CT fluoroscopy compared with the single-image CT fluoroscopy system (Kataoka et al, 2006; Keat, 2001; Paulson et al, 2001)

The evolution of CT fluoroscopy has now made it possible to acquire dynamic CT images in real time (Fig. 13-4), analogous to dynamic images produced in conventional fluoroscopy.

Imaging Principles Overview

The fundamental principles of real-time CT fluoroscopy are based on three advances in CT technology that have also led to other innovations in CT. The fundamental imaging principles involved in real-time CT fluoroscopy are illustrated in Figure 13-5, which shows three steps that are based on the initial framework of Ozaki (1995): fast continuous scanning, fast image reconstruction, and continuous image display. Each of these is briefly described.

Fast Continuous Scanning

Fast continuous scanning was a major technologic development in CT, which resulted in spiral/helical scanning. Spiral/helical scanning is made possible by slip-ring technology, which allows for continuous rotation of the x-ray tube compared with the stop-and-go scanning characteristic of conventional CT systems, which resulted from cable wraparound. Continuous rotation of the x-ray tube speeds up data collection and allows data to be collected for one rotation (360 degrees) per second.

An important point to note during data acquisition in CT fluoroscopy is that the patient does not move during continuous rotation of the x-ray tube. The patient remains stationary. When data are collected after one rotation (360 degrees), the first image is displayed on the monitor for viewing. Subsequent images are displayed every time a data set has been collected for every 60-degree rotation. The data set for every 60-degree rotation is used to refresh the previous image, which is discarded as new 60-degree data sets are processed. This means that six images per second (360/60) can be displayed as shown in Figure 13-6.

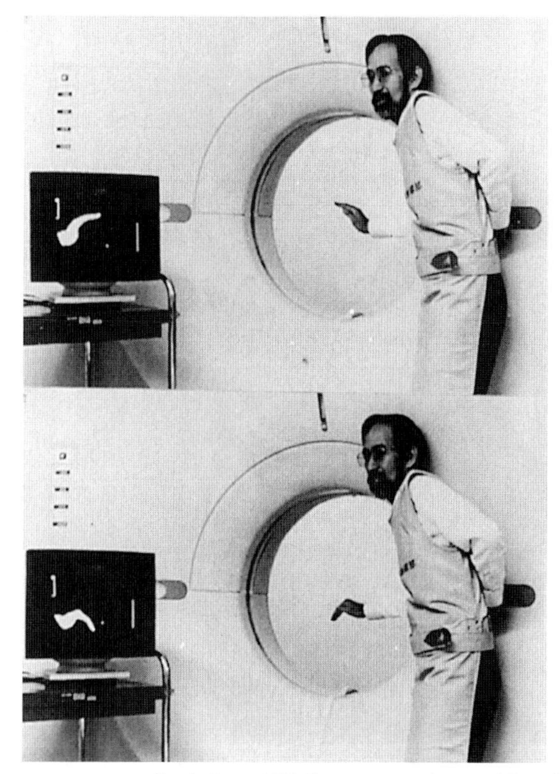

FIGURE 13-4 Real-time CT fluoroscopy is capable of producing dynamic CT images. Images of the hand in both flexion and extension are displayed in real time. (From Katada K: Further innovations in CT technology: CT fluoroscopy and real-time helical scan CT, *Med Rev* 53:1-11, 1995.)

Fast Image Reconstruction

In real-time CT fluoroscopy, fast image reconstruction is made possible by a set of hardware components dedicated to provide fast computations, together with a new image reconstruction algorithm. An important point to note about CT fluoroscopy is that the interpolation algorithm used in spiral/helical CT scanning is not used. The purpose of this algorithm is to compute a planar section from which all other sections can be obtained by interpolation. This process removes artifacts resulting from the simultaneous movement of the patient through the gantry while the x-ray tube rotates continuously during data acquisition.

In CT fluoroscopy motion artifacts are therefore present on the image and appear as streaks; however, these artifacts do not restrict visualization of relevant structures. The dedicated hardware components include a fast arithmetic unit, high-speed memory, and a back-projection gate array. All these components are housed in the image reconstruction unit. Parallel processing of the data is an integral element of real-time CT fluoroscopy.

The other key element of a real-time CT fluoroscopic imaging system is an image reconstruction algorithm, the fundamental elements of which were described earlier by Ozaki (1995) and Katada et al (1996). Conceptually, the fast image reconstruction algorithm for CT fluoroscopy processes six images per second (for a 1-second spiral/helical scanner) by first adding the next 60-degree

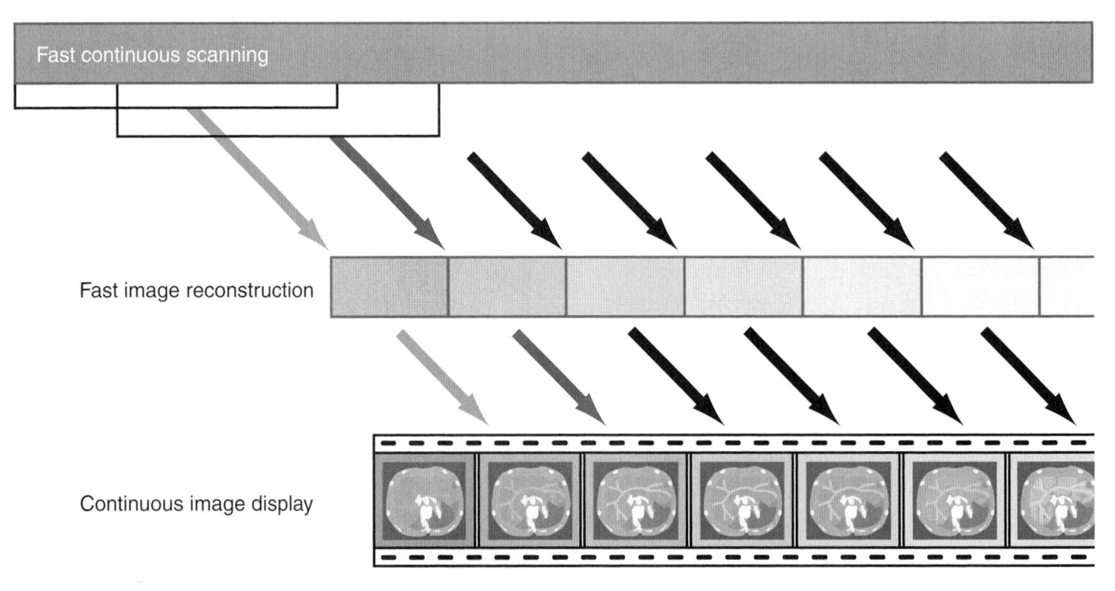

FIGURE 13-5 The principles of real-time CT fluoroscopy are based on three steps: fast continuous scanning, fast image reconstruction, and continuous image display.

data set acquired and subsequently subtracting the previously acquired 60-degree data set from the image as the data set is acquired continuously (see Fig. 13-6).

Continuous Image Display

As data are collected continuously, it is reconstructed by the fast reconstruction unit on a defined matrix size (256 × 256) and subsequently interpolated to larger matrix sizes 768 × 768 (Paulson et al, 2001) or 1024 × 1024 to provide better resolution. Images are subsequently displayed on a monitor in the cine mode (dynamic display) at frame rates that can vary from two to eight images per second (Carlson et al, 2001).

Equipment Configuration and Data Flow

The basic equipment configuration of a CT fluoroscopic imaging system consists of a number of acquisition, image processing, image display, and recording components (Fig. 13-7).

The acquisition components include the scanner, which uses a third-generation spiral/helical data collection geometry with slip-ring technology for continuous data acquisition. The gantry aperture will vary with a variable field of view (FOV) (18 to 40 cm is not uncommon) depending on the type of system. The scanner houses the x-ray generator, x-ray tube, detectors, and associated electronics. The x-ray generator is a high-frequency generator, and the x-ray tube is a high-capacity tube capable of very high heat units.

Once the raw data are acquired, they are sent to a preprocessor and then to the high-speed memory. The first 360-degree data set is processed using convolution and back-projection, and the reconstructed image is displayed on a monitor for viewing. Subsequent CT fluoroscopic data are acquired and processed with the real-time reconstruction unit (as described earlier).

With use of a display interface (I/F), images can be stored and be displayed for viewing and interpretation.

The control console for CT fluoroscopy allows the operator to have full control of the table movement through the gantry, to vary height of the tabletop, and to tilt the gantry during the interventional procedure.

X-Ray Technique Parameters

The x-ray exposure parameters can vary depending on the department and the needs of the examination. In general however, tube currents of 30 to 50 mAs and tube voltages of 80 to 120 kVp are not uncommon. Additionally, in the CT fluoroscopy mode, a special filter is introduced into the dose to the patient. The magnitude of the dose reduction depends on the type of scanner and the exposure parameters used during the examination.

Other technique parameters that must be considered in CT fluoroscopy are slice widths (collimator width), the FOV, and the maximum fluoroscopy time. In addition, a choice of slice widths ranging from say 1, 2, 3, 5, 7, to 10 mm and FOV of 18, 24, 32 or 40 cm is available to the operator, and the maximum fluoroscopy time for continuous imaging is 100 seconds. This timer must be reset after 100 seconds of fluoroscopy.

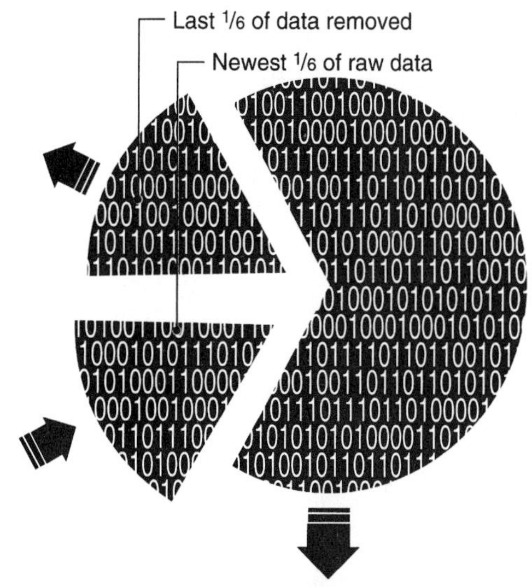

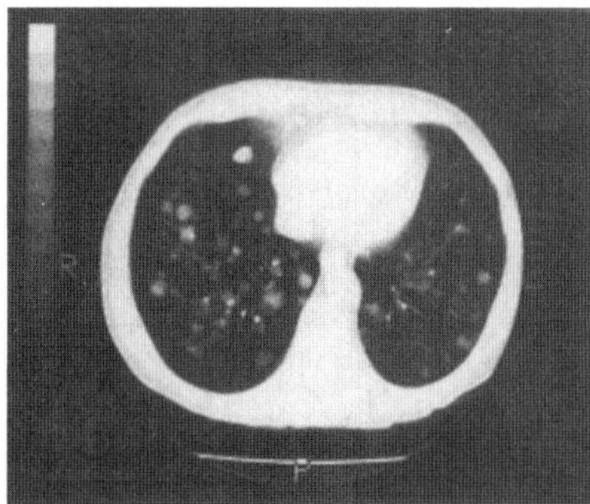

FIGURE 13-6 A diagrammatic representation of fast image reconstruction and display of images in CT fluoroscopy. During continuous scanning of the patient, images are reconstructed and displayed every 1/6 second. (Courtesy Toshiba America Medical Systems, Tustin, Calif.)

Image Quality and Radiation Dose Considerations

Measuring the parameters that affect image quality and radiation dose ascertains the performance of a CT scanner. In CT fluoroscopy, image quality and radiation assessment are ongoing concerns.

Image Quality

Image quality parameters in CT fluoroscopy include spatial resolution, density resolution, image noise, and artifacts. As early as 1995, these parameters were examined by Ozaki (1995), who compared spatial resolution, density resolution, and image noise of CT fluoroscopy with that of conventional CT. These early results demonstrate that the image quality parameters measured for CT fluoroscopy are comparable to those of conventional CT. For example, Ozaki (1995) showed that, although the spatial

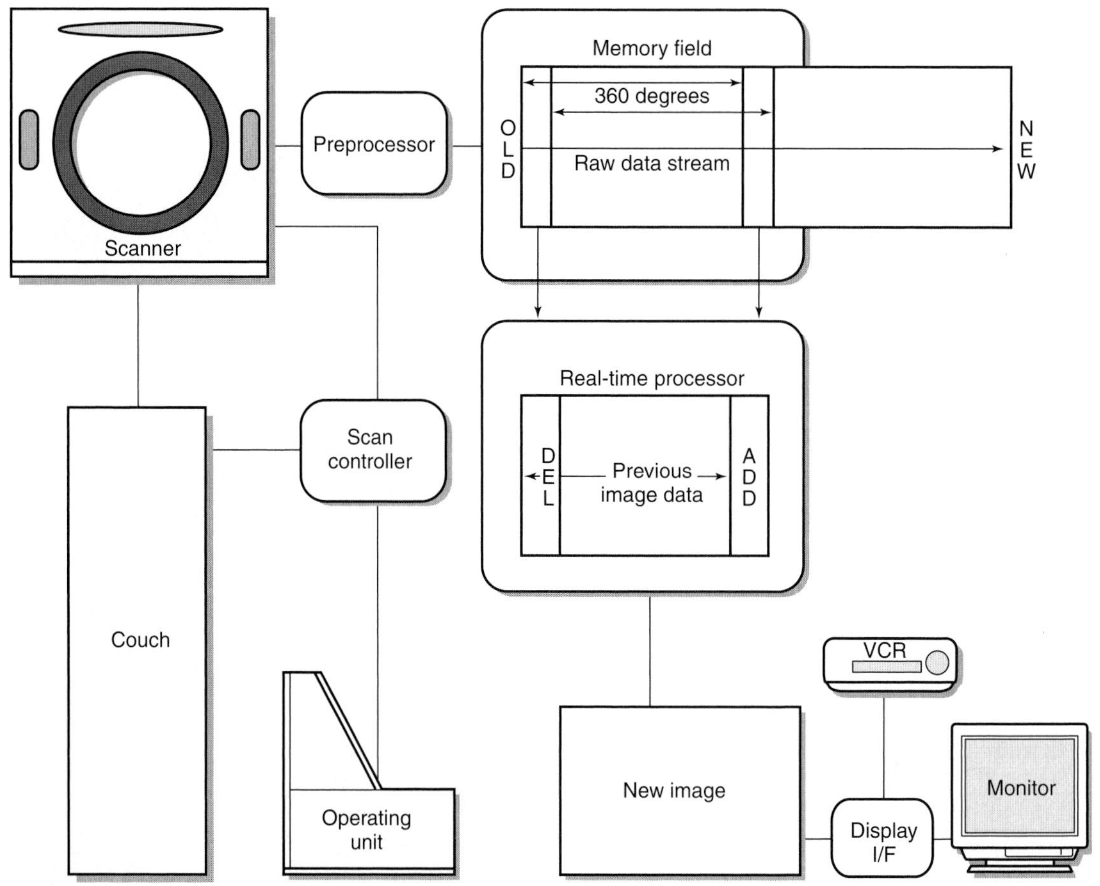

FIGURE 13-7 The basic equipment configuration for CT fluoroscopy. See text for further explanation. (From Katada K et al: Guidance with real-time CT fluoroscopy: early clinical experience, *Radiology* 200:851-856, 1996.)

and density resolution for CT fluoroscopy was 6.8 line pairs per centimeter (lp/cm) and 3 mm at 0.45%, respectively, it was 7.5 lp/cm and 3 mm at 0.41%, respectively, for conventional CT. Although the image noise for a 10-mm slice at 50 mA used for CT fluoroscopy was ±3.9 Hounsfield units (HU), it was the same (±3.9 HU) at 150 mA for conventional CT.

Radiation Dose Considerations

With any new technique that uses x-rays to image the patient, radiation dose is always a primary consideration because the goal of radiology is to operate within the as low as reasonably achievable (ALARA) philosophy. Furthermore, the dose in CT fluoroscopy is also important because personnel are present in the room during the procedure.

A number of factors influence the dose to the patient and operator in CT (Hohl et al, 2008; Kataoka et al, 2006; Keat, 2001). One of the important factors is the length of the time of the exposure because dose is directly proportional to exposure time. For example, in an early dose assessment study, Daly and Templeton (1999) report absorbed doses in the range of 3.53 rad (35.3 milligrays [mGy]) for 50 seconds of exposure at 80 kVp and 30 mA to 19.81 rad (198.1 mGy) for a similar exposure time at 120 kVp and 50 mA.

During the development and early implementation of CT fluoroscopy, the dose to the hands of the operator was of particular concern because they were directly in the x-ray beam during the procedure. Early studies reported excessively high doses to the operator's hands during the procedure (Katada et al, 1996; Kato et al, 1996). The solution to this problem was the development of needle holders, which are intended to keep the hands of the operator out of the x-ray beam. An early study by Kato et al (1996) showed that the needle holders reduced the absorbed dose rate to the operator's hands. Additionally, the needle holders do not produce image artifacts.

Another concern related to the dose in CT fluoroscopy procedures is that of scatter radiation distribution in the room during the procedure and the dose received by the operator resulting from this scatter. One example of an early scattered radiation dose distribution is shown in Figure 13-8.

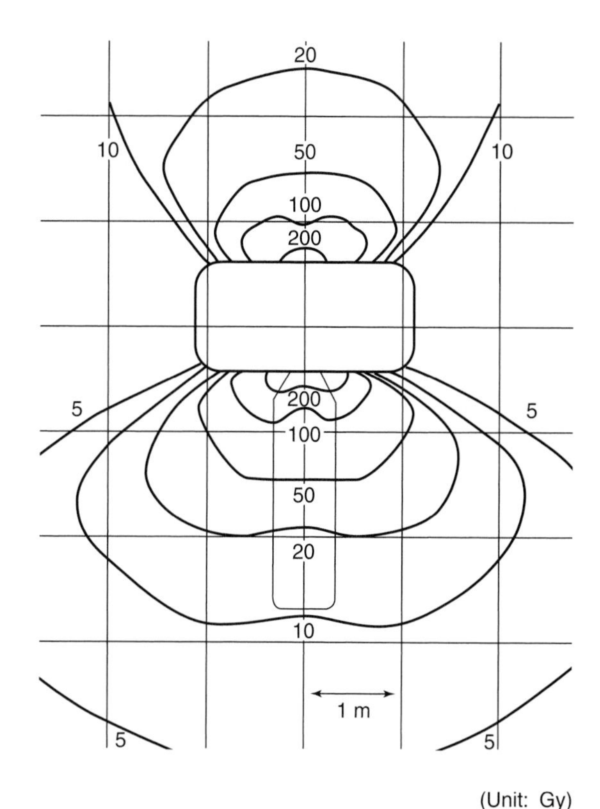

FIGURE 13-8 Scatter radiation dose distribution at CT fluoroscopy.

Wearing a protective apron during the procedure will certainly reduce the effective dose to the operator. Operators standing in the CT room during the procedure must wear protective lead aprons, thyroid shields, and lead glasses or goggles. These protective apparel must be at least 0.5 mm lead equivalent. Additionally, the use of lead drapes in close proximity will result in a marked reduction of exposure to scattered radiation (Nawfel, 2000; Wagner, 2000).

Reducing radiation dose to both patients and personnel is an important goal of radiology. In CT fluoroscopy, one technique that is incorporated in the design of the equipment to reduce the dose to the patient is the use of a special x-ray filter. In addition, lower tube currents and shorter examination times also play a significant role in reducing patient exposures (Paulson et al, 2001). Another technique referred to as the "quick check" technique can be used to reduce the dose in CT fluoroscopy. As described by Paulson et al (2001), the quick check technique is similar to conventional CT and uses single-section CT fluoroscopic spot images to check the location of the needle and ensure that the correct alignment is obtained.

Another useful method to reduce the dose to the patient and operator is the use of a tungsten antimony shielding drape, which hangs near to the scan plane. With a 16-slice volume CT scanner operating in the CT fluoroscopy mode, the dose was measured to adult and pediatric phantoms with a solid-state UNFORS (Billdal, Sweden) dosimeter.

A more recent study by Hohl et al (2008) investigated the use of angular beam modulation (ABM, see Chapter 10) to reduce the dose in CT fluoroscopy. Their prospective study was done with an Alderson-Rando phantom using thermoluminescent dosimeters and a 64-slice volume CT scanner. Their results showed that the ABM technique reduced the effective dose to the patient by 35%, the skin dose by 75%, the breast dose by 47%, and the hand dose by between 27% and 72%. The authors conclude that "ABM leads to significant dose reduction for both patients and personnel during CT fluoroscopy-guided thoracic interventions, without impairing image quality."

APPLICATIONS IN RADIATION THERAPY: CT SIMULATION AND IMAGE FUSION

Radiation therapy is an interdisciplinary field based on not only radiation biology but also on physics, mathematics, and engineering. The goal of radiation therapy is to kill tumor cells (tumor volumes) by delivering maximum radiation dose to these cells with minimum dose to the surrounding healthy tissues, especially those that are highly radiosensitive, such as the gonads, eyes, and thyroid, for example.

Through the years radiation therapy has experienced significant technical developments intended to improve the clinical performance of radiation treatment schemes, including the use of imaging techniques to provide more accurate localization of tumor volumes (Kessler, 2006; Newbold et al, 2006; Schlegel et al, 2006) and guidance (Mah and Chen, 2008) and target delineation (Ahn and Garg, 2008). One such important milestone was the development of the CT scanner that became a significant tool in radiation treatment planning in the late 1970s. The fact that the CT scanner produces 3D images paved the way for 3D treatment planning that has now become an integral tool in radiation therapy. With these 3D images from the CT scanner, the tumor volumes can now be accurately localized with respect to the surrounding healthy tissues. In addition, the physical properties such as the electron densities of the tissues can be extracted from the 3D image data sets and are used to calculate radiation treatment doses.

This section of the chapter outlines the elements of the use of the CT scanner in radiation treatment planning through a technique referred to as *CT simulation*. The physical principles and technology of the CT scanner, image quality, quality assurance, and image processing including 3D imaging techniques, are covered in detail in the rest of this book.

CT Simulation Basics

The CT scanner is now used in the radiation oncology department and plays a role in the radiation treatment planning process. It is an integral part of the CT simulation process (Brunetti et al, 2008; Mutic et al, 2003).

Definition

As defined by Mutic et al (2003), CT simulation "is a geometric simulation process that provides beam arrangements and treatment fields without any dosimetric information." As shown in Figure 13-9, the CT simulator is coupled to the radiation treatment planning system to provide data for radiation dose calculation.

CT Simulator

The CT simulator is a CT scanner characterized by physical devices (hardware) and specialized software.

The hardware is a CT scanner, specifically a multislice CT scanner featuring all the major components (x-ray generator, x-ray tube, detector system, for example) as described in Chapter 12; however, there are several notable features that are different from a CT scanner used in diagnostic CT examinations. For example, this scanner has a flat tabletop with immobilization devices, a large bore (gantry aperture), a registration device, and a laser system. The flat tabletop and immobilization devices ensure that patients are scanned in exactly the same position as they would be when they are

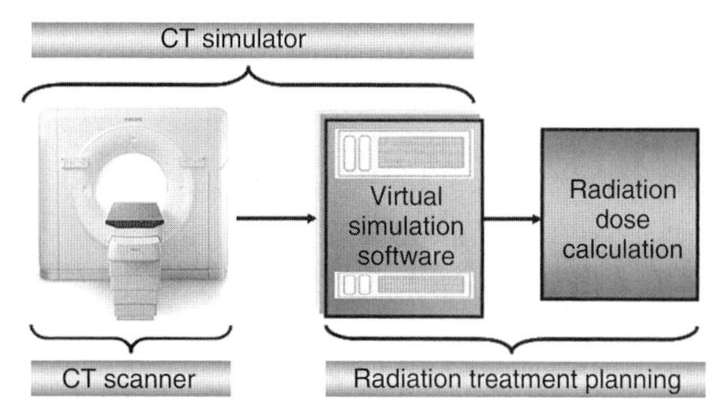

FIGURE 13-9 The CT simulator is coupled to the radiation treatment planning system to provide data for radiation dose calculation.

on the radiation treatment machine, and the large-bore (e.g., 85 cm) of the scanner accommodates patients in specific positions on the tabletop and enables the use of a large scan FOV. The registration device, on the other hand, ensures that the immobilization device on the CT scanner can be moved and used in exactly the same manner on the treatment machine. Finally, the laser system is intended to facilitate accurate positioning with the axes of the CT scanner.

The CT simulator also includes specialized software referred to as *virtual simulation* software. While the CT scanner acquires a volumetric data set from the patient and represents the "virtual" patient (or digital patient), the CT simulation software "provides virtual representations of the geometric capabilities of a treatment machine. This software can be a special virtual simulation program or it can be a component of a treatment planning system. Often CT simulation is referred to as virtual simulation and the two terms are used interchangeably. Virtual simulation is used to define any simulation based on the software created 'virtual simulator' and a volumetric patient scan. The scan does not necessarily have to be a CT and other imaging modalities can be used. A virtual simulator is a set of software which recreates the treatment machine and which allows import, manipulation, display, and storage of images from CT and/or other imaging modalities" (Mutic et al, 2003).

CT Simulation Process

The CT simulation process includes at least three steps (Fig. 13-10) as identified by Mutic et al (2003). These include the following:

1. *Scan the patient in the CT scanner.* The patient is positioned, immobilized, and scanned in exactly the same position that he or she would be on the

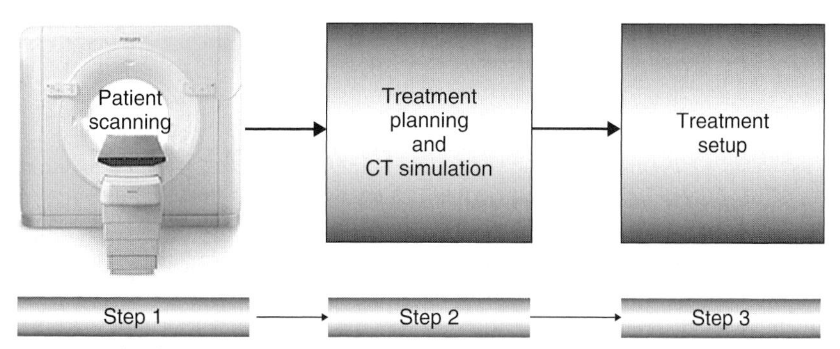

FIGURE 13-10 The three steps of the CT simulation process. See text for further explanation.

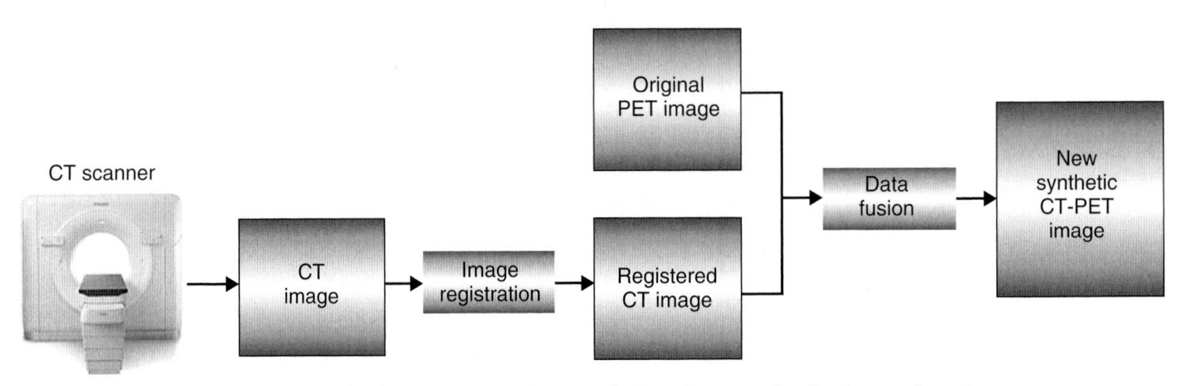

FIGURE 13-11 The basic process of image fusion. See text for further explanation.

treatment machine. The electron densities from the image data set obtained would be used to compute dose distributions.

2. *Plan the treatment and CT simulation.* This is where the beam placement and the treatment design are executed using the virtual simulation software, which includes "contouring of the target and normal structures, placement of the treatment isocenter and the beams, design of the treatment portal shapes" and the production of digitally reconstructed radiographs, and finally documentation. It is not within the scope of this section to describe these procedures; however, the interested reader should refer to Mutic et al (2003) for a description of each procedure.
3. *Treatment setup.* In this final step, the CT simulation software results are used to set up the patient in the treatment machine.

Image Fusion Overview

Anatomical images such as those from the CT scanner or an MRI scanner as well as functional images from nuclear medicine (positron emission tomography [PET]) and single-photon emission computed tomography [SPECT]) are now used in radiation therapy. The overall goal of using these images is to enhance the medical management of the radiation therapy patient (Brunetti et al, 2008; Kessler, 2006; Webb, 2003).

The information from both anatomical and functional images can now be combined using an image synthesis technique called image fusion. Image fusion is computer software that can integrate the image data from CT, MRI, PET, SPECT, and ultrasonography to produce fused images that now contain highly informative data. The basic process is illustrated in Figure 13-11. As can be seen, a technique referred to as *image registration* (establish the geometric relationships between the images) occurs before image fusion. Image registration is a complex process (Maintz and Viergever, 1998) and its principles are not within the scope of this book.

The clinical applications of image registration and image fusion range from treatment planning and treatment delivery to treatment adaptation and customization (Kessler, 2006).

FLAT-DETECTOR CT

The use of flat detectors or flat-panel digital detectors used in digital projection radiography and fluoroscopy is rapidly replacing image intensifier-based C-arm imaging systems that are used in a CT-like fashion in interventional and intraoperative medical imaging. A flat-panel C-arm imaging system is shown in Figure 13-12.

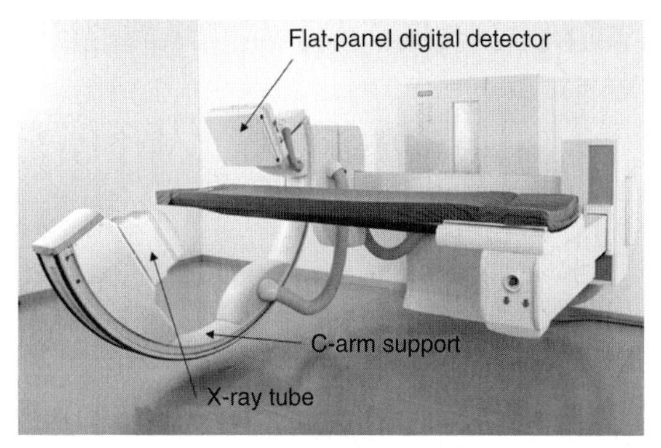

FIGURE 13-12 A C-arm imaging system using a flat-panel digital detector. The digital detector has replaced the image intensifier tube. (Photo courtesy General Electric Healthcare.)

Definition and Use

Flat-detector CT (FD-CT) refers to "CT imaging using C-arm systems built for radiography and fluoroscopy which are equipped with an FD and prepared to take projection data over an angular range of 180° or more" (Kalender and Kyriakou, 2007).

One of the early applications of using the principle of collecting data over 180 degrees (plus the fan angle of the x-ray beam) was with image intensifier-based C-arm units in interventional angiography (Fahrig et al, 2006). Although these units demonstrated high-contrast vascular structures after intra-arterial injection of contrast media with good spatial resolution, they failed to show low-contrast resolution characteristic of soft tissues. This limitation provided the motivational factors for replacing the image intensifier tube with the flat-panel digital detector used in digital radiography imaging systems.

FD-CT systems are now being used in interventional and intraoperative imaging, radiation therapy, maxillofacial scanning, micro-CT imaging (micro-CT scanners are now being used to image small animals), breast CT imaging, and in a physical setup where they are incorporated in a standard CT gantry (Kalender and Kyriakou, 2007). It is not within the scope of this chapter to outline the details of these applications, and the interested reader should refer to the works of Kalender (2005) for more information. The use of FD-CT for breast imaging is reviewed briefly at the end of this chapter.

Technical Elements

Kalender and Kyriakou (2007) present an excellent technical overview of the major components of FD-CT systems. These include the x-ray tube, the digital detectors, image reconstruction, image quality, artifacts, and radiation dose. In summary they identify the following points as being noteworthy:

1. Table 13-2 presents a comparison of the "typical parameters" between MSCT and FD-CT. It is clear that there is a difference between the two technologies with respect to kVp, mA, generator power, focal spot size, rotation time, detector elements, field of measurement, slice thickness, and data rate.
2. Of the two flat-panel digital detectors (indirect and direct conversion detectors graphically illustrated in Fig. 13-13, *A* and *B*. respectively) used for digital radiography, the indirect conversion flat-panel detector is used in FD-CT systems.
3. The indirect conversion detector (Fig. 13-13, *A*) converts x-ray photons to light by using a cesium iodide (CsI) scintillation phosphor coupled to a photodiode thin film transistor (TFT) array. The photodiode receives the light from the CsI phosphor and converts it into electrical charges that are subsequently stored and read out as an electrical signal (analog signal) by the TFT array. This signal is then digitized by the analog-to-digital converters (ADCs) and sent to a digital computer for processing and image creation. As shown in Fig. 13-13, *A*, the CsI phosphor is arranged in

TABLE 13-2 Typical Parameters for Multislice and Flat-Detector Computed Tomography

	MSCT	FD-CT
Tube voltage (kilovolts)	80-140	50-125
Tube current (mA)	10-600	10-800
X-ray power (kilowatts)	20-100	10-80
Focal spot size (mm)	0.6-1.2	0.3-0.8
Rotation time (seconds)	0.33-1	5-20
Detector elements		
In fan direction	512-1024	512-2490
In z-direction	16-64	512-2490
Field of measurement (mm)		
In fan direction	500-700	100-250
In z-direction	2-40	100-200
Minimum slice thickness (mm)	0.6	0.1-0.3
Typical scintillator/thickness (mm)	Gd_2O_2S: 1.4	CsI: (T1) 0.4-0.8
Data rate (megabytes/second)	≤1000	≤60

Kalender WA, Kryiakou Y: Flat-detector computed tomography (FD-CT), *Eur Radiol* 17, 2767-2779, 2007. Reproduced with kind permission of Springer Science and Business Media and the authors.

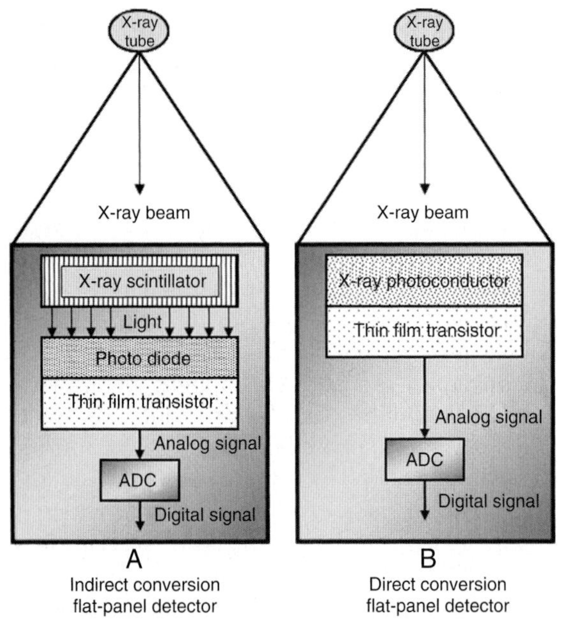

FIGURE 13-13 The basic design structure of two types of flat-panel digital detectors. The indirect conversion detector is shown in **A** and the direct conversion detector is shown in **B**. See text for further explanation.

a needlelike fashion (structured fashion) to reduce the lateral spread of light characteristic of a turbid phosphor. This spread of light (lateral dispersion) destroys the spatial resolution of the image. This problem is solved by the structured phosphor arrangement that improves the spatial resolution of the image.

4. The direct conversion flat-panel digital detector (Fig. 13-13, *B*) converts x-ray photons directly into electrical signals by using amorphous selenium (a-Se). There is no light conversion step. The a-Se detector has been used in some research units; however, it has not become commonplace in clinical FD-CT systems only because they "do not provide the necessary temporal resolution characteristics and dynamic capabilities" (Kalender and Kyriakou, 2007).
5. The beam from the x-ray tube that falls on a two-dimensional (2D) detector is a cone beam, and therefore a cone-beam algorithm, namely, the Feldkamp algorithm (Chapter 12) is used in the image reconstruction process.

6. Image quality can be discussed in terms of spatial resolution, noise, and contrast resolution. Although the spatial resolution for MSCT systems is about 1.2 lp/mm to 1.4 lp/mm (in the high resolution mode), the spatial resolution from FD-CT is about 1.5 lp/mm with a pixel binning (where pixels in a region, say $n \times n$ are combined and read out as one to increase frame rates and reduce noise). With no binning, the spatial resolution is 3.0 lp/mm. This is clearly illustrated in Figure 13-14.
7. Compared with MSCT detectors, the FD-CT detector has higher noise and reduced low-contrast resolution for a given dose. This is visually illustrated in Figure 13-15. To improve low-contrast detectability, the dose must be increased.
8. FD-CT is not an artifact-free imaging system. Artifacts can arise from beam hardening (see Chapter 9), defective detector elements, and metal present in the patient. Other artifacts such as cupping and truncation artifacts (see Chapter 9) are also possible. These artifacts however, can be corrected by using suitable correction algorithms.
9. The radiation dose from an FD-CT system is higher compared with that from a clinical CT study for the same image quality because the detection efficiency of the FD-CT detector is lower (Kalender and Kyriakou, 2007).

BREAST CT IMAGING

Mammography is still considered the best imaging modality for the early detection of cancer of the breast through its use as a screening tool (Boone et al, 2004; Glick et al, 2007). Apart from the screening tool advantage, mammography offers high spatial resolution that is critical in demonstrating microcalcifications and masses located in adipose tissue (Glick et al, 2007), but mammography has some drawbacks. These include its poor performance in imaging dense breasts and the superimposition of structures, which is a common problem in projection imaging where a 3D object (the breast) is projected as a 2D image. Such superimposition can create detection problems for the observer.

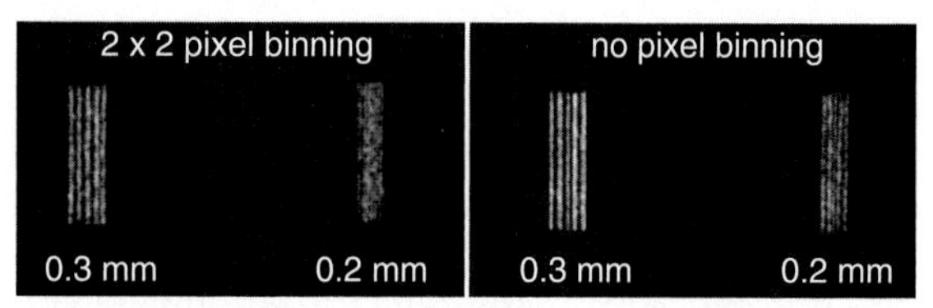

FIGURE 13-14 The visual effect of combining (binning) the pixels on spatial resolution of the FD-CT detector with bar resolution test pattern. No binning of the pixels results in better spatial resolution (sharper bar patterns). (From Kalender WA, Kryiakou Y: Flat-detector computed tomography [FD-CT], *Eur Radiol* 17, 2767-2779, 2007. Reproduced with kind permission of Springer Science and Business Media and the authors.)

Early CT Mammography

In the mid 1970s, General Electric Healthcare (formerly General Electric Medical Systems, Milwaukee, Wis.) built two research prototype CT scanners for mammography (CT/M), one of which was installed at the Mayo Clinic and the other at the University of Kansas Medical Center.

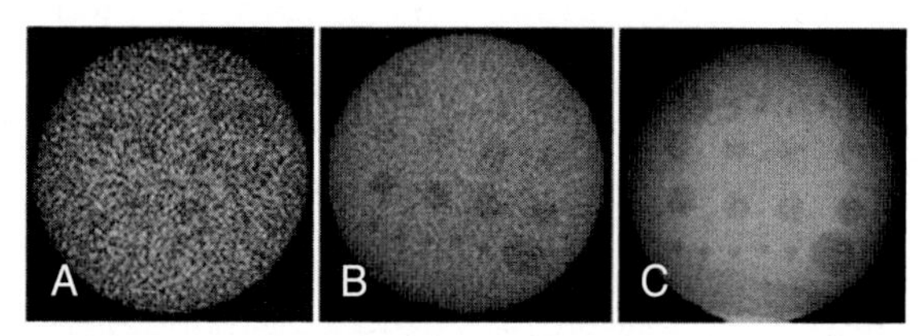

FIGURE 13-15 The detectability of low-contrast details depends on reconstruction parameters and dose. **A** and **B**, High- and low-resolution reconstructions are associated with high and low noise, respectively. **C**, An increase of dose compared with **A** and **B** leads to lower noise and results in improved low-contrast detectability. (From Kalender WA, Kryiakou Y: Flat-detector computed tomography [FD-CT], *Eur Radiol* 17, 2767-2779, 2007. Figure and legend reproduced with kind permission of Springer Science and Business Media and the authors.)

Researchers at these two facilities conducted clinical efficacy studies of the CT/M systems.

The CT/M unit used a continuously rotating fan beam (26 degrees), a water box, and an array of xenon detectors. Operating at 116 kVp and 30 mA, the absorption values from the breast ranged from −127 to +127 with water being assigned the value of zero (Gisvold et al, 1979). The patient was placed in a prone position and the breast inserted into a hole cut into the tabletop. The breast was lowered into the water box and immersed in water for scanning. X-ray transmissions readings were recorded, and images were reconstructed by the already established fan-beam algorithms typical of conventional diagnostic CT scanners in clinical use. Reconstructed images were displayed on a 128 × 128 matrix with pixel dimensions of 1.5 mm × 1.5 mm (Gisvold et al, 1979).

Clinical studies conducted by Gisvold et al (1979) and Chang et al (1979) showed that "the spatial resolution of CT/M was poor and that the main feature used in interpreting results was the attenuation related measure. With infusion of contrast material, CT/M was capable or revealing clinically and mammographically occult malignancy but was not considered suitable for routine screening of asymptomatic women. The reconstructed images of the original CT/M were prone to artifacts caused by the long scanning time: the lower detectability of small lesions was due to the large slice thickness and poor spatial resolution" (Chen and Ning, 2002).

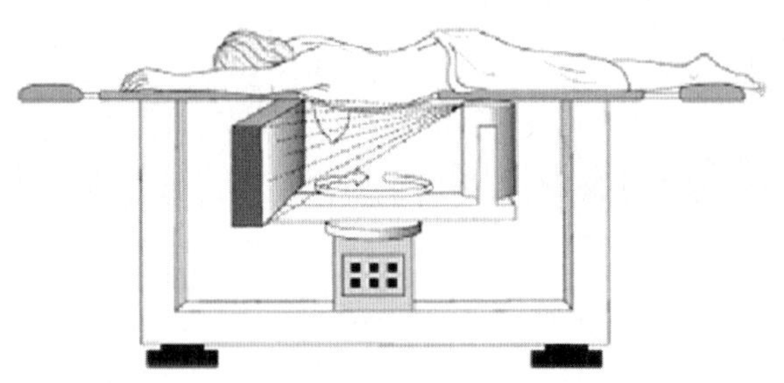

FIGURE 13-16 The basic design framework for an FD-CT scanner for breast imaging on the basis of pendant geometry. See text for further explanation. (From Glick SJ et al: Evaluating the impact of x-ray spectral shape on image quality in flat-panel CT breast imaging, *Med Phys* 34:5-9, 2007. Reproduced by permission of the American Association of Physicists in Medicine.)

Major Technical Components

Interest in developing dedicated breast CT scanners using FD detector technology surfaced as early as 2001 (Boone et al, 2004). The advantages offered by FD technology such as wide dynamic range, high spatial resolution, excellent linearity, high detective quantum efficiency, and no geometric distortion provide a good rationale for using them in the design of FD-CT scanners for breast imaging (Chen and Ning, 2002).

The basic design framework for an FD-CT scanner for breast imaging, shown in Figure 13-16, is based on what is referred to as a pendant geometry cone-beam CT imaging system. The major system components include an x-ray tube coupled to a flat-panel digital detector and a tabletop with a hole cut in it. Although the x-ray tube is designed to produce an x-ray beam optimized for breast imaging with appropriate target materials, filters, and beam intensity (lowered kVp and mAs compared with MSCT scanners) (Boone et al, 2004; Chen and Ning, 2002; Glick et al, 2007; Shaw et al, 2005), the flat-panel detector in most systems is a CsI amorphous silicon TFT digital radiography detector. The FD-CT scanner for imaging the breast shown in Figure 13-17 uses a 14-bit (2^{14}) 40 cm × 30 cm CsI amorphous silicon TFT digital detector.

The patient is placed in a prone position on the tabletop and the breast to be scanned is inserted through the hole to hang during the imaging process by use of a cone beam wide enough to cover the detector, as shown in Figure 13-16. This geometry is referred to as *pendant geometry* (Boone et al, 2007), and it prevents exposure of the chest cavity. The x-ray tube and detector are positioned close to the underside of the tabletop and rotate around the hanging breast. X-ray transmission readings are collected, digitized, and subsequently sent to the computer for image reconstruction with use of the Feldkamp cone-beam algorithm (see Chapter 12).

Research Studies

To date, a number of research studies have been conducted to evaluate the physical imaging parameters of the FD-CT breast scanner, such as the dose and image quality (Boone, 2001; Boone et al, 2004; Chen and Ning, 2002; Glick et al, 2007; Kwan et al, 2007; Shaw et al, 2005). It is beyond the scope of this section to elaborate on the results of these studies, and therefore the interested reader should refer to them for details of the findings with respect to each of these parameters.

In conclusion, Shaw et al (2005) showed that "the 3D nature of the image data may help eliminate interference from overlapping structures and allow lesions to be better defined and localized for biopsy or needle localization procedures. This suggests that cone beam CT breast imaging is a potentially powerful tool for diagnosis and management of breast cancers."

CT SCREENING

Definition

The use of any medical technology for early detection of disease in healthy (asymptomatic) people is referred to as screening. In particular, the use of CT technology for the early detection of diseases in asymptomatic patients is popularly referred to a CT screening (Beinfield, et al, 2005; Brant-Zawadzki, 2002; Brenner, 2006; Furtado et al, 2005; Horton et al, 2004; NY-ELCAP Investigators, 2007).

Rationale

Several investigators have provided the rationale for CT screening; it is fundamentally based on the increased prevalence of various types of high-risk diseases that may cause death to the population (Brant-Zawadzki, 2002). The increasing availability and ease of use of CT imaging has also provided a basis for its use as a screening tool.

Although there are those who support the use of CT as a screening tool, there are others who are vehemently opposed to its use in screening asymptomatic individuals. In this regard, therefore, CT screening "has generated significant controversy" (Horton et al, 2004), and it is not within the scope of this book to outline the elements of the controversy. The interested reader may refer to the various references cited in this section for an elaboration of the controversy.

Applications

The literature exploring the use of CT screening continues to increase from 2002 to the present. CT screening has been used in lung cancer screening, colon screening, coronary artery disease screening, and whole-body screening of healthy individuals. Although clinical efficacy studies have been performed on the first three mentioned previously to provide tangible justification for

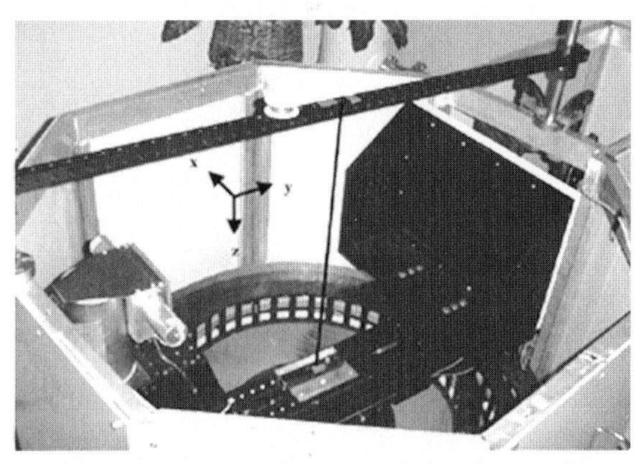

FIGURE 13-17 An inside view of the flat-panel CsI amorphous silicon TFT digital radiography detector used in the FD-CT scanner for imaging the breast. (From Kwan ALC et al: Evaluation of the spatial resolution characteristics of a cone-beam breast CT scanner, *Med Phys* 34:275-281, 2007. Reproduced by permission of the American Association of Physicists in Medicine.)

the use of CT screening, the latter (whole-body screening) remains a highly controversial subject (Brenner, 2006). The reason is that no studies (at the time of writing this chapter) have clearly demonstrated that whole-body CT screening has extended the life of individuals (Brenner, 2006).

Radiation Doses

Personnel working in radiology operate within the ALARA philosophy that requires that the dose to the patient should be kept as low as possible. To operate effectively within this philosophy, operators are now concerned with dose/image quality optimization, a procedure that ensures that the use of low doses does not compromise the image quality needed to make a diagnosis.

In addressing the dose issues in imaging asymptomatic individuals by CT screening, one notable expert, Dr. David Brenner, PhD, DSc, provides the radiological community with the following statement: "...the radiation exposure issues that relate to CT-based mass screening are unique. It is true, of course, that mammography also involves the use of x-rays, but the radiation doses involved are generally much higher for CT-based screening than for mammography. Thus, in addition to the more general efficacy issues discussed... the potential benefits of any CT-based screening procedure must far outweigh any potential harm from repeated low-dose x-ray exposures" (Brenner, 2006).

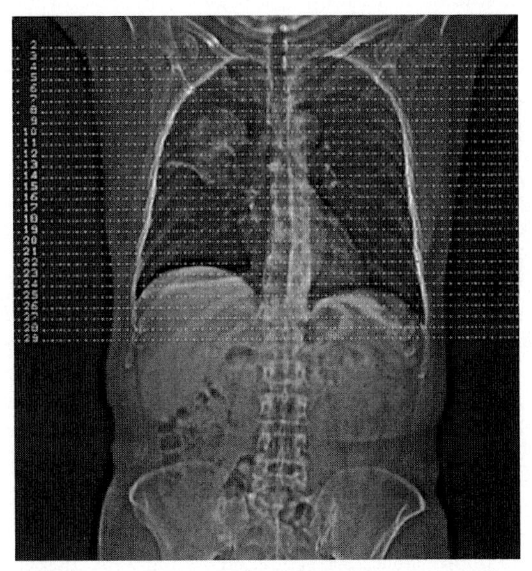

FIGURE 13-18 Prescan localization image produced when the patient moves continuously through the gantry while the x-ray tube and detectors remain in a fixed position. (Courtesy Siemens Medical Systems, Iselin, NJ.)

QUANTITATIVE CT

Quantitative CT is the most sensitive of all x-ray techniques for the measurement of the mineral content of trabecular bone in osteoporosis. This measurement is the bone mineral density (Kalender, 2005). Quantitative CT involves at least seven steps, as follows:

1. A prescan localization image is obtained (Fig. 13-18). This is sometimes referred to as a *scout view* (General Electric), or *topogram* (Siemens). The image is obtained as the patient moves through the gantry aperture while the x-ray tube and detector remain stationary. The computer then builds an image that resembles a conventional radiographic image.
2. The slices are selected from the prescan localization image, and the midvertebral planes are examined.
3. Transverse axial images are obtained. At this time, a reference phantom (Fig. 13-19, *A*) that contains water and bone-equivalent parts is positioned and scanned with the patient (Fig. 13-19, *B*).
4. An automatic contour tracing of trabecular and cortical regions of interest (ROI) is obtained (Fig. 13-20).
5. The computer calculates the mean values of the ROI.
6. The ROI values are converted to bone mineral density values.
7. An image graphics output is obtained, which shows the bone mineral density values plotted as

a function of age. The bone mineral content is then determined and compared with normal values.

PORTABLE MULTISLICE CT IMAGING

Rationale

Several problems are associated with transporting patients to a fixed CT scanner: (1) the risks of transporting unstable patients, (2) the costs associated with the workload of staff who are involved in patient transportation, and (3) the maintenance of the nurse-to-patient ratio in critical care. These problems are solved by using portable CT scanners. These scanners can be transported to critically ill patients in the intensive care unit, for example, to the emergency department, to the operating room, and other areas of the hospital where these patients are cared for. In addition, these scanners can be used in private medical facilities as well, to image ambulatory and other patients seen for various CT examinations.

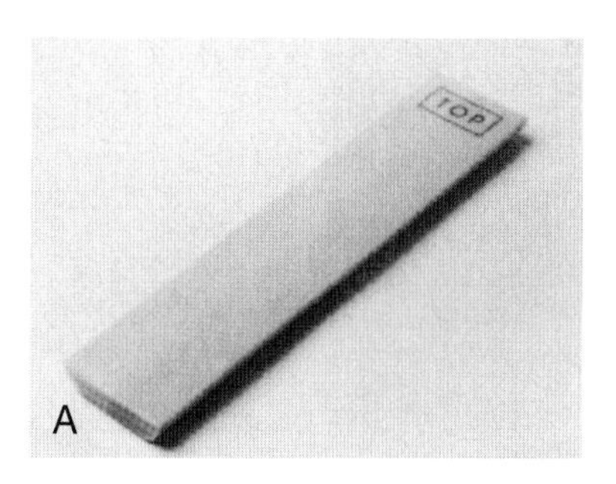

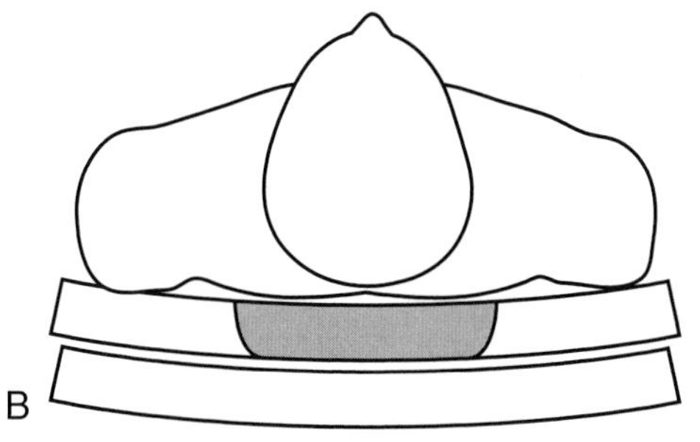

FIGURE 13-19 Reference phantom **(A)** and its position in relation to the patient **(B)** for QCT.

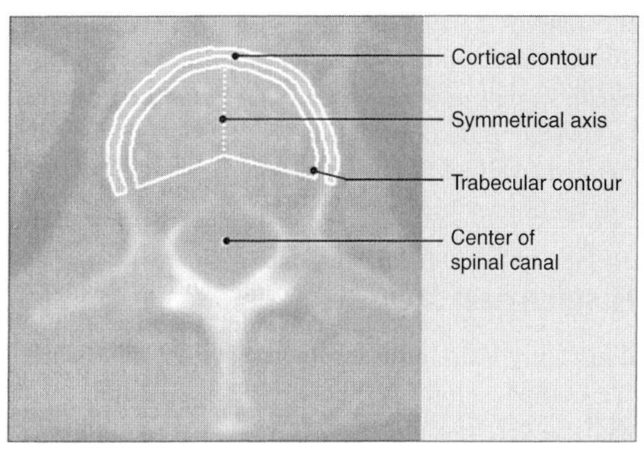

FIGURE 13-20 Automatic contour tracing of trabecular and cortical regions of interest. (From Nagel W et al: Recent clinical results on the use of QCT in diagnosis of osteoporosis, *Electromedica* 55:104-110, 1987.)

Physical Principles

Portable multislice CT scanners are now commercially available from the NeuroLogica Corporation (Danvers, Mass.) specifically for imaging critically ill patients and other patients in the hospital who cannot be easily transported to the radiology department for examination by fixed CT scanners. The NeuroLogica Corporation has developed portable multislice (eight slices/revolution) CT scanners (CereTom) specifically designed for imaging anatomy that can fit into a 25-cm scan FOV, namely, the head and neck. The scanners therefore have been designed to image the brain, the neck up to the fifth cervical vertebrae (C5), and the ear, nose, and throat. In addition, CT perfusion, and xenon CT studies can be done on these portable multislice CT scanners.

The CereTom portable CT scanner is based on the same physical principles as fixed multislice CT scanners with up to eight detector rows (see Chapter 12). The goal of the portable CT scanner is to produce diagnostic quality images that are based on x-ray attenuation data collected from the patient and measured by multirow detectors. The detectors convert the x-ray photons into electrical signals (analog data) that are subsequently converted into digital data by the detector electronics (ADCs). The digital data are then sent to the computer for image reconstruction.

Instrumentation

The CereTom portable multislice CT scanners are compact, lightweight, high speed, battery and wall-powered scanners that can be transported to any point of care. The scanner is characterized by three major equipment components: a compact CT gantry (Fig. 13-21), a silhouette scan board that is made of carbon fiber, and a laptop computer workstation/cart.

General System Requirements

The general system requirements can be described in terms of site requirements (space, room, temperature, and humidity) and installation requirements (power requirements and minimum line current ratings).

The CereTom portable CT scanner does not require any special electrical considerations because it can operate with single-phase alternating current power and 110- to 120-volt wall power outlets operating at 60 Hertz. In case of a power failure, the scanner is equipped with an independent

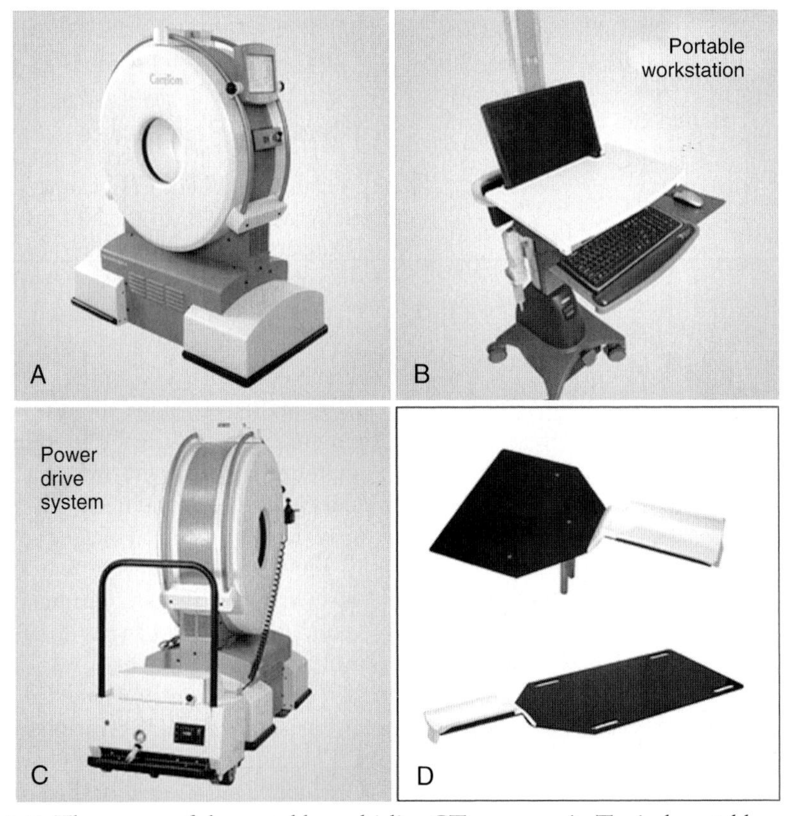

FIGURE 13-21 The gantry of the portable multislice CT scanner. **A,** Typical portable workstation. **B,** Power drive system. **C,** Scan boards to convert the patient's bed into a scanning platform **(D).** (Courtesy NeuroLogica, Danvers, Mass.)

battery power source that can last 2 hours (no scans) when fully charged.

Gantry Characteristics

The CereTom portable CT gantry (see Fig. 13-21) houses the x-ray tube, generator, detectors, and detector electronics. The detector electronics play an important role in analog-to-digital conversion and digital data transmission to the minicomputer system, which is responsible for image reconstruction and image processing.

The gantry characteristics of the CereTom portable CT scanner include the gantry aperture with an opening of 32 cm to accommodate the patient's anatomy. Furthermore, the gantry will not tilt and therefore patient positioning is used to deal with views that require a gantry tilt. As mentioned earlier, the maximum scan FOV is 25 cm to accommodate examinations of the head, face, and neck.

The gantry also houses the x-ray tube with a fixed anode having a focal spot size of 1 mm × 1 mm and a maximum cooling of 2 minutes, and it can operate at tube currents between 1 and 7 mA and at 100, 120, and 140 kVp. The beam emerging from the x-ray tube is a cone beam because an eight-slice multirow solid-state detector system is used. Therefore, image reconstruction follows that described for cone-beam CT scanners using up to eight detector rows, as described in Chapter 12.

The CereTom portable CT scanner is based on the third-generation CT design concept, in which the x-ray tube is coupled to the multidetector row system that can provide slice thicknesses of 1.25, 2.5, 5, and 10 mm. Both the x-ray tube and detectors rotate at the same time during data collection.

Operator's Laptop Computer Workstation

An integral component of the CereTom portable CT scanner system is the operator's console, which is a DICOM (digital imaging and communication in medicine) compliant gigabit Ethernet networked laptop computer workstation with wireless connectivity to PACS (picture archiving and communication system). In addition, a 20-inch liquid crystal display monitor is available with a display matrix of 1920 × 1200. The CT number range with this scanner is between −1024 and 3071, featuring both variable and preset windows.

The workstation allows the operator to select scan protocols and window settings optimized from specific protocols. The operator can also perform several image processing functions such as advanced 3D visualization (targeted, segmentation, MIP) and MPR (sagittal, coronal, axial, curved and sliding slab) and so on, as shown in Figure 13-22.

Imaging Performance

The imaging performance of the CereTom portable CT scanner can be described in terms of spatial resolution, contrast resolution, noise, and radiation dose considerations. NeuroLogica provided the data presented later.

Spatial Resolution

Spatial resolution refers to the ability of the scanner to image fine detail, measured in lp/cm. Several figures for spatial resolution have been reported for the CereTom portable CT scanner and the user should refer to the manufacturer product data for these numbers. For example, spatial resolution has been reported to be 7.4 lp/cm at 10% modulation transfer function (MTF) to 12.2 lp/cm at 10% MTF depending on the reconstruction kernel and the windowing used.

Contrast Resolution

Contrast resolution refers to the ability of the scanner to demonstrate small differences in tissue contrast. The contrast resolution of the CereTom portable CT scanner has been measured by using an 8-inch Catphan phantom with 10-mm slice thickness at 15 mAs and 140 kVp and has been reported to be 3 mm at 0.3%.

Noise

Image quality from the mobile CT scanner is also affected by noise. In CT, *noise* refers to the

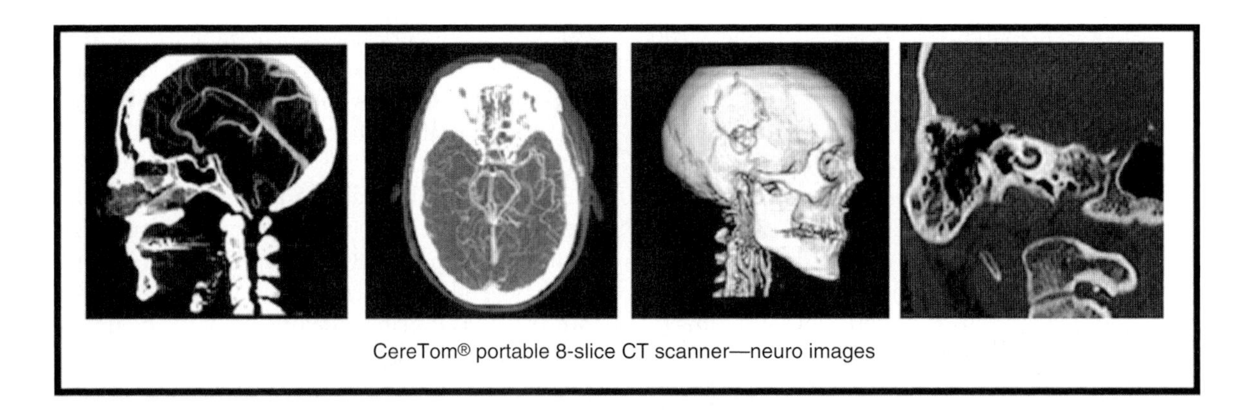
CereTom® portable 8-slice CT scanner—neuro images

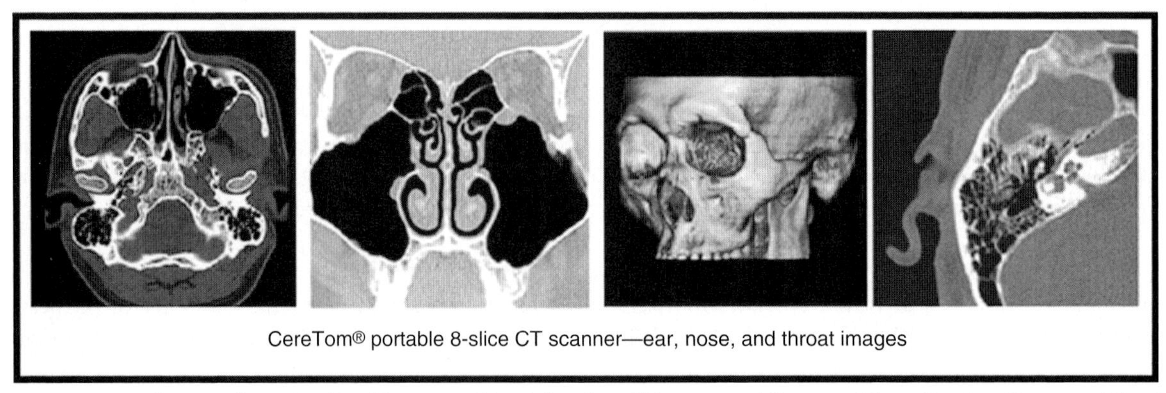
CereTom® portable 8-slice CT scanner—ear, nose, and throat images

FIGURE 13-22 Images from the CereTom portable eight-slice CT scanner. (Courtesy NeuroLogica, Danvers, Mass.)

fluctuation of CT numbers between points in the image for a scan of uniform material such as water. The *noise level* is a percentage of contrast in CT numbers. The noise level of the CereTom portable CT scanner is 0.3% at 15 mAs and 140 kVp with a 10-mm slice thickness.

CT Dose Index

Manufacturers of CT scanners are now required by law to provide the CT dose index (CTDI) for their scanners. For the CereTom portable CT scanner, with a head phantom only (because of the small CereTom patient aperture) at 120 kV, 14 mAs, 2-second scan time, and a 10-mm aperture, the CTDI for the center and surface of the head phantom is 35.8 and 46.64 mGy, respectively.

Scattered Radiation Considerations

As in any portable x-ray imaging procedure, scattered radiation from the portable CT scanner concerns radiation workers and those individuals working in areas in which portable CT examinations are performed. For the CereTom portable CT scanner, the scatter radiation in general at 1 meter from the scanner is about 2 milliroentgens.

REFERENCES

Ahn PH, Garg MK: Positron emission tomography/computed tomography for target delineation in head and neck cancers, *Semin Nucl Med* 38:141-148, 2008.

Beinfield MT et al: Cost effectiveness of whole-body CT screening, *Radiology* 234:415-422, 2005.

Blobel J et al: Heart rate adaptive multisegment image reconstruction in diagnostic cardiac computed tomography, *Visions* 12:12-16, 2008.

Boone JM et al: Dedicated breast CT: radiation dose and image quality evaluation, *Radiology* 221:657-667, 2001.

Boone JM et al: A comprehensive analysis of DgN(CT) coefficients for pendant-geometry cone-beam breast computed tomography, *Med Phys* 31:226-235, 2004.

Brant-Zawadzki MN: Screening CT: rationale, *Radiographics* 22:1532-1539, 2002.

Brenner DJ: Radiation risks in diagnostic radiology. In Huda W, editor: *RSNA categorical course in diagnostic radiology physics: from invisible to visible—the science and practice of x-ray imaging and radiation dose optimization*, pp 41-50, Oakridge, 2006, Radiological Society of North America.

Brunetti J et al: Technical aspects of positron emission tomography/computed tomography fusion planning, *Semin Nucl Med* 38:129-136, 2008.

Carlson SK et al: Benefits and safety of CT fluoroscopy in interventional radiologic procedures, *Radiology* 219:515-520, 2001.

Carlson SK et al: CT fluoroscopy-guided biopsy of the lung or upper abdomen with a breath-hold monitoring and feedback system: a prospective randomized controlled clinical trial, *Radiology* 237:701-708, 2005.

Chang CH et al: Specific value of computed tomography breast scanner (CT/M) in diagnosis of breast diseases, *Radiology* 132:647-652, 1979.

Chen B, Ning R: Cone-beam volume CT breast imaging: feasibility study, *Med Phys* 29:755-770, 2002.

Daly B, Templeton PA: Real-time CT fluoroscopy: evolution of an interventional tool, *Radiology* 211: 309-315, 1999.

Ebert DS et al: Evaluating the potential and problems of three-dimensional computed tomography measurements of arterial stenosis, *J Dig Imag* 11:1-8, 1998.

Fahrig R et al: Dose and image quality for a cone-beam C-arm CT system, *Med Phys* 33:4541-4550, 2006.

Froelich JJ et al: Guidance of non-vascular interventional procedures with real-time CT-fluoroscopy, *Electromedica* 66:50-55, 1997.

Furtado CD et al: Whole-body CT screening: spectrum of findings and recommendations in 1192 patients, *Radiology* 237:385-394, 2005.

Gisvold JJ et al: Computed tomographic mammography (CT/M), *AJR Am J Roentgenol* 133:1143-1149, 1979.

Glick SJ et al: Evaluating the impact of x-ray spectral shape on image quality in flat-panel CT breast imaging, *Med Phys* 34:5-9, 2007.

Gupta R et al: Computed tomography angiography in stroke imaging: fundamental principles, pathologic findings, and common pitfalls, *Semin Ultrasound CT MRI* 27:221-242, 2006.

Hohl C et al: Dose reduction during CT fluoroscopy: phantom study of angular beam modulation, *Radiology* 246:525-530, 2008.

Horton KM et al: CT screening: principles and controversies. In Fishman EK, Jeffrey B, editors: *Multidetector CT: principles, techniques, and clinical applications*, pp 549-559, Philadelphia, 2004, Lippincott Williams & Wilkins.

Hsieh J et al: Step-and-shoot data acquisition and reconstruction for cardiac x-ray computed tomography, *Med Phys* 33:4236-4248, 2006.

Johnson PT et al: Interactive three-dimensional volume rendering of spiral CT data, current applications in the thorax, *Radiographics* 18:165-1987, 1998.

Kalender W: *Computed tomography: fundamentals, system technology, image quality, applications*, GWA, Germany, 2005, Publicis Corp. Publishing.

Kalender WA, Kryiakou Y: Flat-detector computed tomography (FD-CT), *Eur Radiol* 17:2767-2779, 2007.

Katada K et al: Guidance with real-time CT fluoroscopy: early clinical experience, *Radiology* 200: 851-856, 1996.

Kataoka ML et al: Multiple-image in-room imaging guidance for interventional procedures, *Radiology* 239:863-868, 2006.

Kato R et al: Radiation dosimetry at CT fluoroscopy: physician's hand dose and development of needle holders, *Radiology* 201:576-578, 1996.

Keat N: Real-time CT and CT fluoroscopy, *Br J Radiol* 74:1088-1090, 2001.

Kessler ML: Image registration and data fusion in radiation therapy, *Br J Radiol* 79:S99-S108, 2006.

Kuszyk BS, Fishman EK: Technical aspects of CT angiography, *Semin Ultrasound CT MRI* 19:383-393, 1998.

Kuszyk BS et al: Neurovascular applications of CT angiography, *Semin Ultrasound CT MRI* 19:394-404, 1998.

Kwan ALC et al: Evaluation of the spatial resolution characteristics of a cone-beam breast CT scanner, *Med Phys* 34:275-281, 2007.

Lell MM et al: New techniques in CT angiography, *Radiographics* 26:S45-S62, 2006.

Mah D, Chen CC: Image guidance in radiation oncology treatment planning: the role of imaging technologies on the planning process, *Semin Nucl Med* 38:114-118, 2008.

Mahesh M, Cody DD: Physics of cardiac imaging with multiple-row detector CT, *Radiographics* 27:1495-1509, 2007.

Maintz JB, Viergever MA: A survey of medical image registration, *Med Image Anal* 2:1-36, 1998.

Mutic S et al: Quality assurance for computed tomography simulators and computed tomography-simulation process: report of the AAPM Radiation Therapy Committee Task Group No 66, *Med Phys* 30:2762-2792, 2003.

Nawfel RD et al: Patient and personnel exposure during CT fluoroscopy-guided interventional procedures, *Radiology* 216:180-184, 2000.

Newbold K et al: Advanced imaging applied to radiotherapy planning in head and neck cancer: a clinical review, *Br J Radiol* 79:554-561, 2006.

Oldendorf M, Weber P: Postprocessing techniques in CT angiography, *Electromedica* 65:21-26, 1997.

Ozaki M: Development of a real-time reconstruction system for CT fluorography, *Med Rev* 53:12-17, 1995.

Paulson EK et al: CT fluoroscopy-guided interventional procedures: techniques and radiation dose to radiologists, *Radiology* 220:161-167, 2001.

Pomerantz SR et al: Computed tomography angiography and computed tomography perfusion in ischemic stroke: a step-by-step approach to image acquisition and three-dimensional postprocessing, *Semin Ultrasound CT MRI* 29:243-270, 2006.

Prat-Gonzalez S et al: Cardiac CT: indications and limitations, *J Nucl Med Technol* 36:18-24, 2008.

Rawlings LH: Non-invasive cardiovascular imaging: focus on spiral CT angiography, *Appl Radiol* March 12:28-32, 1995.

Schlegel W et al, editor: *New technologies in radiation oncology*, New York, 2006, Springer.

Schoepf UJ et al: Coronary CT angiography, *Radiology* 244:48-63, 2007.

Shaw CC et al: Cone beam breast CT with a flat panel detector—simulation, implementation, and demonstration. In *Proceedings of the IEEE, Engineering in Medicine and Biology 27th Annual Conference*, pp 4461-4464, Hong Kong, China, 2005, The Conference.

Tanenbaum LN: Helical MCCT angiography: tips and techniques, *Appl Radiol* 4:3-10, 2006.

Wagner LK: CT fluoroscopy: another advancement with additional challenges in radiation management, *Radiology* 216:9-10, 2000.

Webb S: The physical basis of IMRT and inverse planning, *Br J Radiol* 76:678-689, 2003.

Three-Dimensional Computed Tomography: Basic Concepts

Chapter Outline

Three-dimensional (3D) imaging in medicine is a method by which a set of data is collected from a 3D object such as the patient, processed by a computer, and displayed on a two-dimensional (2D) computer screen to give the illusion of depth. Depth perception causes the image to appear in three dimensions.

In the past, 3D imaging has created virtual endoscopy, a technique that allows the viewer to "fly through" the body in an effort to examine structures such as the brain, tracheobronchial tree, vessels, sinuses, and the colon (Rubin et al, 1996; Vining, 1996). Additionally, 3D medical reconstruction movie clips are now available on the Internet. Viewers can now "fly through" the colon, skull, brain, lung, torso, and the arteries of the heart. Additionally, 3D imaging unearthed a whole new dimension in examining contrast-filled vessels from volumetric spiral/helical computed tomography (CT) data and CT angiography (CTA), respectively. In radiology, 3D imaging has found applications in radiation therapy, craniofacial imaging for surgical planning, orthopedics, neurosurgery, cardiovascular surgery, angiography, and magnetic resonance imaging (MRI) (Calhoun et al, 1999; Udupa, 1999; Wu et al, 1999). Another use of 3D imaging has been in the visualization of ancient Egyptian mummies without destroying the plaster or bandages (Yasuda et al, 1992). CTA and virtual reality imaging are described in Chapters 13 and 15, respectively.

The advances in spiral/helical CT, such as the introduction of the new multislice CT scanners and MRI technologies, have resulted in an increasing use of 3D display of sectional anatomy. As a result, 3D imaging has become commonplace in most large-scale radiology departments, and researchers continue to explore the potential of 3D applications. For example, as early as 2002, Hoffman et al (2002) used 3D and virtual "fly-through" techniques as a "noninvasive research tool" to evaluate Egyptian mummies, and although Pickhardt (2004) presents research findings on the use of 3D images for the polyp detection in CT colonography, Macari and Bini (2005) review the current and future role of CT colonography. Recently, Dalrymple et al (2005) describe the technical aspects of 3D CT with multislice CT scanners and in particular review the basics of intensity projection techniques (described later in this chapter). In addition, Lawler et al (2005) describe the use of 3D postprocessing, available with multislice CT scanners, in the study of adult ureteropelvic junction obstruction, and Fayad et al (2005) discuss the use of 3D techniques to study musculoskeletal diseases of children. Furthermore, Beigleman-Aubry et al (2005) discuss the use of 3D to assess diffuse lung diseases.

More recently, several workers such as Fatterpekar et al (2006), Lell et al (2006), and Silva et al (2006) report the results of their 3D studies for evaluation of the temporal bone in CTA and virtual dissection at CT colonography, respectively. Additionally, Barnes (2006) reviews the advancement of medical image processing including 3D techniques in a series of three articles. He quotes Dr. Richard Robb, PhD, from the Mayo Clinic in Rochester, Minnesota, who states that "we're in a very exciting generation in medical imaging. We've got very exciting opportunities to contribute to the well-being of humans around the world because of the advances in medical imaging we have available to us."

This chapter describes the fundamental concepts of 3D imaging in CT to provide technologists with the tools needed to enhance their scope and interaction with 3D imaging systems that are becoming more commonplace in imaging and therapy departments in hospitals.

RATIONALE

The purpose of 3D imaging is to use the vast amounts of data collected from the patient by volume CT scanning (and other imaging modalities such as MRI, for example) to provide both qualitative and quantitative information in a wide range of clinical applications. Qualitative information is used to compare how observers perform on a specific task to demonstrate the diagnostic value of 3D imaging; quantitative information is used to assess three elements of the technique: precision (reliability), accuracy (true detection), and efficiency (feasibility) of the 3D imaging procedure (Russ 2006; Udupa and Herman, 2000).

HISTORY

In 1970 Greenleaf et al produced a motion display of the ventricles by using biplane angiography. Soon after, the commercial introduction of CT renewed interest in medical 3D images because it was clearly apparent that a stack of contiguous CT sectional images could generate 3D information. This idea resulted in the development of specialized hardware and software for the production of 3D images and the development of algorithms for 3D imaging.

Technologic developments in 3D imaging continued at a steady pace throughout the 1970s, and by the early 1980s many CT scanners featured 3D software as an optional package. In the early 1980s, 3D imaging was discovered to be useful for clinical applications when several researchers began using the technology in craniofacial surgery, orthopedics, radiation treatment planning, and cardiovascular imaging. The box at the bottom of the page summarizes the major developments in the evolution of 3D imaging to the year 1991. Today, 3D imaging has evolved as a discipline on its own, demanding an understanding of various image processing concepts such as preprocessing, visualization, manipulation, and analysis operations (Russ, 2006; Udupa and Herman, 2000).

FUNDAMENTAL THREE-DIMENSIONAL CONCEPTS

Coordinates and Terminology

To understand how 3D images are generated in medical imaging, it is necessary first to identify

Early History of Three-Dimensional Medical Imaging

- 1969—Hounsfield and Cormack develop the CT scanner.
- 1970—Greenleaf and colleagues report first biomedical 3D display: computer-generated oscilloscope images relating to pulmonary blood flow.
- 1972—First commercial CT scanner introduced.
- 1975—Ledley and colleagues report first 3D rendering of anatomic structures from CT scans.
- 1977—Herman and Liu publish 3D reconstructions of heart and lung of a dead frog.
- 1979—Herman develops technique to render bone surface in CT data sets; collaborates with Hemmy to image spine disorders.
- 1980—A CT scanner manufactured by General Electric features optional 3D imaging software.
- 1980-1981—Researchers begin investigating 3D imaging of craniofacial deformities.
- 1983—Commercial CT scanners begin featuring built-in 3D imaging software packages.
- 1986—Simulation software developed for craniofacial surgery.
- 1987—First international conference on 3D imaging in medicine organized in Philadelphia, Pennsylvania.
- 1990-1991—First textbooks on 3D imaging in medicine published; atlas of craniofacial deformities illustrated by 3D CT images published.

Adapted from Schwartz B: Computerized medical imaging, *Med Devices Res Rep* 1:8-10, 1994.

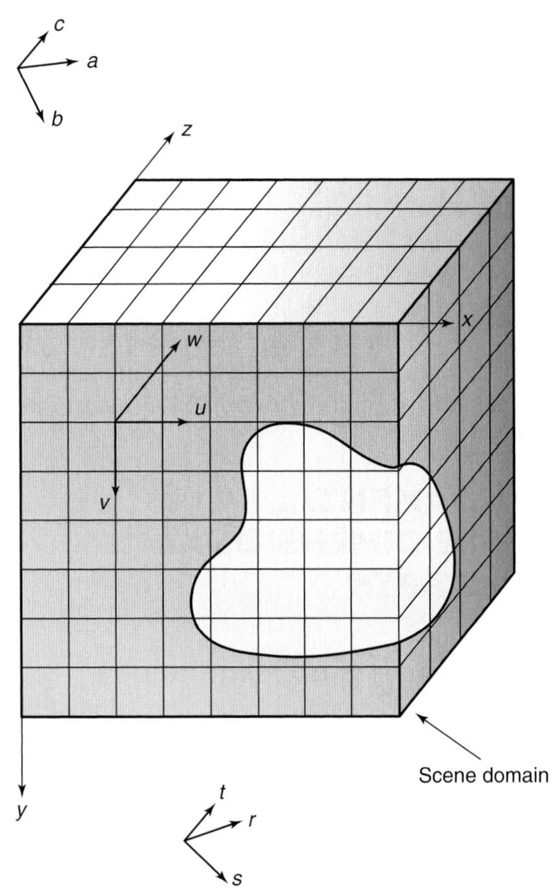

FIGURE 14-1 Drawing provides graphic representation of the four coordinates used in 3D imaging: *abc*, scanner coordinate system; *rst*, display coordinate system; *uvw*, object coordinate system; *xyz*, scene coordinate system.

and outline four coordinate systems that relate to the CT scanner, the display device, the object, and the scene. These coordinate systems are illustrated in Figure 14-1 and include the scanner coordinate system, *abc;* the display coordinate system, *rst;* the object coordinate system, *uvw;* and the scene coordinate system, *xyz*. Each of these is defined in Table 14-1.

The most familiar system is the xyz, the scene or Cartesian coordinate system, as it is commonly called. In this system, the x-, y-, and z-axes are positioned at right angles (orthogonal) to one another. The width of an object is described by the x-axis, whereas the height is described by the y-axis. The z-axis, on the other hand, describes the dimension of depth and adds perspective realism to the image.

Use of the coordinate system allows description of an object by measuring distances from the point of intersection, or zero point. Distances can be positive or negative from the zero point, and images can be manipulated to rotate about the three axes. This rotation occurs in what is referred to as *3D space*, and computer software helps the observer to view 3D space by displaying the front, back, top, and bottom of the object, providing a perspective from the observer's vantage point. The technique is known as *computer-aided visualization* or *3D visualization*, and the application of 3D visualization in medicine is called *3D medical imaging*.

In medicine, 3D imaging uses a right-handed x, y, and z coordinate system (Russ, 2006; Udupa and Herman, 2000) because images are displayed on a computer screen. The x, y, and z coordinates define a space in which multidimensional data (a set of slices) are represented. This space is called the *3D space* or *scene space*. The coordinate system helps to define the voxels (volume elements) in 3D space and allows use of the voxel information such as CT numbers or signal intensities in MRI to reconstruct 3D images.

Transforming Three-Dimensional Space

Generally, 3D space can be subjected to a series of common 3D transformations (Fig. 14-2). The radiologic technologist can manipulate scene, structure, geometric, and projective transformations and control image processing and image analysis. The technologist may transform 3D space in four ways (Table 14-2).

Modeling

The generation of a 3D object using computer software is called modeling. Modeling uses mathematics

TABLE 14-1 Frequently Used Terms in Three-Dimensional Medical Imaging

Term	Definition
Scene	Multidimensional image; rectangular array of voxels with assigned values
Scene domain	Anatomical region represented by the scene
Scene intensity	Values assigned to the voxels in a scene
Pixel size	Length of a side of the square cross-section of a voxel
Scanner coordinate system	Origin and orthogonal axes system affixed to the imaging device
Scene coordinate system	Origin and orthogonal axes system affixed to the scene (origin usually assumed to be upper left corner to first section of scene, axes are edges of scene domain that converge at the origin)
Object coordinate system	Origin and orthogonal axes system affixed to the object or object system
Display coordinate system	Origin and orthogonal axes system affixed to the display device
Rendition	2D image depicting the object information captured in a scene or object system

From Udupa J: Three-dimensional visualization and analysis methodologies: a current perspective, *Radiographics* 19:783-806, 1999.

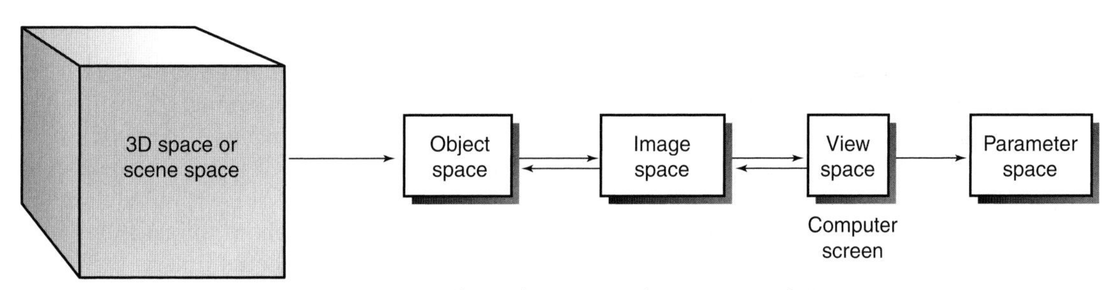

FIGURE 14-2 Sequence of transformations characteristic of 3D imaging.

TABLE 14-2 Transforming Three-Dimensional Space

Space Desired	Task Required
Image space	Translate, rotate, or scale scenes, objects, or surfaces
Object space	Extract structural information about the object from the 3D space
Parameter space	Take measurements from the image's view space on the computer screen
View space	View the 2D screen of the computer monitor

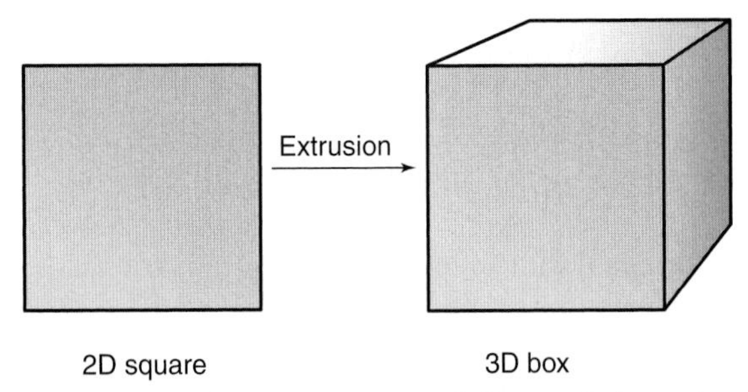

FIGURE 14-3 Extrusion is a modeling technique that generates a 3D object from a 2D profile on a computer screen.

to describe physical properties of an object. According to one definition, modeling is "a computer simulation of a physical object in which length, width, and depth are real attributes. A model, with x, y, and z axes can be rotated for viewing from different angles" (Microsoft Press, 2002).

Several modeling techniques are used. In extrusion, one of the most common techniques, computer software is used to transform a 2D profile into a 3D object. In Figure 14-3, for example, a square is changed into a box. Extrusion can also generate a wireframe model from a 2D profile. The wireframe is made up of triangles or polygons often referred to as *polygonal mesh*. Wireframes were common during the early development of 3D display in medicine, and they are still being used today in other applications.

During the next step of modeling, a surface is added to the object by placing a layer of pixels (image mapping) and patterns (procedural textures) on top of the wireframes. The radiologic technologist can control various attributes of the surface, such as its texture.

Shading and Lighting

Shading and lighting also add realism to the 3D object. There are several shading algorithms, including wireframe shading, flat shading, Gouraud shading, and Phong shading. Each technique has its own set of advantages and disadvantages; however, a full discussion of shading algorithms is outside the scope of this chapter. The interested reader should refer to Russ (2006) for detailed descriptions of these algorithms.

Although shading determines the final appearance of surfaces of the 3D object, lighting helps us to see the shape and texture of the object (Fig. 14-4). Various lighting techniques are available to enhance the appearance of the 3D image; one of the most common is called *ray tracing*, which is described later in this chapter.

Rendering

Rendering is the final step in the process of generating a 3D object. It involves the creation of the simulated 3D image from data collected from the object space. More specifically, *rendering* is a computer program that converts the anatomical data collected from the patient into the 3D image seen on the computer screen. With most 3D software, the object must be rendered before the effects of lighting and other attributes can be observed. Rendering therefore adds lighting, texture, and color to the final 3D image.

Two types of 3D rendering algorithms are used in radiology: surface rendering and volume rendering. Surface rendering uses only contour data from the set of slices in 3D space, whereas volume rendering makes use of the entire data set in 3D space. Because it uses more information, volume rendering produces a better image than surface rendering, but it takes longer and requires a more powerful computer. Rendering is described subsequently.

CLASSIFICATION OF THREE-DIMENSIONAL IMAGING APPROACHES

Udupa and Herman (2000) have identified three classes of 3D imaging approaches: slice imaging, projective imaging, and volume imaging.

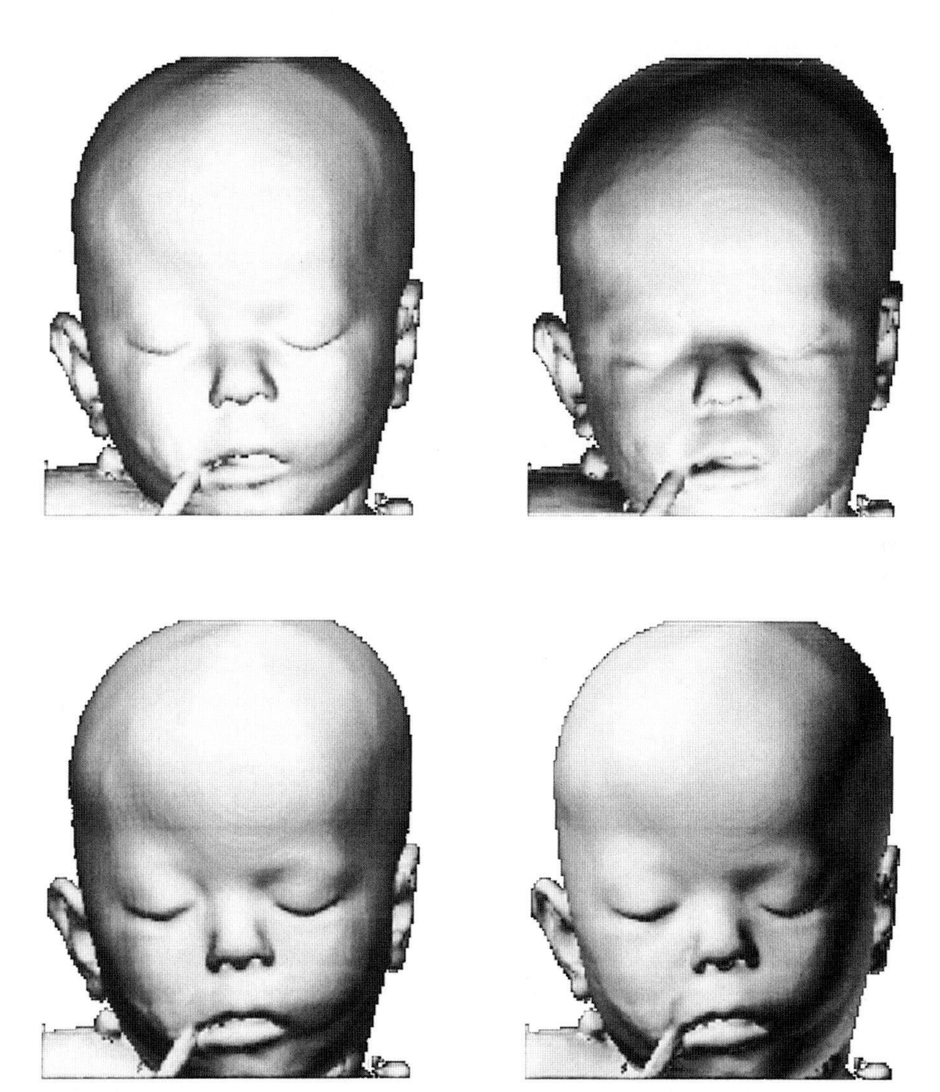

FIGURE 14-4 The effects of lighting in a surface-rendered 3D image. As the light source is moved to different locations, various features of the image become clearly apparent.

Slice Imaging

Slice imaging is the simplest method of 3D imaging. In 1975 CT operators generated and displayed coronal and sagittal images from the CT axial data set. This technique is known as *multiplanar reconstruction* (MPR). In the past, other researchers such as Herman and Liu (1977), Marvilla (1978), and Rhodes et al (1980) also used slice imaging to produce coronal, sagittal, and paraxial images from the transaxial scans. Today, MPR is available on all CT and MRI scanners. However, MPR does not produce true 3D images but rather 2D images displayed on a flat computer screen (Dalrymple et al, 2005).

Projective Imaging

Projective imaging is the most popular 3D imaging approach. However, it still does not offer a true 3D mode; it produces a "2.5 D" mode of visualization, an effect somewhere between 2D and 3D. As Udupa and Herman (2000) explain:

> Projective imaging deals with techniques for extracting multidimensional information from the given image data and for depicting such information in the 2D view space by a process of projection. Surface rendering and volume rendering are two major classes of approaches available under projective imaging.

The technique of projection is illustrated in Figure 14-5. The contiguous axial sections represent the volume image data. Information from this volume image data is projected at various angles into the 2D view space.

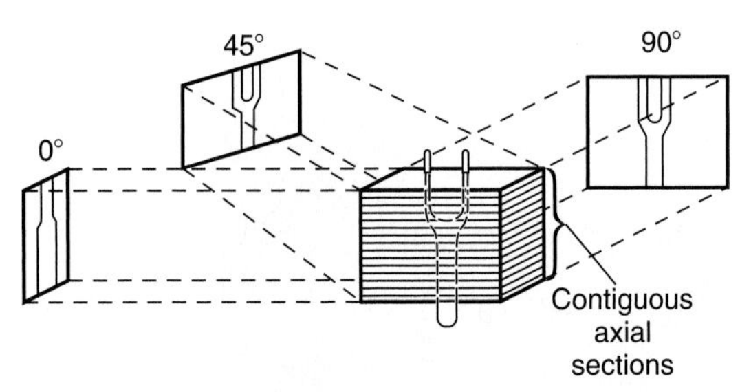

FIGURE 14-5 The technique of projection used in 3D imaging. This is a major characteristic of projective imaging (one class of 3D imaging techniques).

Volume Imaging

Volume imaging must not be confused with volume rendering. Volume rendering belongs to the class of projective imaging, whereas volume imaging produces a true 3D visualization mode. Volume imaging methods include holography, stereoscopic displays, anaglyphic methods, varifocal mirrors, synthalyzers, and rotating multidiode arrays (Jan, 2005). These methods are beyond the scope of this book.

GENERIC THREE-DIMENSIONAL IMAGING SYSTEM

In a recent article describing the current perspective of 3D imaging, Udupa and Herman (2000) provides a framework for a typical 3D imaging system (Fig. 14-6). Four major elements are noted: input, workstation, output, and the user. *Input* refers to devices that acquire data. Imaging input devices, for example, would include CT and MRI scanners. The acquired data are sent to the workstation, which is the heart of the system. This powerful computer can handle various 3D imaging operations. These operations include preprocessing, visualization, manipulation, and analysis. Once processing is completed, the results are displayed for viewing and recording onto output devices. Finally, the user can interact with each

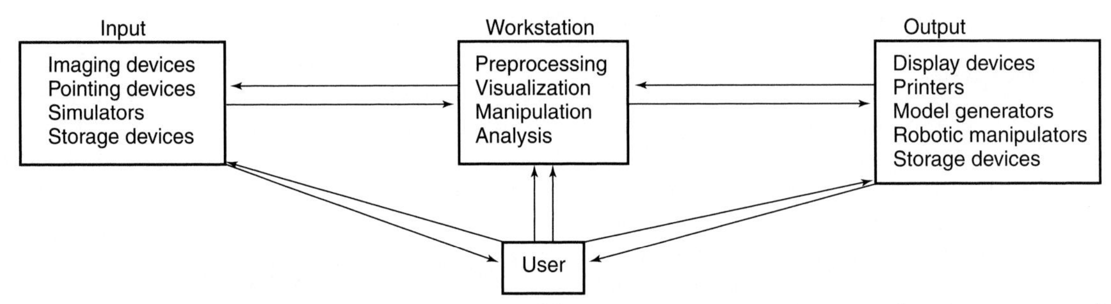

FIGURE 14-6 A typical 3D imaging system consists of four major components: input, workstation, output, and the user.

of the three components—input, workstation, and output—to optimize use of the system.

The goals of each of the four major 3D imaging operations and the commonly used processing techniques are summarized in Table 14-3.

TECHNICAL ASPECTS OF THREE-DIMENSIONAL IMAGING IN RADIOLOGY

Definition of Three-Dimensional Medical Imaging

Dr. Gabor Herman of the Medical Image Processing Group at the University of Pennsylvania defines 3D medical imaging as "the process that starts with a stack of sectional slices collected by some medical imaging device and results in computer-synthesized displays that facilitate the visualization of underlying spatial relationships" (Herman, 1993). Additionally, Udupa and Herman (2000) emphasize that the term *3D imaging* can also refer to the four categories of 3D operations: preprocessing, visualization, manipulation, and analysis.

Four steps are needed to create 3D images (see Fig. 14-6):

1. Data acquisition. Slices, or sectional images, of the patient's anatomy are produced. Methods of data acquisition in radiology include CT, MRI, ultrasound, positron emission tomography, single photon emission tomography, and digital radiography and fluoroscopy.
2. Creation of 3D space or scene space. The voxel information from the sectional images is stored in the computer.
3. Processing for 3D image display. This is a function of the workstation and includes the four operations listed previously.
4. 3D image display. The simulated 3D image is displayed on the 2D computer screen.

These four steps vary slightly depending on which imaging modality is used to acquire the data. Each of the four steps is described in detail, using CT as the method of data acquisition.

TABLE 14-3 Goals of Various Operations for Three-Dimensional Medical Imaging

Classes of 3D Operations	Goals	Commonly Used Operations	Goals
Preprocessing	To take a set of scenes and output computer object models or another set of scenes from the given set, which facilitates the creation of computer object models	Volume of interest	To reduce the amount of data by specifying a region of interest and a range of intensities of interest
		Filtering	To enhance wanted (object) information and suppress unwanted (noise) background, other object information in the output scene
		Interpolation	To change the level of discretization (sampling) of the input scene
		Registration	Takes two scenes or objects as input and outputs a

*Modified from Udupa J: Threeimensional visualization and analysis methodologies: a current perspective, *Radiographics* 19:783-806, 1999.

Continued

TABLE 14-3 Goals of Various Operations for Three-Dimensional Medical Imaging—cont'd

Classes of 3D Operations	Goals	Commonly Used Operations	Goals
			transformation that when applied to the second scene or object matches it as closely as possible to the first
		Segmentation	To identify and delineate objects
Visualization	To create renditions from a given set of scenes or objects that facilitate the visual perception of object information	Scene-based visualization • Section mode • Volume mode	To create renditions from scenes
		Object-based visualization • Surface rendering • Volume rendering	To create renditions from defined objects
Manipulation	To create a second object system from a given object system by changing objects or their relationships	Rigid manipulation	Operations to cut, separate, add, subtract, move, or mirror objects and their components
		Deformable manipulation	Operations to stretch, compress, bend, and so on
Analysis	To generate a quantitative description of the morphology, architecture, and function of the object system from a given set of scenes or object system	Scene-based analysis	Quantitative descriptions obtained from scenes to provide region of interest statistics and measurements of density, activity, perfusion, and flow
		Object-based analysis	Quantitative descriptions obtained from objects on the basis of morphology, architecture, change over time, relationships with other objects in the system, and changes in these relationships

Modified from Udupa J: Three-dimensional visualization and analysis methodologies: a current perspective, *Radiographics* 19:783-806, 1999.

Data Acquisition

In CT, data are collected from the patient by x-rays and special electronic detectors. Data can be acquired slice by slice with a conventional CT scanner or in a volume with a spiral/helical CT scanner. During *slice-by-slice acquisition*, the x-ray tube and detectors rotate to collect data from the first slice of the anatomical area of interest; then the data are sent to the computer for image reconstruction. After the first slice is scanned, the tube and detectors stop, the patient is moved into position for the second slice, and scanning continues. The data from the second slice are transferred to the computer for image reconstruction. This "stop-and-go" technique continues until the last slice has been scanned.

One of the fundamental problems of slice-by-slice CT scanning is that certain portions of the anatomy may be missed because motion caused by the patient's respiration can interfere with scanning or be inconsistent from scan to scan. This problem can lead to inaccurate generation of 3D and multiplanar images. The final 3D image can have the appearance of steplike contours known as the *stairstep artifact*.

In volume data acquisition, a volume of tissue rather than a slice is scanned during a single breath-hold. This means that more data are sent to the computer for image reconstruction. Volume scanning is achieved because the x-ray tube rotates continuously as the patient moves through the gantry. One advantage of this technique is that more data are available for 3D processing, improving the quality of the resultant 3D image.

Creation of Three-Dimensional Space or Scene Space

All information collected from the voxels that compose each of the scanned slices goes to the computer for image reconstruction. The voxel information is a CT number calculated from tissue attenuation within the voxel. In MRI the voxel information is the signal intensity from the tissue within the voxel. The result of image reconstruction is the creation of 3D space, where all image data are stored (see Fig. 14-7).

Data in 3D space are systematically organized so that each point in 3D space has a specific address. Each point in 3D space represents the information (CT number or MRI signal intensity) of the voxels within the slice.

Processing for Three-Dimensional Image Display

Processing, which is a major step in the creation of simulated 3D images for display on a 2D computer screen, is accomplished on the workstation. Although it is not within the scope of this chapter to address these operations in detail, it is important that technologists have an understanding of how sectional images are transformed into 3D images as illustrated in Figure 14-7.

In 1990, Mankovich et al (1990) identified two classes of processing to explain 3D image display: voxel-based processing and object-based processing. *Voxel-based processing* "makes determinations about each voxel and decides to what degree each should contribute to the final 3D display," whereas *object-based processing* "uses voxel information to transform the images into a collection of objects with subsequent processing concentrating on the display of the objects."

Voxel-based processing was used as early as 1975 as a means of generating coronal, sagittal, and oblique images from the stack of contiguous transverse axial set of images—the technique of MPR. Although MPR is not a true 3D display technique, it does provide additional information to enhance our understanding of 3D anatomy (Beigleman-Aubry et al, 2005; Lell et al, 2006). In MPR, the computer scans the 3D space and locates all voxels in a particular plane to produce that particular image (Fig. 14-8).

Object-based processing involves several processing methods to produce a model (called an *object model* or *object representation*) from the 3D space and transforms it into a 3D image displayed

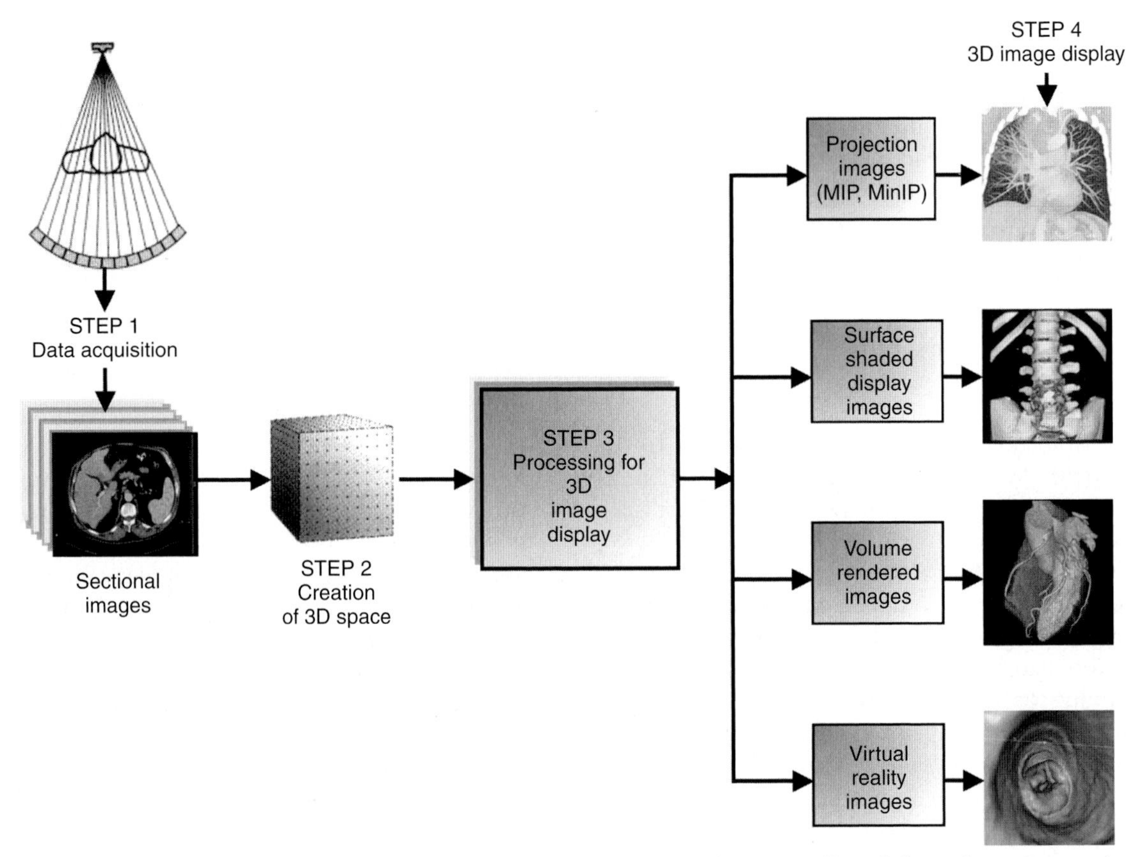

FIGURE 14-7 The major steps in creating 3D images. In Step 1, data are collected from the patient and reconstructed as sectional images, which form 3D space or scene space (Step 2). In Step 3, 3D space can be processed to generate simulated 3D images displayed on a computer screen (Step 4).

on a computer screen. According to Russ (2006) and others (Dalrymple et al, 2005; Lell et al, 2006; Udupa and Herman, 2000), the processing of an object model into a simulated 3D image involves steps such as the following:

1. Segmentation is a processing technique used to identify the structure of interest in a given scene. It determines which voxels are a part of the object and should be displayed and which are not and should be discarded. Thresholding is a method of classifying the types of tissues, such as, say bone, soft tissue, or fat, represented by each of the voxels. The CT number is used for assigning thresholds to tissues.
2. Object delineation is portraying an object by drawing it. It involves boundary and volume extraction and detection methods. Although boundary extraction methods search the 3D space for only those voxels that define the outer or inner border or surface of the object called the object contour, volume extraction methods find all the voxels in 3D space and its surface.
3. Rendering is the stage when an image in 3D space is transformed into a simulated 3D image to be

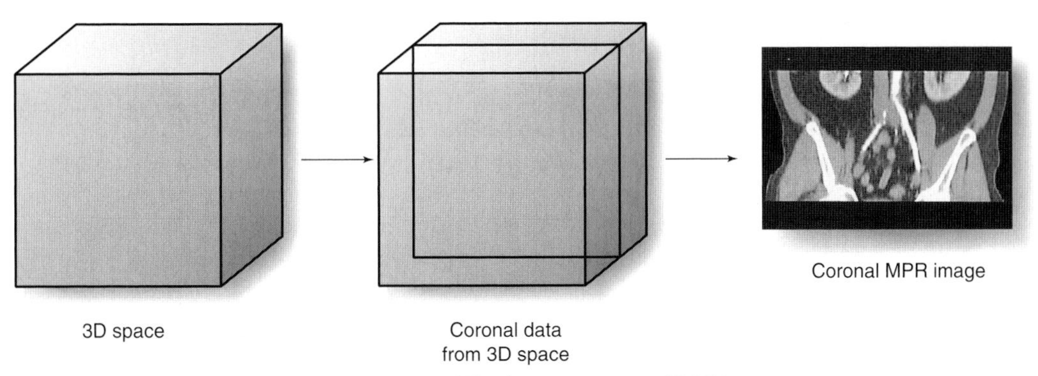

FIGURE 14-8 The basic concept of MPR.

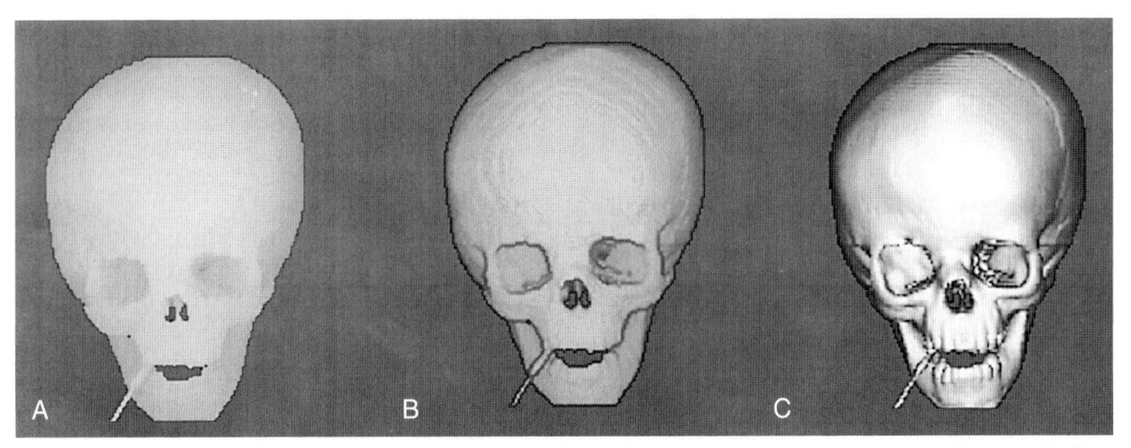

FIGURE 14-9 The evolution of surface rendering technique, demonstrating the improvement in image quality. **A,** Older processing methods. **B,** Recent methods. **C,** Current techniques.

displayed on a 2D computer monitor. Rendering is a computer display technology-based approach (computer program) and therefore requires specific hardware and software to deal with millions of points identified in 3D space.

RENDERING TECHNIQUES

Two classes of rendering techniques are common in radiology: surface rendering and volume rendering (Beigleman-Aubry et al, 2005; Dalrymple et al, 2005; Fishman et al, 2006; Kalender, 2005; Lell et al, 2006; Pickhardt, 2004; Silva et al, 2006; Udupa and Herman, 2000).

Surface Rendering

Surface rendering, or shaded surface display (SSD), has evolved through the years with significant improvements in image quality (Fig. 14-9). In surface rendering, the computer creates "an internal representation of surfaces that will be visible in the displayed image. It then 'lights' them according to a standard protocol, and displays an image according to its calculation of how the light rays

Steps for Surface Rendering

1. Scan the 3D space or scene space for all voxel information relating to the object to be displayed.
2. Create the surface of the object by using contour information (segmentation) obtained by thresholding. The threshold setting determines whether skin or bone surfaces will be displayed. The 3D images of the skull shown in Figure 14-9 are examples of surface rendering.
3. Select the viewing orientation to be processed for 3D image display and assign the position of one or more lighting sources. A standard set of views is shown in Figure 14-10.
4. Surface rendering begins. The pixels of the object to be displayed are shaded for photorealism and particularly to give the illusion of depth. Those pixels farthest away from the viewer are darker than those closer to the viewer.

would be reflected to the viewer's eye" (Schwartz, 1994).

According to Udupa and Herman (2000), surface rendering involves essentially two steps: surface formation and depiction on a computer screen (rendering) (see box above). Surface formation involves the operation of contouring. Rendering follows surface formation and is intended to add photorealism and create the illusion of depth in an image, making it appear 3D on a 2D computer screen. A simulated light source can be positioned at different locations to enhance features of the displayed 3D image (see Fig. 14-4).

The advantage of surface rendering techniques is that they do not require a lot of computing power because they do not use all the voxel information in 3D space to create the 3D image. Only contour information is used. However, this results in poor image information content.

Heath et al (1995) demonstrated this disadvantage when they used surface rendering to image the liver. They reported the following:

> No information about structures inside or behind the surface such as vessels within the liver capsule or thrombus within a vessel is displayed. In medical volume data, which are affected by volume averaging because of finite voxel size, clear-cut edges and surfaces are often difficult or impossible to define. Many voxels necessarily contain multiple tissue types and classifying them as being totally not part of a given tissue introduces artifacts into the image. Surface renderings are very sensitive to changes in threshold, and it is often difficult to determine which threshold yields the most accurate depiction of the actual anatomic structures.

Figure 14-11 illustrates surface rendering numerically. Numbers represent the voxel values for a sample 2D data set. An algorithm is applied to locate a "surface" within the data set at the margin of the region of voxels with intensities ranging from 6 to 9. Standard computer graphics techniques are then used to generate a surface that represents the defined region of voxel values (Heath et al, 1995).

Volume Rendering

Volume rendering is a more sophisticated technique and produces 3D images that have a better image quality and provide more information compared with surface rendering techniques (Neri et al, 2007). Volume rendering overcomes several of the limitations of surface rendering because it uses the entire data set from 3D space. Because of this, volume rendering requires more computing power and is more expensive than surface rendering.

Udupa and Herman (2000) describe the conceptual framework of volume rendering:

> The scene is considered to represent blocks of translucent colored jelly whose color and opacity

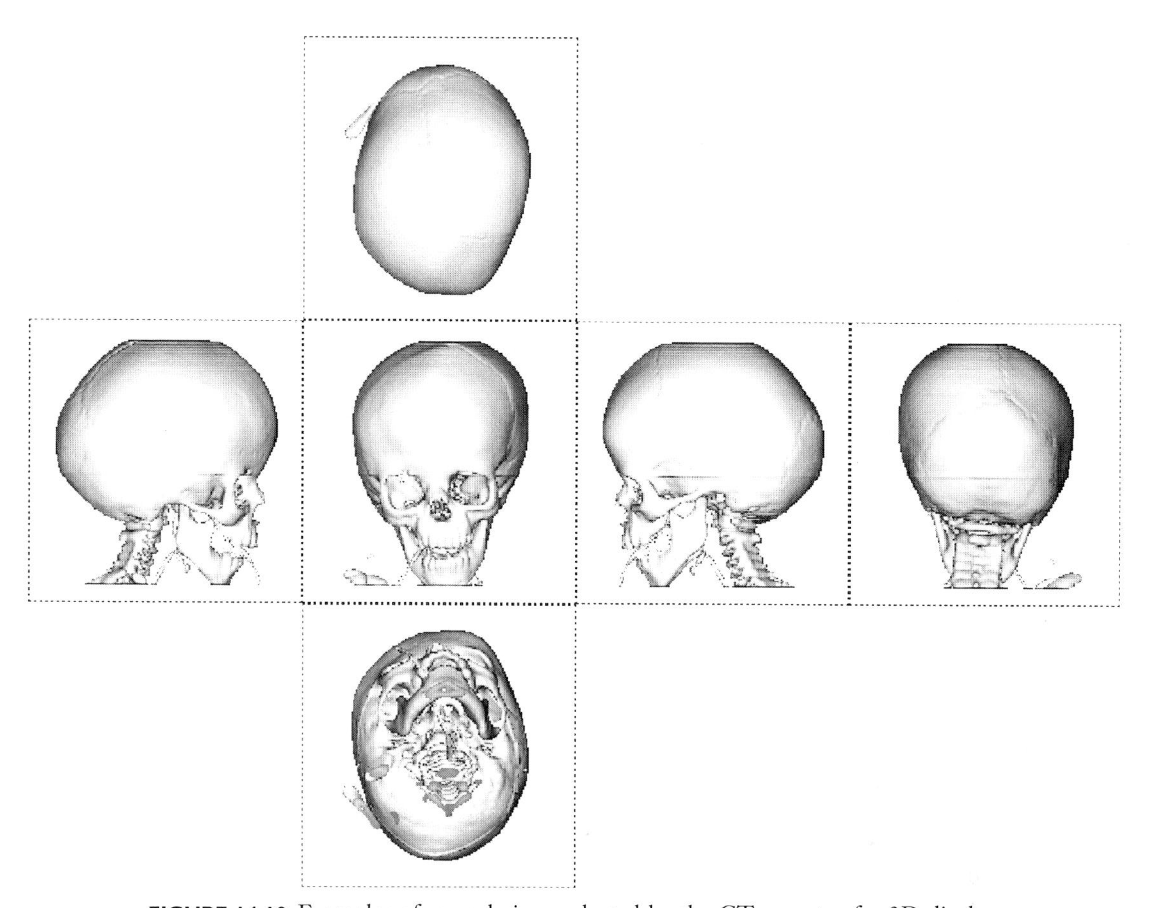

FIGURE 14-10 Examples of several views selected by the CT operator for 3D display.

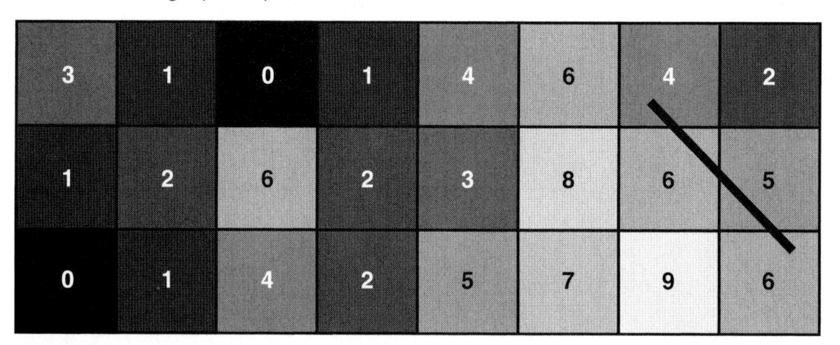

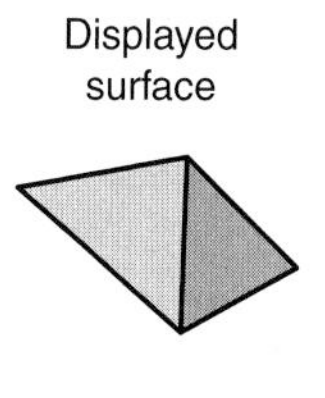

FIGURE 14-11 A numerical illustration of the surface rendering technique or SSD technique. It is important to note that the higher numbers are white and the lower numbers (for example, 0 for air) are dark with 0 shaded black.

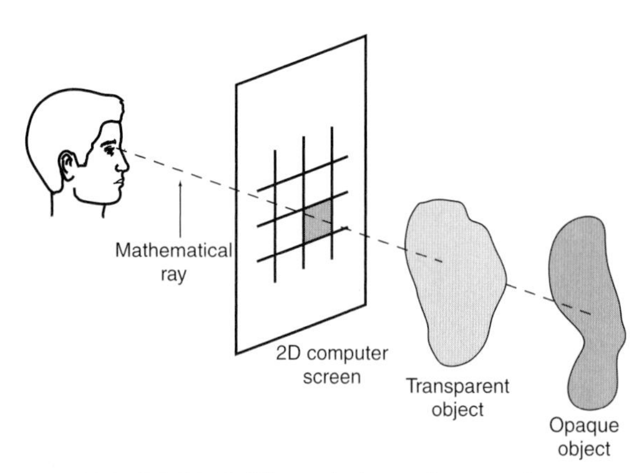

FIGURE 14-12 The technique of ray tracing.

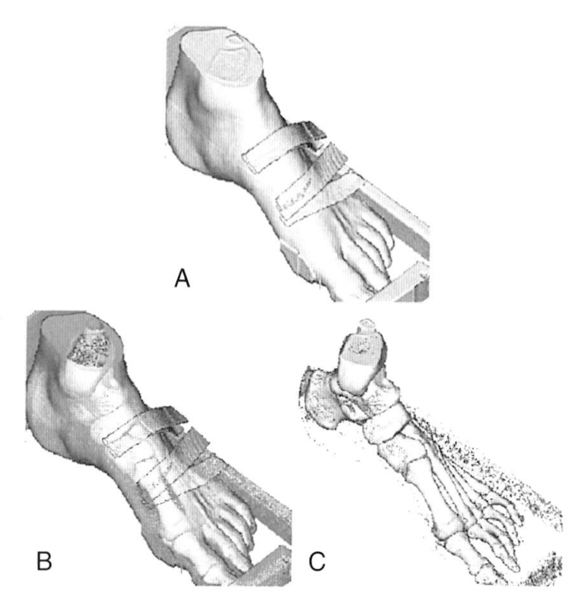

FIGURE 14-13 A, A surface-rendered image. **B,** An example of volume rendering, in which the soft tissues have been made transparent; it allows the viewer to see both the skin and bone surfaces at the same time. **C,** The entire surface is removed.

> (degree of transparency) are different for different tissue regions. The goal of rendering is to compute images that depict the appearance of this block from various angles, simulating the transmission of light through the block as well as its reflection at tissue interfaces through careful selection of color and opacity.

The two stages to volume rendering are preprocessing the volume and rendering.

Preprocessing

Preprocessing involves several image processing operations, including segmentation, also referred to as *classification*, to determine the tissue types contained in each voxel and to assign different brightness levels or color. In addition, a partial transparency (0% to 100%) is also assigned to different tissues that make up 3D space. Three tissue types—fat, soft tissue, and bone—are used for voxel classification.

Rendering

Rendering is stage two of the volume-rendering technique. It involves image projection to form the simulated 3D image. One popular method of image projection is ray tracing, illustrated in Figure 14-12. During *ray tracing*, a mathematical ray is sent from the observer's eye through the 2D computer screen to pass through the 3D volume that contains opaque and transparent objects. The pixel intensity on the screen for that single ray is the average of the intensities of all the voxels through which the ray travels. As Mankovich et al (1990) explain, "If all objects are opaque, only the nearest object is considered, and the ray is then traced back to the light source for calculation of the reflected intensity. If the nearest object is transparent, the ray is diminished and possibly refracted to the next nearest object and so on until the light is traced back to the source."

Unlike surface rendering, volume rendering offers the advantage of seeing through surfaces, allowing the viewer to examine both external and internal structures (Fig. 14-13). A numerical illustration of how this is accomplished is shown in Figure 14-14. Opacities of 0% and 100% are assigned for values of 5 or lower and 9 or higher, respectively. The resulting intermediate opacities for values 6, 7, and 8 are 25%, 50%, and 75%, respectively. The lower portion of the diagram

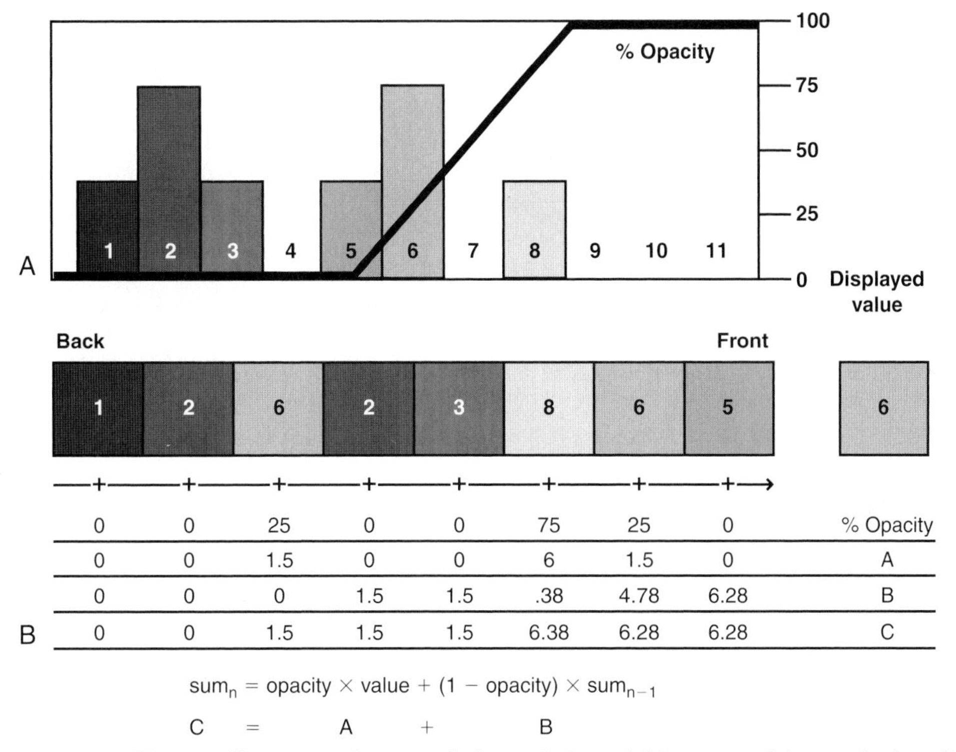

FIGURE 14-14 Diagram illustrates volume-rendering technique. A histogram of the voxel values **(A)** in the data "ray" **(B)**.

shows the equation and progressive computational results used to determine weighted summation along the "ray" through the volume. The resulting displayed value (6) is affected by both opacity (as determined in the graph at the top) and the value of underlying voxels (Calhoun et al, 1999).

The effect of SSD and volume-rendering techniques on image details is clearly illustrated in Figure 14-15.

Intensity Projection Renderings

As noted in Figure 14-8, processing of image data from 3D space can also generate intensity projection images. These images, as Kalender (2005) points out, are "an extension of MPR techniques and consists of generating arbitrary thick slices (slabs) from thin slices reducing the noise level and possibly also improving the visualization of structures, for example, vessels present in the several thin slices.... The term sliding thin slabs is known for this technique...." In addition, Dalrymple et al (2005) note that "multiplanar images can be 'thickened' into slabs by tracing a projected ray through the image to the viewer's eye, then processing the data encountered as the ray passes through the stack of reconstructed sections along the line of sight according to one of several algorithms." This is clearly illustrated in Figure 14-16.

The algorithms for sliding thin slabs (STS) (or thickening of MPR images) include average intensity projection (AIP), maximum intensity projection (MIP), and minimum intensity projection (MinIP).

Average Intensity Projection

The AIP technique is an algorithm that is intended to create a thick MPR image by using the average

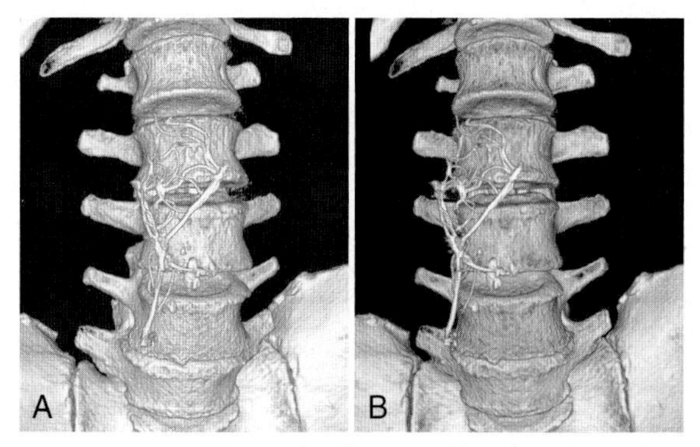

FIGURE 14-15 SSD and volume-rendered images of an inferior vena cava filter overlying the spine. **A,** SSD creates an effective 3D model for looking at osseous structures in a more anatomical perspective than is achieved with axial images alone. It was used in this case to evaluate pelvic fractures not included on this image. **B,** Volume rendering achieves a similar 3D appearance to allow inspection of the bone surfaces in a relatively natural anatomical perspective. In addition, the color assignment tissue classification possible with volume rendering allows improved differentiation of the inferior vena cava filter from the adjacent spine. (From Dalrymple NC et al: Introduction to the language of three-dimensional imaging with multidetector CT, *Radiographics* 25:1409-1428, 2005. Figure and legend reproduced by permission of the Radiological Society of North America and the authors.)

of the attenuation through the tissues of interest to calculate the pixel viewed on the computer, as is clearly illustrated in Figure 14-17. The effects of the AIP algorithm on an image are shown in Figure 14-18.

Maximum Intensity Projection

MIP is a volume-rendering 3D technique that originated in magnetic resonance angiography (MRA) and is now used frequently in CTA. In MIP, the algorithm is such that only the tissues with the greatest attenuation will be displayed for viewing by an observer, as is illustrated in Figure 14-19.

MIP does not require sophisticated computer hardware because, like surface rendering, it makes use of less than 10% of the data in 3D space. Figure 14-20 details the underlying concept of MIP.

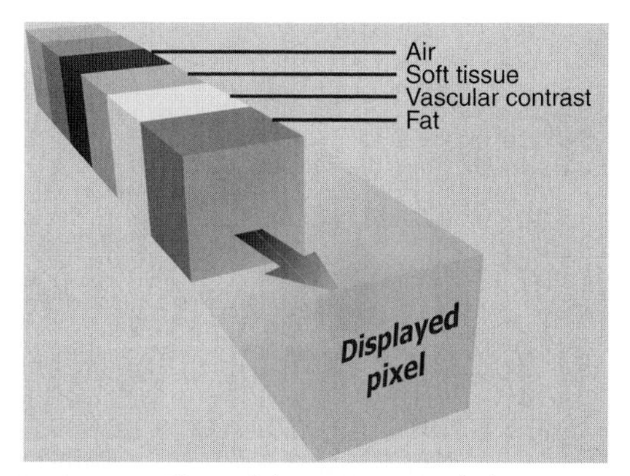

FIGURE 14-16 Row of data encountered along a ray of projection. The data consist of attenuation information calculated in Hounsfield units. The value of the displayed 2D pixel is determined by the amount of data included in the calculation (slab thickness) and the processing algorithm (MIP, MiniIP, or AIP or ray sum). (From Dalrymple NC et al: Introduction to the language of three-dimensional imaging with multidetector CT, *Radiographics* 25:1409-1428, 2005. Figure and legend reproduced by permission of the Radiological Society of North America and the authors.)

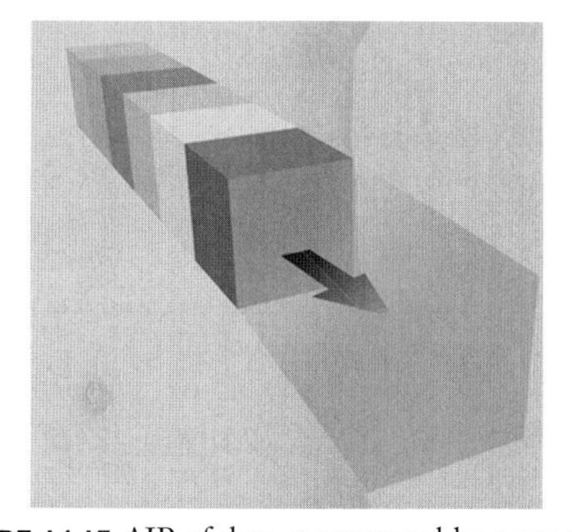

FIGURE 14-17 AIP of data encountered by a ray traced through the object of interest to the viewer. The included data contain attenuation information ranging from that of air (black) to that of contrast media and bone (white). AIP uses the mean attenuation of the data to calculate the projected value. (From Dalrymple NC et al: Introduction to the language of three-dimensional imaging with multidetector CT, *Radiographics* 25:1409-1428, 2005. Figure and legend reproduced by permission of the Radiological Society of North America and the authors.)

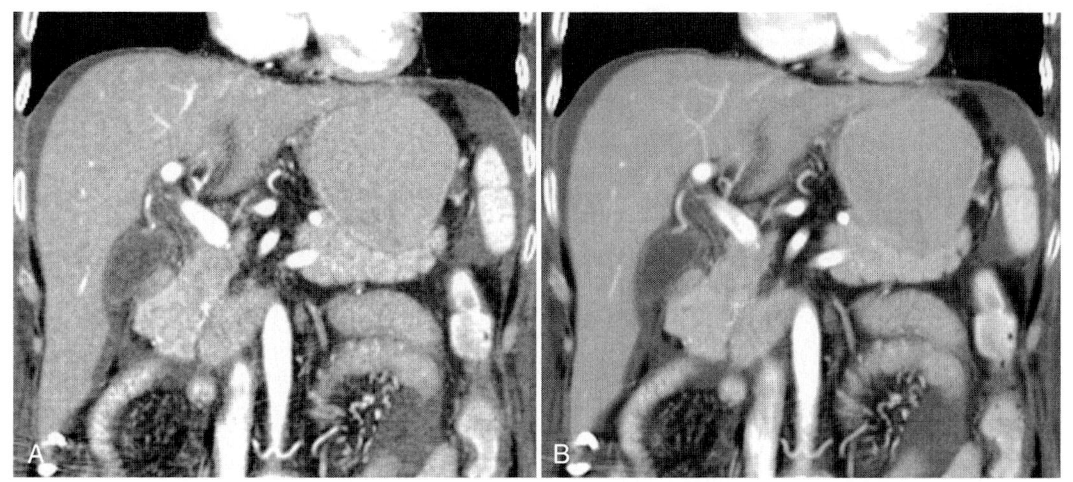

FIGURE 14-18 Effects of AIP on an image of the liver. **A,** Coronal reformatted image created with a default thickness of 1 pixel (approximately 0.8 mm). **B,** Increasing the slab thickness to 4 mm by using AIP results in a smoother image with less noise and improved contrast resolution. The image quality is similar to that used in axial evaluation of the abdomen. (From Dalrymple NC et al: Introduction to the language of three-dimensional imaging with multidetector CT, *Radiographics* 25:1409-1428, 2005. Figure and legend reproduced by permission of the Radiological Society of North America and the authors.)

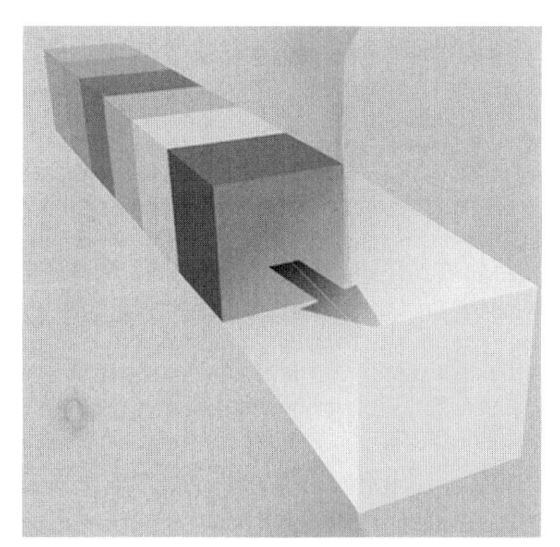

FIGURE 14-19 MIP of data encountered by a ray traced through the object of interest to the viewer. The included data contain attenuation information ranging from that of air (black) to that of contrast media and bone (white). MIP projects only the highest value encountered. (From Dalrymple NC et al: Introduction to the language of three-dimensional imaging with multidetector CT, *Radiographics* 25:1409-1428, 2005. Figure and legend reproduced by permission of the Radiological Society of North America and the authors.)

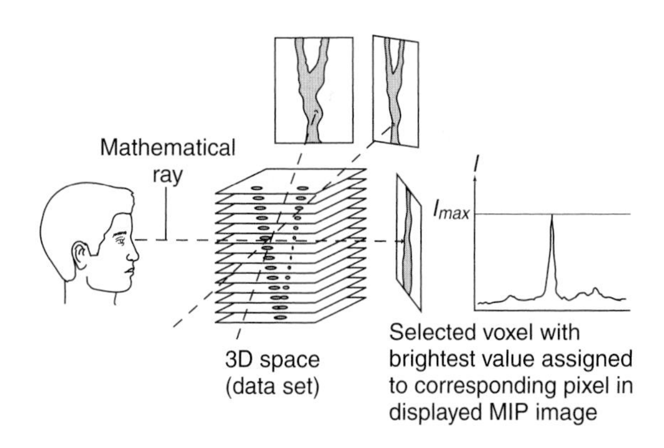

FIGURE 14-20 MIP. The intensity, *I*, is plotted as function of slice number.

Essentially, the MIP computer program renders a 2D image on a computer screen from a 3D data set (slices) as follows:

1. A mathematical ray (similar to the one in ray tracing) is projected from the viewer's eye through the 3D space (data set).
2. This ray passes through a set of voxels in its path.
3. The MIP program allows only the voxel with the maximum intensity (brightest value) to be selected.
4. The selected voxel intensity is then assigned to the corresponding pixel in the displayed MIP image.
5. The MIP image is displayed for viewing (Fig. 14-21).

A numerical illustration the MIP technique is clearly shown in Figure 14-22.

MIP images can also be displayed in rapid sequence to allow the observer to view an image that can be rotated continuously back and forth to enhance 3D visualization of complex structures with postprocessing techniques. Figure 14-23 shows multiple projections that vary only slightly in degree increments.

In the past, one of the basic problems with the MIP technique is that "images are three-dimensionally ambiguous unless depth cues are provided" (Heath et al, 1995). To solve this problem, a depth-weighted MIP can be used to deal with the intensity of the brightest voxel, depending on its distance from the viewer. Other limitations include the inability of the MIP program to show superimposed structures because only one voxel (the one with the maximum intensity) in the set of voxels traversed by a ray is used in the MIP image display. Additionally, MIP generates a "string of beads" artifact because of volume averaging problems with tissues that have lower intensity values (Heath et al, 1995) and artifacts arising from pulsating vessels and respiratory motion.

A significant advantage of the MIP algorithm is that it has become the most popular rendering technique in CTA (Dalrymple et al, 2005; Fishman et al, 2006; Lell et al, 2006) and MRA (Dalrymple et al, 2005) because vessels containing contrast medium are clearly seen. Additionally, because MIP uses less than 10% of the volume data in 3D space, it takes less time to produce 3D simulated images than do volume-rendering algorithms.

Minimum Intensity Projection

The MinIP algorithm ensures that only the tissues with the minimum or lowest attenuation will be displayed for viewing by an observer. This is illustrated in Figure 14-24. Of the three intensity projection techniques, the MinIP is the least used; however, MinIP images may be useful in providing a "valuable perspective in defining lesions for surgical planning or detecting subtle small airway diseases" (Dalrymple et al, 2005).

Virtual CT Endoscopy

The CT image data from 3D space can be processed in such a way by using sophisticated computer algorithms to generate what has been referred to as virtual endoscopic images. These images are based on both 2D and 3D CT image data sets by using a technique known as perspective volume rendering (pVR) (Kalender, 2005). pVR is used to examine hollow structures such as the colon (CT colonoscopy) and the bronchi (CT bronchoscopy), for example. Furthermore, pVR can create an approach that allows the operator to "fly-through" the hollow structure. Virtual CT endoscopy is described in detail in Chapter 15.

Comparison of Three-Dimensional Rendering Techniques

One early comprehensive comparison of surface and volume rendering techniques was performed in 1991 by Udupa and Herman. They concluded that the surface method had a minor advantage over the volume methods with respect to display ability, clarity of the display, smoothness of ridges and silhouettes, computational time, and storage requirements. It had a significant advantage with its time and storage requirements.

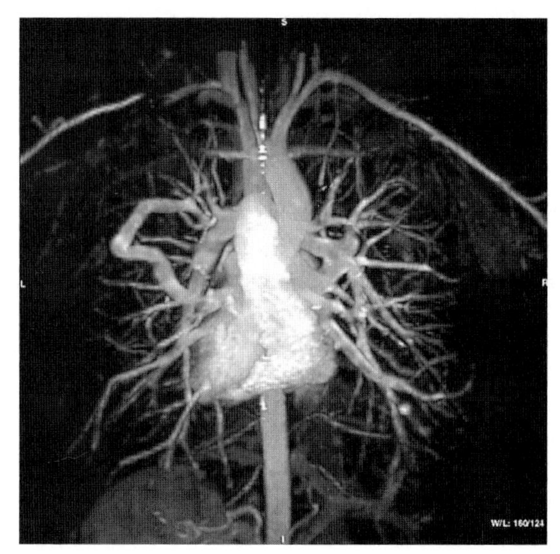

FIGURE 14-21 Example of an MIP image. (Courtesy Vital Images, Minneapolis, Minn.)

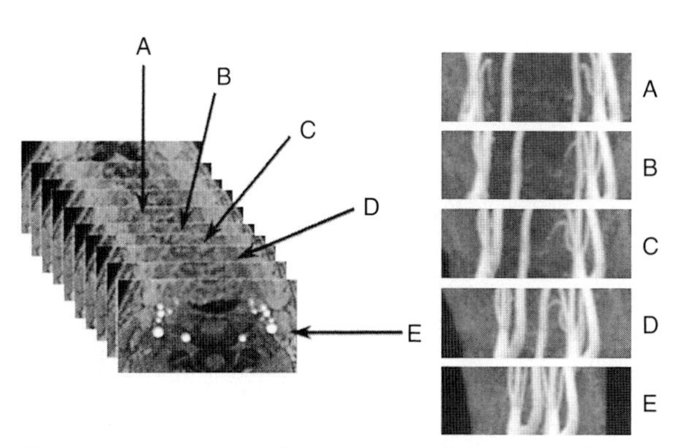

FIGURE 14-23 A complete projection image at different viewing angles. Postprocessing of the 3D data set can generate different views to allow the observers to rotate the image back and forth to enhance the perception of 3D relationships in the vessels. (From Laub G et al: Magnetic resonance angiography techniques, *Electromedica* 66:68-75, 1998.)

Later in 1995, Heath et al (1995) compared surface rendering, volume rendering, and MIP with spiral/helical CT during arterial portography. They compared the techniques with respect to seven parameters: depiction of 3D relationships, edge delineation, demonstration of overlapping structures, depiction of vessel lumen, percentage of data used, artifacts, and computational cost. Their results are summarized in Table 14-4. It is clearly apparent that volume rendering is superior in all parameters compared; however, it has the highest computational cost.

One of the characteristic features of the MIP technique is that it removes discarded data having low values. The SSD technique removes all data with the exception of the data that are associated with the surface and, as mentioned in Table 14-4, typically uses less than 10% of the data. The effect of this data limitation is illustrated in Figure 14-25.

Although volume-rendered images may look similar to images generated by the SSD technique, the use of 100% of the acquired data set and "assigning a full spectrum of opacity values and separation of the tissue classification and shading

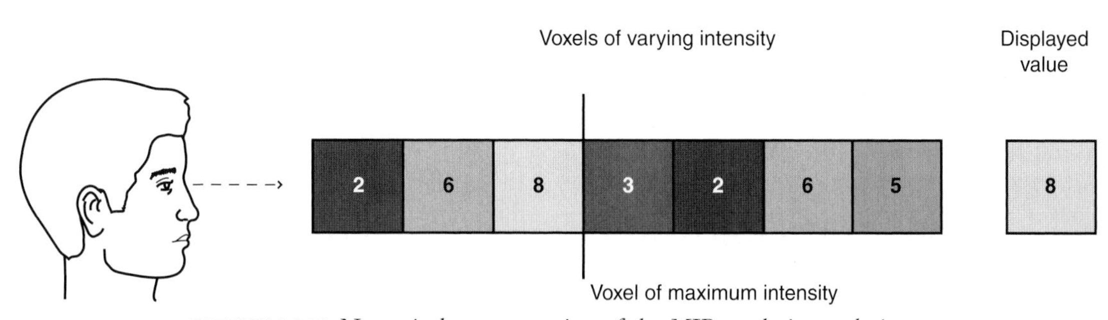

FIGURE 14-22 Numerical representation of the MIP rendering technique.

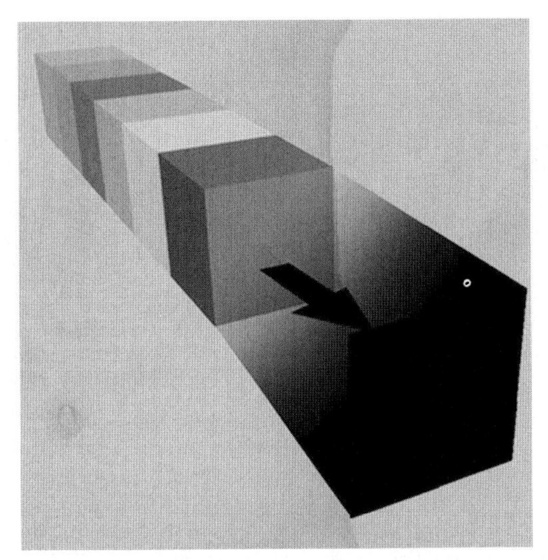

FIGURE 14-24 MinIP of data encountered by a ray traced through the object of interest to the viewer. The included data contain attenuation information ranging from that of air (black) to that of contrast media and bone (white). MinIP projects only the lowest value encountered. (From Dalrymple NC et al: Introduction to the language of three-dimensional imaging with multidetector CT, *Radiographics* 25:1409-1428, 2005. Figure and legend reproduced by permission of the Radiological Society of North America and the authors.)

processes provide a much more robust and versatile data set than the binary system offered by SSD" (Dalrymple et al, 2005). This is clearly shown in Figure 14-26.

In the past years, 3D volume rendering has been shown to be useful in a wide range of clinical applications (Calhoun et al, 1999), including the thoracic aorta (Christine et al, 1999) and in evaluating carotid artery stenosis (Leclerc et al, 1999).

More recent discussions of the use of 3D rendering techniques for clinical imaging using the data obtained from Multislice CT scanners have been reported by several authors, including Kalender, 2005; Dalrymple et al, 2005; Silva et al, 2006; Lell et al, 2006; and Fishman et al, 2006, and the interested student should refer to these original reports for more information.

Some important considerations to note, however, when these 3D imaging techniques are used are noted by several authors as follows:

- "Appreciation of the strengths and weaknesses of rendering techniques is essential to appropriate clinical application and is likely to become increasingly important as networked 3D capability can be used to integrate real-time rendering into routine image interpretation." (Dalrymple et al, 2005)

TABLE 14-4 Comparison of Three-Dimensional Rendering Techniques in Medical Imaging

	Surface Rendering	MIP	Volume Rendering
Depiction of 3D relationships	Good	Fair	Good
Edge delineation	Good	Good	Fair
Demonstration of overlapping structures	No	No	Yes
Depiction of vessel lumen	No	Depicts section that is 1 pixel thick	Yes
Percentage of data used	Typically <10%	Typically <10%	Up to 100%
Artifacts present in medical images	Many false surfaces	MIP artifact and background enhancement	Few if properly segmented
Computational cost	Low	Low	High

From Heath DG et al: Three-dimensional spiral CT during arterial portography: comparison of three rendering techniques, *Radiographics* 15:1001-1011, 1995.

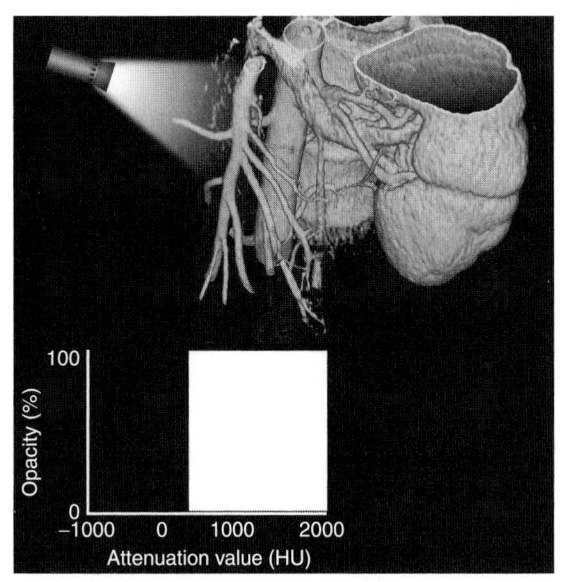

FIGURE 14-25 Data limitations of SSD. Surface data are segmented from other data by means of manual selection or an attenuation threshold. The graph in the lower part of the figure represents an attenuation threshold selected to include the brightly contrast-enhanced renal cortex and renal vessels during CTA. The "virtual spotlight" in the upper left corner represents the gray-scale shading process, which in reality is derived by means of a series of calculations. To illustrate the "hollow" data set that results from discarding all but the surface rendering data, the illustration was actually created by using a volume-rendered image of the kidney with a cut plane transecting the renal parenchyma. Subsequent editing was required to remove the internal features of the object while preserving the surface features of the original image. *HU,* Hounsfield units. (From Dalrymple NC et al: Introduction to the language of three-dimensional imaging with multidetector CT, *Radiographics* 25:1409-1428, 2005. Figure and legend reproduced by permission of the Radiological Society of North America and the authors.)

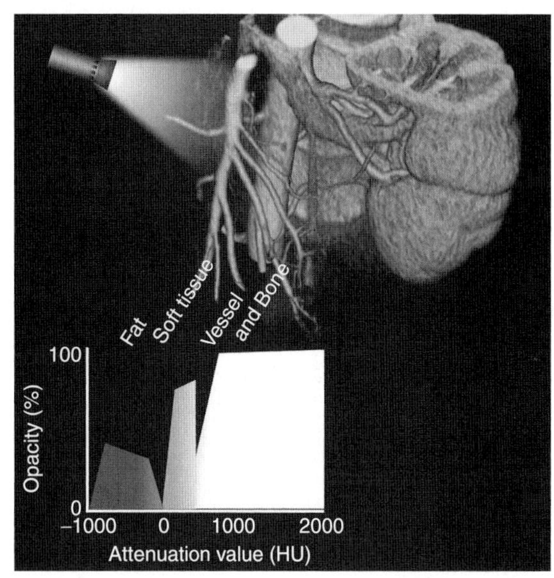

FIGURE 14-26 Data-rich nature of volume rendering. The graph in the lower part of the figure shows how attenuation data are used to assign values to a histogram-based tissue classification consisting of deformable regions for each type of tissue included. In this case, only fat, soft tissue, vessels, and bone are assigned values, but additional classifications can be added as needed. Opacity and color assignment may vary within a given region, and the shape of the region can be manipulated to achieve different image effects. Because there is often overlap in attenuation values between different tissues, the classification regions may overlap. Thus, accurate tissue and border classification may require additional mathematical calculations that take into consideration the characteristics of neighboring data. *HU,* Hounsfield units. (From Dalrymple NC et al: Introduction to the language of three-dimensional imaging with multidetector CT, *Radiographics* 25:1409-1428, 2005. Figure and legend reproduced by permission of the Radiological Society of North America and the authors.)

- "My own expectation is that volume rendering with user friendly, preset evaluation protocols and intelligent editing tools will prevail as the method of choice in 3D display forms. However, they will only supplant and augment, but not replace 2D displays." (Kalender, 2005)
- "Generating 'boneless' 3D images became possible with modern postprocessing techniques, but one should keep in mind the potential pitfalls of these techniques and always double-check the final results with source or MPR images." (Lell et al, 2006)

- "Although different systems have unique capabilities and functionality, all provide the options of volume rendering and maximum intensity projection for image display and analysis. These two post processing techniques have different advantages and disadvantages when used in clinical practice, and it is important that radiologists understand when and how each technique should be used." (Fishman et al, 2006)
- "To avoid potential pitfalls in image interpretation, the radiologist must be familiar with the unique appearance of the normal anatomy and of various pathologic findings when using virtual dissection with two-dimensional axial and 3D endoluminal CT colonographic image data sets." (Silva et al, 2006)

EDITING THE VOLUME DATA SET

The purpose of editing the volume data set is intended for clarity of 3D image display. This is well described by Fishman et al (2006), and the interested reader should refer to the article for a detailed account of the procedure. In summary, Fishman et al (2006) note the following:

1. The volume-rendered 3D technique is much better than the MIP technique for a clear display of the anatomy of interest in the volume data set. The MIP cannot display the 3D anatomical relationships, only because it is 2D.
2. For better clarity of anatomical details, the volume data set must be edited by using thinner slabs compared with the entire volume data set.
3. Several editing tools are available to change the appearance of the images. These include windowing (window width and window length manipulation), color and shading tools, and tools that allow the operator to change the opacity or the transparency of the image display (Fishman et al, 2006) and segmentation (Dalrymple, 2005; Lell et al, 2006).

EQUIPMENT

Equipment for 3D image processing falls into two categories: the CT or MRI scanner console and stand-alone computer workstations. Both types of equipment use software designed to perform several image processing operations, such as interactive visualization, multi-image display, analysis and measurement, intensity projection renderings, and 3D rendering. Most postprocessing for 3D imaging is done on stand-alone dedicated workstations that are becoming more popular as their costs decrease.

Stand-Alone Workstations

A number of popular CT equipment manufacturers provide 3D packages for their CT and MRI scanners, and many are offering both 3D hardware and software packages for use in radiology. Although the technical specifications of each workstation vary depending on the manufacturer, typical 3D processing techniques include software to perform the following:

- MPR
- Surface and volume rendering
- Slice plane mapping. This technique allows two tissue types to be viewed at the same time.
- Slice cube cuts. This is a processing technique that allows the operator to slice through any plane to demonstrate internal anatomy.
- Transparency visualization. This processing technique allows the operator to view both surface and internal structures at the same time.
- MIP, AIP, MinIP
- Four-dimensional angiography. This technique shows bone, soft tissue, and blood vessels at the same time and allows the viewer to see tortuous vessels with respect to bone.
- Disarticulation. This SSD technique allows the viewer to enhance the visualization of certain structures by removing others.
- Virtual reality imaging. Some workstations are also capable of virtual endoscopy, a processing technique that allows the viewer to look into the

lumen of the bronchus and colon, for example. It is also possible for the viewer to "fly through" the 3D data set. Virtual CT endoscopy is described in Chapter 15.

CLINICAL APPLICATIONS OF THREE-DIMENSIONAL IMAGING

One of the major motivating factors for the development and application of 3D imaging in medicine is to improve the communication gap between the radiologist and the surgeon. 3D imaging can help radiologists locate the condition and identify the best way to demonstrate it. Interestingly, craniofacial surgery was one of the first clinical applications of 3D medical imaging. Today, 3D medical imaging is used for applications ranging from orthopedics to radiation therapy (Calhoun et al, 1999; Dalrymple et al, 2005; Fishman et al, 1992; Fishman et al, 2006; Kalender, 2005; Lell et al, 2006; Silva et al, 2006; Udupa and Herman, 1991; Zonneveld and Fukuta, 1994).

The applications of 3D imaging in CT, MRI, nuclear medicine, and ultrasonography continue to evolve at a rapid rate, with most of the work being done in CT and MRI. For example, 3D imaging has provided the basis for endoscopic imaging, where the viewer can "fly through" CT and MRI data sets with the goal of performing "virtual endoscopy." The most recent clinical application of 3D imaging is virtual dissection, "an innovative technique whereby the three-dimensional (3D) model of the colon is virtually unrolled, sliced open, and displayed as a flat 3D rendering of the mucosal surface, similar to a gross pathologic specimen" (Silva et al, 2006).

To date, clinical applications of 3D imaging in CT have been in the craniomaxillofacial complex, musculoskeletal system, central nervous system, cardiovascular system, pulmonary system, gastrointestinal system, and genitourinary system and in radiation treatment planning for therapy. In the craniomaxillofacial complex, for example, 3D imaging has been used to evaluate congenital and developmental deformities (shape of the deformed skull and the extent of suture ossification) and to assess trauma (bone fragment displacement and fractures).

3D imaging can demonstrate complex musculoskeletal anatomy and is used to study acetabular and calcaneal trauma, muscle atrophy, spinal conditions, and trauma of the spine, knee, carpal bones, and shoulder.

The development of CTA opened up additional avenues for the use of 3D imaging in the evaluation of cerebral aneurysms and arteriovenous malformations. It has been applied in CT of the gastrointestinal system, primarily imaging the liver, and genitourinary systems, primarily in kidney and bladder assessment. 3D volume rendering provides accurate evaluation of the thoracic aorta and internal carotid artery stenosis.

In radiation therapy, 3D imaging is especially used to superimpose isodose curves on sectional anatomy for the purpose of providing a clear picture of tissues and organs that receive various degrees of radiation dose. This is essential to demonstrate that the tumor receives maximum dose with minimum dose to the surrounding healthy tissues.

The student should refer to the reports by Dalrymple et al, 2005; Silva et al, 2006; Lell et al, 2006; Fatterpekar et al, 2006; Beigleman-Aubry et al, 2005; Fayad et al, 2005; Lawler et al, 2005; Pickhardt, 2004, and Fishman et al, 2006, for more recent applications of 3D imaging in clinical practice.

FUTURE OF THREE-DIMENSIONAL IMAGING

The first two decades of 3D imaging have generated a new and vast knowledge base on the technology of 3D imaging and on its clinical role in medicine. It has provided additional information that has helped in the diagnostic interpretation of images and enhanced communication between radiologists and surgeons and other physicians.

As research and development in 3D imaging continue, experts predict promising gains for radiology. Additionally, developments can be expected in computer architecture that will boost processing power and speed. Software developments will include improvements in segmentation techniques, for example. Also the cost of dedicated computer hardware and software will decrease, and personal computer–based workstations will become available. 3D rendering is now possible on the Internet.

As the technology for 3D imaging becomes increasingly sophisticated and better refined, clinical applications will expand and 3D imaging will be applied to other areas of the body. Applications in CT, MRI, and other imaging modalities will expand with the goal of providing additional information to support and validate diagnostic interpretation.

3D imaging involves digital image postprocessing techniques. The series of articles by Barnes (2006) entitled "Medical Image Processing has Room to Grow" point out that this is an area of active research, and there will be increasingly new applications for use in medicine, particularly in medical imaging.

ROLE OF THE RADIOLOGIC TECHNOLOGIST

As 3D imaging technology expands and becomes commonplace in medical imaging and radiation therapy, it is likely that radiologic technologists will play an increasing role in image processing and analysis techniques. Radiologic technologists may need to expand their knowledge base to include a basic understanding of 3D imaging concepts. Educational programs in the radiologic technology may need to offer courses that prepare students to perform 3D imaging and various image postprocessing for digital images in medical imaging.

To perform quality 3D medical imaging, the technologist and the radiologist must work as a team. Technical ability in performing CT or MRI examinations and an understanding of the 3D imaging process and other postprocessing digital techniques are equally important. In addition, effective communication between the technologist and radiologist is vital in performing 3D medical imaging and will become even more important as the technology expands to provide new clinical applications.

REFERENCES

Barnes E: Medical image processing has room to grow: parts 1, 2, and 3 (2006): AuntMinni.com. Accessed December 2006.

Beigelman-Aubry C et al: Multi-detector row CT and postprocessing techniques in the assessment of diffuse lung disease, *Radiographics* 25:1639-1652, 2005.

Calhoun PS et al: Three-dimensional volume rendering of spiral CT data: theory and method, *Radiographics* 19:745-764, 1999.

Dalrymple NC et al: Introduction to the language of three-dimensional imaging with multidetector CT, *Radiographics* 25:1409-1428, 2005.

Fayad LM et al: Multidetector CT of the musculoskeletal disease in the pediatric patient: principles, techniques, and clinical applications, *Radiographics* 25:603-618, 2005.

Fishman EK et al: Volume rendering versus maximum intensity projection in CT angiography: what works best, when, and why, *Radiographics* 26:905-922, 2006.

Heath DG et al: Three-dimensional spiral CT during arterial portography: comparison of three rendering techniques, *Radiographics* 15:1001-1011, 1995.

Herman GT, Liu HK: Display of three-dimensional information in computed tomography, *J Comput Assist Tomogr* 1:155-160, 1977.

Herman GT: 3D display: a survey from theory to applications, *Comput Med Imag Graph* 17:131-142, 1993.

Hoffman H et al: Paleoradiology: advanced CT in the evaluation of Egyptian mummies, *Radiographics* 22: 377-385, 2002.

Jan J: *Medical image processing, reconstruction and restoration (signal processing and communications)*, Boca Raton, 2005, CRC Press.

Kalender W: *Computed tomography: fundamentals, system technology, image quality, applications*, Munich, Germany, 2005, Publicis.

Lawler LP et al: Adult uteropelvic junction obstruction: insights with three-dimensional multi-detector row CT, *Radiographics* 25:121-134, 2005.

Leclerc X et al: Internal carotid artery stenosis: CT angiography with volume rendering, *Radiology* 210:673-682, 1999.

Lell MM et al: New techniques in CT angiography, *Radiographics* 26:S45-S62, 2006.

Macari M, Bini EJ: CT colonography: where have we been and where are we going? *Radiology* 237:819-833, 2005.

Mahoney DP: The art and science of medical visualization, *Comput Graph World* 14:25-32, 1996.

Mankovich NJ et al: Three-dimensional image display in medicine, *J Digit Imaging* 3:69-80, 1990.

Marvilla KR: Computer reconstructed sagittal and coronal computed tomography head scans: clinical applications, *J Comput Assist Tomogr* 2:120-123, 1978.

Microsoft Press: *Computer dictionary*, ed 5, Redmond, Wash, 2002, Microsoft Press.

Neri E et al, editors: *Image processing in radiology*, New York, 2007, Springer.

Pickhardt PJ: Differential diagnosis of polypoid lesions seen at CT colonoscopy (virtual colonoscopy), *Radiographics* 24:1535-1559, 2004.

Rhodes ML et al: Extracting oblique planes from serial CT sections, *J Comput Assist Tomogr* 4:649-657, 1980.

Rubin GD et al: Perspective volume rendering of CT and MR images: applications for endoscopic imaging, *Radiology* 199:321-330, 1996.

Russ JC: *The image processing handbook*, ed 5, Boca Raton, 2006, CRC Press.

Schwartz B: 3D computerized medical imaging, *Med Device Res Rep* 1:8-10, 1994.

Silva AC et al: Three-dimensional virtual dissection at CT colonography: unraveling the colon to search for lesions, *Radiographics* 26:1669-1686, 2006.

Udupa JK: Three-dimensional visualization and analysis methodologies: a current perspective, *Radiographics* 19:783-803, 1999.

Udupa J, Herman G: *3D imaging in medicine*, Boca Raton, 1991, CRC Press.

Udupa JK, Herman GT, editors: *3D imaging in medicine*, ed 2, Boca Raton, Fla, 2000, CRC Press.

Vining DJ: Virtual endoscopy flies viewer through the body, *Diagn Imaging* 3:127-129, 1996.

Wu CM et al: Spiral CT of the thoracic aorta with 3D volume rendering: a pictorial review, *Cardiaovasc Intervent Radiol* 22:159-167, 1999.

Yasuda T et al: 3D visualization of an ancient Egyptian mummy, *IEEE Comput Graphics Appl* 2:13-17, 1992.

Zonneveld FW, Fukuta K: A decade of clinical three-dimensional imaging: a review, 2: clinical applications, *Invest Radiol* 29:574-589, 1994.

Virtual Reality Imaging

Chapter Outline

CT IMAGE DATA SETS

The increasing size of computed tomography (CT) image data sets (axial images) obtained from multislice CT scanners has created a range of technical applications including CT fluoroscopy, CT angiography (CTA), three-dimensional (3D) imaging, and CT virtual reality imaging.

Multislice CT scanners produce very large volume data sets of the anatomy under investigation. Hundreds of images can be obtained and presented to the radiologist for interpretation and diagnosis. In general, these images are examined one at a time, and observers must rely on their mental reconstruction abilities to visualize the anatomy in three dimensions by using the two-dimensional (2D) images. The perception of 3D anatomy from 2D images often is difficult for some individuals because of the complexity of the structures in terms of their geometrical shapes. One solution is a 3D image processing technique referred to as *virtual reality (VR) imaging*.

The technical developments in multislice CT scanners have led to the acquisition of increasing amounts of isotropic image data sets (see Chapter 1), leading to improvements in applications such as CT fluoroscopy, CTA, and 3D imaging as described in Chapters 13 and 14, respectively.

Radiologists now use various image display techniques including the display of 2D axial images, 2D multiplanar reformatted (MPR) images, 3D images, and even computer-assisted detection and diagnosis (CAD) and more recently virtual dissection (described subsequently) to assist in image interpretation of VR images.

OVERVIEW OF VIRTUAL REALITY IMAGING

VR is a branch of computer science that immerses users in a computer-generated environment and allows them to interact with 3D scenes. The use of VR concepts to the creation of inner views of tubular structures is called *virtual endoscopy* (Vining, 1996). As explained by Higgins et al (1998):

A virtual endoscope is a graphics-based software system used for simulating endoscopic exploration inside a 3D image. In virtual endoscopy, a 3D image acts as a "copy" or virtual environment, representing the scanned anatomy. With the use of computer-based rendering tools, a virtual endoscope produces endoluminal surface views inside the virtual environment similar to those from a real endoscope. A virtual endoscope permits essentially unrestricted exploration because it cannot traumatize the virtual environment.

A real endoscope uses optical video-assisted technology to help physicians interactively examine the inside of tubular anatomical structures. Because of the nature of the physical device, the patient may feel some discomfort, and other risks may also exist.

Recently, the topic of VR imaging received significant attention at the 2006 Computer Assisted Radiology and Surgery conference held in Osaka, Japan, where researchers presented their work on VR imaging applications. At the conference, Dr. Naoki Suzuki described a number of projects at Japan's Institute of Medical Imaging at the Jikei University School of Medicine in Tokyo and made an important comment that "our vision is to utilize VR techniques to improve medical simulation and navigation" (Barnes, 2006). VR applications in medicine, surgery, and four-dimensional (4D) imaging range from diagnosis using 3D and 4D image data sets, image fusion, and virtual surgery to treatment simulation, human body dynamics and medical education in virtual space (Barnes, 2006).

TECHNICAL CONSIDERATIONS

Several technical requirements must be taken into account when CT virtual endoscopy is considered. The four fundamental requirements are data acquisition, image preprocessing, 3D rendering, and image display and analysis (Fig. 15-1). Each of

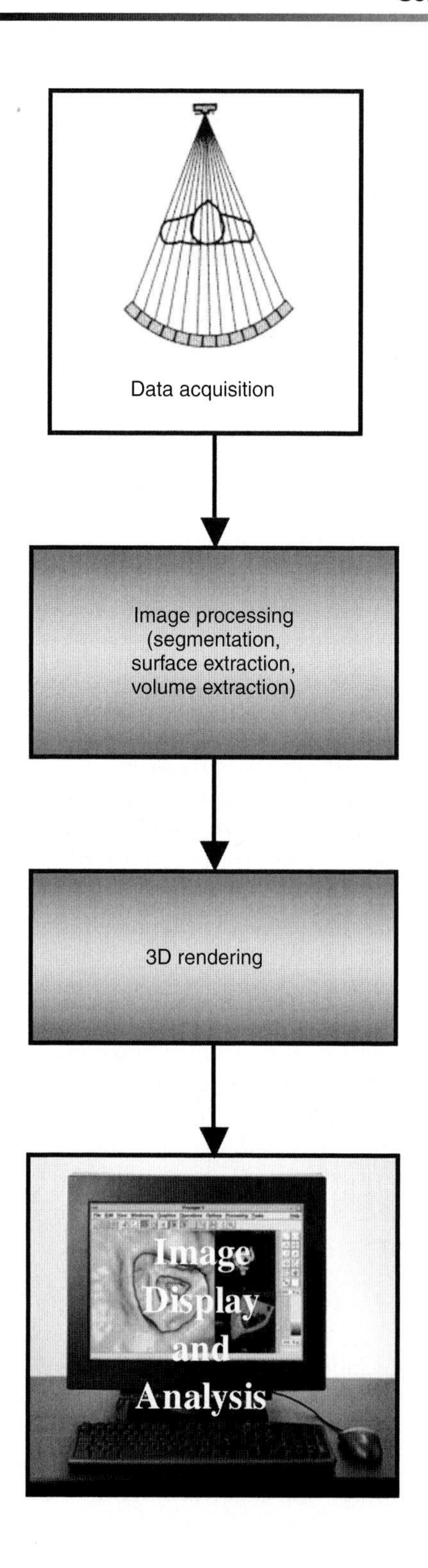

FIGURE 15-1 Technical requirements for CT virtual endoscopy.

these techniques is currently being researched in an effort to improve the performance of virtual CT colonoscopy, although some controversy still exists among physicians such as gastroenterologists and radiologists, for example (Macari and Bini, 2005).

Data Acquisition

The first step in virtual endoscopy imaging is careful selection of the scan parameters to be used for creating the data set. These parameters, which optimize image display while reducing the radiation dose to the patient, include slice thickness, spiral/helical pitch, slice reconstruction overlap, and the scanning exposure technique (i.e., peak kilovolts [kVp], milliamperes [mA]/revolution, and scan time/revolution). In addition, the reconstruction parameters with respect to the type of interpolation algorithm and reconstruction kernel are also vital to the optimization of the procedure (Jolesz et al, 2007).

The selection of these parameters has been discussed in the literature for several virtual endoscopic examinations. For CT bronchoscopy, for example, Hooper (1999) reports that a 2-millimeter (mm) slice thickness, a pitch of 1, and a 75% slice reconstruction overlap produce significantly better virtual images than do a slice thickness of 4 to 8 mm, a pitch of 1.5 to 2, and a 25% to 50% slice overlap. In addition, Jolesz et al (2007) recommends parameters such as 120 kVp, 70 to 165 mA, 20 to 40 seconds' exposure time; 3 to 5 mm collimation, 5 to 6 mm table feed with a pitch of 1 or 2, 512 × 512 matrix size and 180 degrees of linear interpolation algorithm with a standard reconstruction algorithm, and 3 mm table incrementation. In addition, for virtual colonoscopy, proper patient preparation is an essential element of the success of the examination. In this respect, oral colonoscopic preparation

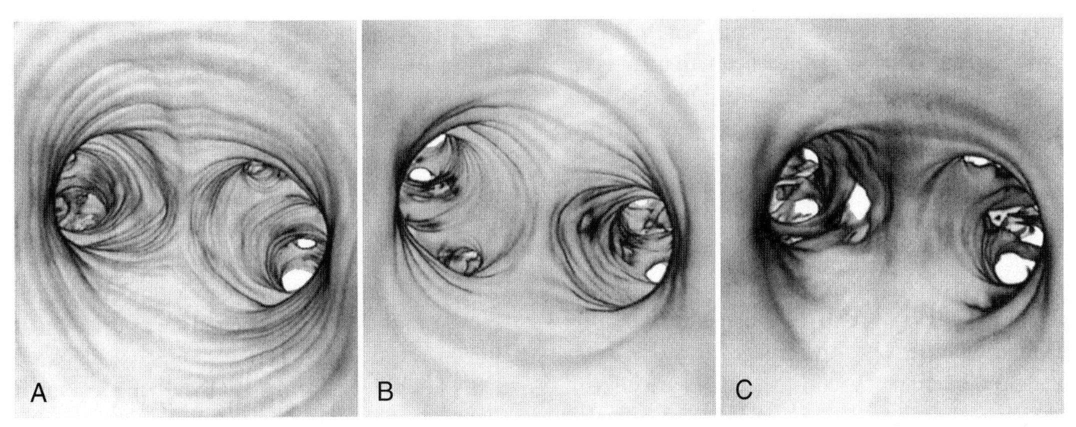

FIGURE 15-2 The effect of slice thickness on image quality in CT virtual endoscopy. Thin (2-mm) slices produce sharper images **(A)** compared with 4-mm **(B)** and 8-mm **(C)** thick slices. These images were obtained with 50% reconstruction overlap using a pitch of 1. (From Hooper KD: CT bronchoscopy, *Semin Ultrasound CT MRI* 20:10-15, 1999.)

and the use of contrast medium should be considered. Additionally, to improve image quality, some individuals may consider the use of glucagons to reduce motion caused by peristalsis of the bowel (Lakarc and Kaufman, 2003).

The imaging parameters represent a tradeoff between radiation dose and image quality. The effect of slice thickness, for example, on image quality is demonstrated in Figure 15-2. Techniques for virtual studies in bronchoscopy, colonoscopy, and angioscopy also require consideration of several parameters such as kilovolts (kV), mA/revolutions, scan time/revolution, pitch, slice thickness, and so forth. The choice of the actual values for each will depend on the clinical facility and radiologists. For example, typical values for a virtual bronchoscopy may include 120 kV, 150 mA/30 revolutions, 1 second/revolution, and a pitch of 1, a slice thickness of, say, 5 mm, and an image index of 1 mm.

Image Preprocessing

Preprocessing of image data is the next step after data acquisition (see Fig. 15-1), and it is intended to optimize the images before they are subject to further processing and analysis. Preprocessing involves the use of various noise filtering algorithms, image segmentation, defining paths through tubular structures, and other tools, such as classification, "cropping," and "cutting."

Image segmentation is an important step in the creation of VR images in CT. Segmentation can be performed by the operator (semiautomatic), or it can be done automatically. In the semiautomatic mode, the user selects objects to include in the data set through the use of windowing. These objects are then prepared for rendering. For bronchoscopy the result of this procedure defines a 3D image mask that, as Higgins et al (1998) explained, "excludes voxels not belonging to the lungs or major airways. All mediastinal structures, bones, and other extraneous structures are removed."

Another preprocessing tool is volume extraction, a technique where 3D surfaces are extracted from a volume (Doi et al, 2002; Takanashi et al, 1997). Another approach to volume extraction is one discussed by Lakarc and Kaufman (2003), a technique where voxels (rather than 3D surfaces) are extracted from a volume into another 3D segmented region. These techniques are beyond the scope of this book.

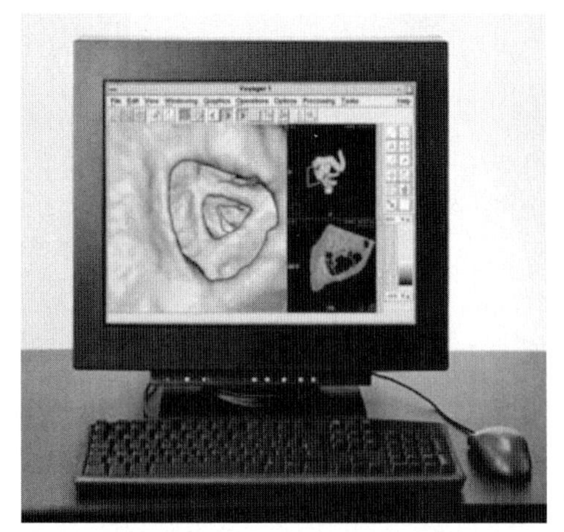

FIGURE 15-3 A workstation for CT virtual reality image display and analysis. (Courtesy Phillips Medical Systems.)

Three-Dimensional Rendering

3D rendering is described in detail in Chapter 14. Two rendering techniques used in virtual CT endoscopy are surface rendering and volume rendering. Both have been used in various virtual CT examinations, but most experts agree that surface rendering is not best suited for use in CT VR imaging (Fleiter et al, 1997; Higgins et al, 1998; Lakarc and Kaufman, 2003) because of problems such as the production of partial volume averaging artifacts.

Volume rendering provides the best results because it produces optimum visualization of the anatomy (e.g., mucosal patterns and lesions), minimizes partial volume averaging artifacts, and adds lifelike reality to images (Hooper, 1999, 2000; Lakarc and Kaufman, 2003; Tomandl et al, 2000; Vining, 1996). Hybrid rendering, or techniques that combine features of both surface and volume rendering algorithms, are under investigation (Vining, 1999).

Image Display and Analysis

Because of the nature of the visualizations and interactivity needed for optimum viewing and evaluation of images, image display and analysis in CT VR imaging require powerful computer workstations (Fig. 15-3) to handle both data acquisition and advanced visualization processing operations.

As an alternative, some CT consoles may also facilitate virtual endoscopy. Virtual CT endoscopy includes image analysis techniques that allow the user to assess images interactively with a wide range of software tools. These tools will allow the user to perform a wide range of operations such as the following, for example:

- Pan through a stack of 2D images (axial CT display mode)
- "Fly through" the 3D-rendered anatomical models (virtual endoscopic mode)
- Navigate the 3D anatomical models by using automated flight path programs
- Split or unfold anatomical models
- Identify pathological conditions through computer-aided detection
- Depict topography of inner colonic surfaces as flattened structures (panoramic endoscopic display mode)

In an early study conducted by Beaulieu et al (1999), the researchers found that panoramic endoscopy is more sensitive than virtual endoscopy for detection of polyps. This has been supported more recently by Silva et al (2006).

APPLICATIONS OF VIRTUAL ENDOSCOPY

Virtual endoscopy is evolving into a clinical tool with a wide range of applications. It has been used to evaluate the colon (virtual colonoscopy) (Vining, 1999), airways (virtual bronchoscopy) (Hooper, 1999), paranasal sinuses, bladder, spinal canal, and, more recently, the pancreatic and common bile ducts (virtual cholangiopancreatoscopy) (Prassopoulos et al, 1998) and the inner ear (virtual labyrinthoscopy) (Tomandl et al, 2000). Figure 15-2 shows an example of images from CT virtual endoscopy of the bronchus.

Of these applications, virtual colonoscopy, or CT colonoscopy as it is popularly referred to, has received much attention in the literature (Macari and Bini, 2005; Pickhardt, 2004; Silva et al, 2006).

CT Colonoscopy: A Brief Overview

The developments in multislice CT scanners have provided the motivation for a number of improvements in CT colonoscopy. Furthermore, CT colonoscopy has become an integral tool for the evaluation of colorectal polyp detection, and it may be used routinely in the future for colorectal screening (Macari and Bini, 2005; Silva et al, 2006; Taylor et al, 2006). In a special review of CT colonography, Macari and Bini (2005) point out that there are two schools of thought with regard to the clinical use of CT colonography. Although some individuals are excited about the noninvasiveness of the technique, others believe that much more work needs to be done to not only demonstrate the sensitivity of CT colonography but also to emphasize that a certain degree of expertise in radiology is required for diagnostic interpretation of the images. Furthermore, the study by Taylor et al (2006) concluded that "for polyps smaller than 1 cm, measurement differences of up to 2.5 mm are within the expected limits of inter- and intraobserver agreement for all measurement techniques. Automated and manual 3D polyp measurements are more accurate than manual 2D measurements."

Display Tools

A typical CT colonoscopy imaging examination may generate a thousand plus images; therefore, it is important that radiologists have the necessary display tools to expedite the viewing of such a large image data set. In this respect, CT manufacturers have provided various software tools for display, viewing, and interpretation. For example, Figure 15-4 shows one manufacturer's workstation display tools for CT virtual colonoscopy, and Figure 15-5 presents another display structure showing several views displayed simultaneously.

Virtual Dissection

A recent report by Silva et al (2006) identifies the work of various researchers who have used display tools such as 2D axial images, 2D MPR images, 3D images, CAD images, and virtual dissection images. They note that virtual dissection "is an innovative technique whereby the three dimensional (3D) model of the colon is virtually unrolled, sliced open, and displayed as a flat 3D rendering of the mucosal surface, similar to a gross pathologic specimen. This technique has the potential to reduce evaluation time by providing a more rapid 3D image assessment than is possible with an antegrade and retrograde 3D endoluminal fly-through. It may also ultimately improve accuracy by reducing blind spots present with endoluminal displays and by reducing reader fatigue" (Silva et al, 2006). Figure 15-6 illustrates the technique of virtual dissection, whereas Figures 15-7 and 15-8 show the 3D volume-rendered image of the colon and the associated virtual dissection image of the same colon, respectively.

ADVANTAGES AND LIMITATIONS

The various features of virtual endoscopy and real endoscopy have been described in the literature (Hooper, 1999; Vining, 1999; Higgins et al, 1998; Blezek and Robb, 1997). Early results indicate that virtual endoscopy offers unique features and advantages for gathering both endoluminal and extraluminal information. (Table 15-1 presents a comparison of the features of virtual and real bronchoscopy.) Virtual endoscopy can also reduce complications (e.g., infection and perforation) that could arise from real endoscopy.

More recently, and as pointed out by Macari and Bini (2005), although CT colonography is a useful tool for the evaluation of colorectal neoplasia, "substantial controversy" still exists as to its clinical efficacy. Silva et al (2006), on the other hand, explain that the technique of virtual dissection can provide radiologists with more information to

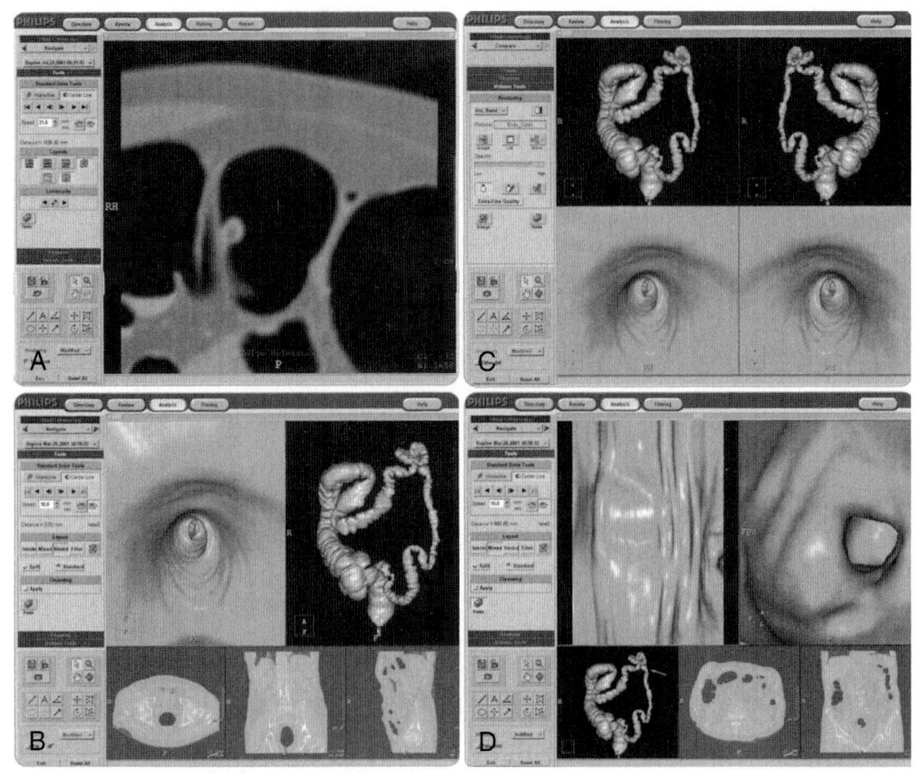

FIGURE 15-4 Examples of various display tools for CT colonoscopy. **A,** 2D/3D mode for primary inspection. **B,** Forward/reverse mode. **C,** Compare mode. **D,** Layout mode with Forward Filet view, 2D, and other reference views. (Courtesy Philips Medical Systems.)

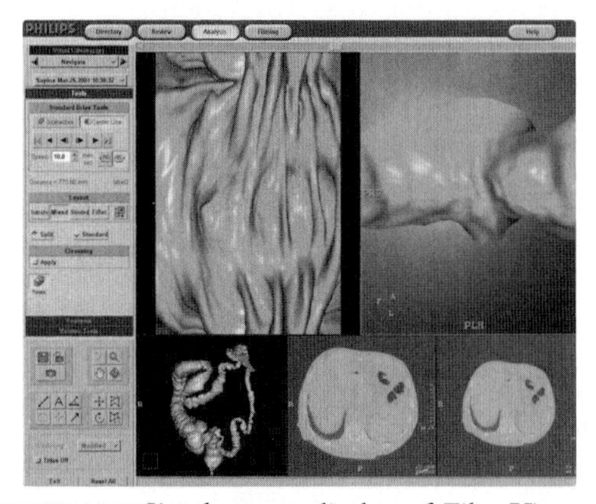

FIGURE 15-5 Simultaneous display of Filet View and split view and the location on the volume-rendered reference view offers optimum flexibility in viewing images obtained in a CT colonoscopy examination. (Courtesy Philips Medical Systems.)

ensure accurate diagnosis compared with 3D endoluminal image displays.

SOFTWARE FOR INTERACTIVE IMAGE ASSESSMENT

A wide range of software tools for interactive image assessment is available. All these packages feature a variety of visual and quantitative tools specifically for use in virtual endoscopy imaging in CT and MRI. For example, in the past, Higgins et al (1998) used QUICKSEE and VIDA in their virtual bronchoscopy studies; Blezek and

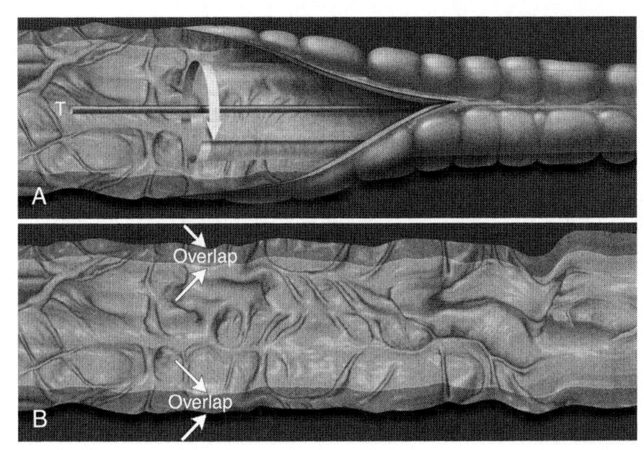

FIGURE 15-6 Virtual dissection schema. **A,** The virtual dissection software slices the colon open and unfolds it longitudinally by reconstructing the axial CT source image data from the perspective of a virtual camera with an orientation perpendicular to the midline of the colonic tract. **B,** A 360-degree view of the inner colonic surface is presented as a flattened 3D panel with a few degrees of overlap at the edges *(arrows)*. (From Silva AC et al: Three-dimensional virtual dissection at CT colonoscopy: unraveling the colon to search for lesions, *Radiographics* 26: 1669-1686, 2006. Figure and legend reproduced by permission of the Radiological Society of North America and the authors.)

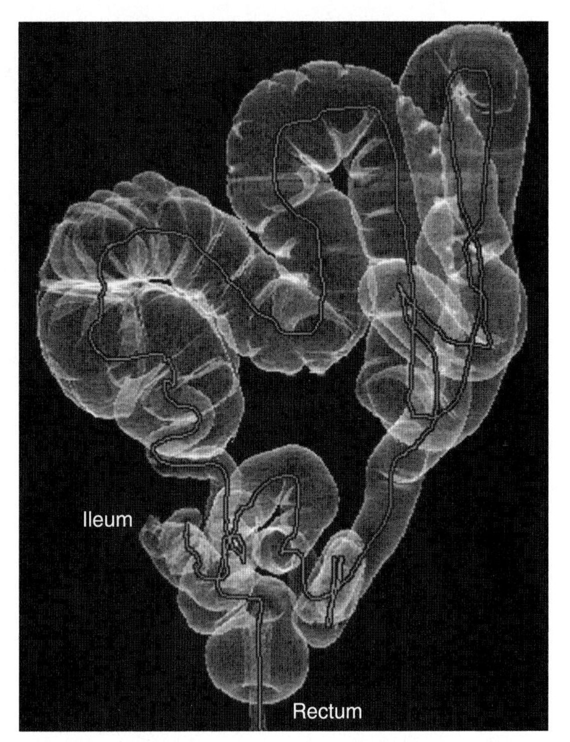

FIGURE 15-7 Normal anatomy and common features in a complete CT colonographic examination. Volume-rendered image of the colon from the rectum to the distal ileum. (From Silva AC et al: Three-dimensional virtual dissection at CT colonoscopy: unraveling the colon to search for lesions, *Radiographics* 26: 1669-1686, 2006. Figure and legend reproduced by permission of the Radiological Society of North America and the authors)

Robb (1997) used ANALYZE software, developed and used at the Mayo Clinic in Rochester, Minnesota.

Other software tools for interactive image assessment have become available, including a CT endoscopy tool (Philips Medical Systems), Navigator (General Electric Healthcare), syngo Fly Through (Siemens Medical Solutions), and the V3D System from Viatronix (Stony Brook, NY).

CT Endoscopy Tool

The CT virtual endoscopy tool is an advanced visualization package that can provide real-time "fly through" within and around tubular anatomy in the same manner that a real endoscope is used. The tool features an intuitive user interface that provides considerable flexibility in interactive image assessment. For example, mouse technology is used to guide the user through the anatomy. In addition, this tool can provide movie loop presentations, which can be recorded on videotape and used for remote communications.

A unique feature of the CT endoscopy tool is compositing (a volumetric imaging technique that displays bone, soft tissues, and vessels at the same time), also called *4D angiography*, which provides 3D images with a fourth dimension, opacity. There are other features as well, but they are beyond the scope of this chapter. For example, this tool makes use of an exclusive technology

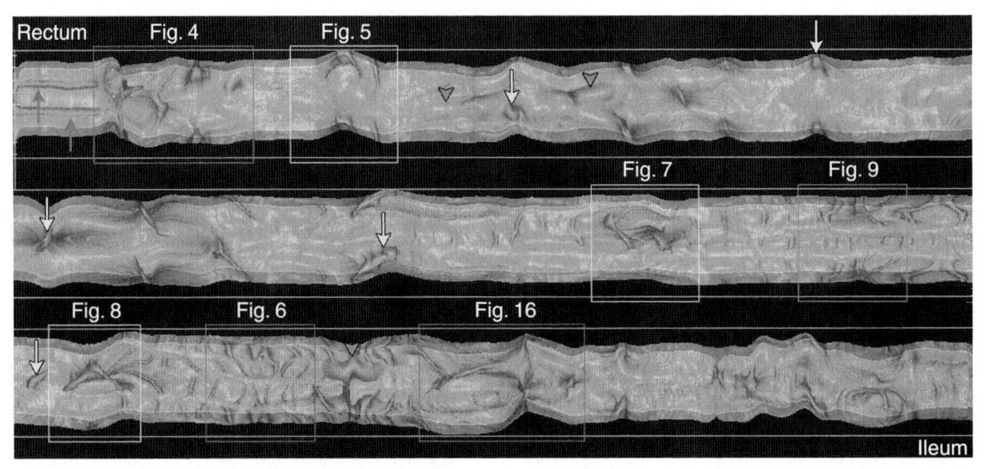

FIGURE 15-8 Virtual dissection image of the same colon shows the rectal tube as an elongated horizontal structure that parallels the midline of the tract *(red arrows)*. The adjacent section outlined in red (Fig. 6 in image) shows the normal appearance of haustral folds in a straight colonic segment. Sections outlined in yellow (Fig. 5, Fig. 7, Fig. 8 in image) and yellow arrows indicate haustral distortions related to the degree of colonic curvature and the relative position of the haustral folds on the virtual dissection image. The section outlined in green (Fig. 9 in image) and the green arrowheads indicate areas of the colon that contain residual fluid. (From Silva AC et al: Three-dimensional virtual dissection at CT colonoscopy: unraveling the colon to search for lesions, *Radiographics* 26: 1669-1686, 2006. Figure and legend reproduced by permission of the Radiological Society of North America and the authors.) Please visit http://evolve.elsevier.com/Seeram/ to view a color image.

TABLE 15-1 Comparison of Features of Virtual and Real Bronchoscopy

Virtual Bronchoscopy	Real Bronchoscopy
Imaging environment is a virtual environment as captured in a 3D CT image.	Imaging environment is illuminated in vivo endoluminal regions.
Awareness is enhanced by the many display tools.	Video is the only display tool.
Many quantitative measurements can be taken.	Quantitation is limited.
Viewing direction is unrestricted.	Only frontal views are possible.
Views inside and outside solid structures are possible.	Only endoluminal views are possible.
Viewing geometry is controllable.	Perspective is fixed.
User can track 3D position during navigation.	User must remember position of scope.
Multiple simultaneous views are possible.	User can see only one view at a time.
Cine sequences can be recorded.	High-quality video can be recorded.
No information on the mucosal surface can be obtained.	Detailed information on the mucosal surface can be obtained.
Performance of interventional procedures with views is not possible without linkage to a real bronchoscope.	Real intervention is possible.
View quality is limited by image resolution.	High-resolution video is used.

From Hooper KD: CT bronchoscopy, *Semin Ultrasound CT MRI* 20:10-15, 1999.

referred to as the *Filet View* that is intended to display all details of the structure in a single view. Figure 15-9 shows Filet Views (Fig. 15-9, *B* and *C*) compared with the typical straight-on colonoscopy view (Fig. 15-9, *A*).

The tool can be used in a wide range of clinical applications, including pre-endoscopic evaluation of lesion screening and planning of endoscopic or surgical procedures. It also can be used to explore hollow anatomical structures such as the bronchus, colon, stomach, blood vessels, upper respiratory tract and larynx, paranasal sinuses, bladder, and spinal canal, for example.

Three-Dimensional Navigator

The Navigator advanced visualization software provides a single icon-driven interface for ease of use and interaction with virtual endoscopic images. For example, it allows real-time navigation of structures, unique "fly through" of tubular structures, enhanced visualization capabilities for viewing inside cavities, smooth or edge detail viewing, and endoluminal viewing of 3D surface-rendered abnormalities of tubular structures (e.g., polyps, tumors, clots, vascular strictures or aneurysms, and blockages). The Navigator also allows the user to "fly around" the outside of the anatomy, such as the circle of Willis.

syngo Fly Through

This interactive image assessment tool allows the user to perform several tasks, including showing the inside of hollow structures, correlating 3D endoscopic and MPR images, and a number of fly modes, for example, to enhance diagnostic interpretation.

V3D Colon

The V3D Colon is yet another example of the types of interactive image assessment tool used for CT colonoscopy. It is intuitive and is intended to provide image visualization of the colon for masses, cancers, polyps and other lesions and allows the user to perform 3D measurements, translucent rendering, automated 2D flights, real-time volume rendering, automatic and interactive navigation, and automatic segmentation, to mention only a few.

Functional and Molecular Imaging Tools

The introduction of image fusion techniques for hybrid imaging such as positron emission tomography (PET)/CT that combines functional or molecular data with anatomical images produced by CT and MRI alone will require new tools to assist radiologists to navigate and interpret multidimensional multimodality images. Recently, one such tool called Osirix was introduced and described by Rosset et al (2006). The tool is also compliant with DICOM (Digital Imaging and Communication in Medicine) software that can be used to navigate through the huge image data sets generated by PET/CT scanners, multislice CT scanners that produce dynamic cardiac images, and MRI scanners that produce functional cardiac images.

FLIGHT PATH PLANNING

Figure 15-10 shows the difference between surface-rendered and volume-rendered images in CT virtual endoscopy. Figure 15-11 shows the use of the navigation tool, one of the visualization tools of the CT endoscopy tool. Three orthogonal projections are created from the image data set sent to the computer workstation to assist the user in navigating through the anatomy. First, the navigation path is outlined by placing markers along the anatomy to be examined. This is followed by a "fly through" of the path. The active virtual image is shown in the middle of the screen.

Navigation

Successful navigation within the hollow anatomical region is essential so that structures of interest can

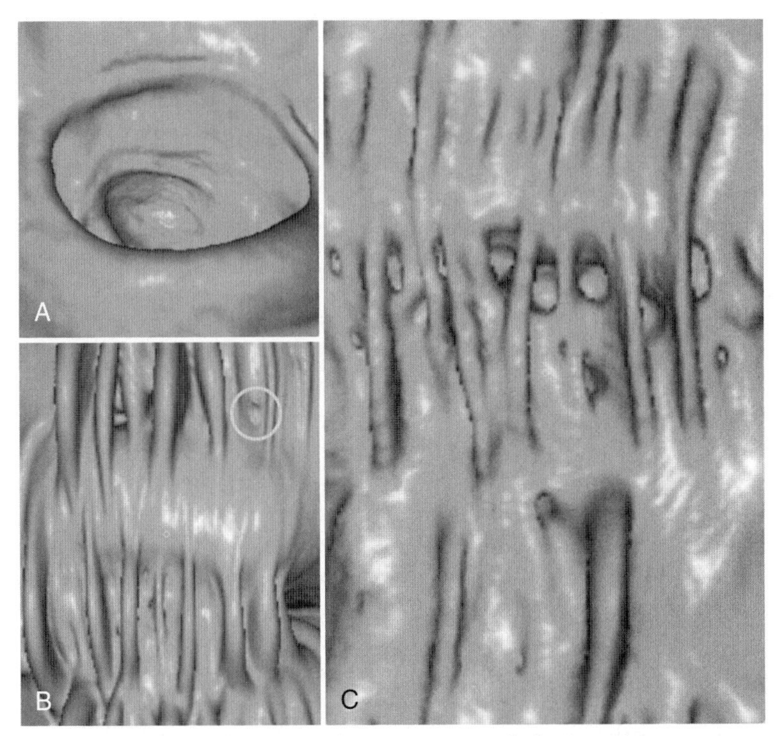

FIGURE 15-9 The effect of the Filet view in demonstrating pathologies of interest compared with the typical straight-on view in CT colonoscopy. Although the straight-on view **(A)** does not show the polyp, the Filet View **(B)** shows not only the polyp *(circle)* but also the entire lumen of the colon on a single view as well as a polyp *(circle)*. **C,** The diverticulosis and the haustral folds are demonstrated. (Courtesy Philips Medical Systems.)

be located and examined; such navigation depends on flight path algorithms. Because manual planning of flight paths can be time consuming, algorithms have been developed that plan the flight paths automatically.

An early algorithm, described by Paik et al (1998), uses a virtual "camera" to fly through the anatomy. First, the camera's position and orientation (straight pointing and angled pointing) are defined. Then a sequence of views along a path can be rendered as a sequence of frames to make a virtual endoscopic movie. Figure 15-12 presents an example of flight path planning. It shows a portion of a hollow anatomical structure in which a path has been defined. The path has three segments: start voxel (V_{start}) to S_1 segment, a segment from S_1 to S_2, and a segment from S_2 to an end voxel (V_{end}). The authors, Paik et al (1998), explain this initial path selection as follows:

> Our algorithm determines the voxel on the surface that is closest to the start voxel, S_1, and the voxel closest to the end voxel, S_2. With a goal voxel of V_{start}, the algorithm computes a Euclidean distance map for the union of the surface and the voxels in the V_{start} to S_1 line segment and the S_2 to V_{end} line segment. This distance map is computed by assigning the goal voxel a distance of zero and iteratively assigning neighbor voxels the minimum Euclidean distance along a voxel path back to the goal voxel in a breadth first traversal until all voxels are reached.

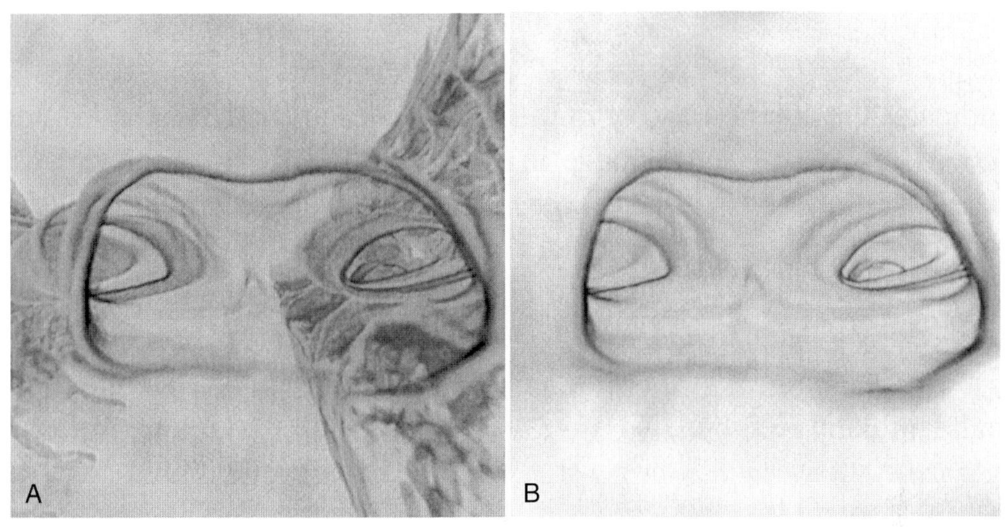

FIGURE 15-10 Visual comparison of a surface-rendered image **(A)** and a volume-rendered image **(B)** in CT virtual endoscopy. Volume rendering not only improves image quality but also reduces artifacts caused by partial volume averaging. (From Hooper KD: CT bronchoscopy, *Semin Ultrasound CT MRI* 20:10-15, 1999.)

The algorithm follows the shallowest descent to find a path connecting V_{end} to V_{start}.

FUTURE OF CT VIRTUAL ENDOSCOPY

CT virtual endoscopy is an evolving diagnostic imaging tool. Investigators involved in research and practical applications of virtual endoscopy have noted that its future is promising. It has great potential as a diagnostic tool for providing better visualization of various anatomic structures such as the colon, airways, and other tubular structures, from both outside and inside perspectives. A special review of CT colonoscopy (Macari and Bini, 2005) indicates that it is a "viable alternative imaging tool for colorectal polyp detection" and

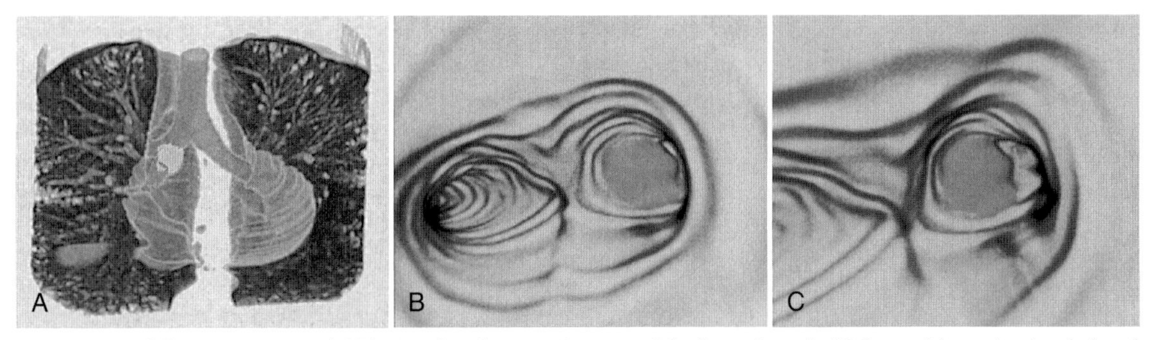

FIGURE 15-11 The appearance of CT virtual endoscopy images of the bronchus. **A,** Holographic projection helps the observer to localize the exact position and shows the "flow in flight path." **B** and **C,** Virtual endoscopic images. (Courtesy Picker International, Cleveland, Ohio.)

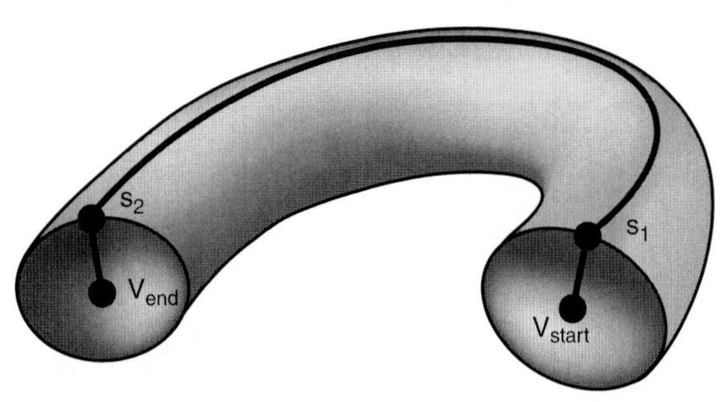

FIGURE 15-12 An example of planning a flight path in virtual endoscopy. (Paik DS et al: Automated flight path planning for virtual endoscopy, *Med Phys* 25:629-637, 1998.)

that a good deal of education in CT colonoscopy techniques will be necessary if it is to have an impact on screening the colon for cancer.

Developments in the technology for virtual endoscopy, such as digital image processing and computer visualization tools and automated techniques, can only lead to improvement of virtual endoscopy as a clinically useful tool. Multislice CT technology will have a significant impact on the accuracy of virtual endoscopy. The vast amount of data sets collected from a multislice CT scanner will generate much better virtual endoscopic images than those obtained with single-slice data sets (Kopecky, 1999). A more recent study indicates that the use of computer software for making 3D measurements and manual 3D measurements provide more accurate results that 2D manual measurements (Taylor et al, 2006).

Already, studies are under way to validate the clinical usefulness of CT virtual endoscopy in a wide range of applications, including colonoscopy and bronchoscopy, which have received more attention in the literature because of the prevalence of colorectal and bronchogenic carcinoma (Higgins et al, 1998; Hooper, 1999; Vining, 1999). Some of these studies have shown that, compared with real endoscopy, virtual endoscopy is much cheaper and risk free and causes the patient less discomfort.

As noted by Vining (1999) and others such as Macari and Bini (2005), Silva et al (2006), and Taylor et al (2006), other factors must be considered before the use of virtual endoscopy becomes commonplace, such as the following:

- It must be better than real endoscopy in detecting various anatomical structures and pathological conditions.
- Radiologists must be well versed in interpreting normal and abnormal features of the anatomy under investigation to make an accurate diagnosis.
- It should be easy to perform on patients and easy for technologists and radiologists to use.
- It should be available on all multislice CT scanners and MRI scanners as well.
- The use of computer software to make measurements provides more accuracy than manual measurements.
- It must be accepted by primary care physicians and insurance companies.
- It must be accepted by the public.

Finally, Brenner (2006) reports that currently, virtual colonoscopy is undergoing clinical trials in the United States and in other countries and will ultimately provide definitive results as to its efficacy as a screening tool for lesions in the colon.

VIRTUAL ENDOSCOPY ON THE INTERNET

The Internet currently offers a number of sites that provide not only 3D images but also virtual endoscopic images. More important, these sites offer the opportunity for "fly through" explorations of various anatomical regions. The reader is encouraged to perform a search on the Internet (a Google search, for example) on virtual colonoscopy or to visit one of the CT manufacturers' sites and experience a "fly-through."

REFERENCES

Barnes E: Medical image processing has room to grow—parts 1, 2, and 3 (2006): AuntMinni.com. Accessed December 2006.

Beaulieu CF et al: Display modes for CT colonography, *Radiology* 212:203-212, 1999.

Blezek DJ, Robb RA: Evaluating virtual endoscopy for clinical use, *J Digit Imaging* 10:51-55, 1997.

Brenner DJ: Radiation risks in diagnostic radiology. In *RSNA categorical course in diagnostic radiology: from invisible to visible—the science and practice of x-ray imaging and radiation dose optimization*, pp. 41-50, Oak Ridge, 2006, Radiological Society of North America.

Doi A et al: 3D volume extraction and mesh generation using energy minimization techniques. In: *Proceedings of the 1st International Symposium on 3D Data Processing Visualization and Transmission*, New York, 2002, IEEE.

Fleiter T et al: Comparison of real-time virtual and fiberoptic bronchoscopy in patients with bronchial carcinoma: opportunities and limitations, *AJR Am J Roentgenol* 169:1591-1595, 1997.

Higgins WE et al: Virtual bronchoscopy for three dimensional pulmonary image assessment: state of the art and future needs, *Radiographics* 18:761-778, 1998.

Hooper KD: CT bronchoscopy, *Semin Ultrasound CT MRI* 20:10-15, 1999.

Kopecky KK: Multislice CT spirals past single-slice CT in diagnostic efficiency, *Diagn Imaging* 21:36-42, 1999.

Macari M, Bini EJ: CT colonography: where have we been and where are we going? *Radiology* 237:819-833, 2005.

Paik DS et al: Automated flight path planning for virtual endoscopy, *Med Phys* 25:629-637, 1998.

Pickhardt PJ: Differential diagnosis of polypoid lesions seen at CT colonography (virtual colonoscopy), *Radiographics* 24:1535-1559, 2004.

Prassopoulos P et al: Development of virtual CT cholangiopancreatoscopy, *Radiology* 209:570-574, 1998.

Rosset A et al: Navigating the fifth dimension: innovative interface for multidimensional multimodality image navigation, *Radiographics* 26:299-308, 2006.

Silva AC et al: Three-dimensional virtual dissection at CT colonoscopy: unraveling the colon to search for lesions, *Radiographics* 26:1669-1686, 2006.

Takanashi I et al: 3D active net-3D volume extraction, *J Inst Image Information Television Eng* 51:2097-2106, 1997.

Taylor SA et al: CT colonoscopy: automated measurement of colonic polyps compared with manual techniques—human in vitro study, *Radiology* 242: 120-128, 2006.

Tomandl BF et al: Virtual labyrinthoscopy: visualization of the inner ear with interactive direct volume rendering, *Radiographics* 20:547-558, 2000.

Vining DJ: Virtual endoscopy: is it reality? *Radiology* 200:30-31, 1996.

Vining DJ: Virtual colonoscopy, *Semin Ultrasound CT MRI* 20(1):56-60, 1999.

Positron Emission Tomography/Computed Tomography Scanners*

Frederic H. Fahey and Matthew R. Palmer

Chapter Outline

*Please visit http://evolve.elsevier.com/Seeram/ and click on the Image Collection link to view color versions of the figures in this chapter.

Computed tomography (CT) of the patient can provide exquisite anatomical detail that is often invaluable for diagnosis. On the other hand, positron emission tomography (PET) provides functional information regarding the patient. For example, malignant tumors tend to be more highly metabolic because of a higher rate of glycolysis than surrounding normal tissue. Therefore, a radioactive pharmaceutical that distributes in the body according to glucose metabolic rate, such as fluorine-18–labeled 2-fluoro-2-deoxy-D-glucose (FDG) can yield additional diagnostic information to that provided by the CT scan. However, the FDG PET scan lacks anatomical detail, and thus it is often difficult to accurately localize features with high uptake. For these reasons, it is extremely useful, if not essential, to correlate the functional information provided by PET with the anatomy shown on CT. In many cases, viewing the PET and CT studies separately is adequate to make the diagnosis, but in a number of cases it is very helpful to "register" the two data sets such that they are displayed as a single "fused" image. Figure 16-1, *A*, shows a small region with high FDG uptake, but it is difficult to discern where within the thorax the feature resides. In Figure 16-1, *B*, the registered PET study is shown overlaid on the CT scan and it is much easier to determine its location. This registration and fusion of the PET and CT data can be performed either by using software approaches that determine the transformation that will best match the PET to the CT or by using a hybrid PET/CT scanner that combines both modalities into a single gantry. This chapter briefly describes the basics behind PET imaging, basic approaches to PET and PET/CT instrumentation, imaging considerations, and a review of some of the clinical applications for PET and PET/CT.

PRINCIPLES OF POSITRON EMISSION TOMOGRAPHY IMAGING

The atomic nucleus contains a number of protons and neutrons. In some instances, there may be too many of one or the other or they may be configured in such a way as to make the nucleus unstable. Such atoms are said to be "radioactive." In these cases, the nucleus may seek to become more stable by undergoing a nuclear transformation with the emission of a particle such as a γ ray or an α or β particle. If the nucleus contains too many protons, the nucleus may transform itself by emitting a positive β particle, also known as a *positron*, or by capturing an orbital electron. A positron is a positively charged β particle. It has the same mass as an electron but a positive rather than

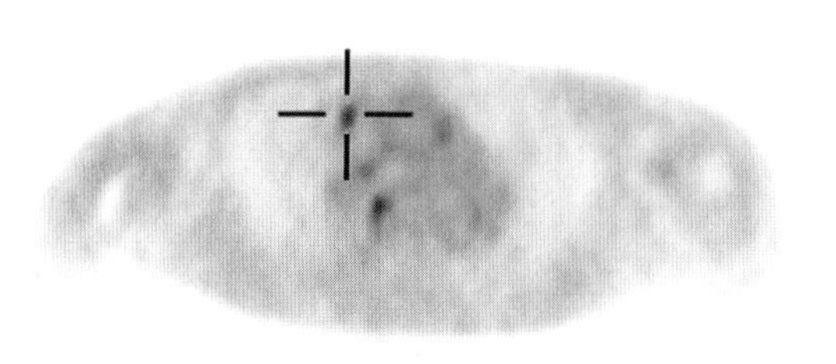

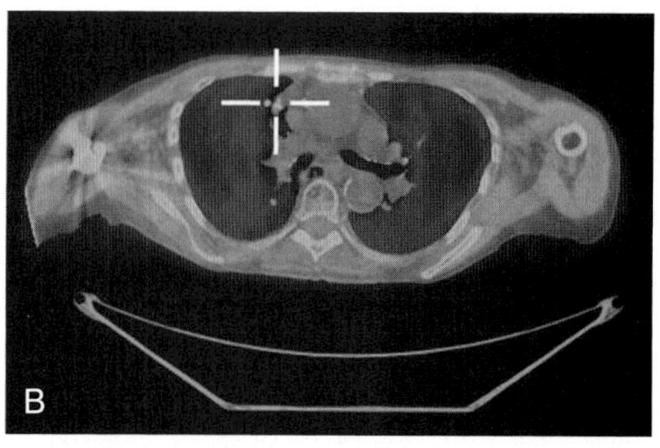

FIGURE 16-1 PET/CT scan of lung tumor. **A,** FDG PET scan of patient with a lung tumor. Although the tumor clearly shows enhanced uptake, it is difficult to localize. **B,** PET is overlaid on the registered CT scan, and the tumor can be localized much more easily.

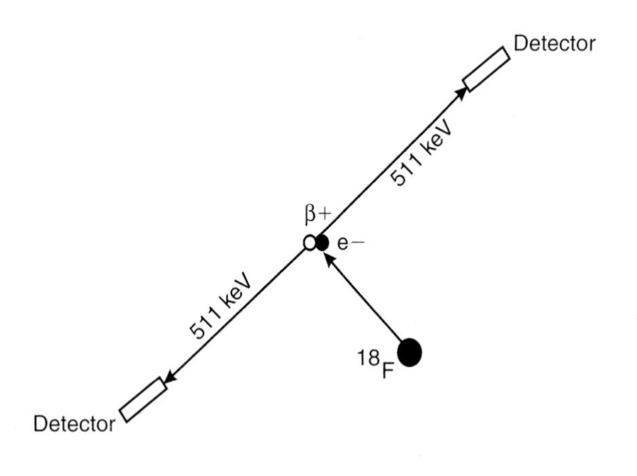

FIGURE 16-2 Annihilation coincidence detection. The positron (or β^+) is emitted from the ^{18}F atom and combines with an electron, and the pair annihilate, leading to two 511-keV photons. The site of the annihilation is assumed to be located along the line that connects the two detectors, the "LOR."

a negative charge (Cherry et al, 2003; Evans, 1982). One of the advantages of PET compared with other nuclear imaging is that many of the radioactive isotopes of elements of biological interest, such as carbon, oxygen, and nitrogen, are positron emitters, and therefore pharmaceuticals incorporating these radioisotopes can be imaged with a PET scanner. In addition, radioactive fluorine can also be very useful because it can often be chemically substituted for a hydrogen atom or a hydroxyl (OH) group. Thus, radiopharmaceuticals such as oxygen-15–labeled water, nitrogen-13–labeled ammonia, carbon-11–labeled methionine, carbon-11–labeled raclopride, or FDG can be produced. These are administered to a patient and the in vivo distribution can be imaged with a PET scanner. Such studies can provide quantitative in vivo images of blood flow, protein synthesis, neuroreceptor site density, or glucose metabolic rate.

Consider an ^{18}F-labeled radiopharmaceutical that has been administered to a patient and one of the ^{18}F atoms has been incorporated into the cell of a tumor. As shown in Figure 16-2, after some time the ^{18}F atom will transform to an oxygen-18 atom by emitting a positron. The positron will travel several millimeters (mm) in the tissue until it loses most of its kinetic energy, at which point it will combine with a neighboring electron to form an entity known as *positronium*. After a very short time ($\approx 10^{-10}$ seconds), the positron-electron pair will "annihilate," converting its mass into two photons that are emitted back to back, almost exactly in opposite directions. The energy of the two photons is determined using Einstein's equation:

$$E = mc^2 \tag{16-1}$$

where m is the mass of the electron (or positron) and c is the speed of light. Therefore, the two photons each have energy of 511 kiloelectron volts (keV).

If each of these photons interact with detectors on opposite sides of the PET scanner and are detected within a short time window (5-15 nanoseconds [i.e., 5-15 $\times 10^{-9}$ seconds]), a "coincidence" detection occurs, and the annihilation event can be assumed to have occurred along the line that connects the two detectors, referred to as the *line of response* (LOR). More accurately, the event can be localized to within the envelope defined by the two detectors and shown as the dotted lines in Figure 16-2. Thus, to a first approximation, the spatial resolution of a PET scanner is determined by the size of the radiation detectors used in the scanner. Therefore, if the scanner uses 4-mm detectors, the spatial resolution can be assumed to be about 4 mm. Modern clinical PET scanners use detectors between 4 and 7 mm in size. On the other hand, even if the annihilation event could be localized exactly, this is really not the locus of interested. One really wants to know from where was the positron emitted (i.e., the location of the ^{18}F atom within the tissue). Because the positron traveled several mm before annihilation (referred to as the *positron range*), the radiopharmaceutical distribution cannot be localized exactly. In addition, the two photons may not be

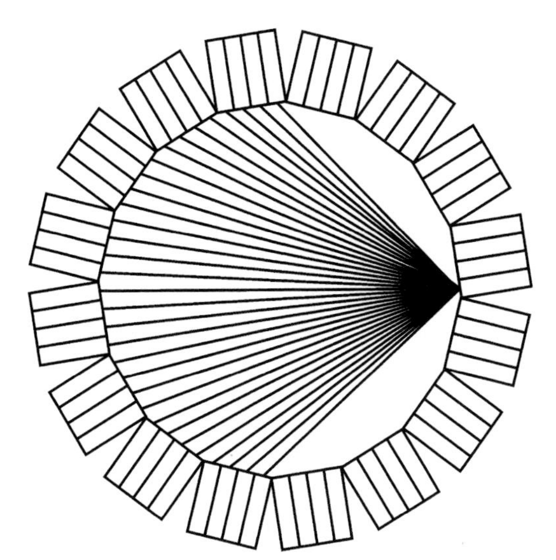

FIGURE 16-3 Ring of detectors. In a modern PET scanner, the object is surrounded by a ring of detectors. A single detector is allowed to be in coincidence with many detectors on the opposite side of the scanner.

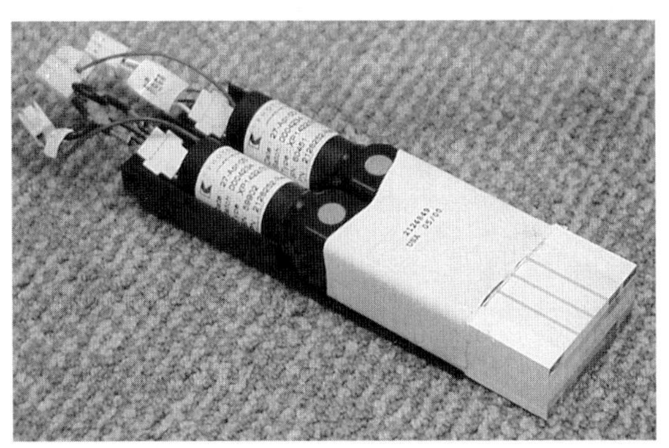

FIGURE 16-4 Block detector module from a PET scanner. A single detector module from a PET scanner consisting of a rectangular array of small detector elements and a photomultiplier tube array.

emitted at exactly 180 degrees to each other. If the positron-electron pair was not completely at rest when annihilation occurred, conservation of momentum would dictate that they would be emitted at an angle slightly different than 180 degrees. These two factors, the positron range and the slight noncolinearity of the two photons, lead to the best possible spatial resolution that could be obtained, even in a perfect PET scanner, of about 3 mm for a whole-body PET scanner and 1 mm for a small-bore animal PET scanner (Levin and Hoffman, 1999; Palmer et al, 2005).

Two small detectors on either side of the patient would not collect very many photons, and thus the placement of a large number of small detectors about the patient is necessary to acquire high-resolution PET data in a reasonable amount of time. In Figure 16-3, a single detector on one side of the patient is not only in coincidence with one detector on the opposite side but with several hundred detectors. In this manner, each detector maps out a fan beam with the detectors on the opposite side with which they are in coincidence. In a single ring, there may be as many as 500 to 700 small detectors. To acquire PET data simultaneously from a number of imaging planes, several detector rings can be placed back to back. Thus, a single detector module becomes a rectangular mosaic of small detectors (Casey and Nutt, 1986). Figure 16-4 shows a detector block from a PET scanner that is a 6×6 array of small scintillating detectors with two dual-channel photomultiplier tubes behind it. In this case, each scintillating detector measures 4×8 mm, so the entire 6×6 array is 24×48 mm. By taking the weighted sum of the signal from the photomultiplier tubes, the system determines within which of the 36 detectors the interaction occurred. A modern PET scanner may have several hundred such blocks of detectors and, thereby, the scanner contains a total of tens of thousands of small scintillating detectors.

Not all coincidence detection events are of the same quality as shown in Figure 16-5. When both annihilation photons exit the patient without incident and are detected in coincidence, this is referred to as a *true* coincidence detection. This is shown at the top of Figure 16-5. However, there is a possibility that one of the photons will undergo Compton scattering before exiting the patient, as shown in the middle of Figure 16-5.

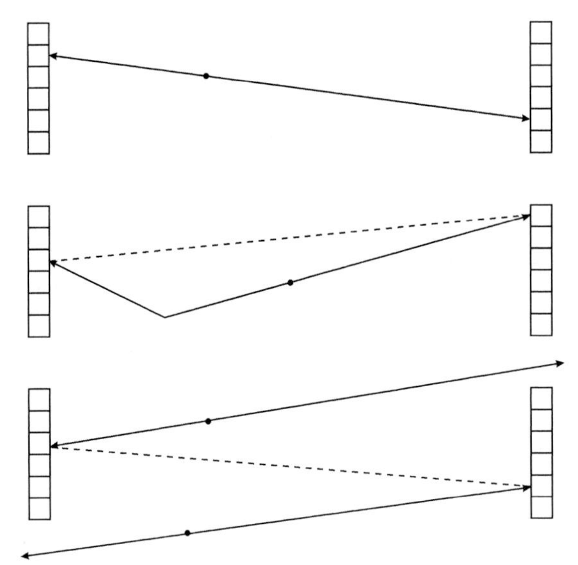

FIGURE 16-5 True, scatter, and random coincidence events. If an annihilation event occurs and the two 511-keV annihilation photons are detected without incident, this is referred to as a "true" coincidence event *(top)*. If one of the photons scatters before detection, this is referred to as a "scatter" coincidence event *(middle)*. If two unrelated events are detected at the same time, this is referred to as a "random" coincidence event *(bottom)*.

In this case the LOR associated with this coincidence detection may not pass through the annihilation event and therefore does not accurately localize the event. This is referred to as a *scatter* coincidence detection. Last, there is a possibility at higher count rates that two independent events occur simultaneously and that two photons are randomly detected in coincidence, as shown at the bottom of Figure 16-5. The resulting LOR does not accurately localize either annihilation event. This is referred to as a *random* or *accidental* coincident detection, and, without compensation, leads to background activity that reduces image contrast. The random coincidence rate can be reduced by either reducing the detector count rates or by reducing the coincidence timing window (Hoffman and Phelps, 1986).

The crystals used in the construction of PET scanner detectors in PET scanners are scintillators. Photons interact in the crystal resulting in the emission of light, which is collected by an array of photomultiplier tubes as shown in Figure 16-4. Table 16-1 lists some common scintillating materials that have been used for PET detectors. Sodium iodide (NaI), the material used in γ cameras, emits the most light per photon, and thereby yields the best energy resolution. However, the lower density and lower effective Z number (the average number of protons per atom) leads to lower detection efficiency (i.e., a smaller fraction of the photons that strike the detector will interact). Bismuth germanate (BGO) has both a higher density and effective Z number, and therefore higher detection efficiency. However, both NaI and BGO emit their scintillation light rather slowly and thus require a 12-nanosecond coincidence

TABLE 16-1 Potential Positron Emission Tomography Scanner Scintillating Materials

Scintillator	NaI	BGO	LSO	GSO
Density (g/mL)	3.67	7.13	7.40	6.71
Photoelectric linear attenuation (cm^{-1})	0.06	0.39	0.23	0.18
Compton linear attenuation (cm^{-1})	0.28	0.52	0.56	0.46
Relative light yield	100	15	75	40
Decay constant (nanoseconds)	230	300	40	50
Peak wavelength (nanometers)	410	480	420	440
Effective Z	51	75	66	59
Index of refraction	1.85	2.15	1.82	1.85
Hygroscopic?	Yes	No	No	No

timing window. Lutetium oxyorthosilicate (LSO) and gadolinium oxyorthosilicate (GSO) are newer scintillating materials that have reasonably high detection efficiency (densities and effective Z numbers almost as high as that of BGO) and emit their light much more quickly (Daghighian et al, 1993; Surti et al, 2000). This allows the coincidence timing window to be reduced by at least a factor of two (from 12 to 5 or 6 nanoseconds). Because the random coincidence rate is proportional to the coincidence timing window, this results in a corresponding reduction in randoms rate.

One approach to reducing scatter coincidences is to introduce absorbing septa between the detector rings. These septa act similarly to the antiscatter grids routinely used in radiography and thereby greatly reduce interplanar scatter within the scanner. In addition, these septa can reduce the contributions to the random coincidence rate attributed to activity that is outside the axial field of view. For example, in imaging the neck of a patient, photons from activity in the brain can increase the detector count rates and thereby the randoms coincidence count rate. However, placement of interplane septa will shield the detectors from this out-of-field activity, leading to a reduction in the random coincidence rate. With the septa in place, detectors are allowed to be in coincidence with either detectors in the same ring or adjacent rings, and thus the data can be reconstructed as a series of two-dimensional (2D) transverse planes. This is referred to as *2D PET acquisition mode*. Removal of the septa will allow detectors in one ring to be in coincidence with detectors from many rings. Acquiring PET data without the use of interplane septa is referred to as three-dimensional (3D) PET acquisition mode because a 3D algorithm must be used for its reconstruction. The use of 3D mode leads to a substantial increase in sensitivity, particularly in the center of the axial field of view. In the center of the scanner, the sensitivity may be as much as ten times higher for 3D mode compared with 2D mode. However, on the periphery of the axial field of view, the sensitivity is not different than for 2D, and thus the overall sensitivity gain is about a factor of 4 or 5. The disadvantage of 3D mode compared with 2D mode is the higher scatter fraction (35%-50% for 3D compared with 10%-20% for 2D) and increased random coincidences from activity out of the field of view. For these reasons, 3D is typically used in brain PET, whereas thoracic or abdominal PET may be performed with either 2D or 3D PET (Badawi et al, 1996; El Fakhri et al, 2002; Lartizien et al, 2004). Some scanners have retractable septa and thus allow the radiologic technician to select either 2D or 3D mode, but other scanners do not have septa and thus acquire data solely in 3D mode.

The ring diameter of most clinical PET scanners is about 1 meter. Thus, it takes about 3 nanoseconds for an annihilation photon to traverse the scanner. If the scintillating material emits its light fast enough and the coincidence electrons are appropriately accurate, one might be able to time the arrival of the annihilation photons and discern not only the LOR of a particular annihilation event, but where along the LOR the event occurred. This approach is referred to as *time of flight* PET. Such localization data could be used by the reconstruction algorithm and lead to a more accurate reconstruction of the PET data. Even localizing this event to within a few centimeters (cm) along the LOR could substantially improve the quality and accuracy of the reconstructed PET data (Kuhn et al, 2004; Lewellen, 1998). Faster scintillating materials are currently being used, and the scanner electronics are constantly being improved; thus PET scanners that can use time-of-flight information are starting to be introduced into the marketplace.

ATTENUATION CORRECTION

The probability of detecting the photons from an annihilation event from the center of an object is less than that for an event on the periphery because at least one of the photons is more likely

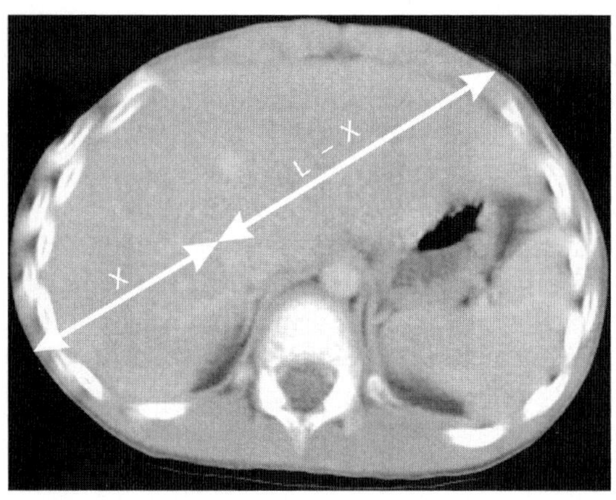

FIGURE 16-6 Photon attenuation in PET. This figure illustrates an annihilation event in the abdomen of a patient. The photon going in one direction must traverse a distance of x, whereas the photon going in the opposite direction must traverse $L - x$. The total probability that both photons will escape the body is given by $e^{-\mu L}$, which depends only on the total thickness of the patient along the LOR and not on the location of the event along the LOR.

to be absorbed or scattered if it has to travel through more material. Thus, if there are two features, each with exactly the same amount of activity, the one on the periphery will have a much higher signal than the one at the center. To achieve uniform quantitative accuracy, the spatial variation in attenuation must be corrected (Cherry et al, 2003).

Consider two PET detectors in coincidence and the intersection of the LOR and an object of uniform attenuating material where L is the length of the LOR within the object. Also consider an annihilation event that occurs at a point within the object along this LOR. This is shown in Figure 16-6. If the distance from this point to the edge of the object in one direction is x and in the other direction it is (L – x), the probability of one of the annihilation photons escaping the object without being attenuated is $e^{-\mu x}$ and in the other direction it is $e^{-\mu(L - x)}$, where μ is the linear attenuation coefficient for the material in question and e is equal to about 2.718 and is the base of the natural logarithm. Thus, the probability of both photons escaping without being attenuated is the product of these two probabilities:

$$P = (e^{-\mu x}) \times \left(e^{-\mu(L-x)}\right) = e^{-\mu L} \quad (16\text{-}2)$$

Thus the total probability that both photons escape without attenuation does not depend on where along the LOR the event occurs. It only depends on the thickness of the object along the LOR, L. If x is small, photons traveling in the x direction are less likely to be attenuated, but those moving in the other direction are more likely and the total probability remains the same. So, to know how many annihilation events would have been detected along this LOR if there were no photons attenuated, it is necessary to divide the number of detected events by $e^{-\mu L}$ or, alternatively, multiply the number of detected events by $e^{\mu L}$. If the attenuating material is uniform and the object outline can be defined, then the value of L can be determined for each LOR and the previous formula used to apply corrections to each LOR before reconstruction. The resultant reconstructed data would be free of the attenuation artifact. This process is referred to as *calculated attenuation correction*.

The object is considered to consist of materials of varying attenuation coefficients. For example, in a thoracic PET scan, LORs may pass through varying amounts of soft tissue, bone (in the spine), and lung. In this case, it is necessary to determine the degree of attenuation along each LOR rather than just the extent. In transmission tomography it is this variation in attenuation that makes the CT scan possible, but for emission imaging, this confounds the data and therefore a correction for it must be applied. One approach is to use an external, photon-emitting source that rotates about the patient to acquire a "transmission scan." First, a transmission scan is acquired without the object (or patient) in place, referred to as a *blank scan*. Then the patient is placed within the scanner and another transmission scan is acquired. For each LOR, the number of counts in the blank scan is divided by the number of counts in the transmission scan to determine the attenuation correction factor. A separate attenuation correction factor is calculated for LOR. Later, after the PET emission scan is acquired, the number of events along each LOR is multiplied by the attenuation correction factor for that LOR and the resultant data are reconstructed. Note that this approach need not make any assumptions about the attenuation material along the LOR, be it soft tissue, bone, or lung. It only looks at the ratio of events acquired with and without the patient in place, that is, the transmission and blank scans, respectively. This approach is referred to as *measured attenuation correction*.

With measured attenuation correction, two sets of noisy data (the blank and transmission scan) are taken and used to correct a third noisy data set. Thus, its application can lead to a substantial increase in the noise in the final reconstructed PET scan. One approach to reducing this noise is to process a reconstructed version of the attenuation correction factors in such a way that the radiologist determines which pixels are most likely bone, which are most likely soft tissue, and which are lungs and applies a single value depending on the type of material for that particular tissue. This is referred to as *image segmentation* because the pixel values are categorized into tissue segments. This greatly reduces the noise associated with the attenuation correction and allows the transmission data to be acquired for a shorter amount of time. The second approach is to use a single photon-emitting source rather than a positron-emitting source.

CT–BASED ATTENUATION CORRECTION

A third approach to attenuation correction in PET is to use the data from a CT scan that is registered to the PET data; that is, it is the same size and in the same orientation and sliced along the same planes as the PET scan (Kinahan et al, 2003). Such registration can be achieved by acquiring both data sets with a hybrid PET/CT scanner or by applying a software registration algorithm to PET and CT data that were acquired on separate machines.

CT inherently provides images of the attenuation properties of the object being imaged. The pixel values are recorded in CT or Hounsfield units (HU) where

$$\mathrm{HU} = \frac{\mu - \mu_{\mathrm{water}}}{\mu_{\mathrm{water}}} \qquad (16\text{-}3)$$

where μ and μ_{water} are the linear attenuation coefficients, at the CT x-ray energy, of the material within the pixel and water, respectively. HU for water is zero, for air −1000, for soft tissue −100 to 100, and for bone about 1000. Therefore, if CT data are available, it is reasonable to use these data for PET attenuation correction. However, there are several major differences between the attenuation data available from CT and that necessary for PET attenuation correction. First, photons used in CT have substantially lower energy than the annihilation photons from PET. The tube voltages typically used in CT are between 80 and 140 peak kilovolts (kVp), leading to mean energies in the 35 to 50 keV range compared with the 511 keV photons used in PET. In Figure 16-7, *A* the linear attenuation coefficients for soft tissue, air, bone, and iodine are plotted as a function of energy, and there is a substantial difference between those in the CT energy range (35-140 keV) and those at 511 keV. Thus, a transformation must be applied between CT HU values and the linear attenuation coefficient suitable for 511 keV. One such transformation is shown in Figure 16-7, *B*. The linear attenuation coefficient for soft tissue at 511 keV is 0.0925 cm^{-1} which corresponds to the value of the transformation at HU equals 0. For HU values between −1000 and 0, the material is assumed to be a mixture of air and soft tissue, which on a per-density basis have very similar attenuation properties, and thus there

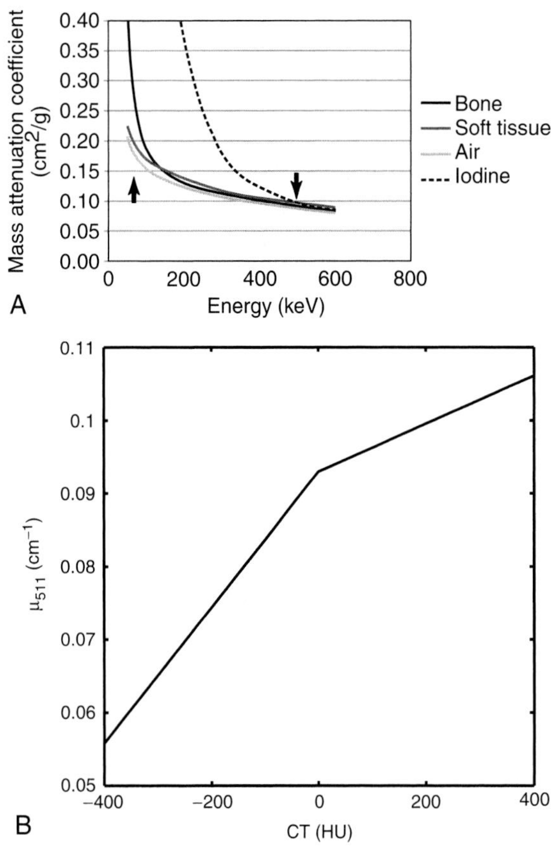

FIGURE 16-7 CT-based attenuation correction for PET. **A,** The mass attenuation coefficients (that is, the linear attenuation coefficient per unit mass) for bone, soft tissue, air, and iodine as a function of photon energy. The arrow on the left of the figure denotes the mean energy range for CT, whereas the arrow on the right indicates 511 keV. **B,** Multilinear transformation from CT HU to the linear attenuation coefficient for 511 keV for PET attenuation correction.

is a single linear slope in this region. For HU values greater than 0, the material is assumed to be a mixture of soft tissue and bone and therefore the linear transformation has a different slope (Lonn, 2003).

There is also a substantial difference in the spatial resolution between CT (on the order of 1.0 mm) and PET (6-8 mm). Applying a very sharp CT correction to smoother PET data can lead to artifacts at the edge of structures within the object. To compensate for this, the transformed CT data are smoothed to a spatial resolution more typical of PET. The resultant transformed, smoothed CT data are subsequently reprojected into an array of attenuation correction factors that can be applied to the PET emission data on reconstruction. Compared with traditional PET measured attenuation correction, the CT data have substantially less noise, and thus the application of CT-based attenuation correction adds very little additional noise to the reconstructed image. Also, the CT data are acquired in a very short amount of time (less than 1 minute) compared with the PET transmission scan (typically 3 minutes per bed position and 18 minutes for a six-bed whole body study).

INSTRUMENTATION

The majority of state-of-the-art PET scanners use the block design previously described. Typically, the individual scintillation detectors are 4 to 7 mm in the transverse direction (around the ring) and 6 to 8 mm in the axial direction (into the ring) and 20 to 30 mm thick. The scanner may consist of 18 to 40 detector rings over a 15-cm axial field of view with a total of 500 to 700 small detectors per ring. Therefore, a modern PET scanner may consist of 9000 to 25,000 small scintillation detectors. The spatial resolution of modern scanners ranges from 4.8 to 6.5 mm depending on the detector size. A scintillation material with high detection efficiency such as BGO, LSO, or GSO is used. Scanners using scintillators that emit their light more quickly (such as LSO and GSO) can reduce their coincidence timing window and thereby reduce the number of random coincidences when imaging high activity concentrations (Fahey, 2001; Fahey 2003).

The availability of interplane septa allows for the acquisition of PET data in 2D mode, which substantially reduces the amount of interplane scatter and random coincidences from activity

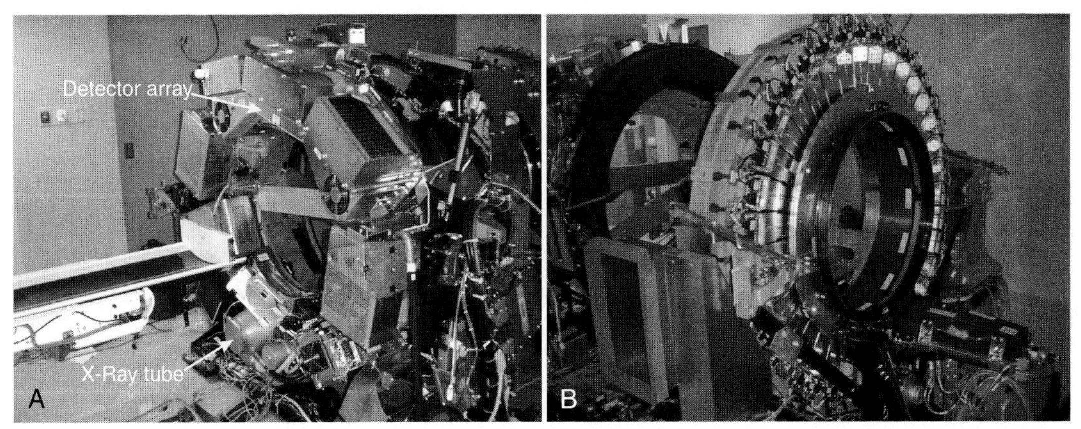

FIGURE 16-8 PET/CT scanner. **A,** CT portion of a modern PET/CT scanner with the covers removed. The detector array and the x-ray tube are noted. **B,** PET component of the PET/CT scanner. Note the ring of block detector modules with photomultiplier tubes.

that is outside the axial field of view. Alternatively, 3D mode leads to an increase by a factor of 4 or 5 in sensitivity. Some modern scanners have retractable septa that provide the option of acquiring data in 2D or 3D mode, whereas other scanners do not have septa and can only be operated in 3D mode. The use of scintillating material with higher and faster light output may reduce scatter and random coincidences so that 3D PET can provide whole body studies with excellent image quality.

All new scanners are now hybrid PET/CT scanners. The CT portion of hybrid PET/CT systems takes advantage of recent developments in multidetector CT technology. Early PET/CT systems used single-detector or four-detector helical CT systems, but modern hybrid scanners may incorporate CT with 8, 16, 64, or even more slices. Figure 16-8 shows two views of a PET/CT system. As is typical, Figure 16-8, *A*, shows the CT component of the system, and Figure 16-8, *B*, shows the PET component. In reality, PET/CT scanners are two separate machines in close proximity with a single bed that moves the patient between the two. The PET and CT data are acquired sequentially.

CLINICAL PET AND PET/CT DATA ACQUISITION

The following describes a typical workflow of a clinical PET procedure. The patient arrives in the PET center, is taken to a preparatory/injection room and injected with the PET radiopharmaceutical. The patient may wait in this room while the radiopharmaceutical distributes within the body. The amount of waiting time will depend on the biokinetics associated with that particular tracer. The patient is then escorted to the scanner room and placed on the imaging table, and the PET emission scan is acquired. In a hybrid scanner, the CT scan is typically acquired just before the PET emission acquisition. In that manner, the CT scout view can be used to position the study anatomically. In a PET-only scanner, a transmission scan may also be acquired, typically just before or just after emission acquisition in each bed position. These data are then reconstructed and processed, and the resultant images are interpreted and analyzed by the physician. Each part of this workflow is briefly reviewed.

One of the great advantages of PET is the fact that many of the elements that are considered biologically pertinent (e.g., carbon, nitrogen, and oxygen) have isotopes that are positron emitters. Therefore, many naturally occurring substrates can be made into radiopharmaceuticals by the simple substitution of a nucleus with a positron-emitting isotope. Some examples are ^{15}O-labeled water, ^{15}O carbon monoxide, ^{13}N ammonia, and ^{11}C methionine. Additionally, ^{18}F can often be substituted for a hydrogen or an OH group such as with ^{18}F FDG or ^{18}F fluorothymidine. However, the disadvantage of the use of these isotopes is their relatively short half-lives, that is, 2, 10, 20, and 110 minutes for ^{15}O, ^{13}N, ^{11}C, and ^{18}F, respectively. Although ^{18}F has a sufficiently long half-life that its radiopharmaceuticals can be produced in regional radiopharmacies and delivered to clinical PET centers, the other three radioisotopes must be produced on site with the use of a medical cyclotron. These cyclotrons typically can generate accelerated charge particle beams in excess of 10 megaelectron volts (MeV) and can be used for the routine production of ^{11}C, ^{13}N, ^{15}O, and ^{18}F.

In some cases, a radiopharmaceutical generator system, similar to the molybdenum-99 (^{99}Mo)–technetium-99m (^{99m}Tc) generator routinely used in conventional nuclear medicine, can be used to deliver PET radioisotopes. For example, the strontium-82 (^{82}Sr)–rubidium-82 (^{82}Rb) generator can be used to provide ^{82}Rb to the PET clinic. ^{82}Sr (25-day half-life) decays to ^{82}Rb (75-second half-life). The ^{82}Sr is chemically bound to a ceramic column. Some of the ^{82}Sr will decay to ^{82}Rb, which has different chemistry and, thereby, will no longer be bound to the column. The column is eluted with saline solution and ^{82}Rb is washed away into a vial, where it is available to be administered to the patient. ^{82}Rb distributes to the myocardium in a manner similar to that of thallium-201 (^{201}Tl) and thus provides a PET alternative to measuring myocardial perfusion and viability. Its use has been shown to be of significant clinical value, particularly in larger patients. The PET clinic can purchase a generator every 4 to 6 weeks and have ^{82}Rb available every day without relying on a regional radiopharmacy.

By far, the most commonly used radiopharmaceutical for PET imaging is FDG, which is a radioactive analog of glucose and thereby distributes in tissues that are actively metabolizing glucose. This makes FDG a useful radiopharmaceutical for a number of very different clinical applications, including neurology, cardiology, and oncology. More specifics of the clinical use of FDG are presented in a later section. Although some PET clinics have their own medical cyclotrons, most receive delivery of their FDG in unit doses from a regional radiopharmacy. They contact the radiopharmacy the previous day and inform them of which types of studies will be performed and how much activity they need for each examination. On the day of the examination, the clinic receives a shipment of the syringes needed for that day. Before injection, the syringe is assayed in the dose calibrator to ensure that the appropriate amount of activity is in the syringe for that study.

Consider, as an example, a whole-body FDG scan. Once the patient arrives at the clinic and is registered, he or she is taken to the preparatory/injection room. The patient is injected with the FDG and then must wait for the radiopharmaceutical to distribute within the body. This uptake waiting period is typically 40 to 60 minutes and 45 to 90 minutes for brain and whole-body imaging, respectively. Because most of the time the patient will be sitting in this room with radioactivity on board, the room should be sufficiently removed from the PET scanner and other γ-counting or imaging equipment or appropriately shielded. After the uptake period, the patient is moved to the imaging room and placed on the imaging table. Because the imaging session will take at least 30 minutes, it may be helpful to secure the patient with hook-and-loop (Velcro) wraps or tape.

Most modern PET scans have an axial field of view of at least 15 cm. If the portion of the patient to be scanned is larger than that, multiple scans are acquired at different axial offsets by moving the couch in precisely controlled steps. The resultant reconstructed images will be formatted so that they can be reviewed as one continuous study. The time to acquire the emission scan at each position may range from 3 to 10 minutes depending on the equipment used and the diagnostic task at hand. If measured attenuation correction is to be applied, a transmission scan (3 to 5 minutes per position) will be acquired at each position. It is desirable to acquire the transmission scan as close as possible to the time of the emission scan and, because it takes time to move the radioactive sources used for the transmission scan in and out of their shielded housings, the emission and transmission scans might be interleaved as follows: emission—transmission—move bed—transmission—emission—move bed—emission—transmission until the study is complete. A whole-body PET scan typically incorporates data from the patient's thighs up to the eyes and, thus, on a machine with a 15-cm axial field of view, would be composed of as many as six or seven bed positions. With both emission and transmission scans, such a study may take an hour or more to acquire. If a CT scan is used rather than transmission scan data for attenuation correction, the CT acquisition takes less than a minute to acquire, so this would reduce the time to complete the study by 20 minutes or so.

ADVANTAGES AND LIMITATIONS OF POSITRON EMISSION TOMOGRAPHY/CT

Hybrid PET/CT scanners were introduced in the 1990s, but the technology did not reach clinical acceptance until more recently (Steinert and von Schulthess, 2002; Wahl, 2004). From the very first use of the early commercial units, it became clear that the combination of these two modalities provided a number of significant advantages over the PET-only devices. The advantages of PET/CT include precise, accurate, and rapidly measured attenuation correction and anatomical correlation for the functional PET scans. However, there are some limitations to the technology that also need to be considered. These include expense, additional radiation dose to the patient, and potential attenuation artifacts that can confound the interpretation of the scans. Although the advantages, in most cases, far outweigh the limitations, it is prudent to be cognizant of their extent and nature.

As described previously, CT-based attenuation correction enables precise and accurate attenuation correction of PET emission data. The number of photons that comprise a CT scan is far in excess of those acquired in a transmission scan using a rotating rod source. For this reason, the magnitude of the noise in the CT scan is substantially lower than in the transmission scan, and thus the noise in the reconstructed CT-based attenuation corrected PET scan is substantially lower. Figure 16-9 shows the effect of various approaches to attenuation correction on a 20-cm-diameter cylindrical phantom uniformly filled with activity. The images are of the same slice reconstructed with no attenuation correction (Fig. 16-9, *A*), calculated attenuation correction (Fig. 16-9, *B*), CT-based attenuation correction (Fig. 16-9, *C*), and conventional measured attenuation correction measured by transmission scanning (Fig. 16-9, *D*). In Figure 16-9, *A*, the effect of not applying attenuation correction can be seen, with the center of the phantom appearing to have a much lower activity concentration than the periphery. In Figure 16-9, *B*, a calculated attenuation correction was applied and thereby no additional noise was added to the data. The quantum noise present in the reconstructed image is solely due to the emission data. In Figure 16-9, *C*, CT-based attenuation correction was used, and it is noted that this figure is almost identical to Figure 16-9, *B*. The very slight additional noise added to the resultant corrected image is virtually imperceptible with CT-based attenuation correction. In Figure 16-9, *D*, the measured attenuation correction was performed by acquisition of a 3-minute transmission scan using rotating rod sources of an equilibrium mixture of germanium-68 and gallium-68. It is noted that substantially more noise is added to the subsequent reconstruction from this measured attenuation correction than from the CT-based approach. In addition, the use of CT-based attenuation correction

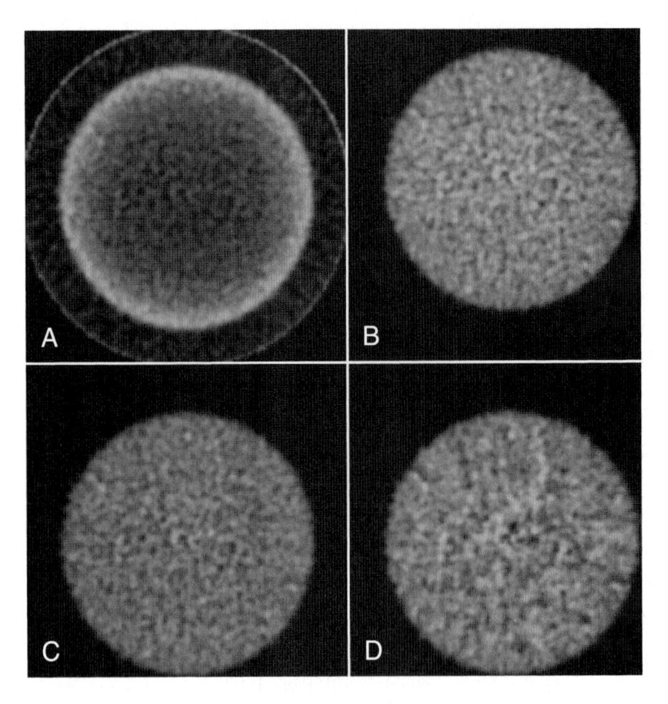

FIGURE 16-9 Attenuation correction of a uniform phantom. A cylindrical phantom filled with ^{18}F was imaged in a PET/CT scanner and reconstructed without applying attenuation correction as well as with three types of attenuation correction. **A,** No attenuation correction was applied. **B,** Calculated attenuation correction was applied. **C,** CT-based attenuation correction was applied. **D,** Measured attenuation correction using rotating rod sources of $^{68}Ge/^{68}Ga$ was applied.

substantially reduces the time necessary for the overall PET study. Conventional measured attenuation correction requires a transmission scan be acquired at each bed position, potentially adding 3 to 5 minutes for each bed position. On the other hand, the entire CT scan can be acquired in under a minute, thus reducing the scan time by 15 to 20 minutes.

As illustrated in the clinical examples in a later section, the combination of the anatomical information from the CT scan with the functional information provided by PET can be invaluable for the diagnosis of the patient's condition. In some instances it can be extremely valuable in localizing and determining the extent of the pathology. Conversely, the CT scan can better help to define normal anatomy with high uptake and rule out pathological conditions. A good example of this is in identifying brown fat. Brown fat is adipose tissue containing a dark pigment present more commonly in small children and related to the regulation of body temperature that can have a very high FDG uptake and thus could be confused with either tumor or metastatic disease located in lymph nodes. The CT scan can often identify those areas of brown fat as distinct from disease. In some cases, the CT acquired in conjunction with the PET is only used for anatomical correlation, whereas in other cases it can be acquired as a diagnostic CT scan. Acquiring the PET scan together with a diagnostic CT scan in the same imaging session can be an efficient use of the imaging equipment and usually much more convenient to the patient.

Despite the substantial advantages of hybrid PET/CT, one disadvantage is the higher radiation dose delivered to the patient. The radiation dose delivered by CT depends on a number of factors, including tube voltage, tube current, and exposure time (Fahey et al, 2007). In addition, the effective dose to the patient would depend on the region of the body that is scanned. Typical effective doses for helical CT of the chest and abdomen/pelvis are 7.5 to 12.9 and 12.4 to 16.1 millisieverts (mSv) (750 to 1290 and 1240 to 1610 millirads), respectively (Cohnen et al, 2003). Because the CT portion of a PET/CT is acquired over an extended part of the body, it is reasonable to assume that the effective dose for this is closer to 20 mSv. This can be compared with the typical effective dose for a FDG PET study involving a 520 megabecquerels (MBq) injection of 10 mSv (International Committee on Radiation Protection, 1998). Therefore, the effective dose to the patient arising from the CT portion of the study can be double that from the PET portion. In some cases, a diagnostic CT scan may not be indicated for this type of study (e.g., for brain imaging, where magnetic resonance imaging (MRI) is the anatomical imaging modality of choice), and thus the CT scan is only used for attenuation correction. Even if CT is indicated, a diagnostic CT scan may be acquired in addition to the PET/CT scan. In some instances, if the patient has moved between the acquisition of the CT scan and the PET scan, then another CT scan may have to be acquired. In all these cases, the acquisition of a CT scan with a much lower radiation dose may be appropriate. A CT scan adequate for attenuation correction can be obtained with a much reduced tube current (10 milliamperes [mA] instead of 200 mA or more) and in the case of smaller patients, lower tube voltages (as low as 80 kVp) can be used. Lowering the tube current from 200 to 10 mA reduces the radiation dose by a factor of 20, and reducing the tube voltage from 120 to 80 kVp can lead to a further reduction by at least a factor of 3 (Fahey et al, 2007). Although such reduction in tube current and voltage would still lead to an adequate attenuation correction, the utility of the resultant CT images for anatomical correlation would be limited because of the excessive quantum noise.

In some cases, the use of CT-based attenuation correction can lead to artifacts in the reconstructed PET data. There are two assumptions associated with CT-based attenuation correction, and if either one of these is not met, notable artifacts can occur that can sometimes affect the ability to interpret the study. The first assumption is that the patient is in exactly the same position and state during the acquisition of both the CT and PET scans. The second assumption is that the transformation used to convert CT HU values to the linear attenuation coefficient at 511 keV is appropriate for all materials within the field of view. Typically, the CT scan is acquired first, starting at the head and moving toward the feet. As previously noted, this acquisition can take less than 1 minute. The PET scan is then acquired, starting below the bladder and moving toward the head. This acquisition can take 20 to 40 minutes to acquire. Thus for the head and neck in a whole body PET scan, there can be 30 to 40 minutes between the time the CT scan was acquired and when the PET scan was acquired. It is possible that the patient could move in this time so that the CT and PET scans are no longer registered. This can lead to an artifact in the reconstructed PET data. For example, if the CT scan is shifted laterally relative to the PET scan, then one side of the patient will be undercorrected and the other side will be overcorrected. The asymmetry introduced could be interpreted as being the result of a pathological condition. Therefore, it is crucial to keep the patient immobilized from the beginning of the CT scan until the end of the PET scan. In addition, the final reconstructed data should be visually evaluated for the presence of this artifact. If this artifact is suspected, the PET data can be reconstructed without attenuation correction to see whether the asymmetry exists in the underlying emission data. If this artifact is noted and the patient is still on the imaging table, it might be possible to acquire a low-dose CT scan to be used for attenuation correction of this part of the body, or a calculated attenuation correction could be applied.

Even if the patient is kept very still, the motion of internal organs from breathing can also lead to artifacts in the reconstructed PET data. It is routine practice in conventional CT of the chest to have the patient hold the breath during the acquisition of the helical CT scan. However, because it takes 30 to 40 minutes to acquire the PET emission scan, it is impossible to have the patient hold the breath for that period of time, so the patient is typically instructed to breathe quietly during the PET scan. The attenuation in the area of the diaphragm during the PET study will be an average over the entire breathing cycle and over many cycles. Applying attenuation correction from the CT data acquired during a particular instant over the liver and diaphragm can lead to substantial overcorrections in regions of the lung, resulting in regions of apparent high uptake in the lungs that could either be confused for tumor or obscure actual conditions. Several approaches have been used to better control breathing during the data acquisition to help minimize these artifacts (Goerres et al, 2003). One approach is to allow the patient to breathe during the acquisition of the CT scan. The patient can also be instructed to hold the breath at mid or end expiration rather than at end inspiration. This probably leads to the diaphragm being in about the same position in the two studies. A more complicated technical approach is to gate the CT and PET acquisitions on the respiratory cycle and use these data to better register the two data sets. In these studies, an apparatus is used to monitor the breathing cycle during the data acquisition. This leads to a number of scans acquired at different parts of the respiratory cycle. The resultant data can be averaged over the breathing cycle before attenuation correction so that it more closely matches the PET data. In addition to providing better registration between the CT and the PET data for artifact-free attenuation correction, respiratory gating can also improve the quantification of lung tumors by reducing the blurring resulting from breathing motion.

The use of contrast material in CT can also lead to artifacts in the reconstructed PET data. Barium contained in oral contrast media and iodine contained in intravenous contrast media are high atomic number elements (Z of 56 and 53, respectively). At CT photon energies (less than 140 keV), on a per unit mass basis, barium and iodine attenuate x-ray photons to a much greater degree than does tissue. This is precisely why they are used as contrast materials in diagnostic CT. At 511 keV, however, attenuation per unit mass of barium, iodine, and all the tissue components is virtually the same. The attenuation map obtained by transforming HUs from a CT image containing contrast material is therefore inaccurate. The transformed attenuation coefficient for 511-keV photons will be too high because of the presence of contrast material leading to an overcorrection of the PET emission image. This can be either focal hot spots that might be misinterpreted as pathological conditions or larger regions or structures that may be recorded with higher uptake values in quantitative analyses.

Increased activity in PET images as a result of contrast material being present in high concentrations in the CT images used for attenuation correction are typically on the order of 10% to 20%. The advantages of using contrast materials and the improvement in diagnostic quality probably outweigh the problems associated with these errors. For this reason, the routine use of oral and intravenous contrast materials in conjunction with PET/CT is becoming more common. One method to reduce these errors is to use alternative transformation curves that compensate for the presence of contrast media. This option is available on commercial PET/CT scanners. It must be understood, however, that this solution is a compromise because the revised curve must assume some typical mix of water, bone, and now iodine, for example, to explain higher-density pixels. Another method is to have available routinely the uncorrected emission images and use them to rule out false-positive findings that might appear in areas where contrast material pools. This latter method has the advantage that it can also be used to rule out a number of artifacts introduced by attenuation correction errors, such as motion between CT and PET acquisitions and the presence of metallic prostheses (Antoch et al, 2002).

CLINICAL EXAMPLES

Oncology—Lung

PET with FDG is a powerful imaging modality for use in the initial diagnosis, staging, and follow-up of lung cancer. Most lung cancer nodules are FDG avid and are generally surrounded by tissue with relatively low FDG uptake. Figure 16-10 illustrates a case of lung cancer in a 66-year-old man. Panels *A* through *C* contain transaxial CT, PET, and PET/CT fusion images, respectively, through the primary lung tumor mass (labeled *p* on the PET image). A collapsed portion of the lung adjacent to the mass is also clearly visible on the CT scan. Panels *D* through *F* contain transaxial sections inferior to the previous set and illustrate a metastasis in the adrenal gland *(a)*. High activity seen in the kidney *(k)*, however, is a normal finding.

Oncology—Lymphoma

Another disease where PET is invaluable is lymphoma. Figure 16-11 contains images of a 17-year-old female patient with Hodgkin's lymphoma acquired for initial staging (*A* and *B*) and follow-up about 6 weeks later at mid treatment (*C* and *D*). Transaxial sections through the primary site of involvement are shown in panels *A* and *C*. Panels *B* and *D*

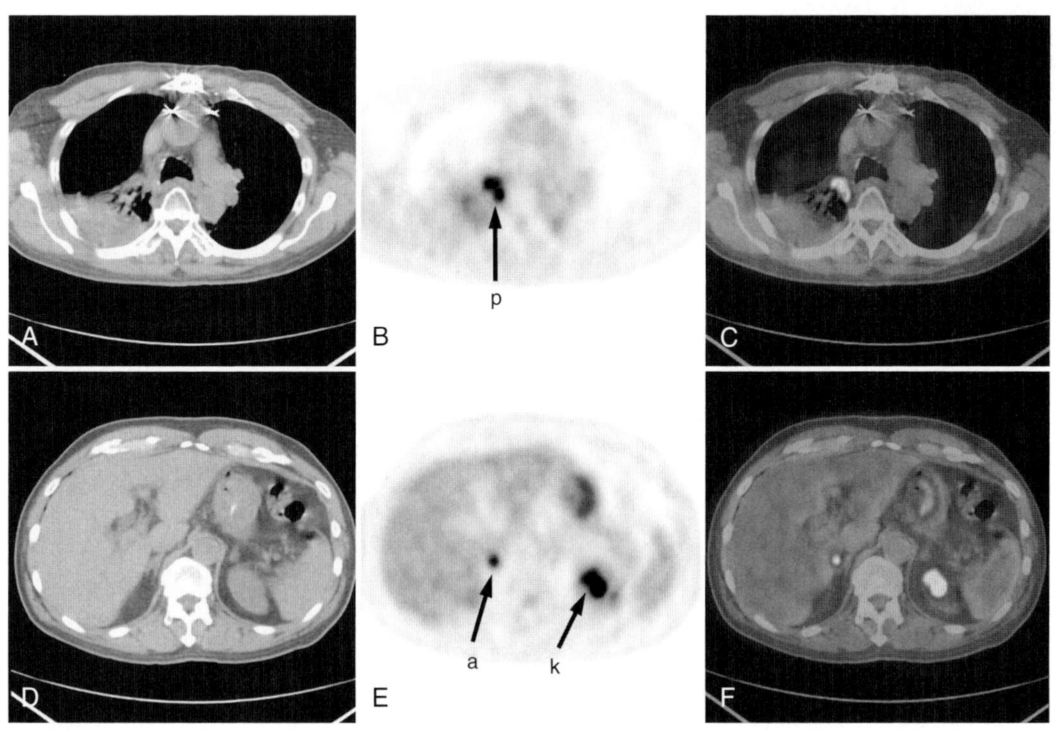

FIGURE 16-10 FDG PET/CT scan in patient with lung cancer. FDG PET/CT scan for 66-year-old man with lung cancer. **A,** Transaxial CT scan. **B,** Transaxial PET scan. **C,** Fused PET/CT fusion images. The primary lung tumor mass is labeled *p* on the PET image. **D, E,** and **F,** Transaxial sections inferior to the previous set illustrating a metastasis in the adrenal gland *(a)*. High activity seen in the kidney *(k)* is a normal finding.

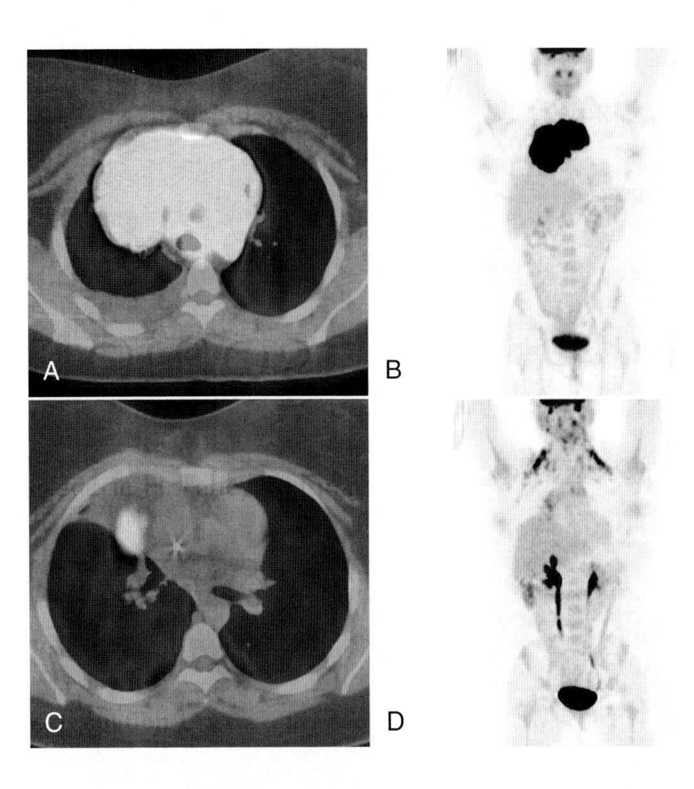

FIGURE 16-11 FDG PET/CT scan in a patient with lymphoma. FDG PET/CT scan of a 17-year-old female patient with Hodgkin's lymphoma. **A,** Transaxial slice at initial staging. **B,** MIP image at initial staging. **C,** Transaxial slice at mid treatment 6 weeks later. **D,** MIP image at mid treatment.

contain the whole-body maximum intensity projection (MIP) images. These images document a dramatic reduction in FDG avidity from initial scan to follow-up. The whole-body MIP images also show other areas of normal high FDG uptake in the brain, bladder, kidneys, and ureters. Also visible at the base of the neck in panel *D* are areas of high FDG uptake corresponding to metabolically active brown fat.

Cardiac Fluorine-18–Labeled 2-Fluoro-2-Deoxy-D-Glucose

Although the clinical mainstay of PET with FDG is in oncology, there is growing interest in cardiac applications. The myocardium is normally quite variable in its affinity for FDG, but it can be made to be FDG avid to assess myocardial viability. In an FDG myocardial viability study, the patient is first given a drink high in glucose followed by a series of insulin injections. When blood glucose has returned to normal, the FDG is injected. Figure 16-12 shows coronal reconstructions through the chest of a 72-year-old man who was administered 500 MBq (14 millicuries) of FDG 45 minutes before image acquisition. The PET images clearly show little or no uptake in the inferior myocardial wall, which indicates the lack of viable tissue there. Often this study would be performed and interpreted in conjunction with a myocardial perfusion single-photon emission CT study.

Epilepsy

FDG PET has also been shown to be useful in the localization of epileptic seizures (Ollenberger et al, 2005). Seizure foci tend to be hypometabolic on the interictal PET scan, that is, a scan acquired when the patient is not having a seizure.

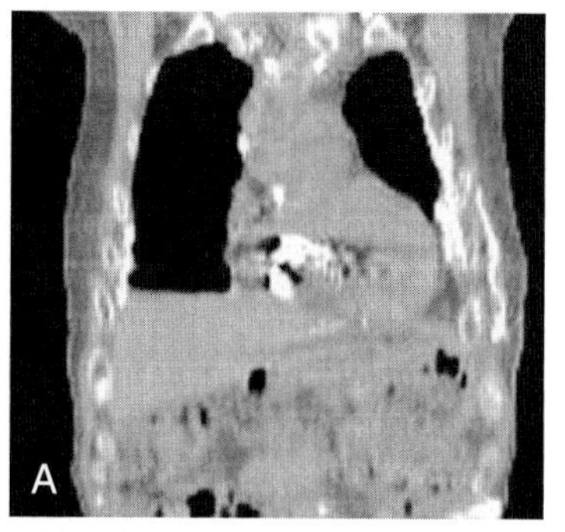

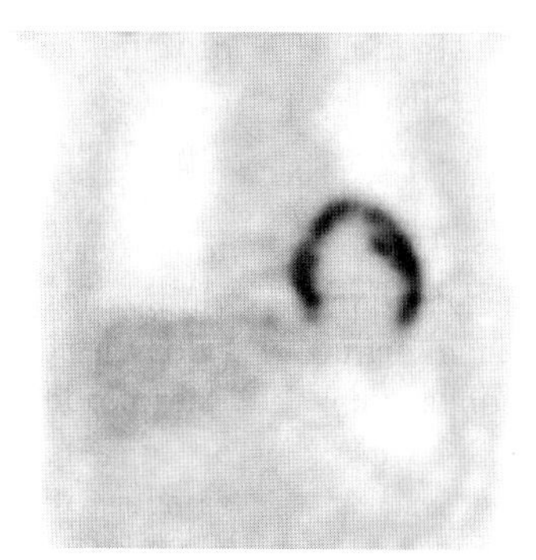

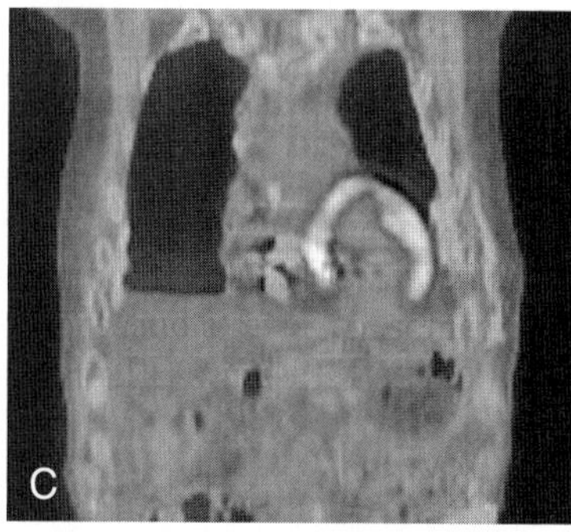

FIGURE 16-12 FDG PET/CT scan of myocardium. Coronal reconstructions through the chest of a 72-year-old man. The PET images clearly show little or no uptake in the inferior myocardial wall, which indicates the lack of viable tissue there.

Figure 16-13 shows a transverse and coronal slice through the FDG PET scan of a patient with right-sided intractable temporal lobe epilepsy. It is clearly shown that the patient's right temporal lobe (on the viewer's left) has substantially reduced signal on the FDG PET compared with the left temporal lobe. This information can be invaluable to the neurosurgeon treating this patient. For example, this scan indicates that this patient has unilateral disease that is limited to the right temporal lobe, indicating that this is an appropriate candidate for surgical intervention.

SUMMARY

In the past 10 years, PET has become an invaluable clinical tool, particularly in oncology but also in cardiology and neurology. PET can provide outstanding images of function and metabolism that augments the anatomical information provided by CT and MRI. For these reasons, it is very useful to register the functional and anatomical data to each other to provide a more complete view of the patient. Thus, in the past 5 years, hybrid PET/CT scanners have been developed that can

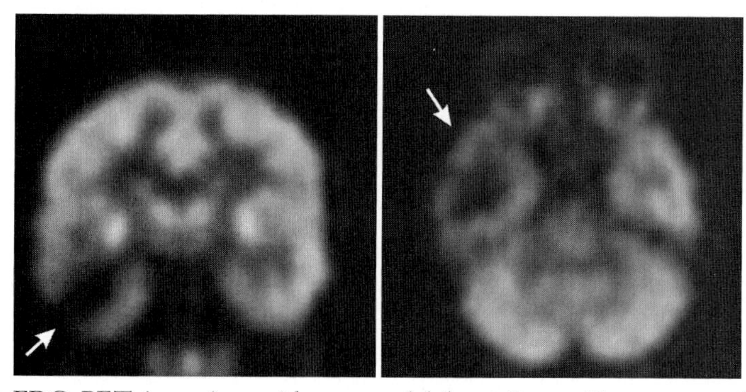

FIGURE 16-13 FDG PET in patient with temporal lobe epilepsy. Transverse and coronal slices through an interictal FDG PET scan of a patient with temporal lobe epilepsy. The seizure focus is hypometabolic and noted by arrows.

provide both anatomical and functional imaging in a single setting. Although there are many advantages to this hybrid approach, there are also some limitations of which the technologist needs to be cognizant to more optimally use these devices and to better interpret their data. In the near future, further advancements in imaging technology along with the development of novel radiopharmaceuticals will continue the rapid growth of PET and PET/CT in the new era of molecular medicine.

REFERENCES

Antoch G et al: Focal tracer uptake: a potential artifact in contrast-enhanced dual-modality PET/CT scans, *J Nucl Med* 43:1339-1342, 2002.

Badawi RD et al: Optimization of noise-equivalent count rates in 3D PET, *Phys Med Biol* 41:1755-1776, 1996.

Casey ME, Nutt R: A multicrystal 2-dimensional BGO detector system for positron emission tomography, *IEEE Trans Nucl Sci* 33:460-463, 1986.

Cherry SR et al: *Physics in nuclear medicine*, ed 3, Philadelphia, 2003, WB Saunders.

Cohnen M et al: Effective doses in standard protocols for multi-slice CT scanning, *Eur Radiol* 13:1148-1153, 2003.

Daghighian P et al: Evaluation of cerium doped lutetium oxyorthosilicate (LSO) scintillation crystal for PET, *IEEE Trans Nucl Sci* 40:1045-1047, 1993.

El Fakhri G et al: Impact of acquisition geometry and patient habitus on tumor detectability in whole-body FDG-PET: a channelized hotelling observer study, In *IEEE Nuclear Science Symposium Conference Record*, Piscataway, NJ, 2002, Institute of Electrical and Electronics Engineers, pp 1082-3654.

Evans RD: *The atomic nucleus*, New York, 1982, Kreiger.

Fahey FH: Positron emission tomography instrumentation, *Radiol Clin North Am* 39:919-929, 2001.

Fahey FH: Instrumentation in positron emission tomography, *Neuroimag Clin North Am* 13:659-669, 2003.

Fahey FH et al: Dosimetry and adequacy of CT-based attenuation correction for pediatric PET, *Radiology* 243:96-104, 2007.

Goerres GW et al: Respiration-induced attenuation artifact at PET/CT: technical considerations, *Radiology* 226:906-910, 2003.

Hoffman EJ, Phelps ME: Positron emission tomography: principles and quantitation. In Phelps ME, et al, eds: *Positron emission tomography and autoradiography: principles and applications for the brain and heart*, New York, 1986, Raven.

ICRP Report 80: radiation dose to patients from radiopharmaceuticals, pp. 49-110, Oxford, 1998, International Commission on Radiation Protection.

Kinahan PE et al: X-ray-based attenuation correction for positron emission tomography/computed tomography scanners, *Semin Nucl Med* 33:166-179, 2003.

Kuhn A et al: Design of a lanthanum bromide detector for time-of-flight PET, *IEEE Trans Nucl Sci* 51:2550-2557, 2004.

Lartizien C et al: A lesion detection observer study comparing 2-dimensional versus fully 3-dimensional whole-body PET imaging protocols, *J Nucl Med* 45:714-723, 2004.

Levin CS, Hoffman EJ: Calculation of positron range and its effect on the fundamental limit of positron emission tomography system resolution, *Phys Med Biol* 44:781-799, 1999.

Lewellen TK: Time-of-flight PET, *Semin Nucl Med* 28:268-275, 1998.

Lonn A: Evaluation of method to minimize the effect of x-ray contrast attenuation correction. In *2003 IEEE Nuclear Science Symposium: Conference Record-19-25*, October 2003, Portland, Oregon, vol 3, Piscataway, NJ: Institute of Electrical and Electronics Engineers, 2004, pp. 2220-2221.

Ollenberger GP et al: Assessment of the role of FDG PET in the diagnosis and management of children with refractory epilepsy, *Eur J Nucl Med Mol Imaging* 32:1311-1316, 2005.

Palmer MR et al: Modeling and simulation of positron range effects for high resolution PET imaging, *IEEE Trans Nucl Sci* 52:1392-1395, 2005.

Steinert HC, von Schulthess GK: Initial clinical experience using a new integrated in-line PET/CT system, *Br J Radiol* 75:S36-S38, 2002.

Surti S et al: Optimizing the performance of a PET detector using discrete GSO crystals on a continuous lightguide, *IEEE Trans Nucl Sci* 47:1030-1036, 2000.

Wahl RL: Why nearly all PET abdominal and pelvic cancers will be performed as PET/CT, *J Nucl Med* 45:82S-95S, 2004.

Computed Tomography of the Head, Cerebral Vessels, Neck, and Spine

Jocelyne S. Lapointe

Chapter Outline

Beginning in 1972, computed tomography (CT) has provided anatomical information about the body in ways that have greatly increased the diagnosis of pathological conditions in a noninvasive fashion. Neuroradiology is the subspecialty of radiology that deals with the central nervous system and conditions affecting the head and neck. It was revolutionized by CT scanning. It became possible to see inside the brain (i.e., inspect the gray and white matter without the need for a brain biopsy) and to see inside the spinal canal and evaluate disks.

With the advent of multiple detector CT scanners at the beginning of the twenty-first century, visualizing the entire vascular tree in a few seconds after an intravenous contrast injection has become feasible. More uses will follow, with further technical developments.

INDICATIONS

Head and Face

CT is valuable for assessing intracranial pathological conditions, especially in the acute stage. It is performed to guide further investigations and therapy. It is fast and causes no security concerns, in contrast to magnetic resonance imaging (MRI). (Patients must be screened before being positioned in the MRI machine, which causes delays.) Motion can cause artifacts, but it is less of an issue than with MRI. (Terminology commonly found on imaging requests is written in *italics*, to help the student identify conditions. Not all the conditions mentioned later are illustrated.)

A common indication for CT scanning is acute neurological dysfunction, often presenting as paralysis *(stroke)* or transient ischemic attack *(TIA)*. The neurological deficit can be caused by a cerebral infarction from blockage of a blood vessel in the neck or head, by a spontaneous brain hemorrhage caused by hypertension or an underlying blood vessel abnormality such as an aneurysm, by an infection (*viral encephalitis* or *bacterial abscess*), or by a *primary or metastatic tumor*.

Cerebral infarction is the result of loss of adequate blood supply to a portion of the brain. In the early stages, it may be difficult to see the location of the infarcted tissue on CT. Early edema (as seen in Fig. 17-1, *A*) causes loss of gray-white matter differentiation, which is the earliest CT sign of infarction. As the infarct matures, it becomes more obvious and better defined. Because of the increased water content of the infarcted tissue, the density is decreased (i.e., dark) (Fig. 17-1, *B*).

Hemorrhage in the brain substance (Fig. 17-2, *A*) can occur spontaneously, either because of an underlying vascular anomaly, such as a tumor or an *arteriovenous malformation* (*AVM*) or because the patient's hypertension has weakened the walls of the capillary vessels. Hemorrhage can also occur in the subarachnoid space (Fig. 17-2, *B*), resulting in bloody cerebrospinal fluid (CSF) (from a leaking aneurysm) or between the brain and its meninges (epidural and subdural spaces). Acutely extravasated blood is of increased density (i.e., white). The degree of mass effect caused by the hematoma is reflected in the amount of brainstem compression from the shift of the midline structures. This affects the patient's level of consciousness, which is measured by the *Glascow Coma Scale* (range 3-15). A normal score is 15 and the lowest score is 3. Delay in scanning any patient with a score less than 13 or 14 after a head injury should be avoided because this score can change in less than 5 minutes in the presence of an expanding intracranial hematoma. The technologist should always advise the medical personnel immediately if a dramatic change in level of consciousness is seen while the patient is in the scanner. (This is one type of patient who should not be left unsupervised, while waiting for transport, for example.)

Hematomas evolve in density over time, becoming less and less dense and finally approaching CSF in density. The clot will be jellylike in the acute phase and will eventually liquefy and shrink. *Chronic subdural hematoma* is the most

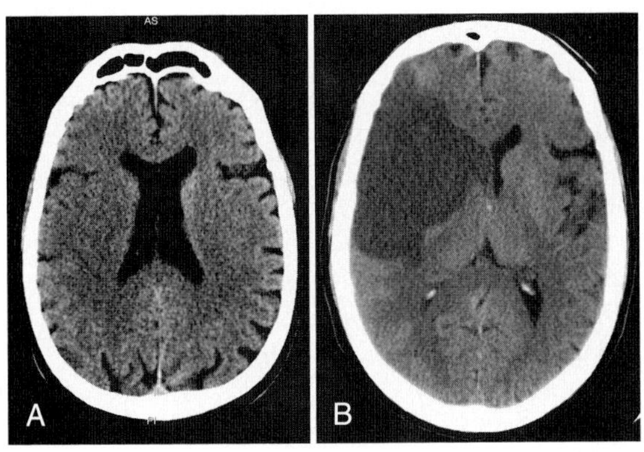

FIGURE 17-1 **A,** Early subtle infarction. **B,** Late well-defined cerebral infarction. Subtle loss of the distinction between the gray and the white matter is present on the early CT, in the right middle cerebral artery territory, with good delineation of the affected area on the later CT.

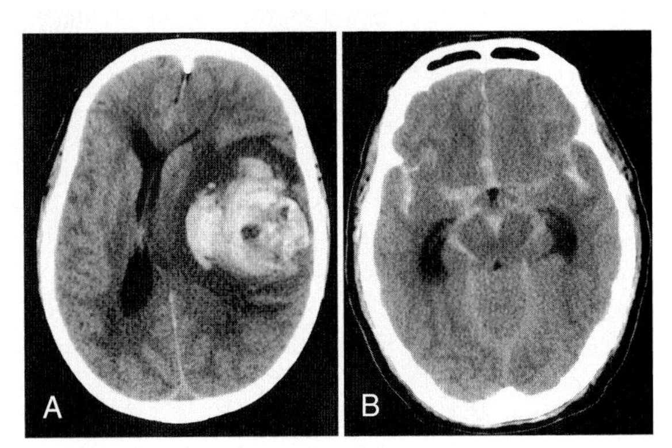

FIGURE 17-2 **A,** Large left parenchymal hematoma causing a marked midline shift to the right. **B,** Severe *subarachnoid hemorrhage* outlining all the cisterns of the skull base.

common condition followed up by repeated CT scanning to document its complete disappearance. Reaccumulation of a chronic subdural hematoma is also common, requiring repeated drainage.

When a traumatic brain or facial injury is suspected, CT provides rapid information about *contusions* (brain bruise) and *hematomas* (blood clot) in the brain and in the spaces between skull and brain (*epidural and subdural hematomas*). Facial and skull *fractures* are easily seen (Fig. 17-3, *A*), except linear cranial vault fractures coursing in the plane of section. The depth of depressed bone fragments can be measured (Fig. 17-3, *B*). The results of corrective surgery and the location of metallic hardware in the face, as well as the degree of healing callus, are easily appreciated on follow-up examinations.

The most common brain tumor is a *metastasis*; metastases are often multiple (Fig. 17-4, *A*). Common primary brain tumors are *meningioma* and *glioblastoma multiforme* (GBM) (Fig. 17-4, *B*). Their location and pattern of enhancement is used to predict their histological grade preoperatively.

Stereotaxic procedures by various methods are commonplace in neurosurgery. They are used to accurately localize the lesion before biopsy or resection. The preoperative studies can be obtained with fiducial markers applied to the scalp or with the head in a stereotaxic frame. Different systems are available, with some frames attaching to the CT table, in place of the head holder. Newer systems are frameless, using a combination of computer programs to superimpose the images and correlate them to the patient's anatomy.

In the case of *meningitis* or *encephalitis*, it is useful to analyze the CSF for the presence of cells and various compounds, such as glucose, proteins, antibodies, and bacteria and viruses. A lumbar puncture (LP) can only be safely performed if the possibility of an intracranial mass (hydrocephalus [Fig. 17-5, *A*], tumor or abscess) has been ruled out. Many physicians prefer the certainty of CT before proceeding with the LP because signs of an intracranial mass are not always present. Brain atrophy can also result in large ventricles and must be distinguished from hydrocephalus (Fig. 17-5, *B*).

Many *congenital brain abnormalities* are diagnosed in childhood, whereas others are only recognized in adulthood. Some types of *seizure* disorders are caused by localized arrested brain development (for example, *cortical dysplasia*). Surgery may alleviate the seizures. Some brain anomalies remain asymptomatic and are an imaging curiosity

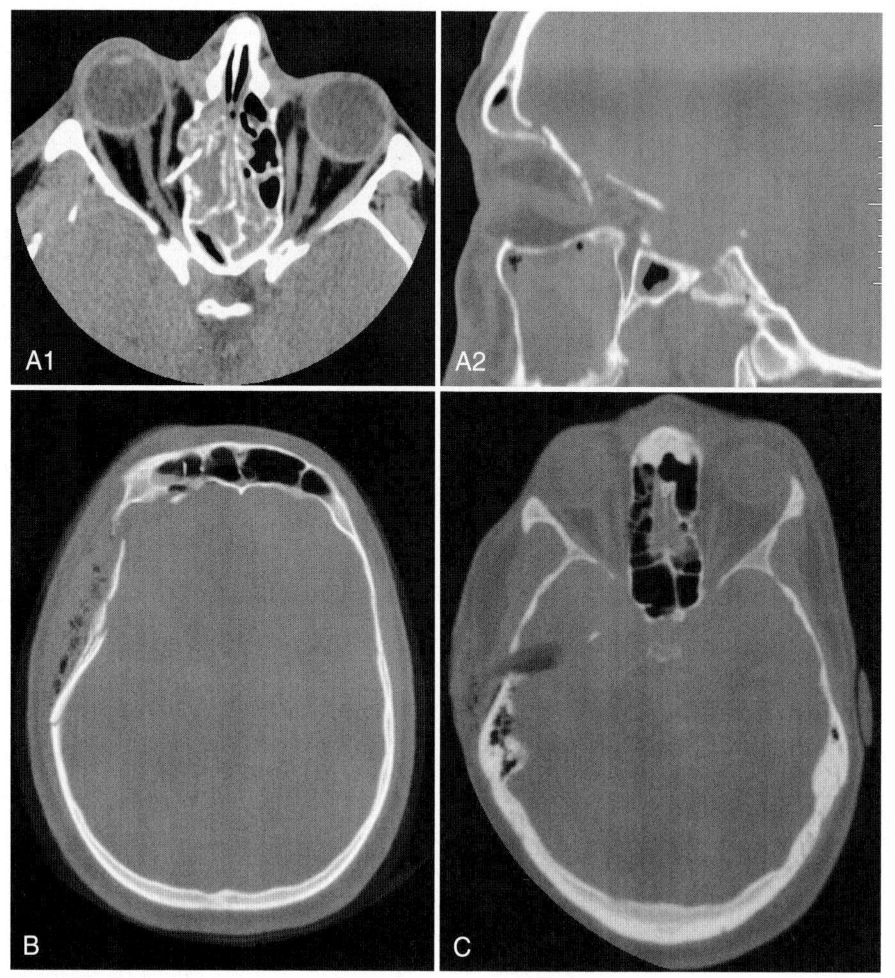

FIGURE 17-3 **A,** Orbital roof fractures; the transverse image on orbit settings shows the bone fragment spearing the right medial rectus muscle and the sagittal image on bone windows shows the rotation of this fragment. **B,** Comminuted depressed skull fracture with *subcutaneous emphysema* and fluid in the right frontal sinus. **C,** Wooden stick piercing the right temporal bone and lobe, displacing a fragment of bone into the brain, better appreciated on wide windows (it mimics air on routine brain windows, not shown).

(for example, cavum of the septum pellucidum, cisterna magna).

Apart from the brain, conditions affecting other components of the head, such as the sinuses, temporal bones, and orbits are commonly evaluated by CT scanning.

Sinus disease (*sinusitis*, tumor) is readily seen with CT (Fig. 17-6, *A*). Sinus anatomy shows many variations important to the ear, nose, and throat surgeon. To avoid complications such as entering the brain or orbit inadvertently, sinus surgery is often performed with direct correlation with the CT images, a procedure known as functional endoscopic sinus surgery, or FESS.

The mandible, being a curved bone, is not optimally assessed for pathological conditions with

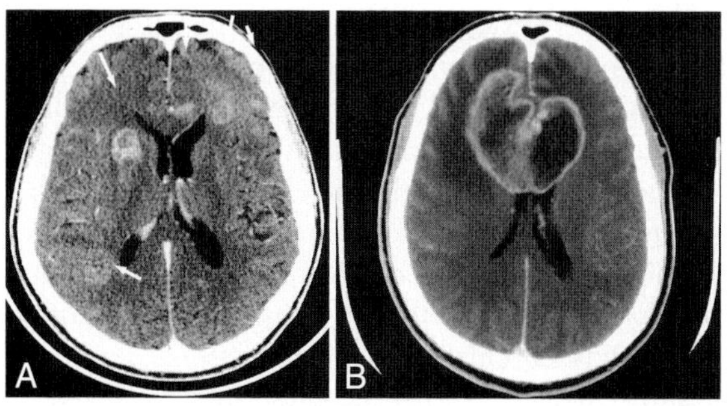

FIGURE 17-4 **A,** Multiple ring enhancing metastases in both frontal lobes. **B,** Enhancing bifrontal (butterfly) GBM; it is surrounded by edema, causing mass effect on the frontal horns.

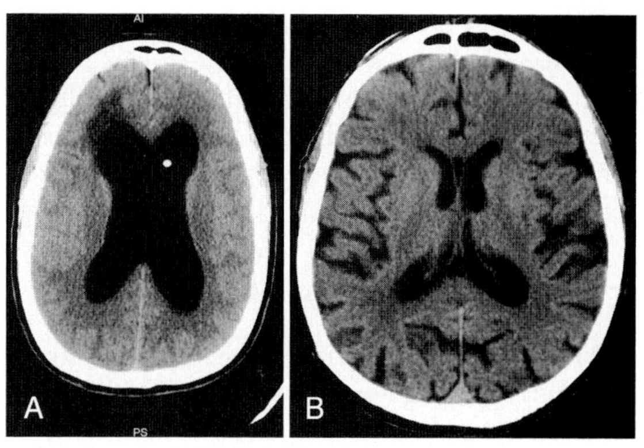

FIGURE 17-5 **A,** Shunted *hydrocephalus* (enlarged ventricles caused by obstruction to CSF flow) can fail, requiring shunt revision. **B,** Brain *atrophy* can also result in large ventricles, without CSF obstruction.

plain films; it is easily evaluated with CT by using two-dimensional and three-dimensional (3D) reformatted images; a 3D reformatted mandible is shown in Figure 17-6, *B*.

Orbital CT scan images should always be available in at least two planes (transverse and coronal) because of the pyramidal shape of the bony orbit. The intraorbital fat delineates the optic nerve, extraocular muscles, and superior ophthalmic veins. For example, CT accurately localizes radiopaque *foreign bodies* for the surgeon. Wood is not radiopaque and may mimic air, so bone windows should be available (shown in Fig. 17-3, *C*). Although orbital ultrasonography is used widely to study the ocular globe, CT is better at characterizing orbital mass lesions and identifying the cause of *proptosis* (displacement of the globe).

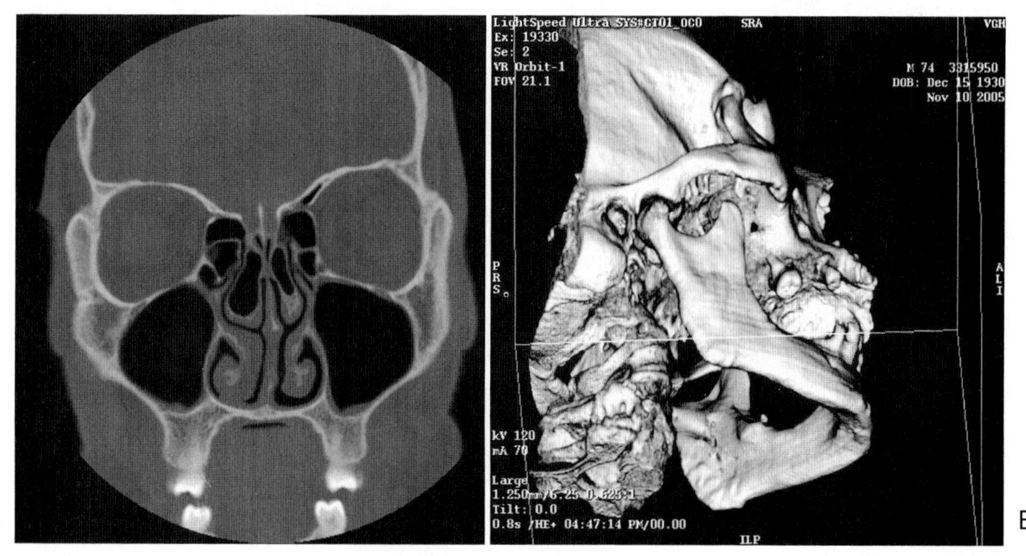

FIGURE 17-6 **A,** Paranasal sinuses obtained prone to better see the drainage pathways of the maxillary sinuses (known as the ostia). **B,** Reformatted three-dimensionl image of the mandible. The image can be rotated on the computer to evaluate all the margins of this curved bone.

Other uses of CT include looking for pituitary *microadenoma* in the pituitary gland situated in the sella turcica (cause of many endocrine problems) and masses in the middle ear (*cholesteatoma*) and internal auditory canal (*acoustic neuroma*) as causes for hearing loss (Fig. 17-7).

Cerebral Blood Vessels

Helical scanning makes it possible to image structures during the continued intravenous (IV) injection of a bolus of iodinated contrast medium. Multislice CT scanners extend the length of the vascular tree that can be imaged with one contrast injection; because of the speed of image acquisition, a pump is used to inject the contrast. A greater scan length (i.e., length of travel of the tabletop) is possible with a greater number of simultaneous slices. At this time, the artifacts caused over the carotid arteries by metal in the mouth (dental fillings, caps, braces) cannot be completely eliminated. Magnetic resonance angiography (MRA) or catheter angiography may be necessary to rule out or confirm a vascular abnormality suggested by CT angiography (CTA).

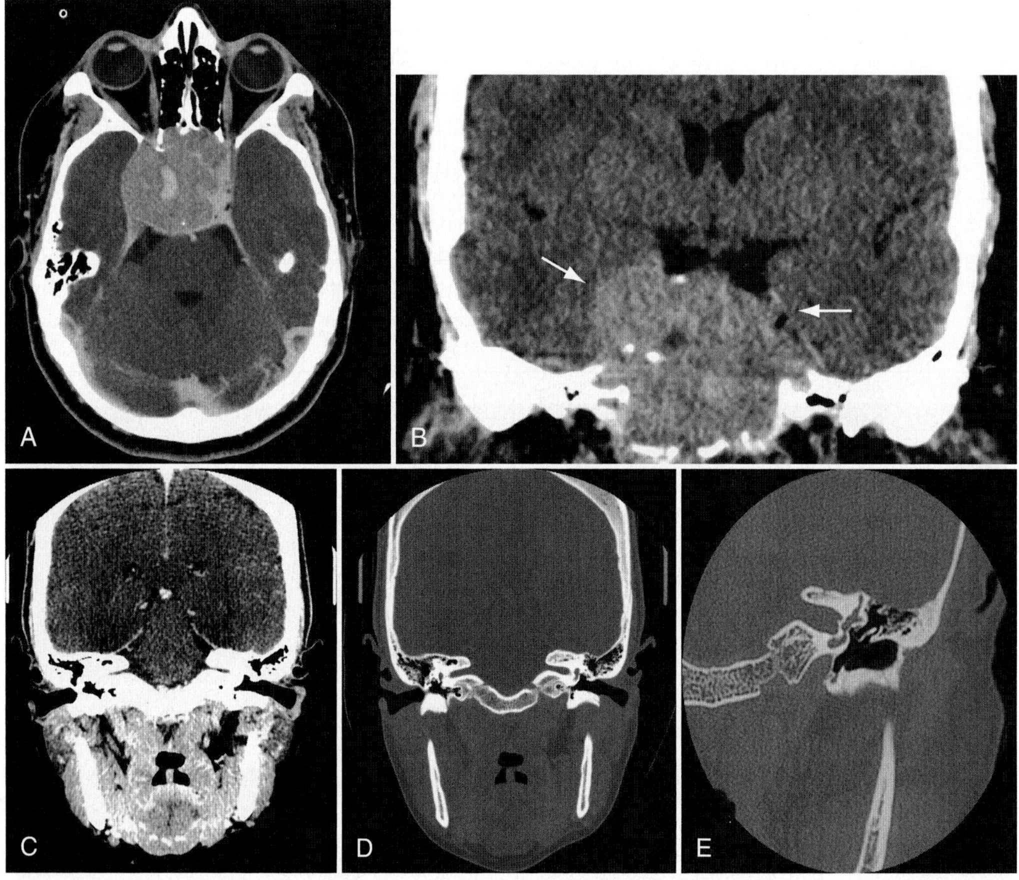

FIGURE 17-7 **A** and **B**, Very large pituitary adenoma, filling the sphenoid sinus but not abutting on the optic chiasm, imaged in transverse plane and reformatted in coronal plane. **C** and **D**, Direct (i.e. with neck extension) coronal images of the internal auditory canals (IAC), on soft tissue **(C)** and bone **(D)** algorithms. **E**, Left petrous bone, acquired in direct coronal plane, showing the ossicles in the middle ear, surrounded by air.

CTA can outline the cerebral blood vessels from their origin on the aortic arch to their various intracranial branches, as shown in Figure 17-8, *A* and *B*. Because of the ease and convenience of CTA, the number of patients being investigated for vascular conditions has multiplied. The vessels supplying the brain originate from the aortic arch (the innominate or brachiocephalic trunk, left common and left subclavian arteries). Both the subclavian and the vertebral arteries, the common carotid artery bifurcations (site of most *stenoses*), the internal carotid arteries, the intracranial arteries (anterior, middle and posterior cerebral, basilar, and cerebellar) arteries (aneurysm sites) are readily visible (Fig. 17-9).

A delay of a few seconds between injection and acquisition of images of the entire brain increases the visualization of the jugular veins and dural sinuses (sagittal and transverse sinuses), sites of possible *thrombosis*. This is known as a CT venogram (CTV) (not shown).

An important use of CTA is in suspected acute cerebral infarction because rapid intervention may result in lessening the extent of brain damage. After a non contrast CT of the brain to rule out hemorrhage, CT perfusion (CTP) at the level of the suspected infarct is obtained (in some centers) to delineate the amount of brain at risk for permanent damage; CTA of the cerebral vessels follows to identify the presence of clot in a major intracranial artery (usually the middle cerebral or the basilar artery) before a "clot-busting" drug, known as a thrombolytic agent (such as thrombin plasminogen activator, or TPA) is administered.

Patients with a hemorrhage caused by, for example, a suspected aneurysm or an AVM can undergo a CTA to confirm the diagnosis before being transferred to a more specialized treatment center. This is particularly useful in smaller or more remote localities where a neurosurgeon or neurologist is not available.

Spine and Neck

In many centers CT has replaced plain films of the cervical spine in cases of trauma because it shows injuries not detectable otherwise (see examples of fractures in Fig. 17-10). A certain amount of

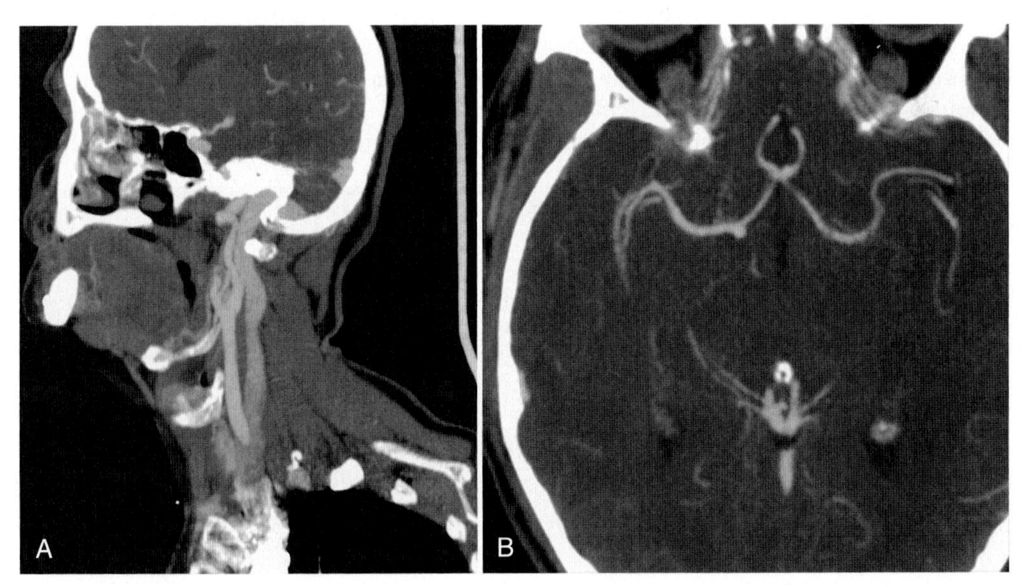

FIGURE 17-8 **A,** Normal CTA of the common carotid bifurcation, showing the Y-shaped arteries and the large jugular vein posterior to it. **B,** Normal CTA of the circle of Willis, showing the anterior communicating artery and both middle cerebral arteries.

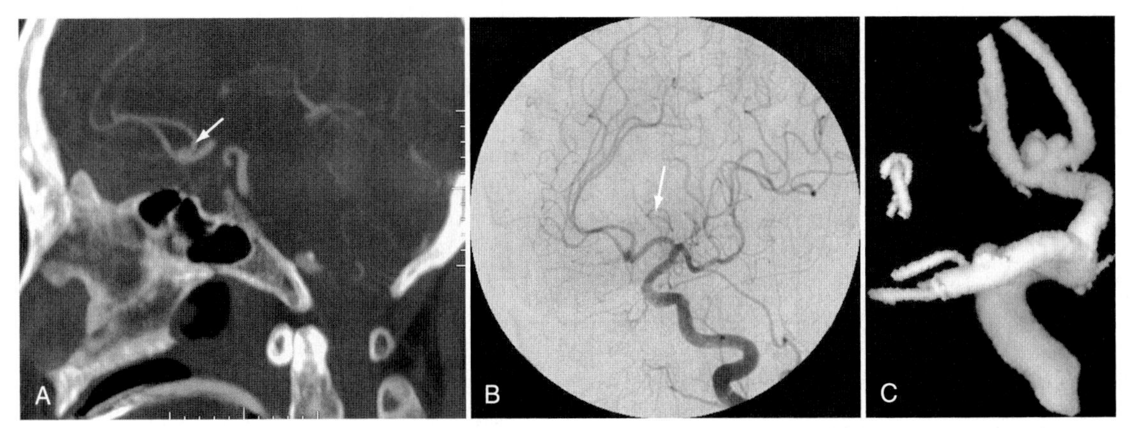

FIGURE 17-9 **A** to **C**, The same *anterior communicating artery aneurysm* is shown on the CTA, the cerebral angiogram, and the 3D model constructed from this angiogram.

"pathology" overlap is seen in the cervical region because conditions affecting the vessels, the bones, and the soft tissues are often found when one type of cervical examination is being carried out. This is most evident when the study is a CTA covering the neck; in addition to bone and vessels, abnormalities of the thyroid gland, the salivary glands, lymph nodes, and neck muscles can be appreciated.

In the case of trauma, the carotid or vertebral arteries may be injured (resulting in a *dissection* or *occlusion*) during the violent neck motion that caused a spinal fracture or *dislocation*. Patients with *carotid stenosis* caused by arteriosclerosis are usually older; the cervical spine often shows *disk herniation* or osteophytes causing nerve root compression or *spinal stenosis*. The converse is also true. Studies looking for cervical disk herniation may also show carotid bifurcation calcification, a possible cause of symptomatic carotid artery disease and a potential cause of stroke or TIA.

Masses can occur along the chains of lymph nodes in the neck (for example, *lymphoma*, *Hodgkin's disease*), along nerves (such as vagus nerve *schwannoma*), or adjacent to the vessels (*carotid body tumor*; Fig. 17-11, *A*). Tumors occurring in the salivary glands, nasopharynx, tongue, and floor of the mouth can

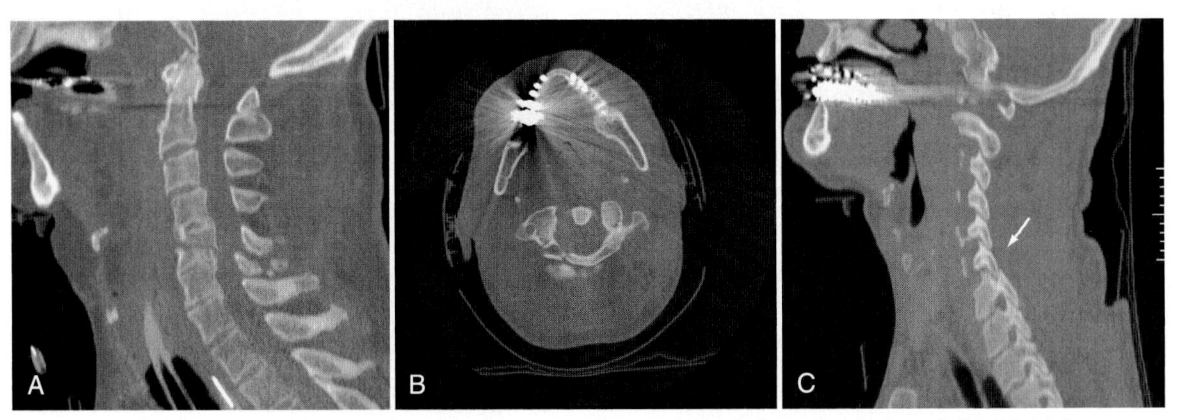

FIGURE 17-10 **A,** Reformatted image of the cervical spine showing fractures of C2 and C5. Multiple *spinal fractures* are not uncommon. **B,** Metal causes streak artifacts but still demonstrates the C1 fracture. **C,** Alignment is a critical component of spinal assessment. A *facet lock* is present.

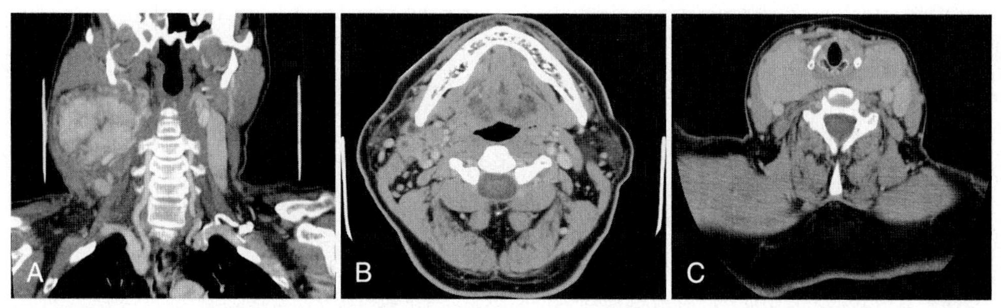

FIGURE 17-11 **A,** Large vascular mass (carotid body tumor) shown on CTA. **B,** Metastatic ring enhancing necrotic lymph nodes, abutting on the right submandibular gland. **C,** Large thyroid goiter encircling the trachea.

metastasize to the neck nodes, changing the tumor grade and treatment protocol and the survival rate (Fig. 17-11, *B*).

Preservation of the voice can be achieved in localized laryngeal cancers when treatment consists of a partial laryngectomy. This emphasizes the need for accurate delineation of tumor.

Enlargement of the thyroid gland as the result of a *goiter* is a frequent incidental finding when the neck is imaged for any reason (Fig. 17-11, *C*). When large, a goiter can plunge into the superior mediastinum and cause airway obstruction. Thyroid hormone production can be abnormal, resulting in various symptoms.

Many infections start in the disk space (*diskitis, osteomyelitis*) at any level of the spine; they can spread to the epidural space (*epidural abscess*), resulting in spinal cord compression and paralysis. Other infections extend into the prevertebral or paraspinal tissues; in the neck, they can obstruct the airway or cause difficulty swallowing and drooling. An acutely swollen neck can be life threatening because of the potential for obstruction of the airway, particularly in children.

Tumors affecting the spine or spinal cord can originate as primary tumors or metastasize from other sites to bone or soft tissue, affecting the vertebral bodies, the pedicles, laminae, and facet joints. Their treatment often requires removal of much bone, resulting in possible instability of the spine. Bone grafts and metallic instrumentation are frequently inserted to preserve patient mobility. Metallic instrumentation may fail, requiring frequent follow-up by imaging (plain films/CT) and occasionally surgical revision.

Instrumentation of the spine is also used in treating atlantoaxial (C1-2) instability in *rheumatoid arthritis* and in treating *scoliosis*, spine fractures, *spinal stenosis* and *spondylolisthesis*. It requires accurate placement of pedicle screws, hooks, wires, and plates. CT accurately depicts the position of the instrumentation. In some cases, screws may traverse a foramen and impinge on a nerve root or a vertebral artery; a neurologic deficit or pain can ensue (Fig. 17-12, *A*).

Another type of spinal procedure is vertebroplasty. Radiopaque cement (methylmethacrylate) is injected under fluoroscopic control into spinal compression fractures to reduce pain and in some cases to decrease the kyphosis.

Postprocedure CT scans of the many types of spinal interventions described previously are common to assess the results (Fig. 17-12, *B* and *C*).

ROLE OF CT COMPARED WITH OTHER IMAGING MODALITIES

The recent advent of multislice CT scanners with the capacity to image multiple organ systems at one sitting, without having to move the patient, has revolutionized the evaluation of a number of

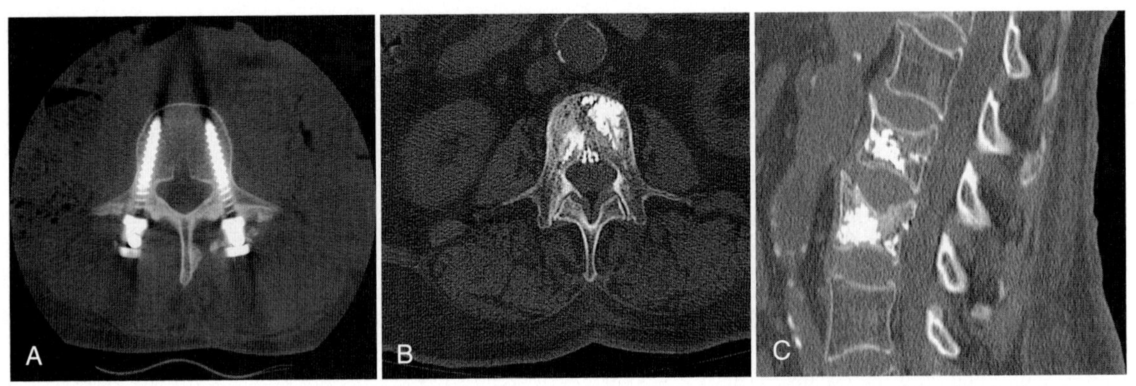

FIGURE 17-12 **A,** Pedicle screws in the lumbar spine, with bone graft material around the head of the left screw. **B** and **C,** Vertebroplasty: radiopaque cement is injected through the pedicles into the vertebral body: transverse and sagittal images.

acute conditions. Multiple trauma patients in particular are being assessed from head to toe by CT scan, in many cases replacing plain radiographs and catheter angiography. The sequencing of these examinations is important to increase diagnostic accuracy while minimizing the radiation dose and the volume of IV contrast. Ideally, the sequence should evaluate the patient for the most life-threatening conditions first on the basis of the initial assessment.

The noncontrast head CT (using thin slices for later reformatted images if facial fractures are readily apparent) should be followed by CTA of the thoracic aorta (to rule out a dissection) and CT of the chest, abdomen, and pelvis (to look for solid and hollow organ injury). CTA of the neck vessels can be obtained last.

Reformatted images of the entire spine on bone algorithm in three planes, obtained from the previous series, are used to rule out spine fractures and evaluate alignment. Reformatted facial bone and mandible images, also on bone algorithm, are produced if required.

More subtle fractures can be diagnosed with CT than with plain films. Nursing practices (for example, turning the patient in the intensive care unit to avoid bed sores) can be influenced by the presence of spine fractures not visible on plain films.

Such multiple studies can easily result in 2000 to 2500 images in total. Better quality images are obtained if the patient's arms can be moved (down for the head and neck CTA and up for the chest-abdomen) (i.e., if the patient has no clavicle, scapula, or humeral fractures). Some trauma cases also require other orthopedic scans (e.g., pelvis, hips) or a CT cystogram.

CTA can complement duplex ultrasonography. It is not hampered by calcification, unlike ultrasonography. Also unlike ultrasonography, it cannot determine direction or velocity of blood flow. The CTA can image the cervical blood vessels over a longer segment than can duplex ultrasonography.

Transcranial Doppler imaging (another form of ultrasonography) can be used to evaluate flow in intracranial vessels, but it is not widely available. The CTA images are more "user friendly" than ultrasonography for most clinicians. MRA currently does not provide the same rapid answers as CTA in acute stroke, in most institutions.

Enlarged thyroid glands can indicate an increased or decreased production of thyroid hormone, resulting in symptoms affecting various organ systems. Initial evaluation of a thyroid goiter by ultrasonography allows for fine-needle aspiration. Gadolinium-enhanced MRI of the neck does not affect thyroid iodine metabolism. It can be used as a substitute for CT when iodine therapy of a thyroid nodule is planned.

Although MRI is the preferred imaging technique for the spinal cord and the intervertebral disks, CT scanning continues to provide valuable information about calcification and the bones. Similar to brain CT, spine lesions such as tumor and infection will enhance with IV contrast. CT can thus be used when MRI is dangerous, as in the presence of a cardiac pacemaker or the older types of cerebral aneurysm clips.

In the absence of trauma, CT (or MRI) can be used when acute spinal cord compression is diagnosed by the sudden loss of sensation, motor function, or bowel or bladder function. Common causes include *epidural abscesses* in IV drug users and *spinal metastasis*. (Symptoms caused by metastasis to the brain or spine are often the presenting complaint in individuals with no known primary cancer; up to half of new cases of cancer are discovered because of their metastases.)

CT-guided procedures such as nerve root blocks, facet blocks, and spine biopsies require scanning the same levels repeatedly. Some CT scanners have a "fluoroscopy" option to assist in these procedures. These procedures are also performed on the usual fluoroscopic units.

Patients with spinal instrumentation sometimes need reevaluation of the contents of their spinal canal. Metallic artifacts can impede CT and MRI diagnosis because the spinal canal is obscured or distorted by the artifact. Some newer CT scanners can reduce this metallic spray artifact by extending the Hounsfield units thanks to a special metal artifact reduction software program.

Another way around this problem is a myelogram followed by a CT scan: water-soluble contrast medium specific for subarachnoid use is injected under fluoroscopy by LP or C1-2 puncture into the subarachnoid space by the radiologist. After suitable fluoroscopic images are obtained, CT images are acquired on bone algorithm (kernel) and reformatted in the appropriate planes. Adhesions of spinal cord or nerve roots *(arachnoiditis)*, spinal cord cavities *(syrinx)*, and other conditions obscured by the metallic artifacts can be diagnosed and treated appropriately (Fig. 17-13).

SECTIONAL ANATOMY: A REVIEW

R. A Nugent, revised by J. S. Lapointe

Image acquisition is obtained in the transverse (axial) plane with the patient in a (usually) supine position or (occasionally) in a prone or decubitus position. Knowledge of sectional anatomy is mandatory. A readily available reference text is an invaluable tool.

Because the acquisition of images with most CT scanners now in use is multiplanar (i.e., 4 to 64 slices), the review of coronal and sagittal reformatted images is now commonplace. These planes, by presenting the anatomy in a more traditional fashion, illustrate variations in the expected anatomy and the spread of disease. The student gains a better understanding of sectional anatomy by correlating transverse images with reformatted images in the other two planes. The angle of an oblique structure, such as the lateral wall of the orbit, is subsequently easier to appreciate.

As with plain radiographs, such as a chest x-ray, transverse (axial) images and coronal reformatted images are viewed with the patient's right side on the viewer's left (i.e., as if facing the individual). Local preference (usually the radiologist) dictates whether the transverse (axial) images are viewed from top to bottom or vice versa and if the sagittal images are viewed from right to left or left to right. Labeled scout (topogram, scanogram) images must be available, to decrease uncertainty about slice location and for accurate reporting.

Head

Transverse Sections

The anatomical structures of the normal appearance of the brain by use of a standard algorithm are shown in Figure 17-14. Slices through the skull base (Fig. 17-15) give exquisite detail of the foramina, facial structures, pituitary fossa, and temporal bones. CSF in the basal cisterns and ventricles helps define the anatomy, as does calcium

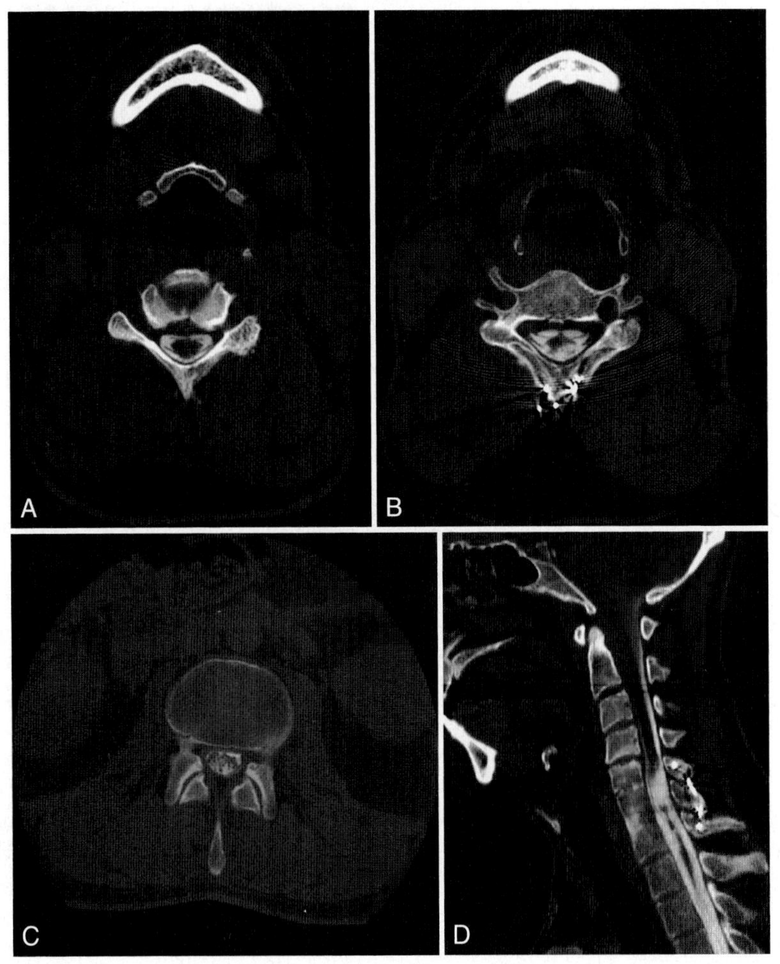

FIGURE 17-13 **A,** CT myelogram delineates a normal cervical spinal cord and nerve roots. **B,** The cervical spinal cord (outlined by contrast) is distorted by injury. **C,** The normal lumbar nerve roots are outlined by the intrathecal contrast. **D,** A sagittal reformatted image shows how using the bone algorithm (or equivalent) minimizes the artifact caused by the posterior metallic wiring of the spine.

in normal structures such as the choroid plexus, pineal gland, and falx cerebri. Differentiation of white and gray matter allows for definition of the basal ganglia, thalamus, and external and internal capsules.

Coronal Sections

Coronal images (Figs. 17-16 through 17-19) are particularly useful for assessing bone when the plane of the bone runs parallel to the axial slice. Coronal images therefore are valuable for scans of the floor and roof of the orbit, the skull base, and the top of the cranial vault. The pituitary gland is well defined as a fairly rectangular structure within the sella turcica that is intersected in the midline, slightly posteriorly, by the pituitary stalk. The cranial nerves in the cavernous sinus can be identified on either side of the pituitary gland.

Coronal images of the temporal bone can highlight the relationships of the ossicles and structures

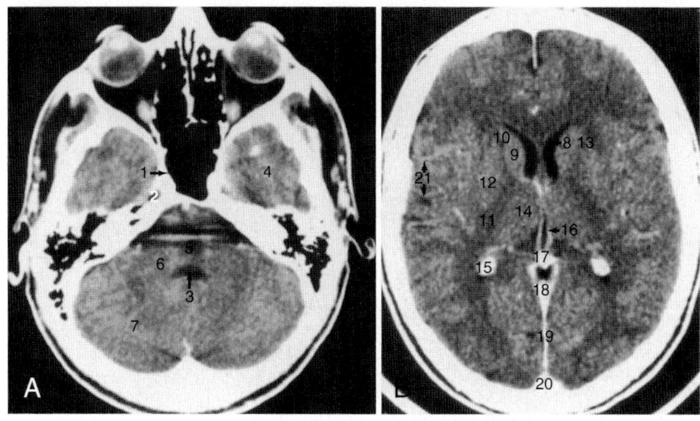

FIGURE 17-14 **A** and **B**, Brain. The normal appearance of the brain using a standard algorithm and 5-mm thick images, obtained with IV contrast enhancement. *1*, Sphenoid sinus; *2*, trigeminal ganglion; *3*, fourth ventricle; *4*, temporal lobe; *5*, pons (partly obscured by streak artifact); *6*, middle cerebellar peduncle; *7*, cerebellar hemisphere; *8*, frontal horn of the lateral ventricle; *9*, head of the caudate nucleus; *10*, anterior limb of the internal capsule; *11*, posterior limb of the internal capsule; *12*, lentiform nucleus; *13*, external capsule; *14*, thalamus; *15*, calcified choroid plexus; *16*, internal cerebral vein; *17*, pineal calcification; *18*, straight sinus; *19*, falx cerebri; *20*, superior sagittal sinus; *21*, branches of the middle cerebral artery. The use of a standard algorithm with a relatively narrow window (80 units) results in good contrast between white and gray matter.

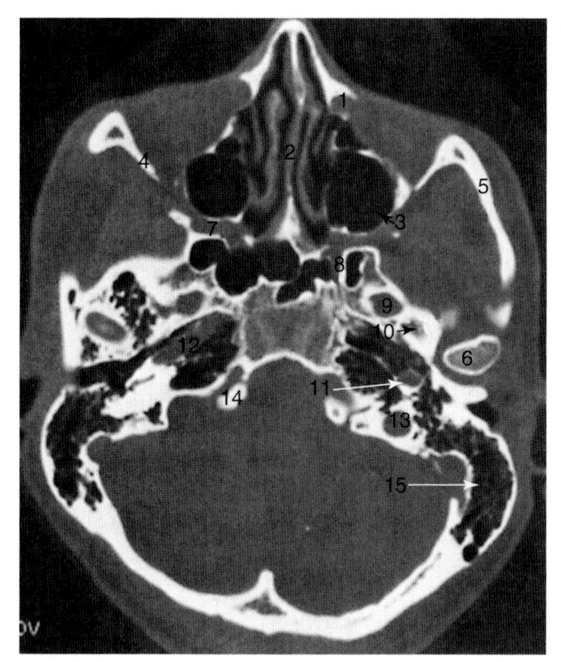

FIGURE 17-15 A 1.5-mm thick axial slice through the base of the skull using the bone algorithm shows excellent spatial resolution. *1*, Opening of the nasolacrimal duct; *2*, nasal septum; *3*, maxillary sinus; *4*, lateral orbital wall; *5*, zygomatic arch; *6*, mandibular condyle; *7*, pterygopalatine fossa; *8*, vidian (pterygoid) canal; *9*, foramen ovale; *10*, foramen spinosum; *11*, ascending carotid canal; *12*, horizontal carotid canal; *13*, jugular fossa; *14*, jugular tubercle; *15*, mastoid air cells.

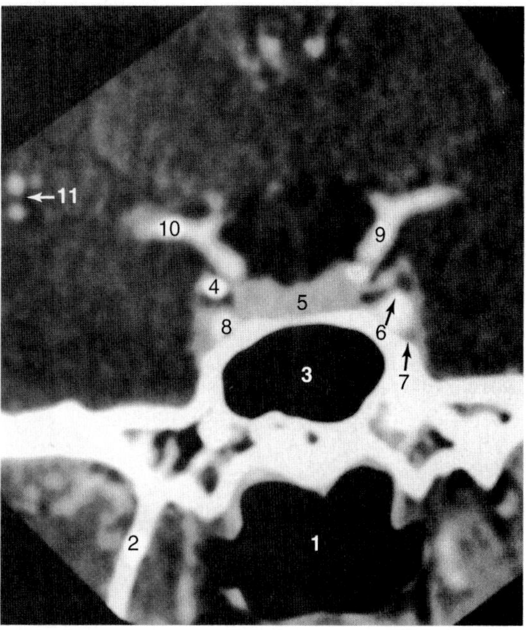

FIGURE 17-16 Sella turcica. A 1.5-mm thick coronal slice through the sella turcica, obtained with IV contrast enhancement, demonstrates these structures: *1*, oropharynx; *2*, lateral pterygoid plate; *3*, sphenoid sinus; *4*, anterior clinoid; *5*, pituitary gland; *6*, cranial nerve III; *7*, cranial nerve VI; *8*, cavernous portion of the internal carotid artery; *9*, supraclinoid portion of the internal carotid artery; *10*, middle cerebral artery; *11*, branches of the middle cerebral artery.

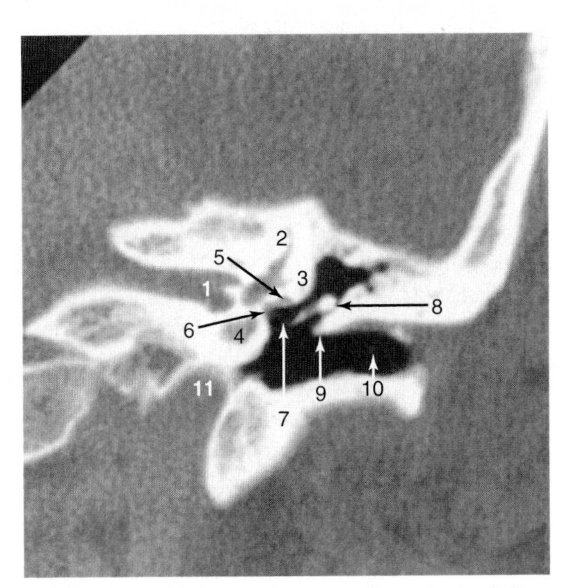

FIGURE 17-17 Temporal bone. A 1-mm coronal image through the left temporal bone using the high-resolution bone algorithm is demonstrated. The thinness of the slice, as well as the smaller FOV, helps maximize the spatial resolution. *1*, Internal auditory canal; *2*, superior semicircular canal; *3*, lateral semicircular canal; *4*, cochlea; *5*, horizontal portion of the facial canal; *6*, oval window; *7*, stapes; *8*, malleus; *9*, Chausse spur; *10*, external auditory canal; *11*, carotid canal.

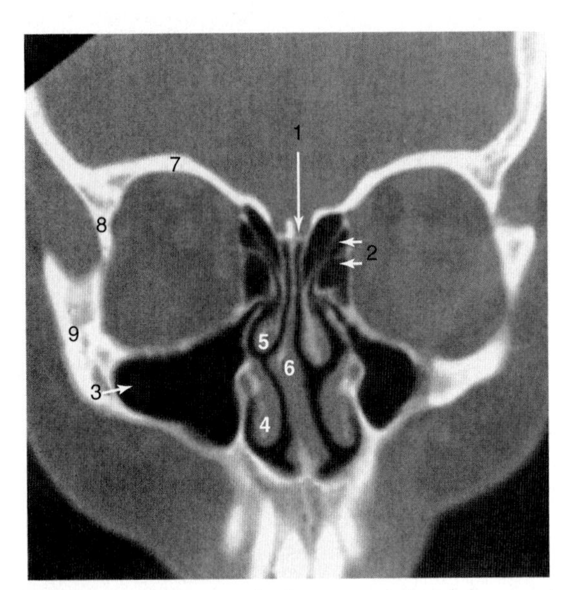

FIGURE 17-18 Paranasal sinuses and facial bones. A 3-mm thick coronal image using the bone algorithm demonstrates the air-containing paranasal sinuses and nasal airway. *1*, Cribriform plate; *2*, ethmoid sinuses; *3*, maxillary sinus; *4*, inferior turbinate; *5*, middle turbinate; *6*, nasal septum; *7*, roof of the orbit; *8*, lateral orbital wall; *9*, zygoma.

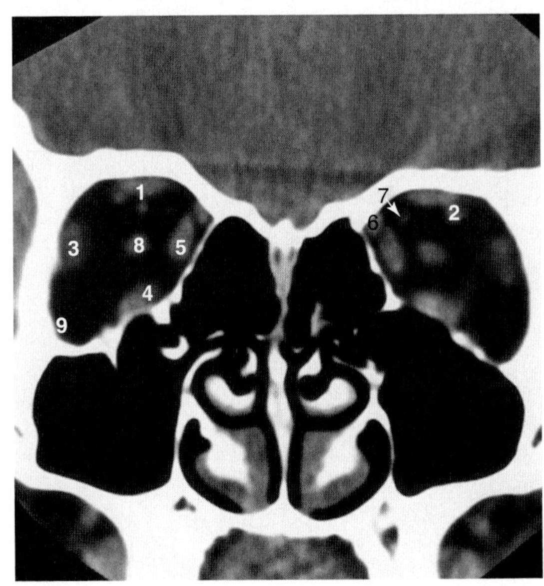

FIGURE 17-19 Orbits. A 3-mm thick coronal view of the orbits, obtained without IV contrast enhancement, demonstrates that orbital fat produces excellent contrast, resulting in good definition of the extraocular muscles and optic nerve. *1*, Superior rectus muscle; *2*, superior ophthalmic vein; *3*, lateral rectus muscle; *4*, inferior rectus muscle; *5*, medial rectus muscle; *6*, superior oblique muscle; *7*, ophthalmic artery; *8*, optic nerve.

along the medial wall of the middle ear, including the facial canal, oval window, and lateral semicircular canal. Coronal images intersect the tentorium and demonstrate its tentlike appearance. They help define whether a lesion is supratentorial or infratentorial, which aids in surgical planning.

A tumor that abuts a ventricle can be assessed in the coronal plane to determine whether it arises from or is extrinsic to the ventricle.

Sagittal Sections

Sagittal sections are not used routinely in most institutions, but are now easier to obtain with multislice scanners. They are particularly helpful in evaluating the midline structures.

Neck

When an IV contrast medium is used to enhance images, major vascular structures such as the carotid arteries and jugular veins can be identified. Both the superficial mucosa and the submandibular glands enhance. The parotid gland, with its high fat content, demonstrates an intermediate density between those of fat and muscle (Fig. 17-20).

Thin sections of the larynx show the relationship of the cartilages to the adjacent soft tissue. The level of the true vocal cords is defined by the position of the arytenoid cartilages (Fig. 17-21).

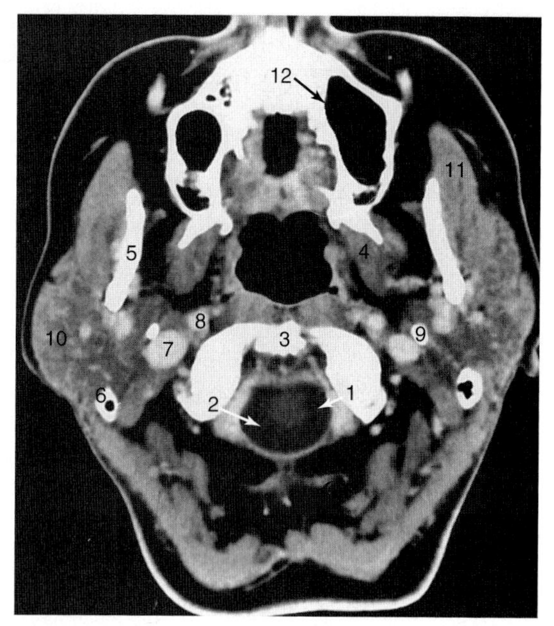

FIGURE 17-20 Neck. This 3-mm thick axial slice through the upper neck was obtained with IV contrast enhancement. *1*, Spinal cord; *2*, cerebrospinal fluid; *3*, top of the odontoid; *4*, pterygoid muscles; *5*, mandible; *6*, tip of the mastoid; *7*, internal jugular vein; *8*, internal carotid artery; *9*, styloid process; *10*, parotid gland; *11*, masseter muscle; *12*, maxillary sinus.

Spine

The sectional anatomy of the lumbar and cervical spines is illustrated in Figures 17-22 and 17-23, respectively. Spine images are acquired in the transverse plane, either helically or by varying the gantry tilt. Coronal or sagittal images can now be obtained easily with multiplanar CT scanners. CT differentiates the disk from the adjacent ligamentum flavum, thecal sac, intraspinal fat, and bone. The nerve roots are easily identified as they exit through the intervertebral foramina. Epidural veins can be seen, particularly in the lumbar spine, but are better visualized with contrast medium enhancement.

PATIENT PREPARATION

Little preparation is needed in most cases. Attention to the following details will minimize artifacts, ensure patient safety and comfort, and produce a study of optimal diagnostic quality.

- *Metallic objects*: The area to be scanned should be free of all jewellery, hairpins, metal gown snaps, wires attached to the patient, and other devices. They can be moved out of the field when they are noted on the scout (scanogram, topogram) images, without having to repeat the scout in most cases. Glasses are removed but contact lenses remain in place for brain scanning.

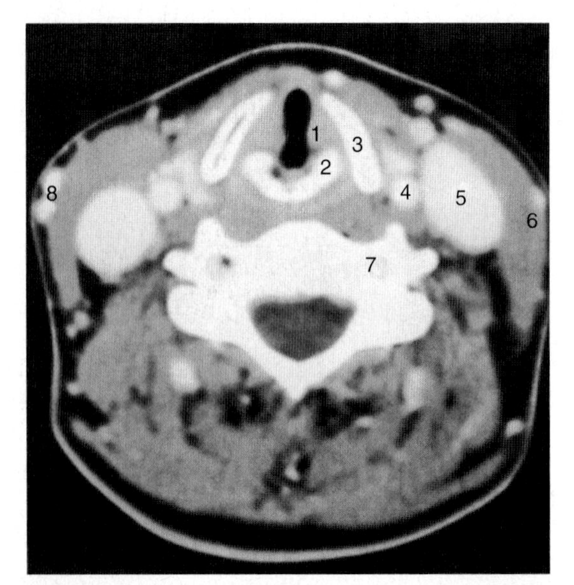

FIGURE 17-21 Larynx. A 3-mm thick axial slice through the larynx obtained at the level of the vocal cords demonstrates prominent enhancement of the vascular structures. The laryngeal cartilages are better defined on the bone setting, which is not included here. *1*, True vocal cord; *2*, arytenoid cartilage; *3*, thyroid cartilage; *4*, common carotid artery; *5*, internal jugular vein; *6*, sternocleidomastoid muscle; *7*, vertebral artery; *8*, superficial veins.

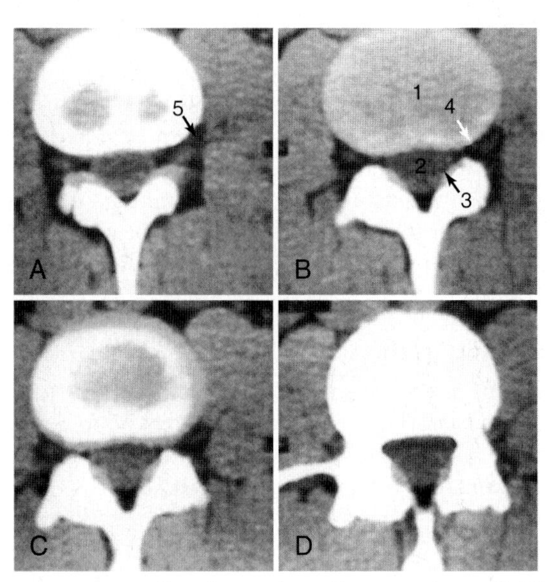

FIGURE 17-22 Lumbar spine. Four sections **(A-D)** through the L3-L4 disk space were obtained every 4 mm using a slice thickness of 5 mm. The disk *(1)* is slightly higher in density than the adjacent paravertebral muscle and the thecal sac *(2)*. The ligamentum flavum *(3)* is also slightly more dense than the thecal sac. Fat in the spinal canal and intervertebral foramen *(4)* helps define the root sleeve *(5)*.

- *Fasting* is not required. However, if IV contrast is being used, a large meal immediately before the CT scan is discouraged in case the contrast causes nausea or vomiting.
- An *empty bladder* is important, especially if the time in the CT scan may be prolonged, as for a CT-guided biopsy or nerve root block.
- *Patient anxiety* may be eased by the technologist's calm demeanor. After confirming the patient's identity, the technologist introduces himself or herself, gives a short explanation of the procedure and the reason for using contrast, and describes expected sensations (heat, noise, table movement, need for staying still).
- *Contrast injection* requires a review of known drug/contrast allergies and of the renal function to minimize contrast reactions and kidney impairment resulting from contrast-induced nephropathy. (This step may be done before the study is scheduled, but the technologist should be aware of this information before contrast is administered.) The appropriate needle size and injection site for the requested study can then be chosen.
- *Cardiac medications* may indicate poor cardiac function. This is relevant information for CTA.
- A *comfortable position* on the scanning table, with holding straps and warm blankets or cushions under the knees and elbows, may result in less motion, reducing image repetition and radiation dose.
- The *eyes* should be closed when the laser positioning light is used near the eyes.

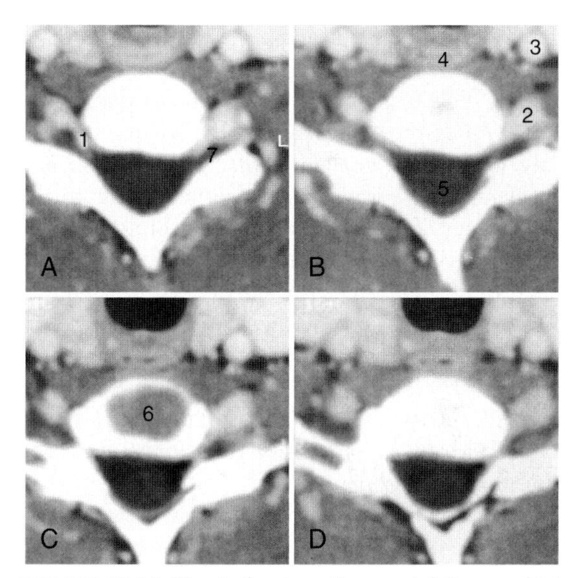

FIGURE 17-23 Cervical spine. Sequential 3-mm thick images **(A-D)** obtained every 2 mm through the C6-C7 disk space demonstrate prominent enhancement of the epidural veins *(1)*, vertebral artery *(2)*, and carotid artery *(3)*, as well as the esophagus *(4)*, spinal cord *(5)*, and disk *(6)*. The dorsal root ganglion *(7)* is outlined by the epidural veins.

The following may be helpful when the technologist is faced with challenging patients:

- *Combative or uncooperative patients* (because of, for example, head injury, psychiatric problems, dementia, and alcohol) require special precautions. More restraints than usual may be needed to obtain a diagnostic study. Use of rapid helical scanning (for example, 800 milliseconds, instead of the usual 1000 to 2000 milliseconds) reduces the resolution between gray and white matter, but the study will be of sufficient quality to demonstrate life-threatening lesions, such as an intracerebral hematoma and the degree of midline shift it has caused, necessitating urgent surgical intervention. The technologist must be very vigilant to avoid personal injury.
- *Body fluid protection* should always be observed (the minimum is gloves when dealing with a trauma patient). When appropriate, the patient or the technologist will need to wear a mask and gown (e.g., carriers of antibiotic-resistant bacteria, termed MRSA (for methicillin-resistant *Staphylococcus aureus*) or VRE (for vancomycin-resistant *Escherichia coli*).

POSITIONING

Image acquisition is obtained with the patient in a supine position. Occasionally, the prone position is required, as for paranasal sinuses, sella turcica, and some CT-guided procedures such as biopsies or nerve root or facet blocks.

A decubitus position, which is seldom used, is reserved for patients who cannot tolerate the supine position. The images can be rotated to a correct position on the reporting console. However, proper annotation of the images, as to side, is necessary for accurate reporting.

Patients with ankylosing spondylitis may present a special positioning challenge because of their severe kyphosis. Stabilizing the patient with cushions or folded blankets minimizes motion. If tilting the gantry to the desired plane is not feasible, helical images reformatted in the usual plane are often diagnostic. Severe scoliosis can be assessed in a similar fashion.

The technologist must center the area to be scanned in the center of the gantry, both horizontally and vertically. Choosing the correct field of view (FOV) to encompass the anatomy in question ensures a quality study. The reference detectors must not receive interference from equipment or coverings, such as restraints or blankets, to produce accurate CT numbers.

SCANNING PROTOCOLS

CT scanners are equipped with preset protocols/techniques and a variety of slice thicknesses, which may vary depending on the model and the manufacturer. Adjustments to radiation dose can be made on the basis of patient size. Locally developed protocols can also be used. This usually consists of choosing a slice thickness and a plane of section for the organ or structure in question, as well as determining the route of contrast administration and dose.

Standardized departmental protocols, developed in collaboration with the radiologists, help to ensure image quality and facilitate patient throughput. Technological changes/updates will require protocol adjustments from time to time.

The following information is based on current usage at a single institution, which has four different types of helical CT scanners (single slice, eight slice, 16 slice, and 64 slice scanners). Protocols are adjusted to approximate results from each of the four scanners for the sake of uniformity. Some studies are only carried out on certain scanners to optimize the images (for example, temporal [petrous] bone).

Circumstances such as excessive motion may require changing the technique (milliamperage, time). Image quality will be decreased when a shorter scanning time is used, but the study should be adequate to rule out a surgical emergency.

Head and Its Contents

Two transverse scanning planes are widely used in brain imaging. In adults, the orbitomeatal baseline (OM line, also called Reid's baseline or RBL) joining the infraorbital rim to the superior border of the external auditory meatus is favored because it results in better images of the orbits, sella turcica, posterior fossa, and brainstem. Some centers use the canthomeatal line (CM line), which joins the lateral canthus of the eye to the center of the external auditory canal. The angle measured between these two lines is 10 degrees.

In children, a steeply angled plane, commonly 20 to 25 degrees to the OM or CM line is used to scan the brain to avoid radiating the ocular lens leading to early cataracts (see Fig. 17-26, *A*, later in this section).

The transverse plane is still the most used plane for image interpretation of the skull and its contents. If reformatted images are required, it is better to acquire thin slices initially and to reformat the images. This technique is useful when scanning the orbits; for example, the lenses of the eyes are scanned only once, dental amalgam artifact is eliminated, and images in true coronal plane (perpendicular to the hard palate) are generated. Patient comfort is also increased compared with direct coronal imaging, when the neck must be hyperextended to achieve a near coronal position and the gantry tilted appropriately. Coronal sections are particularly useful when structures that run parallel to the transverse plane are assessed, such as the floor and roof of the orbits, the sella turcica and adjoining cavernous sinuses, and the skull base and vertex.

Exceptions to this approach exist. Direct coronal images of the temporal petrous bones/internal auditory canals and sella turcica are preferred because the resolution of the 0.6 to 1.25 millimeter (mm) slices is greater than with reformatted images and the orbits are avoided. Prone direct coronal images are also preferred in some centers for the study of paranasal sinuses because air-fluid levels tend to pool away from the path of drainage, known as the ostia, resulting in a better study than the supine transverse or hyperextended (supine coronal) positions. Thin transverse images with sagittal and coronal reformatted images are used when extension of the neck is not possible.

Sagittal images have not been used routinely in the past but are gaining in popularity. They are particularly useful when assessing midline structures and midline abnormalities of the brain and spine.

The algorithm (or kernel) chosen will affect the resolution of the images. In some cases, it may be possible to acquire diagnostic images using a low milliamperage, as with paranasal sinuses or facial bones. Fractures, *sinusitis*, and *nasal polyps* can easily be assessed this way, using only a bone algorithm or equivalent kernel. Temporal (petrous) bones, on the other hand, need a higher milliamperage to get accurate detail of the densest bone in the body and its small structures, such as the cochlea, semicircular canals, and ossicles.

Contrast enhancement is not visible on bone algorithm or bone windows. When contrast is used, images on soft tissue algorithms (standard or equivalent) are also required to see the enhancing tissue, such as with sinus tumors and chronic sinus infections.

Neck, Spine, and Cerebral Blood Vessels

Traditionally, the transverse plane was the preferred plane for interpretation. However, multiplanar reconstructions in coronal, sagittal, and oblique planes greatly enhance the radiologist's ability to diagnose conditions affecting these areas, which contain bony curves (cervical lordosis, mandible), soft tissue curves (carotid bifurcation, cervical disk), and many overlapping organ systems (salivary glands, airway, lymph nodes).

To avoid artifacts on soft tissue algorithm caused by dental amalgam and capped teeth, when possible, transverse angled images on either side of the teeth can be obtained by tilting the gantry. The artifacts are not as distracting if only a bone algorithm (kernel) is needed, for example, to study only the bones; in that case, a single set of images may be acquired. Newer computer software allows reformation of images scanned with a different gantry tilt. This software may be on the scanner workstation or on the PACS (picture archiving communications systems) unit used for reporting.

The Neck

The face and neck contain salivary glands, chains of lymph nodes, and blood vessels. Fat delineates many compartments in the neck. Neck studies usually include images from the nasopharynx to the manubrium/jugular notch. IV contrast is used to help distinguish blood vessels from lymph nodes and muscles because *metastatic lymph nodes* are common in head and neck cancer.

Patients with neck masses may have difficulty breathing in the supine position. This presents a special challenge in positioning the patient. Some patients require a tracheostomy to lie supine, often resulting in the presence of subcutaneous emphysema marring some images.

Transverse images acquired in the same plane as the cervical disks are preferred because they are in the same plane as the true vocal cords, which are situated at the level of the small bilateral arytenoid cartilages. Sequential, rather than helical, acquisition is used because it improves resolution.

Special phonation techniques are occasionally used to assess the mobility of the vocal cords. After the routine image acquisition, the level of the true vocal cords is determined. A limited number of slices are then acquired while the patient vocalizes EEEEEE (in expiration) or a reversed EEEE (in inspiration).

The larynx is surrounded by a number of cartilages (Fig. 17-24).They can be fractured or dislocated with a blow to the front of the neck, affecting the airway and the voice. This is why bone algorithm of the cartilages of the neck is sometimes requested. The thyroid cartilage is larger and more calcified in men than in women. Reformatted sagittal and coronal images depict the cartilaginous abnormality to best advantage before repair.

The salivary glands include the parotid glands, the submandibular glands, the sublingual glands, and minor salivary glands scattered throughout the mouth. Benign and malignant tumors arise in them (Fig. 17-25). *Calculi* can obstruct salivary gland ducts.

The Spine

Spine imaging is acquired either perpendicular to the tabletop or by tilting the gantry to align the plane of section with the vertebral body end plate, as seen on the lateral scout image (Fig. 17-26, *B*).

The use of sequential versus helical scanning depends on the type of equipment available as well as the need for reformatted images. The equipment may or may not allow a gantry tilt with helical scanning. Depending on the indication for spine imaging, bone algorithm (kernel), with or without soft tissue algorithm is obtained.

Disk disease, spinal stenosis, and trauma do not require IV contrast. The disk, as shown in Figure 17-27, *A*, can be differentiated from the dural sac

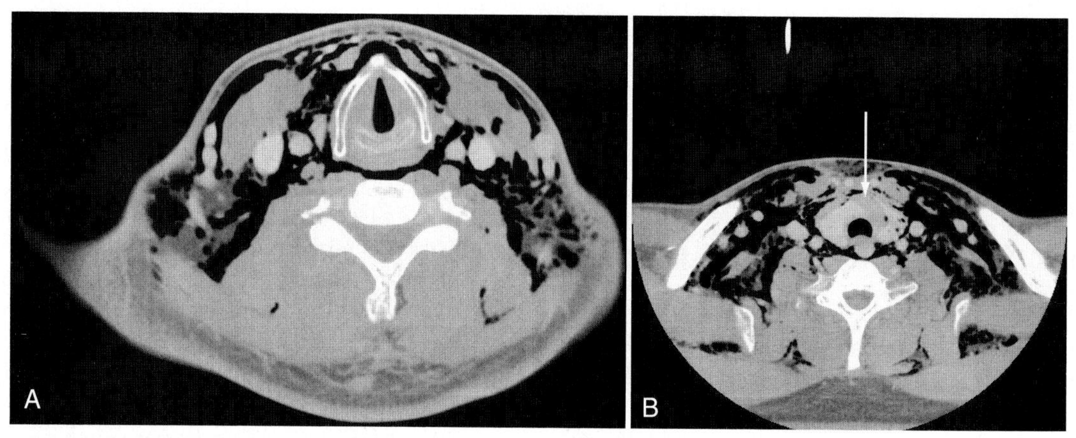

FIGURE 17-24 **A,** Extensive *subcutaneous emphysema* outlines a normal thyroid cartilage. **B,** The thyroid gland is lacerated in the same patient.

(filled with spinal cord, nerves, and CSF), intraspinal fat, ligaments (ligamentum flavum, posterior longitudinal ligament), and bones.

Reformatted sagittal and coronal images help in the assessment of the alignment and the evaluation of *scoliosis* and *spondylolisthesis*. They show the nerves in the intervertebral foramina; they help to determine whether the nerves are being compromised by *disk herniation* or osteophytes. Quality coronal images are produced when the curves (*kyphosis* and *lordosis*) seen on the sagittal images are taken into account.

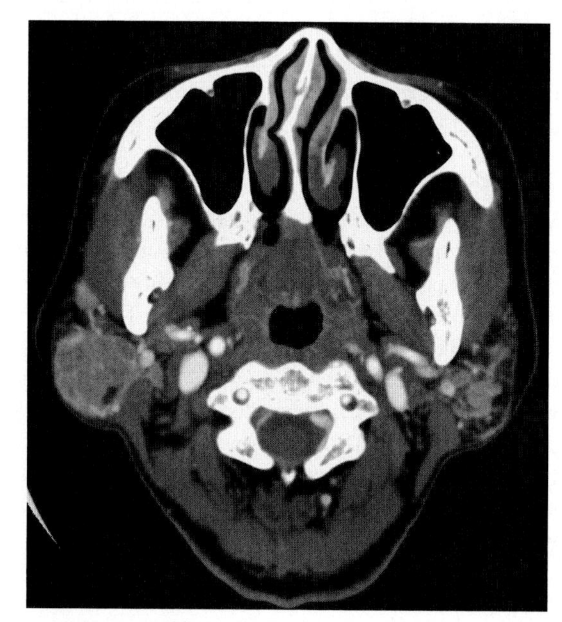

FIGURE 17-25 Bilateral parotid tumors.

Because of its curved outline and smaller size, a cervical disk herniation is more difficult to diagnose than a lumbar disk herniation. Because IV contrast highlights the epidural veins and a herniated disk will displace these veins, IV contrast is used frequently (but not by everyone) to better outline a cervical disk herniation (Fig. 17-27, *B*). A continuous drip infusion or preferably a pump injection will highlight these veins.

Cerebral Blood Vessels

CTP is one form of CTA used in suspected acute brain infarction to determine the amount of brain tissue at risk of permanent damage. The perfusion study is usually followed immediately by the CTA study. The CTP and CTA each require injection of a bolus of contrast. The amount of contrast is adjusted to limit the total amount used in this instance. Our current practice is to use 50 milliliters (ml) of contrast for the CTP and 100 ml for the CTA. A CTA without CTP receives 100 to 150 ml of contrast, our limit for a single dose study (see Contrast Media Usage later).

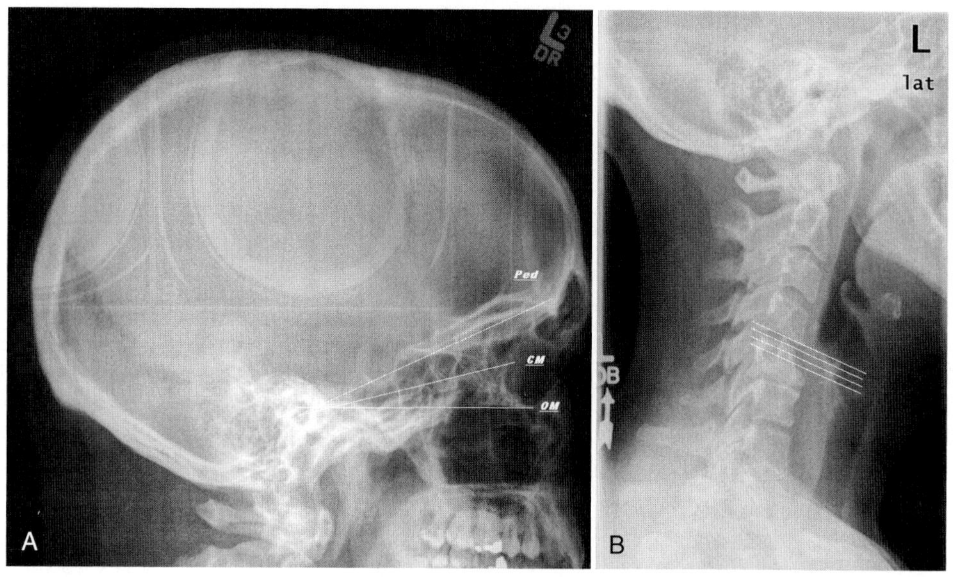

FIGURE 17-26 A, Lateral scout of skull with a selection of scanning planes: orbitomeatal *(OM)*, canthomeatal *(CM)*, and steeper "pediatric" angle to avoid the lens. **B,** Lateral scout of the cervical spine shows the optimum plane of section for imaging the cervical disks and larynx/vocal cords.

A limited area of brain is repeatedly scanned (two-four locations currently) during the first contrast bolus for the CTP. These levels are determined by the radiologist or neurologist from the findings on the unenhanced CT and from the presumed area of infarction on the basis of the neurological examination.

Bolus tracking is used for the CTA to time the image acquisition to the peak of contrast in the cervical vessels by sampling the carotid just below the skull base. This is immediately followed by the second bolus (if a CTP preceded the CTA) and acquisition of images from the aortic arch to the circle of Willis.

The technologist can produce maximum intensity projection (MIP) reformatted images or 3D surface-shaded images while the radiologist evaluates the CTP study on an independent workstation using a CTP software program provided by the manufacturer. Values of cerebral blood flow, blood volume,

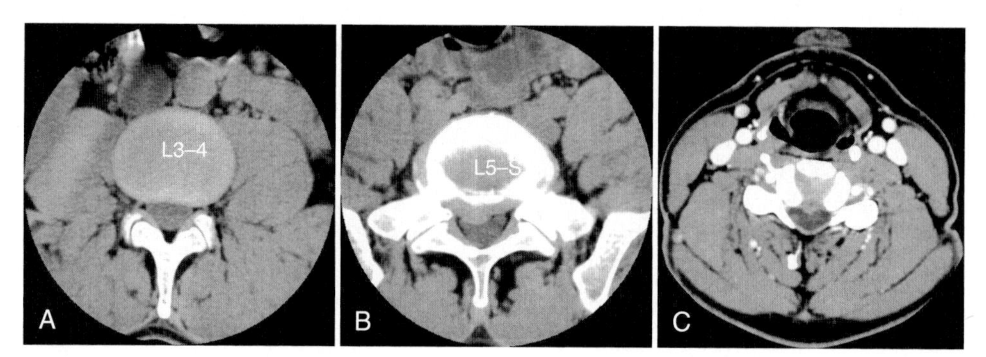

FIGURE 17-27 A, Normal lumbar disk (no contrast used). Lumbar **(B)** and cervical disk **(C)** herniations: the herniation of the smaller cervical disk is better seen when IV contrast is used.

and mean transit time are determined by the radiologist to further evaluate the brain infarction and the amount of potentially salvageable brain.

A CTV images the head from the skull base to the vertex to look for thrombus in the dural (sagittal and transverse) sinuses and in the cortical veins. An 8- to 10-second delay is added to the CTA protocol before images are acquired. Sagittal and coronal reformatted images delineate the patency of these channels.

RADIOGRAPHIC TECHNIQUE

Milliamperage, Kilovoltage, Helical Pitch, and Rotation Time

The preset techniques and protocols supplied by manufacturers are helpful. However, the technologist must be able to manipulate milliamperage, kilovoltage, helical pitch, scan time, and slice thickness to suit the circumstances.

Increasing the milliamperage and the kilovoltage will improve the signal-to-noise ratio. Sufficiently high technique is necessary for contrast resolution of soft tissue in the brain (gray-white matter differentiation). Similarly, spine imaging in large patients can be improved by increasing the technique (by using the maximum kilovoltage and increasing the scan time).

Increasing the scan rotation time will result in better resolution because each image is generated from more projections.

Increasing the helical pitch results in a shorter scan time but reduces the overall image quality because of more interpolation in the scan data and vice versa.

Longer scan times can result in longer tube cooling and the possibility of patient motion (often a result of back pain).

Slice Thickness

Slice thickness should be adapted to the area of interest. Studies requiring reformatted images are acquired helically, with thin slices. Sequential image acquisition is preferred for brain, petrous bones, and neck masses, for better resolution.

Thin transverse sections show the base of the skull well, giving excellent definition of the temporal bones, pituitary fossa, facial bones, and foramina. Thicker slices increase the definition of gray and white matter in the brain.

The low density of various brain tissues, such as fat (in the myelin of white matter) and CSF, outlines components of the brain such as frontal and temporal lobes, basal ganglia, and ventricles. The high density of calcium is found in many normal structures inside the skull (pineal gland, choroid plexus) and must be differentiated from pathological calcium (tumor, AVM).

Spatial resolution is improved with thinner slices, at the cost of a decreased signal-to-noise ratio. Increasing the milliamperage and kilovoltage will improve the signal-to-noise ratio but will also increase the radiation dose.

The average slice thickness has decreased over the years, with the old 10-mm slice of the brain now being 2.5 to 5 mm. Our current practice for a routine head scan consists of 2.5- to 3-mm sequential slices in the posterior fossa and 5-mm slices for the rest of the head.

Orbits are studied with 1- to 2-mm helical slices and a small FOV (13-15 cm).

Temporal bone images are sequential 0.6 to 1 mm thick with a 10-cm field of view.

CTA image acquisition is 1-mm helical. CTP, on the other hand, uses cine mode and 5- to 10-mm thick slices; the tabletop may toggle back and forth during CTP image acquisition, depending on the scanner.

The cervical spine is imaged with helical 1- to 2-mm slices every 1 to 2 mm when good bone detail is needed. On the other hand, 2.5- to 3-mm sequential slices overlapped every 2 mm are used to look for a disk herniation. Wide shoulders present a challenge. Enlarging the field of view and increasing the technique may not always be successful in preventing overrange artifacts from the humeral heads. A swimmer's position is used in some settings to decrease these artifacts.

Lumbar images consist of 3- to 5-mm sequential slices every 3 to 4 mm. One method uses overlapping thicker slices (for example, 7-mm slices every 4 to 5 mm) to improve visualization of herniated lumbar disks, for example, when scatter radiation is increased because of a large girth.

Matrix Size and Reconstruction Algorithms

Matrix size is predetermined at 512 × 512 on most current equipment. Some systems have a 1024 × 1024 matrix (e.g., Philips).

Many reconstruction algorithms are available. The three basic algorithms used for the brain, neck, and spine are the standard, the bone, and the detail algorithms (General Electric) or the Siemens kernels (31, 70, and 45 seconds).

The standard algorithm (and its equivalents) is chosen for most soft tissue imaging, such as the brain and the intervertebral disk, because it provides good contrast resolution. It is important to distinguish gray from white matter when looking for acute cerebral infarction.

The detail algorithm is useful when studying the soft tissues of the neck. It increases edge definition, especially when good definition of lymph nodes and fat planes is required.

The bone algorithm is used to increase the sharpness of the bony detail. This algorithm optimizes spatial resolution; contrast resolution is poor. This is why it should not be used in isolation when IV contrast is administered because tissue enhancement is not visible on bone windows or bone settings. However, bone algorithm is the preferred technique when subarachnoid (intrathecal) contrast has been injected by LP. This is true whether the imaging is of the spine (post myelography CT) or of the brain (CT cisternography).

CONTRAST MEDIA USAGE

Intravenously injected iodinated contrast media have been used since the early days of CT scanning to improve visualization of normal and abnormal structures. In recent years, safer nonionic and iso-osmolar contrast media have become available. Iodinated contrast does not interfere with MRI studies done on the same day.

By further attenuating the x-ray beam, structures containing the iodinated contrast are denser and thus more visible. In the brain, a number of normal structures enhance, including the blood vessels, the choroid plexus, the pineal gland, the pituitary stalk, and the meninges.

In the spine, the enhanced epidural veins, situated along the posterior margin of the vertebral bodies outline the disk margin along the spinal canal and adjoining nerve roots; the ability to diagnose a small disk herniation by the displacement of these veins is increased. In the neck, the enhanced vessels make the lymph nodes distinct because the nodes run chainlike along the vessels.

Abnormal tissue can enhance, either because the blood-brain barrier has been breached (e.g., malignant tumor or abscess in the brain) or because of an inflammatory response (e.g., scarring in the postoperative spine). The degree of enhancement is related to the method of contrast administration (drip infusion versus pump injection) and the dose and concentration of contrast received, as well as the delay between contrast administration and image acquisition.

In the brain and spine, most studies are performed with the IV drip method. This allows the contrast to "percolate" and enhance lesions such as meningioma and metastasis. At least 3 to 5 minutes is required after most of the contrast has been injected to reach satisfactory enhancement. A delay in image acquisition (up to 1 hour) can result in more pronounced enhancement. Because enhancement persists for hours, at least 6 to 8 hours should elapse after a contrast scan before an unenhanced CT is obtained. This will confirm that the enhancement is real and not the result of calcification or hematoma.

CT angiography (CTA and CTP) requires the opposite method. Images are acquired during rapid contrast injection by a pump to best opacify the cerebral blood vessels.

An antecubital vein and a large-bore needle (18 to 20 gauge) help deliver the contrast efficiently, at a rate of 3 to 5 ml per second. Care to avoid contrast extravasation in the arm is required. The volume injected per second in the vein should take its size in consideration. (Skin necrosis caused by extravasation may require a skin graft.) Specific instructions on what to do in such a case must be available to the technologist.

Use of indwelling catheters, such as percutaneous indwelling central venous catheter lines, is not recommended for pump infusion because their small size cannot handle the rate (volume/second) of injection. Site-specific instructions should be respected.

Pump injection is also used in studying the pituitary gland (sella turcica) for the presence of a microadenoma and the cervical spine for disk disease (to best outline the epidural veins) and neck masses.

Nonionic contrast media have decreased the number of mild and moderate contrast reactions (nausea, vomiting, urticaria, rigor) but have not altered the risk of anaphylactic reaction and death. Efforts to minimize contrast use and contrast volume are encouraged.

A standard dose of contrast is administered for each type of examination on the basis of patient weight up to a maximum. For example, our adult-only practice uses 3 ml of nonionic contrast per kilogram (kg), to a maximum of 150 ml for both the drip and pump methods. The current contrast concentration is 320 milligrams (mg) per ml of iodine. A single dose of iodine is thus 48 grams (gm) of iodine and a double dose is limited to 200 ml of contrast or 68 gm of iodine.

Variations do occur. Sella turcica studies use a bolus of 100 ml of contrast (32 gm of iodine).

Postoperative lumbar studies looking for epidural fibrosis (scar) use 200 ml of contrast, by the drip method (unless the patient weighs less than 100 pounds/45 kg.) because enhancement can be quite subtle with a single dose.

In younger patients with lung carcinoma, a workup for brain metastasis consists of 200 ml of contrast and at least a 30-minute delay to allow the contrast to enhance small (< 3 to 5 mm) metastases. Patients older than 75 years of age receive a single dose to protect their renal function.

Great care must always be exercised when iodinated contrast is administered. *Contrast induced nephropathy* (deteriorated kidney function as a result of iodine-based contrast) has been shown to significantly increase morbidity (and length of stay in hospital) and mortality rates. Patients at risk of having borderline or poor renal function, such as diabetics, heart patients, hypertensives, and the elderly, should have documented laboratory values such as a creatinine and estimated glomerular filtration rate (eGFR) before the contrast CT. A creatinine level in the normal range does not mean that the renal function is normal. The eGFR is a better indicator of normal function.

Our current practice is to look for alternative imaging if the creatinine is greater than 120 micromoles per liter (normal in our laboratory is 45-110 micromoles per liter) or the eGFR is less than 60 ml per minute per 1.73 square meters (normal >59).

Exceptions include acute trauma, when life is in danger from bleeding, and acute stroke, when "time is brain."

Contrast media can be used (cautiously) in patients with multiple myeloma and a normal renal function. Reevaluation of the kidney function in the days after the CT is desirable. Good hydration after the CT may help prevent worsening of kidney function.

All our patients are encouraged to increase their intake of water or juice (but not coffee or cola, which are diuretic) in the hours before and after the examination.

Other types of central nervous system contrast media include air and subarachnoid iodinated contrast. Both are types of intrathecal (subarachnoid) contrast media.

Air was used, by an LP, to outline the internal auditory canal before the advent of MRI to look for an intracanalicular acoustic neuroma as a cause of deafness. When air is found today in the brain or spinal canal, it indicates that a communication exists between the environment and the central nervous system (such as a penetrating injury), raising the possibility of meningitis, or that a recent LP has been performed.

Iodinated subarachnoid contrast is used to look for leakage of CSF from the nose or ear (*rhinorrhea, otorrhea*) or in the spine (*intracranial hypotension*) and to study instrumented spines (postmyelogram). This type of contrast remains visible on CT for hours, even when it is no longer visible on fluoroscopy or plain films, so CT can be used to "rescue" a myelogram. A CT study in the first hour after intrathecal contrast injection is preferable. Occasionally, repeat CT scans after 6-, 12-, or 24-hour delays are used to detect clearance or accumulation of contrast, for example, in a spinal cord *syrinx*.

A CT of the brain obtained less than 24 hours after a myelogram will have an unusual appearance because of the reabsorption of the contrast by the brain before excretion by the kidneys; it will show greater gray-white matter differentiation than normal. This finding is most puzzling when the history of a myelogram performed at another institution in the prior 24 hours is not provided.

The assistance of CT technologists Donna Lopez and Ron Chitsaz in the preparation of the manuscript is very much appreciated. Any inaccuracy is entirely my own.

Computed Tomography of the Body

Borys Flak

Chapter Outline

In the early years of computed tomography (CT), many were skeptical about its usefulness outside the central nervous system (CNS). Earlier scanners were unsuitable for examining the body because of the image degradation that occurred with patient motion and movement of internal organs during the 2 to 5 minutes required for a single slice. Within several decades, however, astonishing technologic advances including helical scanning techniques, multidetector arrays, subsecond scan times, near real-time reconstruction of images, and advanced viewing workstations have completely revolutionized CT. The latest generation of scanners can obtain up to 64 slices simultaneously at 0.5-millimeter (mm) collimation with 400 millisecond scan times. This enables extended ranges of coverage with thinner collimation and increased speed, allowing for large volume data acquisitions during single short breathholds. The resultant three-dimensional (3D) and multiplanar reformations (MPRs) are outstanding. CT of the body has therefore not only fulfilled but in fact surpassed the expectations of its early supporters and has become an important means of evaluating many pathological conditions. Magnetic resonance imaging (MRI) has replaced CT as the primary method of investigation for most diseases of the cranium, spinal cord, and musculoskeletal system; however, CT is still superior to MRI for most clinical indications in the chest and abdomen.

CLINICAL INDICATIONS

In addition to CT, a wide variety of radiological techniques are available for studying diseases of the body, including plain radiographs, barium studies, angiography, nuclear medicine, ultrasonography, and MRI. Clinicians are faced with the dilemma of which imaging method or methods to use and in what order. Often too many examinations are requested or studies are performed in the wrong sequence before a diagnosis is reached. For these reasons, the use of algorithms or flowcharts has become popular. The suggested approach, however, may not be the most appropriate for the individual institution when the limitations of available equipment and expertise are considered. The radiologist, acting as a consultant, should discuss the clinical problem with the referring physician and choose the most expeditious and cost-effective method or methods for answering the clinician's questions. This chapter presents the major indications for CT of the body.

Chest and Mediastinum

Mediastinum

Almost all mediastinal abnormalities detected on chest radiographs (typically suspected masses) or suspected from clinical evidence can be confirmed with CT (Gamsu, 1992). CT is most commonly used to detect lymphadenopathy in patients suspected of having bronchogenic carcinoma, lymphoma, or other malignancies (Fig. 18-1). Although highly sensitive, CT and MRI have some limitations; they are less efficient at detecting tumors within normal-size nodes or differentiating between enlarged hyperplastic nodes without a tumor and tumor-containing nodes. CT is useful in patients known to have or suspected of having bronchogenic carcinoma; in these cases, CT is used to determine the extent of invasion of the chest wall, mediastinum, and diaphragm and to detect extrathoracic metastases in the liver and adrenal glands. MRI better demonstrates chest wall invasion and is more accurate in detecting mediastinal invasion and staging apical tumors (Manfredi et al, 1996; Tateishu et al, 2003).

With enhancement of vascular structures in the mediastinum by use of intravenous (IV) contrast medium, an aneurysm can be differentiated from other mediastinal masses (Posniak et al, 1989) (Figs. 18-2 and 18-3). CT is highly accurate and comparable to MRI and transesophageal echo in detecting and defining the extent of traumatic aortic ruptures and aortic dissections (Sommer et al, 1996). Angiography is now rarely used to confirm these diagnoses.

In patients with myasthenia gravis, CT can detect thymic masses not evident on chest radiographs (Fon et al, 1982). Cysts and fatty deposits are distinguished by their characteristic CT numbers. A specific diagnosis cannot be made with most other masses, but the relationship of the mass to surrounding structures and its location and extension within the mediastinum can be readily defined and a differential diagnosis suggested.

Lung

CT is the most sensitive technique for detecting pulmonary metastases (Muhm et al, 1978; Schaner et al, 1978). However, the increased sensitivity is achieved at the price of decreased specificity.* Benign lesions such as subpleural lymph nodes and granulomas can be detected, as well as a greater number of metastatic lesions. CT therefore is most useful in patients being evaluated for resection of metastatic pulmonary nodules, such as patients with osteogenic sarcoma. In the appropriate clinical setting, high-resolution CT (HRCT) can be diagnostic for lymphangitic carcinomatosis (Munk et al, 1988). CT also can be used to detect occult primary lung tumors in patients who show malignant cells on sputum cytological studies but who have normal chest x-ray films. Some investigators have used nodule densitometry (i.e., the measurement of nodule density with Hounsfield numbers) (Zerhouni et al, 1986) or the degree of contrast enhancement (Swensen et al, 1996) on CT to evaluate solitary pulmonary nodules that are indeterminate for malignancy on conventional radiographs.

Helical CT is more sensitive than ventilation/perfusion scans and of equal specificity in detecting pulmonary emboli (Mayo et al, 1997). Emboli are seen as filling defects in the enhanced pulmonary arteries (Fig. 18-4). CT will miss clots in the smaller subsegmental branches, but this may not be clinically significant unless the patient has severe underlying cardiac or pulmonary disease (Stein et al, 1995).

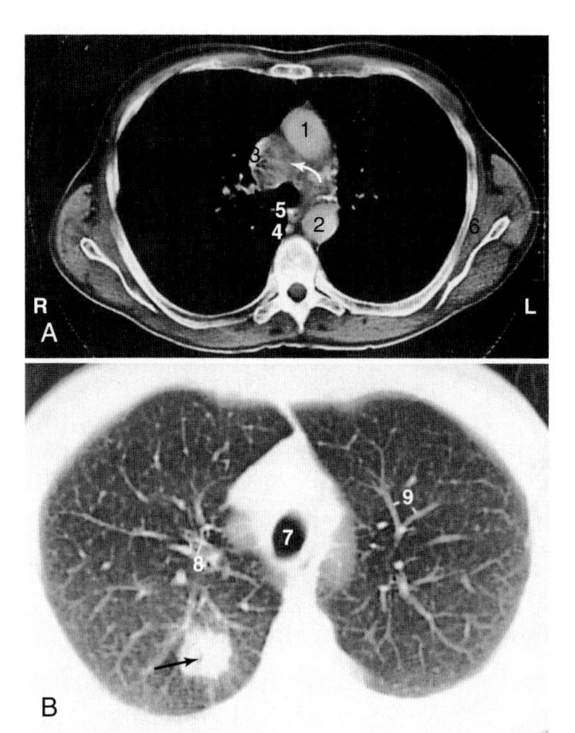

FIGURE 18-1 Bronchogenic carcinoma *(black arrow)* with pretracheal mediastinal lymphadenopathy *(white arrow)*. *1*, Ascending aorta; *2*, descending aorta; *3*, superior vena cava; *4*, azygos vein; *5*, esophagus; *6*, subscapular muscle; *7*, trachea; *8*, segmental bronchi; *9*, pulmonary vessels.

HRCT using thin sections has become the established method for evaluating diffuse lung diseases (Muller, 1991) (Fig. 18-5). When the CT findings are analyzed in the context of the clinical history, physical findings, pulmonary function tests, and laboratory data, characteristic HRCT findings may allow a confident diagnosis in conditions such as asbestosis, silicosis, and idiopathic pulmonary fibrosis. In some cases such as allergic alveolitis, HRCT findings may preclude the need

*Sensitivity is defined as the likelihood that a test will be positive in an individual who has disease (i.e., the ability to detect disease). Specificity is defined as the likelihood that a test will be negative in an individual who has no disease (i.e., the ability to detect normalcy).

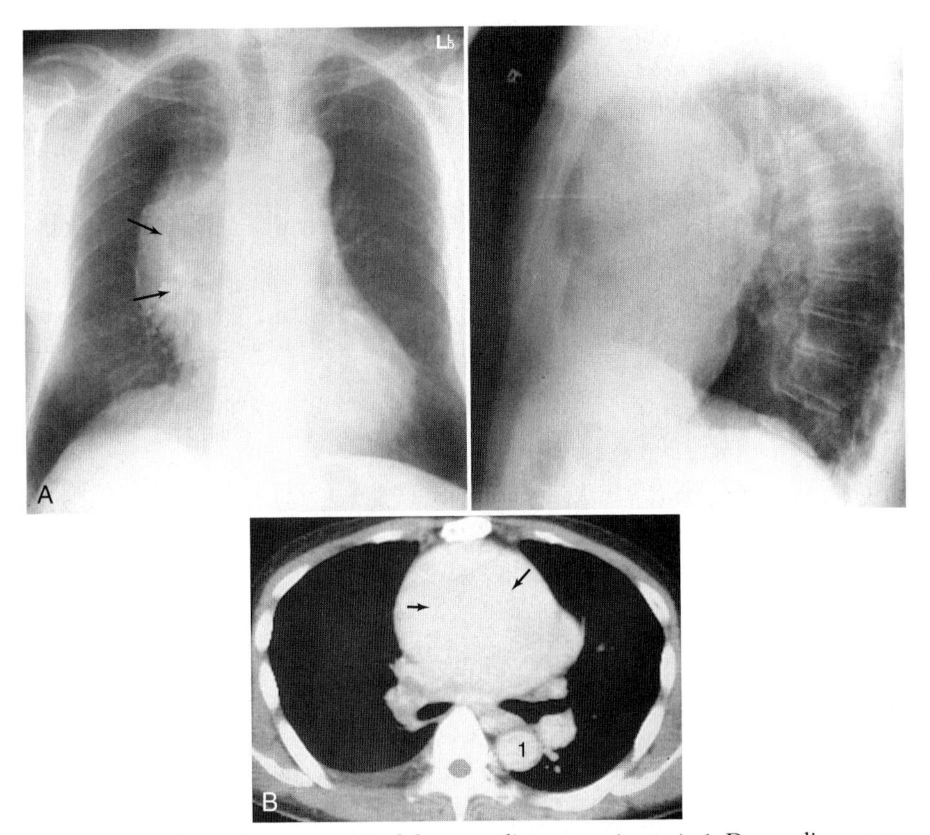

FIGURE 18-2 Dissecting aneurysm of the ascending aorta *(arrows)*. *1*, Descending aorta.

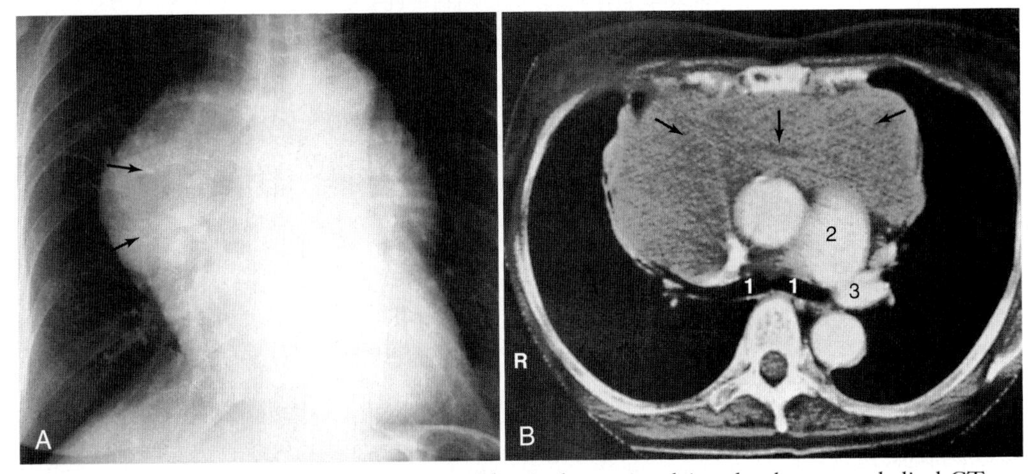

FIGURE 18-3 Lymphoma seen as an anterior mediastinal mass involving the thymus on helical CT scan *(arrows)*. *1*, Right and left main stem bronchi; *2*, main pulmonary artery; *3*, left pulmonary artery.

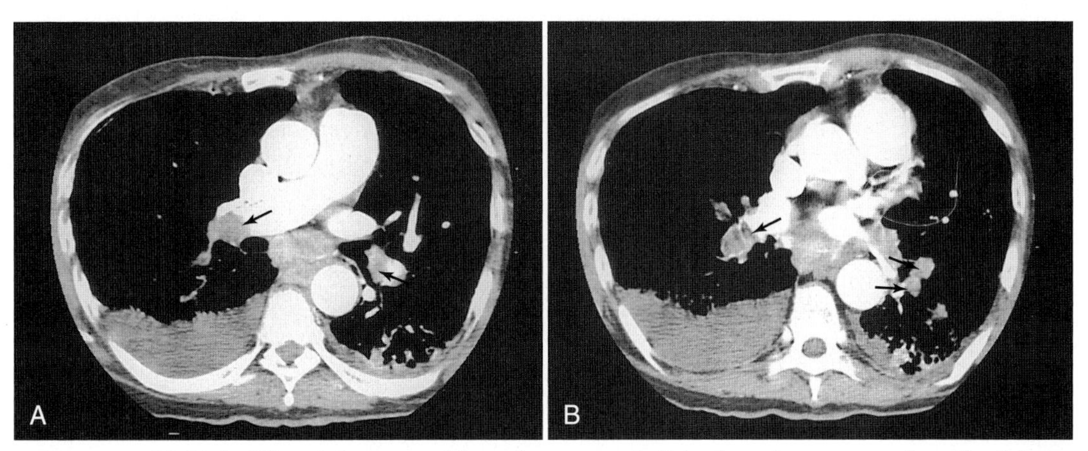

FIGURE 18-4 Multiple filling defects caused by pulmonary emboli in the pulmonary arteries of both lungs *(arrows)*.

for lung biopsy, or it can be used as a guide in selecting the best site for a biopsy. HRCT is more sensitive than chest radiography for detecting emphysema (Fig. 18-6), and it has replaced bronchography as the definitive method for detecting bronchiectasis (Pang et al, 1989).

Multislice CT is the most effective way to image patients after blunt chest trauma, which is second only to CNS injury as a cause of posttrauma death. A myriad of injuries may result, including pulmonary contusion or laceration, pneumothorax, hemothorax, tracheobronchial laceration, diaphragmatic injury, and chest wall and spinal injuries. Although the chest radiograph is useful in detecting a number of potentially life-threatening conditions (e.g., tension pneumothorax, gross hemothorax), chest radiography is simply not sensitive enough to reliably identify or quantify the extent of most thoracic injuries.

Screening CT studies of the lungs to detect nodules has recently become popular, but this remains a highly controversial indication. This is primarily due to the high false-positive rate caused by benign nodules such as granulomas and lymph nodes and current lack of adequate studies to confirm decreased mortality rates from earlier tumor detection (Swensen et al, 2002).

Cardiac

The technology of the latest generation of CT scanners combining very rapid scanning with thin collimation, extended range, and electrocardiographic gating is enabling for the first time the ability to accurately study the coronary arteries noninvasively. It is possible to assess the degree of

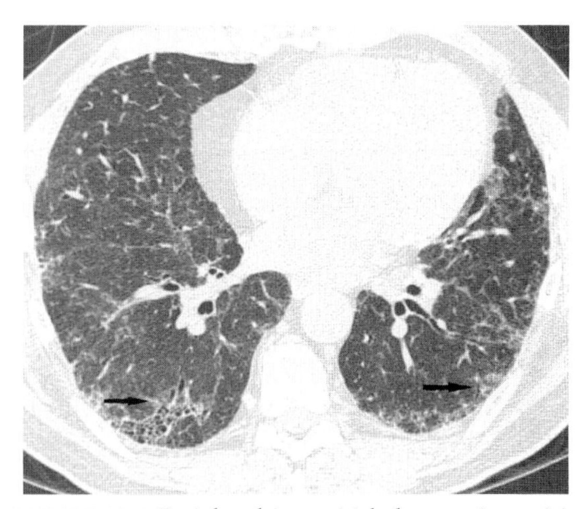

FIGURE 18-5 Peripheral interstitial changes *(arrows)* in both lungs typical of usual interstitial pneumonia. (Image courtesy Dr. Nestor Muller, Vancouver Hospital.)

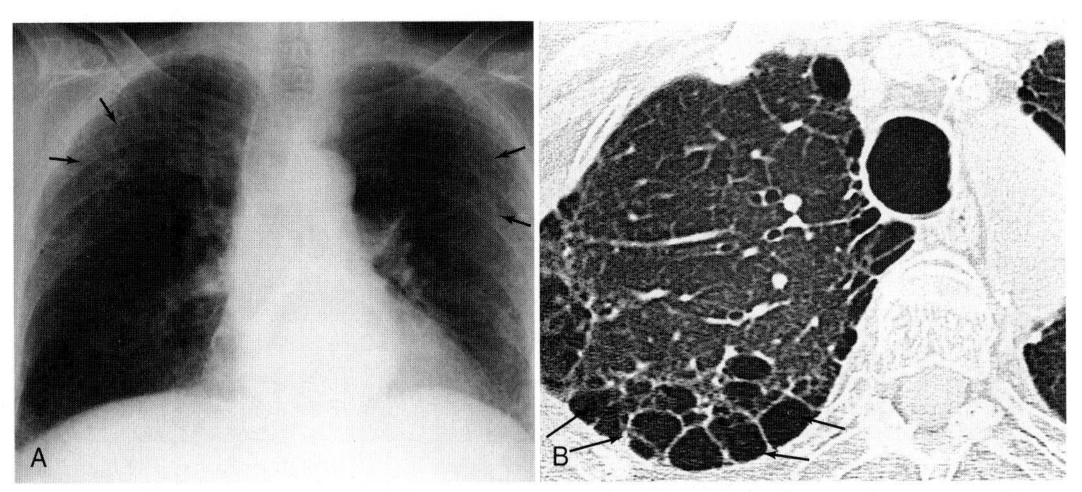

FIGURE 18-6 Additional interstitial changes *(arrows)* on plain films **(A)** are shown to have occurred as a result of paraseptal emphysema on high-resolution thin sections **(B)**.

coronary artery calcification, to obtain angiograms of the coronary arteries, and to display these images in 3D and multiple other projections, in some cases eliminating the need for more invasive and risky catheter angiography. The same technology is also enabling the determination of ventricular volume as a function of time from which cardiac output, ejection fraction, stroke volume, and so forth can be calculated.

Coronary artery calcium scoring examinations are now widely performed to detect the extent of calcification in the coronary arteries and help clinicians manage patients at risk for a myocardial infarction. "Coronary artery disease is the single most important cause of death in North America, but traditional Framingham risk factor assessment* predicts only 60-65% of acute myocardial infarctions or sudden cardiac deaths. Coronary artery calcification has been shown to be an accurate marker for atherosclerotic disease" (Forster and Isserow, 2005). Typically 45 to 65 images are obtained, areas of calcification in the five major coronary branches are marked, and each plaque is assigned a score on the basis of its area and density. All the scores are added and adjusted for age and sex on the basis of existing data files.

The coronary arteries represent the ultimate challenge for CT angiography because of their small size, tortuous course, and pronounced rapid motion. Catheter coronary angiography has been the undisputed gold standard for many years; however, recent studies by Leschka et al (2005) and Raff et al (2005) have shown that CT can reliably identify significant coronary stenoses in vessels as small as 1.5 mm with a sensitivity of 94% to 95%, a specificity of 90% to 97%, and, very important, negative predictive values of 93% to 98%.* The latter indicates that multislice CT angiography (CTA) can be reliably used to noninvasively exclude significant coronary artery disease in patients with chest pain of uncertain etiology or whose other test results may be inconclusive or conflicting. The image quality is truly impressive.

*Framingham risk factor assessment is a predictive algorithm that estimates the risk for development of angina, myocardial infarction, or coronary disease death over the course of 10 years. The factors considered include age, blood cholesterol levels, blood pressure, cigarette smoking, and diabetes mellitus.

*Negative predictive value is defined as the likelihood that a patient with a negative test truly has no disease.

Liver

Although CT is more sensitive than ultrasonography in the initial screening of the liver for focal lesions, ultrasonography continues to play a significant role in this regard because of the large volume of patients. CT is always used when ultrasonography results are inconclusive or when more detailed localization and characterization of lesions are required (Fig. 18-7).

Proper use of an IV contrast medium is important for detecting focal masses in the liver. Helical CT used with power injection boluses of contrast medium, with or without the help of bolus-tracking software, allows a so-called triphasic examination of the liver. This examination includes one series during the early arterial phase, a second during the venous phase, and a delayed scan. Dynamic CT, which involves multiple repeat scans at the same level or several selected levels, is helpful for demonstrating the characteristic contrast medium–enhancement pattern seen with hemangiomas (Freeny and Marks, 1986) (Fig. 18-8). CT hepatic angiography and CT arterial portography are probably still the most sensitive methods available for detecting additional tumor nodules (Hori et al, 1998) and are especially useful for planning hepatic resection. The introduction of multidetector scanners, however, has allowed the use of very thin scans (e.g., 2.5-mm collimation through the entire liver), and a study by Weg et al (1998) confirmed higher rates of detection and improved conspicuity of small liver lesions (less than 10 mm) compared with 5- to 10-mm collimation.

With a few exceptions, diffuse liver disease cannot be diagnosed by CT. Hemachromatosis, amiodarone therapy, and some glycogen storage diseases are associated with dense livers on CT (Goldman et al, 1985), whereas fatty infiltration is evidenced by a liver that is less attenuating than the spleen on unenhanced scans (Alpern et al, 1986).

CT and ultrasonography are equally accurate in demonstrating intrahepatic and extrahepatic bile ducts in jaundiced patients (Baron et al, 1982) (Fig. 18-9). CT is performed only if the ultrasound technique is unsuccessful. If dilated ducts are demonstrated and the obstructing lesion is not delineated, the next investigation usually is direct cholangiography (transhepatic cholangiography or endoscopic retrograde cholangiopancreatography) or MRI cholangiography.

The liver is the second most common solid abdominal organ to be injured in blunt trauma; however, the majority of injuries can be treated conservatively. Contrast-enhanced CT can identify hematomas which may be subcapsular or parenchymal, lacerations, and evidence of active hemorrhage, which could mean the presence of a more severe vascular injury involving the inferior vena cava, portal veins, or hepatic artery (Shanmuganathan, 2004).

Spleen

The spleen is the most commonly injured solid organ in the abdomen, and trauma is the most common indication for scanning the spleen. Contrast-enhanced CT can diagnose the principal types of injury, namely, hematoma, laceration,

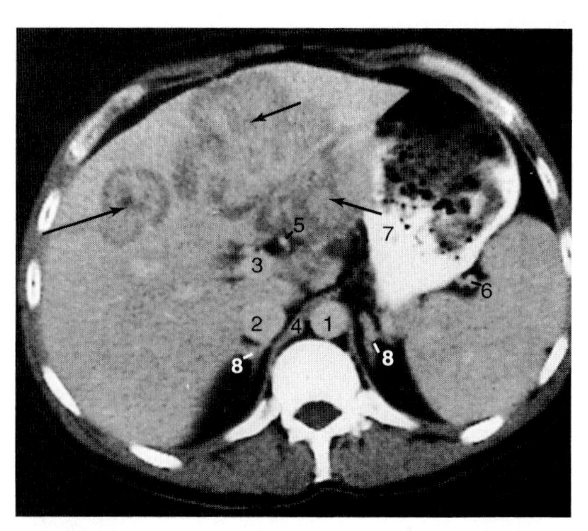

FIGURE 18-7 Hepatoma *(arrows)* involving the lateral and medial segments of the left lobe of the liver. *1*, Aorta; *2*, inferior vena cava; *3*, portal vein; *4*, crus; *5*, hepatic artery; *6*, splenic artery; *7*, stomach; *8*, adrenals.

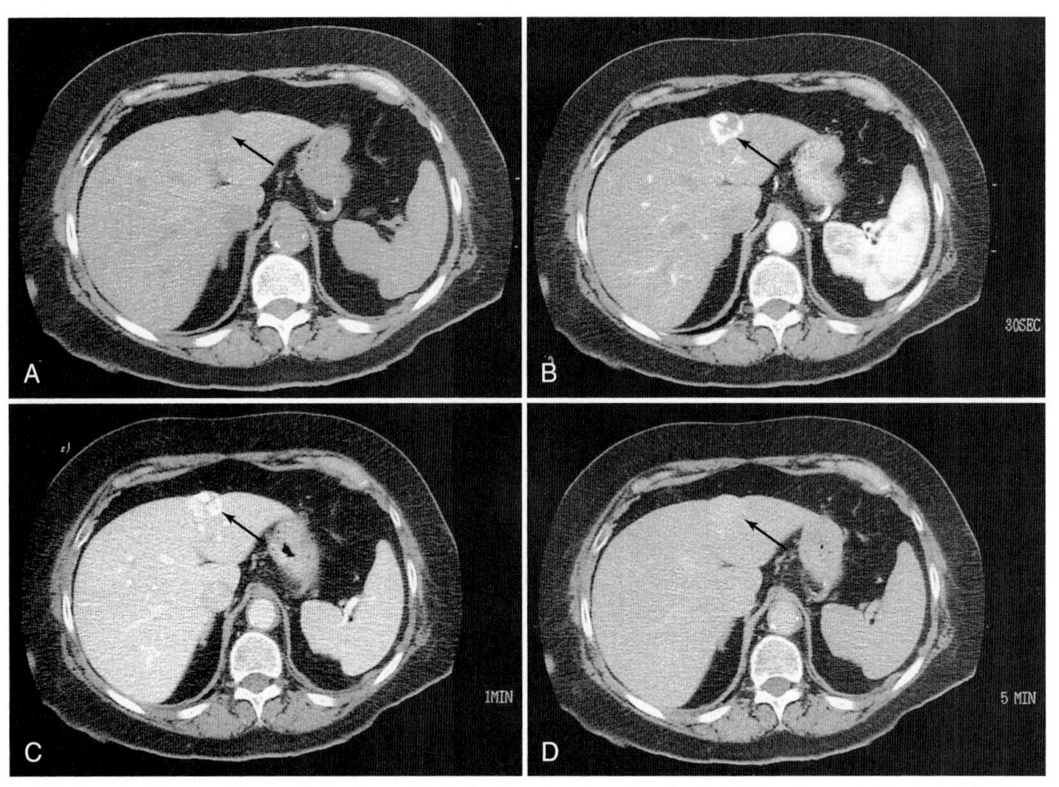

FIGURE 18-8 Hemangioma of the liver. **A,** Low-density mass in the left lobe *(arrow)*. **B,** Arterial phase study demonstrates dense, lobulated peripheral enhancement *(arrow)*. **C,** Venous phase study demonstrates that the lesion is filling in with the contrast medium *(arrow)*. **D,** Delayed scan demonstrates complete filling in of the lesion, which is nearly isodense *(arrow)*.

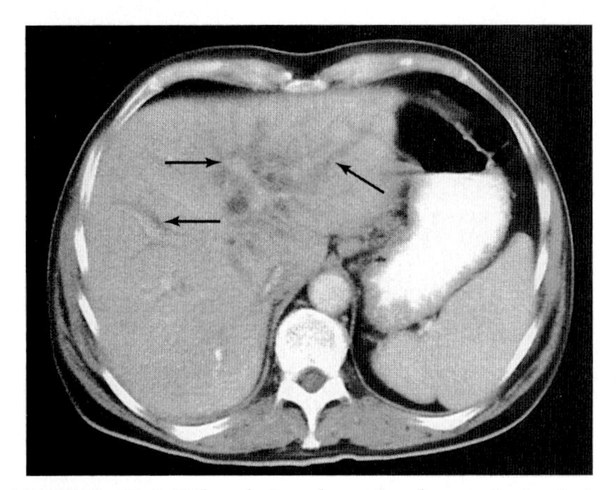

FIGURE 18-9 Dilated intrahepatic ducts *(arrows)* in a jaundiced patient known to have cholangiocarcinoma.

and vascular injury (Fig. 18-10). The latter two more often require surgical intervention (Shanmuganathan 2004). Although focal masses can be seen in the spleen with both CT and ultrasonography, the results of spleen assessment in patients with lymphoma has unfortunately remained poor for both methods (Castellino et al, 1984).

Bowel

Barium studies and endoscopy traditionally have been the mainstays of alimentary tract investigation, CT is assuming an ever-increasing role because of its ability to delineate not only the lumen but also the bowel wall and adjacent structures. Virtual colonoscopy, or CT colonography, is a new development in gastrointestinal (GI) radiology that is challenging the barium enema and even colonoscopy in the detection of colon polyps (Hara et al, 1997). This technique involves cleansing the colon with a standard bowel preparation, insufflating the colon with air or carbon dioxide (or both), performing thin-section helical scans (typically 2-3 mm with overlapping reconstruction in both the supine and prone positions), and subsequently reviewing the images in cine or movie mode, as well as performing MPR. The data also can be volume rendered and displayed in a "fly through" navigation mode simulating colonoscopy (Fenlon et al, 1999). The results of preliminary studies have been extremely encouraging, rivaling or surpassing those of conventional methods (Pickhardt et al, 2003).

Although CT has proved not very accurate for staging of GI malignancies, it is still widely used for this purpose, primarily to prevent unnecessary surgery in cases that demonstrate strong evidence of unresectability because of local invasion or distant metastases, such as to the liver (Davies et al, 1997).

Plain radiographs are diagnostic in only about 50% to 60% of small bowel obstructions, equivocal in 20% to 30%, and normal or nonspecific in 10% to 20% (Mucha, 1987). CT can confirm an obstruction, determine the level and perhaps the cause, and often indicate whether vascular compromise is present in uncertain cases (Fig. 18-11) (Balthazar, 1994).

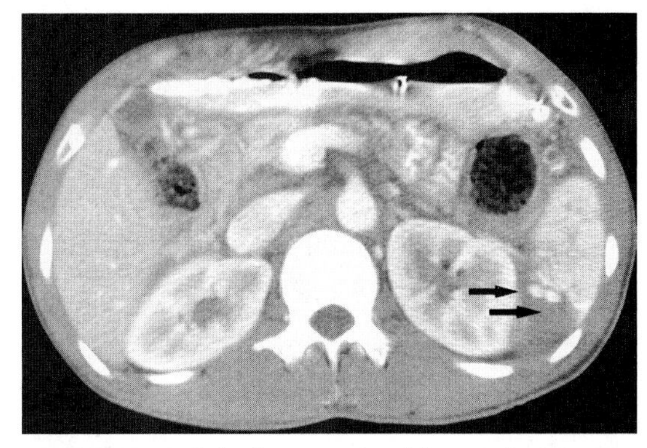

FIGURE 18-10 Splenic rupture with pseudoaneurysms *(arrows)*. (Image courtesy Dr. Luck Louis, Vancouver Hospital.)

Barium studies remain the primary procedure for evaluating patients with inflammatory bowel disease, but CT is the key to studying the mural extent and detecting any extraintestinal involvement or complications such as phlegmons, abscesses, sinus tracts, and fistulas (Gore et al, 1996).

In approximately 20% to 33% of patients suspected of having appendicitis, the clinical presentation is atypical (Berry et al, 1984), requiring imaging. We prefer to perform graded compression sonography as the initial test; however, a

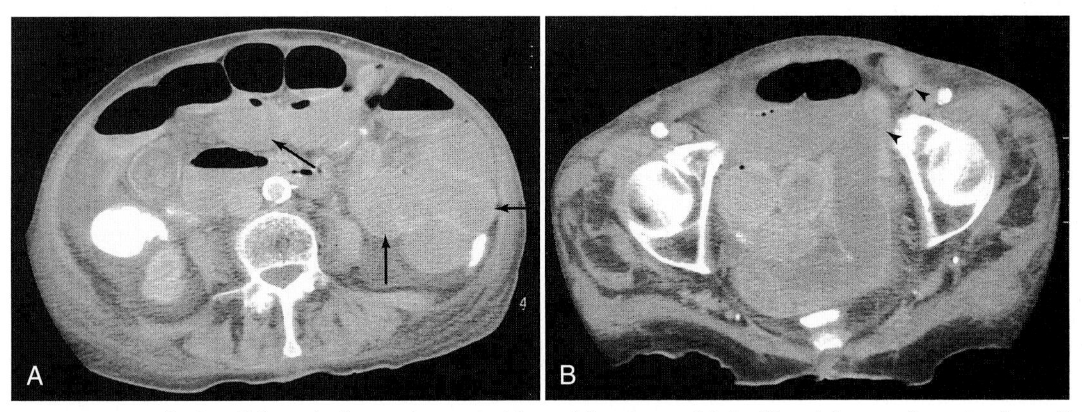

FIGURE 18-11 A, Small bowel obstruction as evidenced by the multiple dilated loops of proximal small bowel *(arrows)*. **B,** A herniated loop in the left groin *(arrowheads)*.

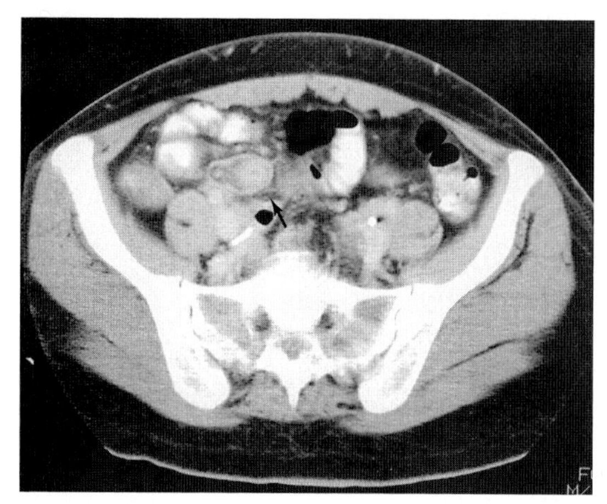

FIGURE 18-12 Thickened, inflamed appendix *(arrow)* in the right lower quadrant.

number of studies have demonstrated greater accuracy with CT and therefore this should be considered an alternative, especially in obese patients or if the sonogram is inconclusive (Lane et al, 1997) (Fig. 18-12). Clinically, patients with diverticulitis typically have a fever and a tender mass in the left lower quadrant. CT can accurately determine the severity of involvement and whether a complicating abscess is present (Ambrosetti et al, 1997).

Although bowel injury resulting from blunt trauma is uncommon, CT can be used to differentiate between a full-thickness bowel wall injury that requires surgery and a less serious bowel wall contusion/hematoma or serosal tear.

Retroperitoneum

Pancreas

Previously the pancreas was a difficult organ to evaluate, clinically or with routine radiological studies. Cross-sectional imaging methods such as ultrasonography, CT, and MRI now permit direct demonstration of the pancreas. The role of MRI in the diagnosis of pancreatic disorders is still questionable, and the technique probably offers no significant advantages over CT. When the pancreas is well visualized on a sonogram, the accuracy is comparable to that of CT. In general, the success rate for delineating the entire pancreas is much higher with CT than with ultrasonography because bowel gas often obscures part or all of the pancreas (Hessel et al, 1982) (Fig. 18-13).

Acute pancreatitis is a clinical diagnosis, and normally neither CT nor ultrasonography is necessary. Imaging should be performed only when the diagnosis is uncertain, when complications are suspected (Siegelman et al, 1980), or when the clinical course is severe or unexpected. With acute pancreatitis CT is preferred mainly because of the high incidence of associated paralytic ileus, which obscures visualization of the pancreatic region by sonogram (Fig. 18-14). Larger pseudocysts can be monitored with ultrasonography, although CT generally provides a more graphic and complete delineation of the extent of involvement, and smaller changes in size and extent can be appreciated. A specific diagnosis of chronic pancreatitis can be made with CT if pancreatic calcification (often not seen on plain films) and pancreatic ductal dilation are noted.

Biphasic or triphasic examinations of the pancreas are helpful when searching for potential solid lesions in the pancreas. The arterial phase study with MPR or 3D reconstruction can delineate the vascular anatomy and help stage lesions by determining whether any vascular invasion is present. The parenchymal phase identifies adenocarcinomas as an area of diminished density because they tend to be hypovascular, whereas islet cell tumors, which are small and often difficult to identify (Rossi et al, 1985), appear as increased in density because of their hypervascularity. Solid pancreatic masses may be caused by a tumor (Fig. 18-15) or by focal inflammation, and differentiation may be difficult unless an ancillary finding such as liver metastases is also present. In most cases percutaneous aspiration or core needle biopsy under CT or ultrasonographic guidance for cytological and histological diagnosis is required (Sundaram et al, 1982) (Fig. 18-16).

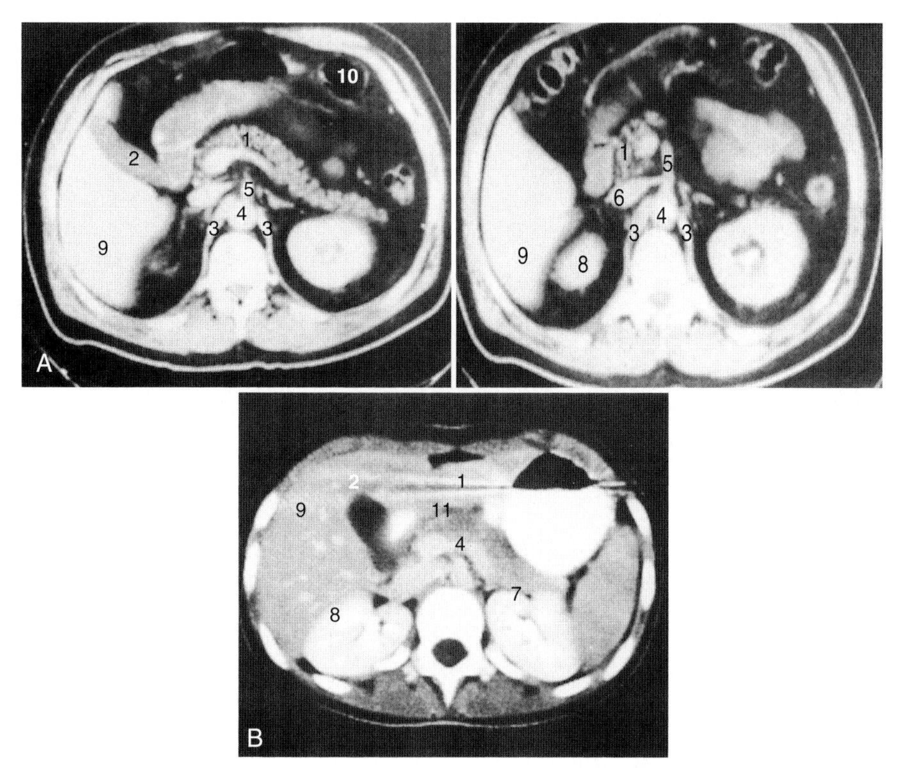

FIGURE 18-13 Normal pancreas in patient with abundant **(A)** and little **(B)** intra-abdominal fat. *1*, Pancreas; *2*, gallbladder; *3*, crus of the diaphragm; *4*, aorta; *5*, superior mesenteric artery; *6*, inferior vena cava with left renal vein; *7*, left kidney; *8*, right kidney; *9*, liver; *10*, bowel; *11*, splenoportal confluence.

Kidneys

Renal ultrasonography and excretory urography (or IV pyelography) traditionally have been the primary means of investigating the kidney, but CT has rapidly gained ground and conventional IV pyelography is now rarely performed. The investigation of renal colic, which was the exclusive domain of the IV pyelogram now is more effectively and rapidly diagnosed with noncontrast CT (Chen and Zagoria, 1999) (Fig. 18-17). CT is more sensitive in detecting stones (Smith et al, 1995), can delineate signs associated with obstruction (Smith et al, 1996), and aids in treatment planning primarily by determining stone size and location (Fielding et al, 1998). Although this study can certainly identify other causes of abdominal pain that may mimic renal colic, it is a limited examination because no

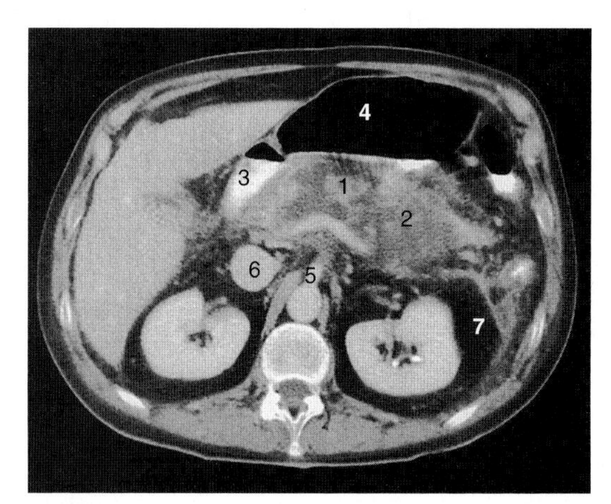

FIGURE 18-14 Acute pancreatitis. Necrotic pancreas *(1)* surrounded by fluid *(2)*, duodenum *(3)*, air-filled stomach *(4)*, superior mesenteric artery *(5)*, inferior vena cava *(6)*, and perirenal fat *(7)*.

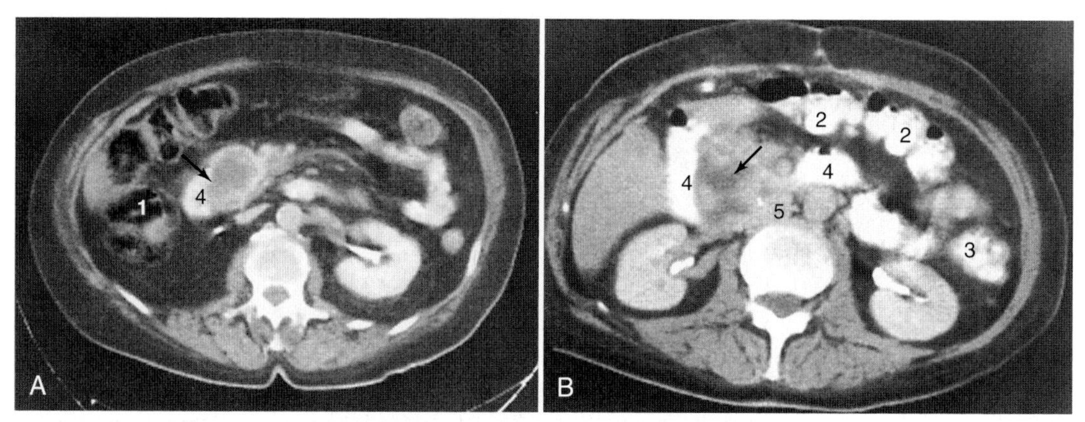

FIGURE 18-15 Enlargement of the head of the pancreas *(arrows)* caused by carcinoma **(A)** and pancreatitis that has occurred as a result of a perforated ulcer **(B)**. *1*, Ascending colon; *2*, transverse colon; *3*, descending colon; *4*, duodenum; *5*, inferior vena cava.

contrast is administered and significant pathological conditions such as renal tumors may be missed. Another concern is the radiation dosage, especially if repeated studies might be needed.

In most cases, ultrasonography can distinguish a cystic from a solid mass. When a solid lesion is identified, CT is useful for preoperative staging (Johnson et al, 1987). It is also useful for detecting local recurrence after a nephrectomy. Bowel loops and displaced normal organs make ultrasonographic evaluation difficult. In patients with polycystic kidneys, the demonstration of cysts with higher attenuation is consistent with a diagnosis of an infected cyst or bleeding into a cyst (Levine and Grantham, 1985). Angiomyolipomas have a characteristic CT appearance demonstrating areas of fatty attenuation (Totty et al, 1981). Occasionally calculi may appear as filling defects in the renal pelvis, mimicking tumors or blood clots on pyelography. In these cases CT may be useful for differentiating a tumor (Fig. 18-18) from a faintly calcified stone, a distinction that may not be evident on plain film (Pollack et al, 1981). CT IV pyelographic examinations that combine two contrast injections with MPRs of the kidneys and collecting system are used to assess patients for unexplained hematuria, which previously required IV or retrograde pyelography studies.

Preoperative assessment of renal donors with 3D CT CTA studies provides the surgeon with a very graphic road map that demonstrates the number and location of renal arteries.

Adrenal Glands

CT has made it possible to delineate healthy adrenal glands easily and reliably, except when the patient is extremely thin (Abrams et al, 1982). If clinical and biochemical evidence of hyperfunction is present, CT usually is the only imaging method necessary. Pheochromocytomas and tumors causing Cushing's and Conn's syndromes that are larger than 5 mm are consistently demonstrated on CT. In adrenal hyperplasia, the adrenals may appear normal in size or may be slightly enlarged. Because small aldosteronomas may be missed on CT, adrenal venous sampling and venography are still important (Geisinger et al, 1983). Adrenal metastases, most commonly seen with bronchogenic and breast carcinomas, are readily demonstrated on CT and can be confirmed by biopsy.

A common clinical problem is the incidentally discovered, nonfunctioning small adrenal mass. These masses most often are nonfunctioning adenomas with a high lipid content. Recent studies have concluded that if the attenuation coefficient of the mass is low (10 or lower) on a noncontrast scan or if there is >50% washout of enhancement on 10-minute delayed scanning compared with an 80-second delayed scan, a confident diagnosis of adenoma can be made (Mayo-Smith et al, 2001) (Fig. 18-19).

Miscellaneous

The other main indications for imaging of the retroperitoneum are detection of lymphomatous or metastatic lymph nodes (Fig. 18-20) and assessment of abdominal aortic aneurysms.

The retroperitoneum often is obscured on a sonogram because of bowel gas, fat, and bony structures. CT therefore is the superior and obvious imaging method of choice. Because the main criterion for abnormality is lymph node enlargement, false-negative CT results may occur when the internal architecture of the lymph node is distorted without any associated enlargement.

Ultrasonography is adequate for sizing and following up on abdominal aortic aneurysms. Preoperative assessment, however, generally requires CT (Siegel et al, 1994) or MRI (Prince et al, 1995) to determine the relationship of the aneurysm to the renal arteries, to precisely size the entire aneurysm, and to assess the iliac arteries, especially if endovascular grafting is considered. CT is also more useful when complications are suspected, such as rupture of an aneurysm (Fig.18-21).

Primary retroperitoneal tumors tend to be large when first suspected clinically. When masses are large enough to be detected on physical examination, an ultrasound examination can differentiate a cystic lesion from a solid one. CT is often performed, however, because it can provide additional information about the extent of disease and the relationship to normal structures.

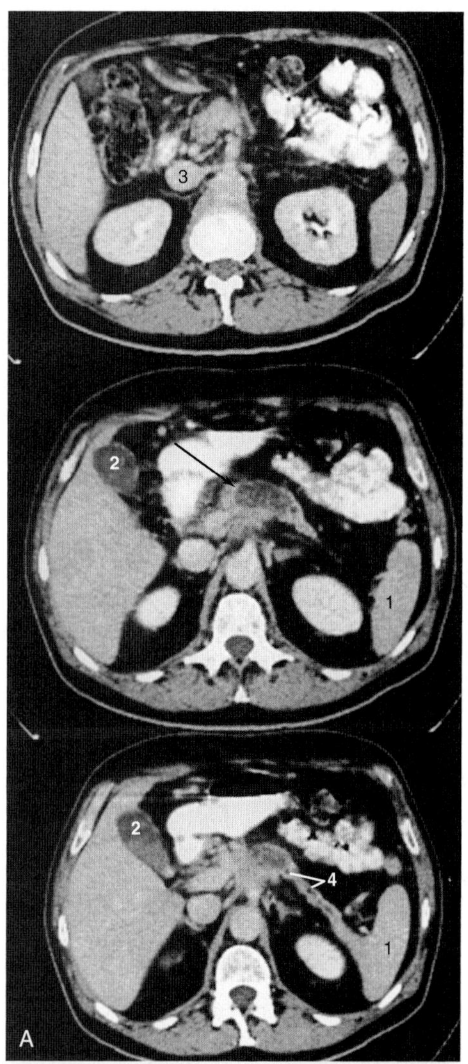

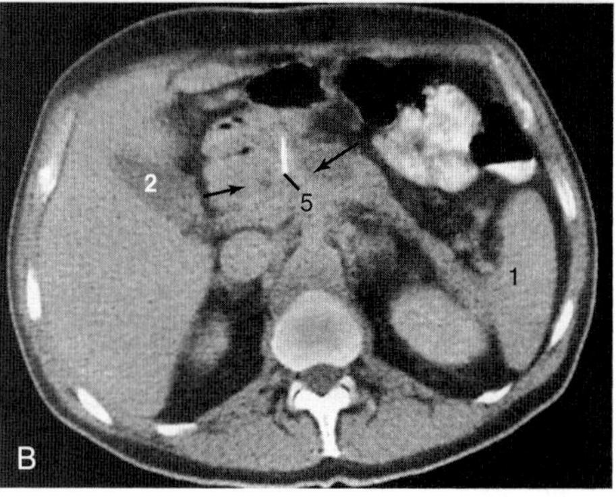

FIGURE 18-16 **A,** Carcinoma of the neck of the pancreas *(arrows)* with associated atrophy and dilation of the pancreatic duct. **B,** Aspiration biopsy of the mass with a 22-gauge needle. *1,* Spleen; *2,* gallbladder; *3,* inferior vena cava with left renal vein; *4,* dilated pancreatic duct with cystic changes; *5,* needle tip.

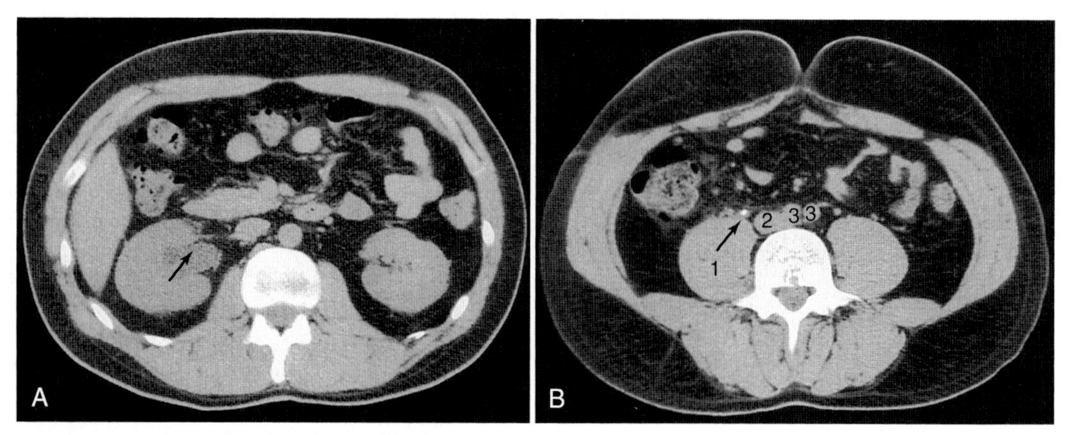

FIGURE 18-17 **A,** Dilated right renal pelvis *(arrow)*. **B,** Calculus *(arrow)* in the right ureter. *1,* Psoas muscle; *2,* inferior vena cava; *3,* iliac arteries.

Pelvis

Ultrasonography remains the primary means of pelvic assessment. The main role of CT in the pelvis, apart from assessment of the bowel and as part of an overall trauma assessment, remains staging the extent of tumor involvement of the bladder (Fig. 18-22), prostate, uterus, and ovaries and documenting any change after treatment. However, MRI, because of its superior soft tissue contrast and multiplanar capability, is assuming a greater role in staging pelvic neoplasms.

Trauma

Trauma is the leading cause of death of individuals less than age 45 years (Novelline et al, 1999). CNS injuries as the cause of death rank the highest, followed by blunt chest trauma and then blunt abdominal trauma. Because of its high sensitivity, specificity, negative predictive value, speed, and ability to provide comprehensive information about not only abdominal injuries but also extra-abdominal injuries such as pelvic, spinal fractures, skull and facial fractures, pulmonary contusions,

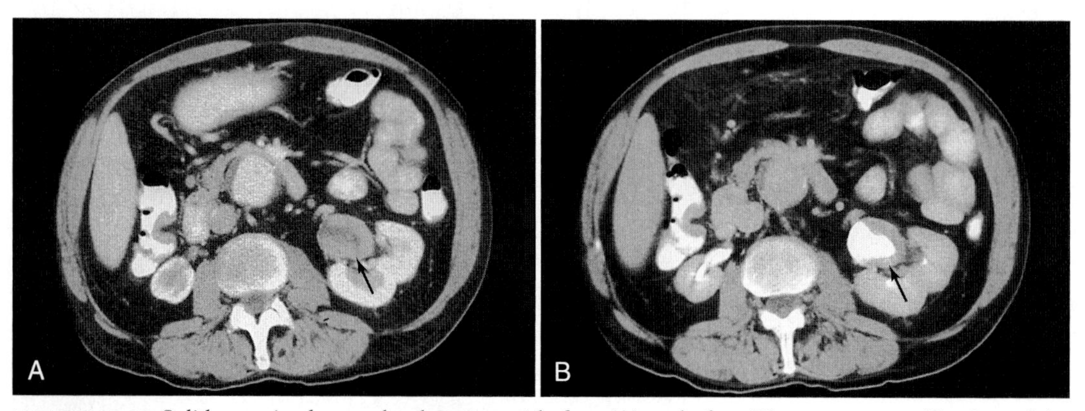

FIGURE 18-18 Solid mass in the renal pelvis *(arrow)* before **(A)** and after **(B)** contrast opacification of the renal pelvis.

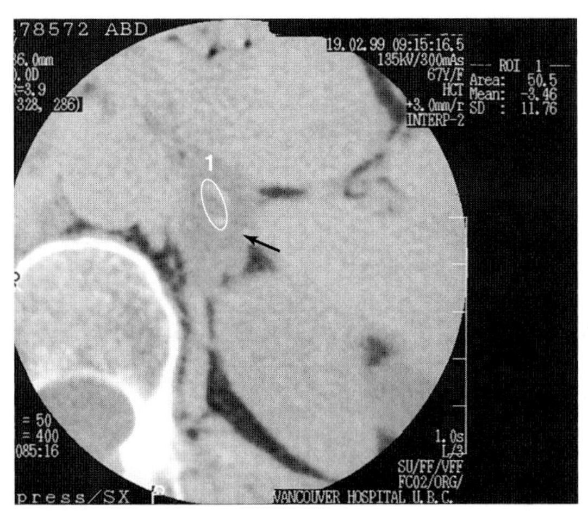

FIGURE 18-19 Region of interest within an adrenal mass *(arrow)* indicating a negative Hounsfield number, confirming the diagnosis of adenoma. *1*, Left kidney; *2*, aorta.

and pneumothorax, CT has become an integral component of the assessment of blunt abdominal and chest trauma, especially in specialized trauma centers (Shuman, 1997). A full-body trauma protocol can be completed in minutes, allowing scanning of all but the most hemodynamically unstable patients, who may require immediate surgery. By acquiring very thin helical axial slices (e.g., 0.5 mm), it is possible to subsequently use this same data to acquire MPR images to specifically

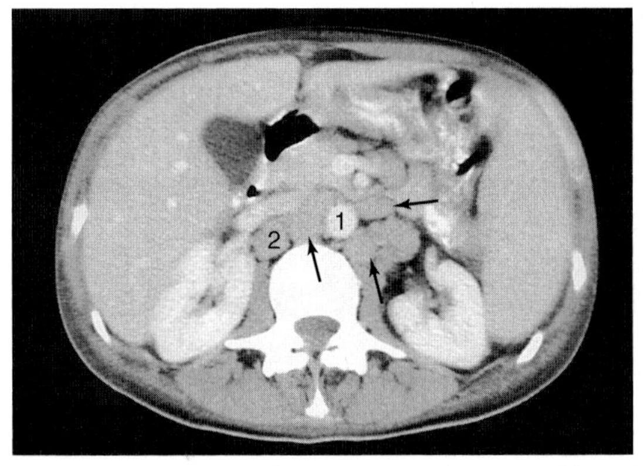

FIGURE 18-20 Enlarged paraaortic and paracaval lymph nodes *(arrows)*. *1*, Aorta; *2*, inferior vena cava.

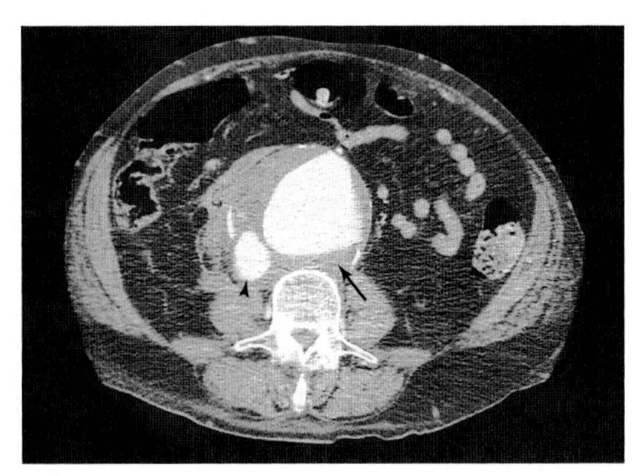

FIGURE 18-21 Large abdominal aortic aneurysm *(arrow)* that has ruptured into the IVC *(arrowhead)*, resulting in abnormally dense contrast within the IVC.

assess the spine or major vascular structures (e.g., aorta). Grading schemes are available to help determine the extent of injury to various organs, which helps determine whether immediate surgery is required or whether conservative management is appropriate. Findings that are worrisome

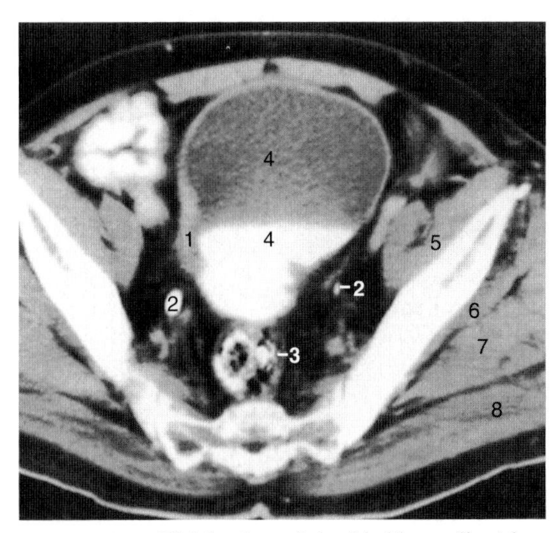

FIGURE 18-22 Thickening of the bladder wall without evidence of extension into the perivesical fat (proven amyloidosis). *1*, Thickened bladder wall; *2*, ureters; *3*, sigmoid colon; *4*, urine and contrast medium in the bladder; *5*, iliac muscle; *6*, gluteus minimus; *7*, gluteus medius; *8*, gluteus maximus.

include evidence of active arterial extravasation, evidence of hypotension such as a collapsed inferior vena cava (IVC) or a small aorta, and the presence of free fluid. Measuring the Hounsfield units (HU) of fluid can be helpful for characterization purposes: extravasated contrast 85 to 350 HU, unclotted blood 25 to 50 HU, clotted blood 40 to 75 HU, and ascites, bile, urine, bowel contents 5 to 10 HU (Rhea, 2004).

CT has largely replaced other imaging methods and considerably reduced the need for exploratory laparotomies. The so-called *FAST ultrasonography* (*f*ocused *a*bdominal *s*onogram in *t*rauma), which is useful in screening for free intraperitoneal fluid, sometimes is performed first to identify patients more likely to have a positive CT result. However, FAST ultrasonography has a limited ability to define the extent and site of injury and cannot assess the retroperitoneal structures thoroughly (Molina et al, 1998).

Vascular System

The use of CT for aortic injury, dissection, coronary arteries, pulmonary arteries, renal arteries, and abdominal aortic aneurysms has already been discussed. CTA has largely replaced standard catheter angiography for the diagnosis of peripheral vascular disease. CTA can provide an angiographic caliber study that includes the entire aorta to the digital arteries in the foot (Fig 18-23). Catheter angiography is now largely reserved for interventional procedures such as angioplasty or stenting.

Interventional Applications

Abscess Drainage

An abscess is a potentially curable condition. Because the morbidity and mortality rates associated with an undrained abscess are high, it is important to

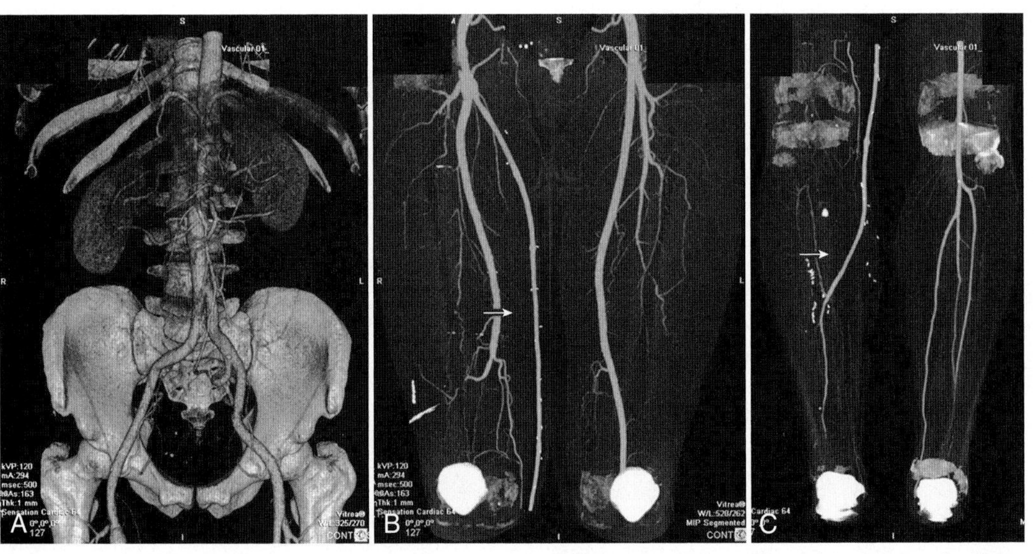

FIGURE 18-23 CT runoff angiogram demonstrating the entire vascular tree from the aorta to the lower calves. 3D reconstruction of the aorta and iliac arteries (**A**). Maximum intensity projection image of the thighs (**B**) demonstrating a femoral graft on the right *(arrow)* replacing the occluded superficial femoral artery. Maximum intensity projection image of the calves (**C**) demonstrating that the graft *(arrow)* has been anastomosed to one of the runoff branches. Most of the bony structures have been segmented and removed. (Images courtesy Dr. Mike Martin, Vancouver Hospital.)

use whatever means are available to localize the abscess accurately, to determine the relationship to adjacent structures, including bowel loops, and to institute prompt treatment through the placement of drainage catheters (Callen, 1979; Gerzof et al, 1981; Halber et al, 1979). The advantage of CT over ultrasonography is that it is not limited by wounds, drains, ostomies, bandages, or bowel gas associated with paralytic ileus, which is common in postoperative patients. Extraluminal gas, although not always present, is the most specific CT sign of an abscess (Fig. 18-24). This may be missed on a sonogram because differentiation from normal bowel gas can be extremely difficult.

Biopsy

Cytological aspiration biopsy and core biopsy have proved to be effective, safe, and simple techniques for establishing a cytological or histological diagnosis for masses anywhere in the body (Ferrucci et al, 1980). The exact location of the needle tip relative to the tumor (see Fig. 18-19, *B*) can be displayed on CT; therefore even small lesions deep in the abdomen can be approached. This capability was enhanced by the introduction of CT fluoroscopy, which allows the radiologist to directly monitor the position of the needle tip by continuous scanning. The biopsy thus can be performed under direct vision rather than using the conventional "blind" approach of advancing the needle and then determining its location. Problems arising from erratic patient breathing are diminished, the procedure time is reduced, and the patient's safety and comfort are improved.

Musculoskeletal System

CT generally is a problem-solving technique. It is often performed after plain films or radionuclide bone scans have already been used. Conventional tomography and arteriography, which formerly were used to determine the extent of disease, are now rarely used. With bony tumors, CT is useful in showing the location of the tumor in the bone, evaluating cortical integrity, articular involvement and intermedullary extent, and defining extraosseous extension (Schreiman et al, 1986). When soft tissues are involved, the relationship of these masses to important neurovascular structures can be determined (Fig. 18-25). However, because of its superior soft tissue contrast resolution (Boyko et al, 1987; Petasnik et al, 1986), MRI has replaced CT for many musculoskeletal applications.

Skeletal trauma generally can be studied by standard radiographs. In complex anatomical regions, however, such as the pelvis, shoulder, foot, and ankle, more precise information about the presence, location, orientation, and relationship of fracture fragments can be obtained with CT (Guyer et al, 1985; Lange and Alter, 1980). In this regard, multiplanar reformations and 3D reconstructions can be extremely useful.

EXAMINATION PREPARATION

Planning

After the radiologist has determined that a CT scan is clinically indicated, the radiologist and technologist must plan the patient preparation, including the potential use of oral or IV contrast media,

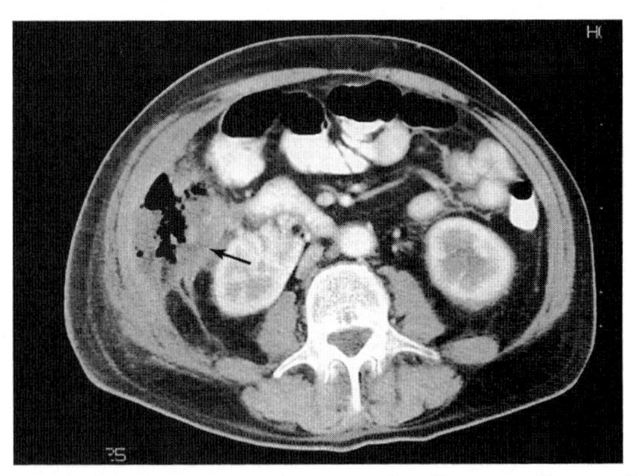

FIGURE 18-24 Abnormal localized collection of gas and fluid *(arrow)* in a right flank abscess that occurred as a result of a ruptured appendix.

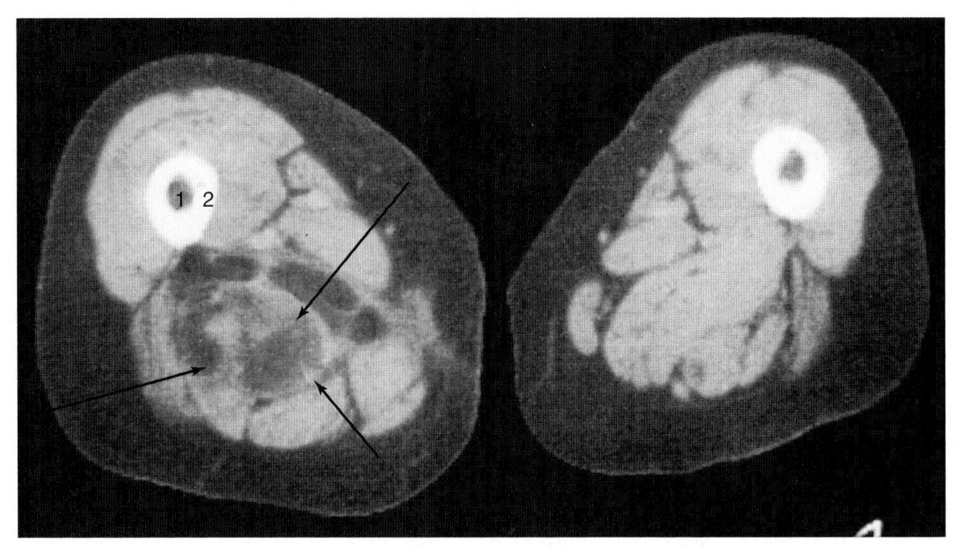

FIGURE 18-25 Liposarcoma *(arrows)* involving the right adductor magnus muscle. *1,* Medullary canal; *2,* cortex.

and the scanning protocol to be used. This can be done verbally or by written instructions. Patients need to be screened for potential contrast allergies and status of renal function. Patients with compromised renal function generally defined as a calculated glomerular filtration rate (GFR) of <60 have a threefold greater risk for development of contrast-induced nephropathy (CIN) compared with healthy individuals (McCullough et al, 1997). Two studies have found that CIN may occur in up to 15% of unselected patients undergoing contrast studies (Iakovou et al, 2003; McCullough et al, 2006). Each site should have in place specific protocols based on the patient's calculated GFR. This may determine whether contrast is administered, which contrast agent is used (i.e., low osmolar or iso-osmolar), whether extra hydration is required, or whether the patient may require N-acetyl cysteine or sodium bicarbonate infusion.

The use of standard protocol sheets may be helpful. When these instructions are different from those routinely followed, it is important for the technologist to discuss the case individually with the radiologist so that the examination can be tailored specifically to the clinical problem. This is even more crucial with helical multislice scanners, which have a myriad of new and very specialized protocols. After reviewing the initial scans, the radiologist may extend, modify, or terminate the examination.

Patient Information

The "high-tech" aspect of CT does not diminish the importance of establishing good rapport with the patient. Patient cooperation can mean the difference between a poor-quality examination and a high-quality result. It is essential that the technologist explain procedures clearly before and during the CT study. The explanations should be brief and given in "lay" terms so that patients know what to expect and what is expected of them. A patient information sheet may be helpful, and pictures of scans may be of interest to the person.

Before the examination, the technologist should:

1. Briefly explain the process of CT.
2. Describe the examination to be performed, including the area of the body to be studied, and give an estimate of the duration of the examination.

3. Emphasize the importance of keeping still because of the image degradation that occurs with motion.
4. Give appropriate breathing instructions.
5. Have the patient empty the bladder immediately before the examination so that the patient is more comfortable and less likely to move, especially if the study involves use of an IV contrast medium.
6. If a contrast medium is to be used, explain the reason for its use and question the patient about allergies. A description of any unpleasant sensations the patient may feel from injection of the contrast material also should be given (this is especially important when mechanical power injectors are used).
7. Reassure the patient that the technologist, although not in the room, will be able to see and talk to the patient.

The patient should always be encouraged to ask questions about the examination. If the questions are more medical in nature, the patient should speak directly with the radiologist. It is important to remember that, although the examination is routine to the staff, it is not for the patient. In addition to being anxious and worried about the results of the examination, patients are fearful and concerned about the examination itself. The staff should try to make the "high-tech" study a "high-touch" experience and constantly be sensitive to the patient's feelings.

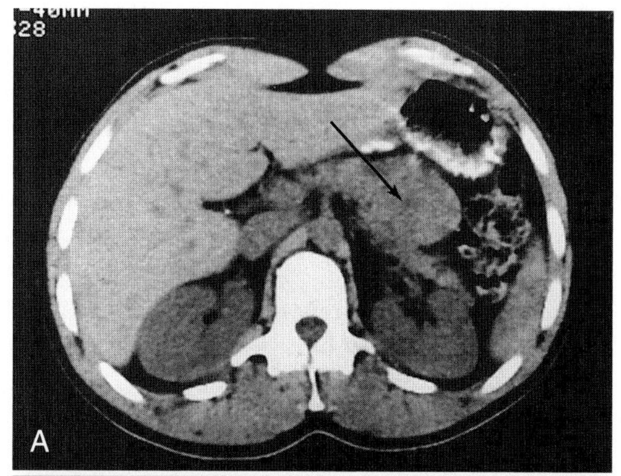

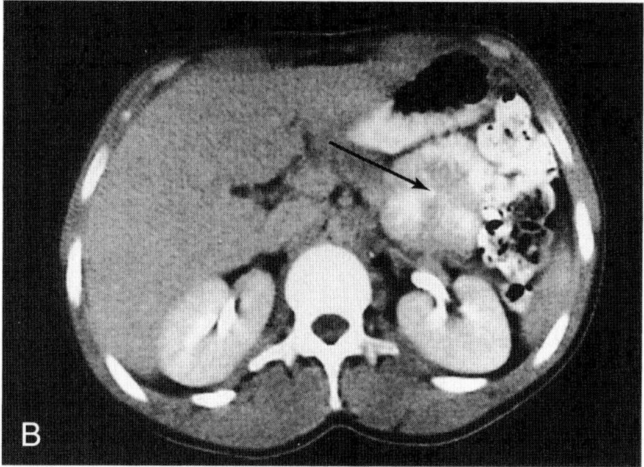

FIGURE 18-26 **A,** An apparent mass of the body of the pancreas *(arrow)*. **B,** When an oral contrast medium is used, the mass is revealed to be multiple small bowel loops *(arrow)*.

Oral Contrast Media

The use of dilute oral contrast material to opacify the entire GI tract has been the typical standard of practice so that homogeneous, fluid-filled bowel loops are not mistaken for masses (Fig. 18-26) or gas-filled loops of bowel for abscesses. Proper opacification of the GI tract can be especially valuable in very thin patients who lack the amount of intra-abdominal fat necessary to outline various structures (see Fig. 18-13, *B*). To simplify the preparation for outpatients by not requiring them to pick up contrast before the scan and because of the improved resolution and multiplanar capabilities of current CT scanners, some radiologists are now satisfied to only administer water as the sole bowel preparation. A typical regimen is 1 liter (L) of water the night before followed by 1.5 L 1 to 2 hours before the scan and 300 to 400 milliliters (ml) immediately before the scan. If positive contrast agents are required, dilute barium sulfate solution (e.g., Readi-Cat 2.0% weight/weight 225 ml mixed with 275 ml of water and ingested the evening before and again 1 hour before the scan) and water-soluble iodinated contrast solutions (e.g., Telebrix 10 ml diluted in 900 ml of water or juice, 400 ml of this mixture ingested 2 hours before, 400 ml 1 hour before, and the remaining 100 ml immediately before the scan) are commonly used. The latter has the advantage of being able to more quickly opacify the entire small and large bowel, and therefore it is especially useful for inpatients who may require somewhat more urgent scanning. Barium sulfate suspension should not be used for patients suspected of having a GI perforation. However, when there is concern about a contrast reaction to iodinated compounds, barium sulfate solution should be used instead. Failure to give the patient the first dose, however, is not a reason to cancel or postpone the procedure; a small-volume contrast enema (150 to 250 ml) can be given to opacify the rectum and distal large bowel. The enema also distends the colon, whereas perioral techniques do not.

For assessment of gastric neoplasms, water alone with or without gas may be given instead of a positive contrast medium to distend the stomach. Some investigators distend the stomach with air or gas alone. An effervescent agent similar to that used in double-contrast upper GI examinations can be administered or a carbonated soft drink can be administered. This method allows good visualization of the gastric wall. If a patient cannot drink the oral contrast medium because of nausea and vomiting, air can be introduced through a nasogastric tube. However, the radiopaque markers used in nasogastric tubes to indicate their position on conventional radiographs can produce artifacts on CT; therefore, these should be removed before the examination, if possible, or at least replaced by ones that are not radiopaque.

If the patient has had a recent barium examination of the GI tract, sufficient time should be allowed for elimination of the contrast medium, or the colon can be cleansed of residual barium. Because residual barium can result in considerable image degradation caused by streak artifacts, the technologist should seek the advice of the radiologist if contrast is detected on the scout scan as the examination may need to be postponed.

CT colonography typically requires the use of purgatives, hydration, and dietary restriction to ensure a clean colon, although some recent studies have shown promising results without a full bowel preparation but instead tagging stool with contrast agents.

Intravenous Contrast Agents

IV contrast material is used for several purposes. The initial vascular opacification may be useful for anatomical localization, distinguishing vessels from a mass, determining the extent of vascular displacement or invasion by a tumor, assessing specific vascular disease such as aneurysms, stenoses, or loss of vascular integrity resulting in extravasation of the contrast medium. The subsequent extravascular distribution of contrast medium into various tissues helps confirm an intact blood supply of body organs and, to a limited extent, provides some functional assessment such as in opacification of the urinary tract. Often tumors and normal parenchyma do not enhance to the same extent or at the same time. This differential enhancement, which increases the attenuation difference between normal and abnormal tissue (Fig. 18-27), can be used to advantage to maximize lesion detectability. However, the timing of the scans and the contrast injection protocols must be chosen carefully because some lesions may be masked by tissue enhancement.

The degree of contrast medium enhancement is the result of a combination of complex factors, including the rate, amount, and concentration of contrast material administered, the speed of injection, the timing of the scans, cardiac output, plasma expansion, extravascular redistribution, and renal filtration and excretion of the contrast material. Various approaches to IV administration of contrast material have been used, reflecting the inadequacies of any one method (Nelson, 1991). Drip infusion of contrast medium usually does not result in ideal enhancement because of inconsistent flow rates, which result in too slow a rise in the plasma iodine concentration. This method has largely been replaced by bolus injections, with some notable exceptions such as routine contrast medium–enhanced head scans and postoperative lumbar spine and cervical spine scans.

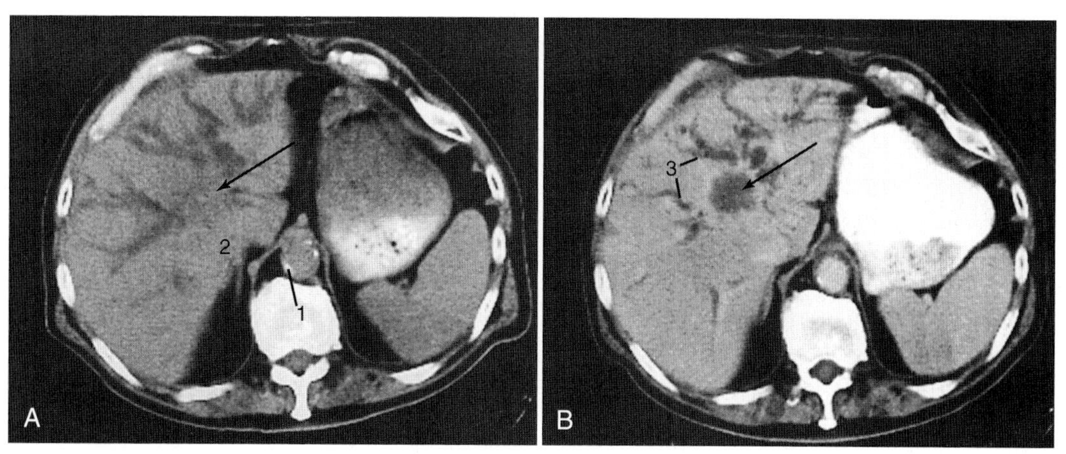

FIGURE 18-27 Cholangiocarcinoma *(arrow)*. **A,** Precontrast scan. **B,** Postcontrast scan. The large mass at the porta hepatis is more evident on the postcontrast scan, which also better differentiates dilated bile ducts from blood vessels. *1,* Aortic calcification; *2,* adrenal gland; *3,* dilated intrahepatic ducts.

A mechanical injector is mandatory for use of injection rates as high as 5 or 6 ml per second and to obtain a sustained, reproducible level of contrast medium enhancement. This usually requires insertion of an 18- or 19-gauge short IV needle catheter into a medially directed antecubital vein connected to tubing capable of withstanding the pressures generated in high-flow injections. It is imperative that any air bubbles in the syringe and tubing be cleared before the final connection is made to the needle to prevent the possibility of a potentially fatal cerebral air embolus. The major disadvantage of a power injector is the slight risk of extravasation of contrast material into the soft tissues. It therefore is imperative that the patient be able to alert the technologist immediately if a local "burning" sensation occurs so that the injection can be stopped, preventing tissue damage. Most often the injector is loaded with 100 to 180 ml of 60% contrast medium, with injection rates varying from 1 to 6 ml per second depending on the specific indication.

Different delay times are used to match scanning with the arrival of contrast medium at the appropriate vessels and organs. These delays can be set empirically on the basis of experience and published data, or they can be tailored individually through the use of bolus tracking or automated techniques such as "SmartPrep" (General Electric) or "SureStart" (Toshiba). With use of helical or spiral volumetric acquisition, a large region (typically 30 centimeters [cm] or more) such as the entire liver can be easily examined in several seconds. The latest generation of scanners, with subsecond and multislice technology, enhances this capability (Berland and Smith, 1998) further by allowing even greater ranges or thinner collimation or both.

With a single bolus injection of contrast medium, the pattern of vascular enhancement during the first circulation and the pattern of vascular and tissue enhancement during recirculation can be studied. This method is useful for studying aortic dissection, in which flow in the false lumen is often delayed, and for evaluation of a possible hemangioma (see Fig. 18-8). In these a specific area may be examined dynamically and repeatedly over a period of time without table movement.

Other, more specialized techniques include selective catheterization and injection of specific vessels followed by CT scanning such as the proper hepatic artery for CT hepatic arteriography and the superior mesenteric artery or splenic artery for CT arterial portography (Nelson, 1991). These studies are reported to be more sensitive for detecting small liver lesions (less than 2 cm) than either MRI or biphasic CT (Hori et al, 1998).

SCANNING PROTOCOLS

Developing routine protocols is helpful. These protocols serve as general guidelines and can be modified as required, tailoring the examination to a particular patient's clinical problem. In addition to the details specific to a region, scanning protocols should optimize the radiographic technique to maximize lesion detection. This requires careful consideration in choosing the appropriate kilovoltage (kV), milliamperage (mA), collimation, reconstruction interval, pitch, range, field of view (FOV), reconstruction matrix, field size, reconstruction algorithm, postprocessing filters, and window widths and levels.

Scanning protocols can vary significantly from site to site, primarily on the basis of the type of scanner that is being used and to some extent on the preference of the radiologists. The following protocols deal exclusively with helical (spiral) multislice scanners. Even among multislice scanners significant variations exist between 4-, 8-, 16-, 32-, and 64-slice scanners. Many centers with multislice scanners, especially 16 slice or greater, will use the narrowest detector collimation possible (typically 0.5 to 0.75 mm) to obtain a volume data set. These initial scans are used to obtain near isotropic voxels that enable excellent quality MPRs and 3D images. According to study requirements and department preferences, scans of varying thickness and in the axial, sagittal, or coronal planes may be reconstructed for diagnosis and documentation. Typically these will consist of contiguous or overlapping 2- to 5-mm thick images that are reconstructed from the initial volume data set.

Thorax

In most thoracic examinations, scanning begins superiorly from the level of the clavicles and extends to the posterior costophrenic angle. When a neoplasm is suspected, the scans should include the liver and adrenal glands. Because detection of liver metastases is maximized when scans are obtained immediately after administration of a contrast medium, it may be more appropriate to scan in a caudocranial direction through the liver and adrenal glands first and then superiorly through the remainder of the chest, where a high plasma iodine concentration is not as critical (Foley, 1989b). This is not necessary with current multislice scanners.

Scans are typically obtained in full inspiration during a single breath-hold therefore misregistration artifacts are no longer a problem (Costello et al, 1991). When the posterior lung base is the region of primary concern, prone scans may be helpful to increase aeration to this area. Lateral decubitus scans also are helpful in rare instances in distinguishing between complex pleural and pulmonary pathological conditions, such as differentiating an empyema from a large lung abscess.

Thoracic CT scans should be viewed with at least two different window width settings (Fig. 18-28). One of these should be optimized for the mediastinum and chest wall and the other for the lungs. If necessary, an additional setting for the bones should be used. The use of higher frequency filters for the lung parenchyma is helpful.

Scans of the chest are generally obtained with the patient supine and the arms elevated. The arms should not be so high as to obstruct the flow of IV contrast material. Therefore some radiologists prefer to leave the arm with the IV line by the patient's side, especially for high flow rate examinations, even though some artifacts will result.

Some radiologists believe that an IV contrast medium need not be used routinely because the anatomy of the mediastinal structures is not complicated and they are generally well delineated by the mediastinal fat. Contrast medium is useful, however, for better defining the mediastinum, for determining the relationship of the mass to the mediastinal vessels, or for checking for vascular abnormalities.

CT examination of the thorax usually begins with a digital localizing radiograph (e.g., scout

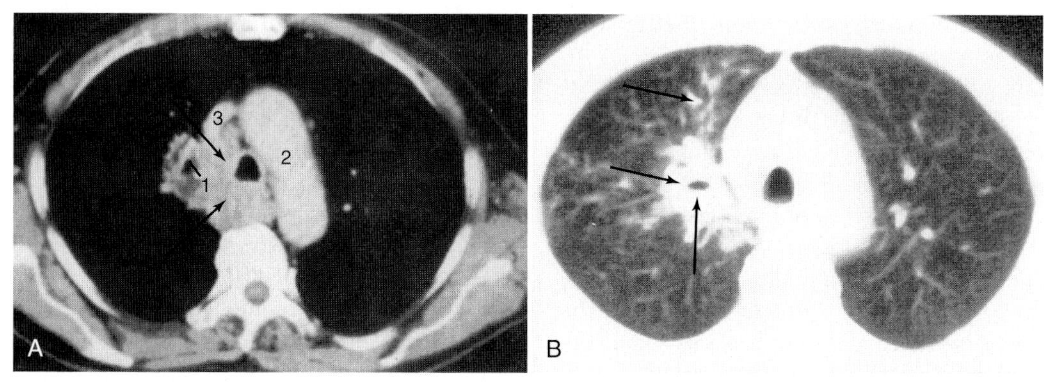

FIGURE 18-28 Bronchogenic carcinoma *(arrows)* involving the right hilum with mediastinal invasion and distal obstructive pneumonitis in the right upper lobe. **A,** Mediastinal window. **B,** Lung window. *1,* Right superior segmental bronchus of the right upper lobe; *2,* aortic arch; *3,* superior vena cava.

view, topogram, or scanogram), typically in the anteroposterior projection. Scan levels can be prescribed from this image, and the scans obtained can be displayed on it. This can be helpful in correlating the CT images with a plain film abnormality and may be of some value in planning radiation therapy and guiding biopsy. Thicker slices (2.5 to 7 mm) obtained at 1.25- to 5-mm slice intervals are routinely used. Thinner sections of 1 to 2 mm may be used to improve spatial resolution, particularly in assessing the hila, fissures, and airways. When HRCT is used for assessing diffuse lung disease, 1- to 2-mm thick sections are used, often with a smaller FOV with target reconstruction and a high spatial frequency algorithm to improve spatial resolution (Mayo, 1991) (see Fig. 18-6).

Before the current generation of multidetector scanners, it was impractical to examine the entire chest by using contiguous thin slices. The examination therefore was tailored to the particular clinical indication. For the assessment of bronchiectasis and diffuse infiltrative lung disease, 1- to 2-mm thick sections obtained at 10-mm intervals was used most often. In assessing asbestos-related disease, a more limited examination consisting of five to eight scans spaced throughout the middle and lower thorax usually was sufficient. With multidetector scanners it is now feasible to examine the entire chest with contiguous thin slices, the main consideration being to balance benefit with risk with respect to radiation exposure, especially with repeated examinations. Because of the high intrinsic contrast, HRCT can be performed by using lower radiation (low mAs) techniques. Occasionally, selected scans obtained in expiration may be useful for determining the presence or extent of air trapping.

Abdomen and Pelvis

Scans are most commonly obtained with the patient supine. Scanning in the prone position may be useful for biopsy of posterior structures, such as the adrenal glands or retroperitoneal lymph nodes. CT kidneys-ureter-bladder (KUB) studies for renal colic are also typically performed in the prone position because bladder stones that are not impacted at the ureterovesical junction will be located in the dependent portion of the bladder.

All abdominal and pelvic scans are acquired helically using the narrowest detector collimation available. A general survey type examination generally consists of axial images reconstructed as 5-mm contiguous or overlapping slices. Adrenal and pancreatic studies are reconstructed at 2- to 3-mm thickness and generally with some overlap. Newer multislice scanners permit extended coverage and reduce scan times to 5 to 10 seconds for an average abdominal examination. Helical data acquisition using detector collimation of 0.5 to 0.75 mm allows retrospective reconstruction of varying slice thickness at closer intervals, including overlapping slices, if the raw data are saved. This provides tremendous flexibility in protocols, largely solves problems of volume averaging and provides excellent multiplanar reformations.

Images obtained without the use of a contrast medium usually are of limited value with the following exceptions: identification and characterization of calcific masses or renal calculi or to localize a hepatic lesion before rapid, contrast medium–enhanced, dynamic scans are obtained at the same level without table movement.

IV contrast medium generally is essential, particularly for evaluating the liver and pancreas. Several factors are important in the detection and differential diagnosis of liver lesions, including (1) the liver has a dual blood supply, from the hepatic artery and the portal vein; (2) arterial inflow occurs earlier than portal inflow; and (3) most neoplasms receive their blood primarily from the hepatic artery, whereas normal hepatocytes primarily receive their blood from the portal vein.

The early "arterial phase" scans with typical scan delays of 20 to 30 seconds best visualize highly vascular lesions, both benign and malignant, such as focal nodular hyperplasia, hepatic adenoma, hepatocellular carcinoma, and hypervascular metastases such as from the kidney, breast, and islet cell tumors (Fig. 18-29). The later "venous phase" scans with scan delays of 70 to 80 seconds are best suited for studying hypovascular lesions such as colon metastases that, lacking a portal venous supply, enhance much less than normal hepatocytes (Baron, 1994). The trend therefore is to perform these so-called *biphasic examinations* for many hepatic studies. In some cases delayed scans (e.g., 10 minutes) may be helpful in studying cholangiocarcinoma, which may show delayed enhancement and hemangioma by demonstrating contrast "filling in."

A biphasic protocol for pancreatic scans is also useful. The earlier arterial phase with injection of 100 to 120 ml of contrast medium at a rate of 4 to 5 ml per second, reconstructing thin (2.5 to 3 mm) overlapping images (every 1.5 to 2.5 mm) and a scan delay set to the time of aortic peak plus 5 seconds, optimally enhances the arteries and pancreatic parenchyma, allowing visualization of small hypodense or hyperdense masses (islet cell tumors) and demonstrating any vascular invasion (Hollett et al, 1995). The later venous phase with a scan delay of 70 seconds and 2.5- to 5-mm overlapping reconstructed images through the liver and pancreas delineates the peripancreatic veins, further helping to stage a pancreatic carcinoma. This phase is also best for detecting hepatic metastases from non-islet-cell tumors, which tend to be hypovascular.

Renal CT typically is performed to further characterize a renal mass or to stage a tumor. This is best done with a three-phase study: examination of the kidneys without a contrast medium (0.5-0.75 mm detector collimation, 2.5- to 5-mm slice thickness, 1.25- to 2.5-mm slice intervals) followed by examination after administration of the contrast medium (100 to 120 ml at 3.5 to 4 ml per second) with an early study in the corticomedullary phase (minimum 70-second delay) and by a later scan (3- to 5-minute delay) in the nephrographic or pyelographic phase (Fig. 18-30). The unenhanced scan is useful for detecting stones and fatty tumors (e.g., angiomyolipomas) and for establishing a baseline for determining whether a mass is enhancing. Performing two studies after administration of the contrast medium improves the detection of masses and provides better characterization and more accurate staging (Kopka et al, 1997).

The protocol for the so-called CT KUB is designed specifically to identify renal and ureteral calculi, typically in the acute phase. Neither oral nor IV contrast material is administered. The range scanned extends from the top of the kidneys to the symphysis pubis. Our preferred protocol is to use 0.6-mm detector collimation with 5-mm thick slices reconstructed every 2.5 mm. The images are transferred to a workstation to be reviewed in cine or movie mode to facilitate interpretation. Only

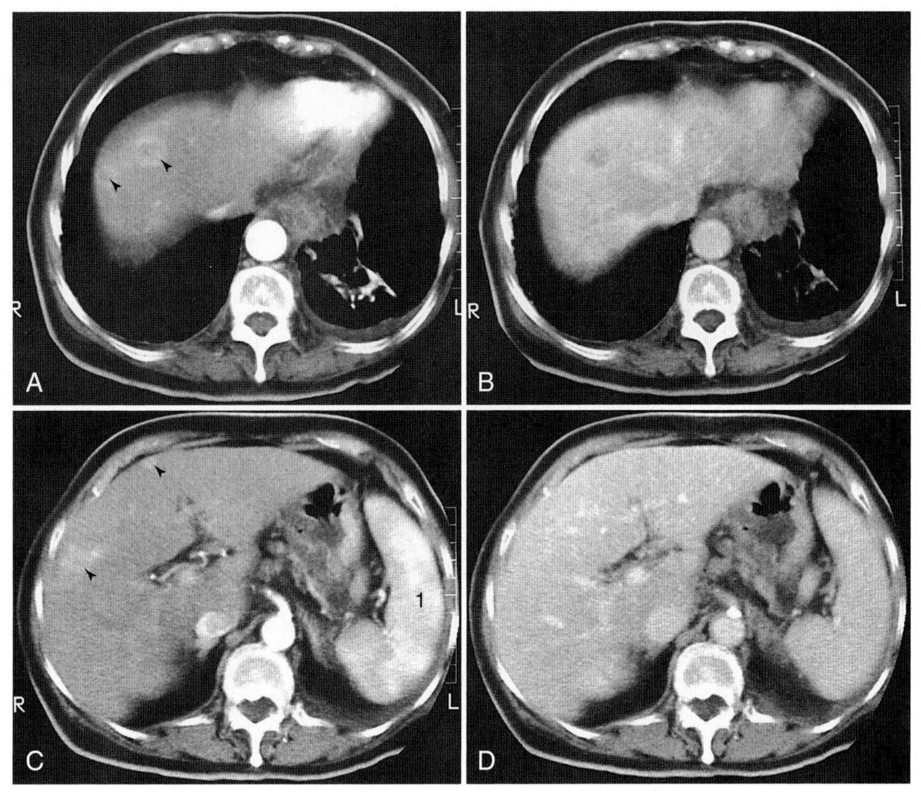

FIGURE 18-29 **A** and **C,** Scans obtained within 2 minutes of administration of a contrast medium reveal four hypervascular lesions. **B** and **D,** In "early delayed" scans (i.e., scans obtained approximately 5 minutes after injection of the contrast medium), two of the lesions have "disappeared" and two others are much less conspicuous. *1,* Normal inhomogeneous appearance of the spleen during early enhancement by the contrast medium.

every third image is filmed. The radiation dosage can be significantly diminished by lowering the mA to 80 to 120 because more noisy images are adequate for the purposes of this examination.

For "routine" abdominal scans with less specific indications, an adequate protocol generally is 2.5- to 5-mm thick scans, administration of 100 to 120 ml of contrast medium at a rate of 2.5 ml per second, and a scan delay of 70 seconds.

The use of oral contrast medium has already been emphasized. When the pelvis is examined, use of a tampon is an easy means of anatomical localization of the vagina.

Musculoskeletal System

Because the anatomy of the musculoskeletal system varies from one region to another, the technique used for each patient should be tailored to the clinical problem. A computed radiograph is helpful for visualizing any bony abnormalities to determine the number, location, and range of images needed and to correlate with plain films.

Precise positioning is important. Whenever possible, the normal extremity should also be examined. The two sides should be symmetrically positioned and displayed to facilitate side-to-side

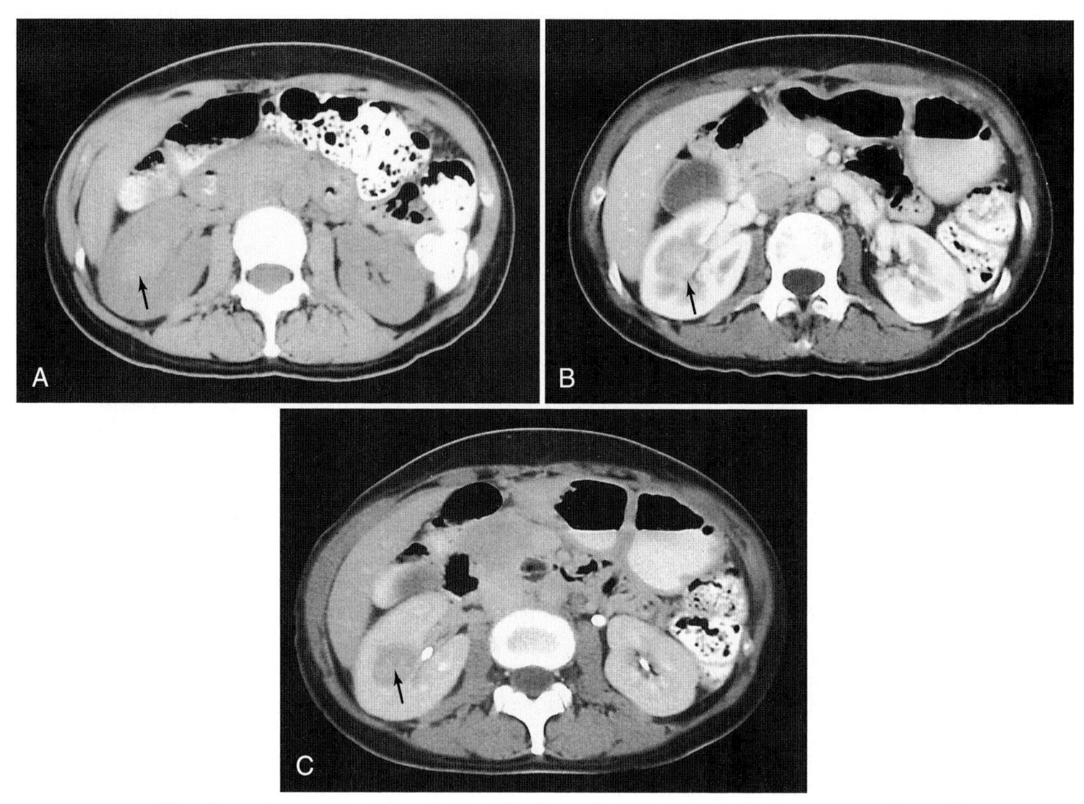

FIGURE 18-30 Renal carcinoma. **A,** Scan obtained before administration of a contrast medium demonstrates a mass of higher density *(arrow)* than renal parenchyma. This is atypical because most renal carcinomas are isodense or hypodense on studies done without use of a contrast medium; the higher density likely indicates recent hemorrhage. **B,** A corticomedullary phase scan demonstrates that the mass *(arrow)* is enhancing, but less than normal renal cortex. **C,** A nephrographic phase scan demonstrates the mass *(arrow)* with greater conspicuity because of the now homogeneous enhancement of the cortex and medulla. Contrast medium is also seen within the collecting system.

comparison. Slice thickness and interval are determined by the clinical problem. For assessing most tumors and masses, 2.5- to 5-mm slices are adequate. Smaller lesions require 1- to 3-mm slices, and examination of smaller structures such as the ankle and wrist often requires 0.5- to 1-mm slices.

Once the images have been obtained, they should always be displayed and viewed at two window settings, soft tissue and bone settings. In some cases reconstruction of the images with higher resolution algorithms and higher spatial frequency filters may be necessary to improve bony detail. Multiplanar and 3D reconstructions can be helpful with complicated anatomy, particularly in the evaluation of fractures.

When tumors and their relationship to neurovascular structures are assessed, bolus injection of IV contrast material is required. Intra-articular injection of a contrast medium or air can be useful when joints are being evaluated, but these arthrographic examinations are now more often performed as MRI studies.

REFERENCES

Abrams HI et al: Computed tomography versus ultrasound of the adrenal gland: a prospective study, *Radiology* 143:121-128, 1982.

Alpern MB et al: Focal hepatic masses and fatty infiltration detected by enhanced dynamic CT, *Radiology* 158:45-49, 1986.

Ambrosetti P et al: Computed tomography in acute left colonic diverticulitis, *Br J Surg* 84:532-534, 1997.

Balthazar EJ: CT of small bowel obstruction, *AJR Am J Roentgenol* 162:255-261, 1994.

Baron RL et al: A prospective comparison of the evaluation of biliary obstruction using computed tomography and ultrasonography, *Radiology* 145:91-98, 1982.

Baron RL: Understanding and optimizing use of contrast material for CT of the liver, *AJR Am J Roentgenol* 163:323-331, 1994.

Berland LL, Smith JK: Multidetector-array CT: once again, technology creates new opportunities, *Radiology* 209:327-329, 1998.

Berry J Jr, Malt RA: Appendicitis near its centenary, *Ann Surg* 200:567-575, 1984.

Boyko OB et al: MR imaging of osteogenic and Ewing's sarcoma, *AJR Am J Roentgenol* 148: 317-322, 1987.

Callen PW: Computed tomographic evaluation of abdominal and pelvic abscesses, *Radiology* 131: 171-175, 1979.

Castellino RA et al: Computed tomography, lymphography and staging laparotomy: correlations in initial staging of Hodgkin's disease, *AJR Am J Roentgenol* 143:37-41, 1984.

Chen MY, Zagoria RJ: Can noncontrast helical computed tomography replace intravenous urography for evaluation of patients with acute urinary tract colic? *J Emerg Med* 17:299-303, 1999.

Costello P et al: Pulmonary nodule: evaluation with spiral volumetric CT, *Radiology* 179:875-876, 1991.

Davies J et al: Spiral computed tomography and operative staging of gastric carcinoma: a comparison with histopathological staging, *Gut* 41:314-319, 1997.

Fenlon HM et al: A comparison of virtual and conventional colonoscopy for the detection of colorectal polyps, *N Engl J Med* 341:1496-1503, 1999.

Ferrucci JT Jr et al: Diagnosis of abdominal malignancy by radiologic fine needle biopsy, *AJR Am J Roentgenol* 134:323-330, 1980.

Fielding JR et al: Unenhanced helical CT of ureteral stones: a replacement for excretory urography in planning treatment, *AJR Am J Roentgenol* 171: 1051-1053, 1998.

Foley WD: Dynamic hepatic CT, *Radiology* 170: 617-622, 1989b.

Fon GT et al: Computed tomography of the anterior mediastinum in myasthenia gravis, *Radiology* 142:135-141, 1982.

Forster BB, Isserow S: Coronary artery calcification and subclinical athersclerosis: what's the score?, *BCMJ Br Columbia Med Assoc Journal* 47:181-187, 2005.

Freeny PC, Marks WM: Hepatic hemangioma: dynamic bolus CT, *AJR Am J Roentgenol* 147: 711-719, 1986.

Gamsu G: The mediastinum. In Moss AA et al, editors: *Computed tomography of the upper body with magnetic resonance imaging*, ed 2, Philadelphia, 1992, WB Saunders.

Geisinger MA et al: Primary hyperaldosteronism: comparison of CT, adrenal venography, and venous sampling, *AJR Am J Roentgenol* 141:299-302, 1983.

Gerzof SG et al: Percutaneous abscess drainage, *Semin Roentgenol* 16:62-71, 1981.

Goldman IS et al: Increased hepatic density and phospholipidosis due to amiodarone, *AJR Am J Roentgenol* 144:541-546, 1985.

Gore RM et al: CT features of ulcerative colitis and Crohn's disease, *AJR Am J Roentgenol* 167:3-15, 1996.

Guyer BH et al: Computed tomography of calcaneal fractures: anatomy, pathology, dosimetry, and clinical relevance, *AJR Am J Roentgenol* 145:911-919, 1985.

Halber MD et al: Intraabdominal abscess: current concepts in radiologic evaluation, *AJR Am J Roentgenol* 133:9-13, 1979.

Hara AK et al: Detection of colorectal polyps with CT colography: initial assessment of sensitivity and specificity, *Radiology* 205:59-65, 1997.

Hessel SJ et al: A prospective evaluation of computed tomography and ultrasound of the pancreas, *Radiology* 143:129-133, 1982.

Hollett M et al: Quantitative evaluation of pancreatic enhancement during dual-phase helical CT, *Radiology* 195:359-361, 1995.

Hori M et al: Sensitivity in detection of hypervascular hepatocellular carcinoma by helical CT with intra-arterial injection of contrast medium and by helical CT and MR imaging with intravenous injection of contrast medium, *Acta Radiol* 39:144-151, 1998.

Iakovou I et al: Impact of gender on the incidence and outcome of contrast-induced nephropathy after percutaneous coronary intervention, *J Invasive Cardiol* 15:18-22, 2003.

Johnson CD et al: Renal adenocarcinoma: CT staging of 100 tumors, *AJR Am J Roentgenol* 148:59-63, 1987.

Kopka L et al: Dual-phase helical CT of the kidney: value of the corticomedullary and nephrographic phase for evaluation of renal lesions and preoperative staging of renal cell carcinoma, *AJR Am J Roentgenol* 169:1573-1578, 1997.

Lane MJ et al: Unenhanced helical CT for suspected acute appendicitis, *AJR Am J Roentgenol* 168: 405-409, 1997.

Lange TA, Alter AJ: Evaluation of complex acetabular fractures by computed tomography, *J CAT* 6: 849-852, 1980.

Leschka S et al: Accuracy of MSCT coronary angiography with 64-slice technology: first experience, *Eur Heart J* 10:1093-1100, 2005.

Levine E, Grantham JJ: High-density renal cysts in autosomal dominant polycystic kidney disease demonstrated by CT, *Radiology* 154:477-482, 1985.

Manfredi R et al: Accuracy of computed tomography and magnetic resonance imaging in staging bronchogenic carcinoma, *MAGMA* 4:257-262, 1996.

Mayo JR: The high-resolution computed tomography technique, *Semin Roentgenol* 26:104-109, 1991.

Mayo JR et al: Pulmonary embolism: prospective comparison of spiral CT with ventilation-perfusion scintigraphy, *Radiology* 205:447-452, 1997.

Mayo-Smith WW et al: State-of-the-art adrenal imaging, *Radiographics* 21:995-1012, 2001.

McCullough PA et al: Acute renal failure after coronary intervention: incidence, risk factors, and relationship to mortality, *Am J Med* 103:368-375, 1997.

McCullough PA et al: Risk prediction of contrast-induced nephropathy, *Am J Cardiol* 98:5K-13K, 2006.

Molina PL et al: Computed tomography of thoracoabdominal trauma. In Lee JKT et al, eds: *Computed body tomography with MRI correlation*, ed 3, New York, 1998, Raven Press.

Mucha P Jr: Small intestinal obstruction, *Surg Clin North Am* 67:597-620, 1987.

Muhm JR et al: Comparison of whole lung tomography and computed tomography for detecting pulmonary nodules, *AJR Am J Roentgenol* 131:981-984, 1978.

Muller NL: Differential diagnosis of chronic diffuse infiltrative lung disease on high-resolution computed tomography, *Semin Roentgenol* 26:132-142, 1991.

Munk PL et al: Pulmonary lymphangitic carcinomatosis: CT and pathologic findings, *Radiology* 166: 705-709, 1988.

Nelson RC: Techniques for computed tomography of the liver, *Radiol Clin North Am* 29:1199-1212, 1991.

Novelline RA et al: Helical CT of abdominal trauma, *Radiol Clin North Am* 37:591-612, 1999.

Pang JA et al: Value of computed tomography in the diagnosis and management of bronchiectasis, *Clin Radiol* 40:40-44, 1989.

Petasnick JT et al: Soft tissue masses of the locomotor system: comparison of MR imaging with CT, *Radiology* 160:125-133, 1986.

Pickhardt PJ et al: Computed tomographic virtual colonoscopy to screen for colorectal neoplasia in asymptomatic adults, *N Engl J Med* 349:2191-2200, 2003.

Pollack HM et al: Computed tomography of renal pelvic filling defects, *Radiology* 138:645-651, 1981.

Posniak HV et al: Computed tomography of the normal aorta and thoracic aneurysms, *Semin Roentgenol* 24: 7-21, 1989.

Prince MR et al: Breath-hold gadolinium-enhanced MR angiography of the abdominal aorta and its major branches, *Radiology* 197:785-792, 1995.

Raff GL et al: Diagnostic accuracy of noninvasive coronary angiography using 64-slice spiral computed tomography, *J Am Coll Cardiol* 46:552-557, 2005.

Rhea JT: CT of abdominal trauma: part 1. In *RSNA categorical course in diagnostic radiology: emergency radiology*, Oak Brook, Ill, 2004, Radiological Society of North America, pp 91-99.

Rossi P et al: CT of functioning tumours of the pancreas, *AJR Am J Roentgenol* 144:57-60, 1985.

Schaner EG et al: Comparison of computed and conventional whole lung tomography in detecting pulmonary nodules: prospective radiologic-pathologic study, *AJR Am J Roentgenol* 131:51-54, 1978.

Schreiman JS et al: Osteosarcoma: role of CT in limb-sparing treatment, *Radiology* 161:485-488, 1986.

Shanmuganathan K: CT of abdominal trauma: part II. In *RSNA categorical course in diagnostic radiology: emergency radiology*, Oak Brook, Ill, 2004, Radiological Society of North America, pp 101-112.

Shuman WP: CT of blunt abdominal trauma in adults, *Radiology* 205:297-306, 1997.

Siegel CL, Cohan RH: CT of abdominal aortic aneurysms, *AJR Am J Roentgenol* 163:17-29, 1994.

Siegelman SS et al: CT of fluid collections associated with pancreatitis, *AJR Am J Roentgenol* 134: 1121-1132, 1980.

Smith RC et al: Acute flank pain: comparison of non-contrast-enhanced CT and intravenous urography, *Radiology* 194:789-794, 1995.

Smith RC et al: Acute ureteral obstruction: value of secondary signs on helical unenhanced CT, *AJR Am J Roentgenol* 167:1109-1113, 1996.

Sommer T et al: Aortic dissection: a comparative study of diagnosis with spiral CT, multiplanar transesophageal echocardiography, and MR imaging, *Radiology* 199:347-352, 1996.

Stein PD et al: Untreated patients with pulmonary embolism, *Chest* 107:931-935, 1995.

Sundaram M et al: Utility of CT-guided abdominal aspiration procedures, *AJR Am J Roentgenol* 139: 1111-1115, 1982.

Swensen SJ et al: Lung nodule enhancement at CT: prospective findings, *Radiology* 201:447-455, 1996.

Swensen SJ et al: Screening for lung cancer with low-dose spiral computed tomography, *Am J Respir Crit Care Med* 165:508-513, 2002.

Tateishu U et al: Chest wall tumors: radiologic findings and pathologic correlation, 2: malignant tumors, *Radiographics* 23:1491-1508, 2003.

Totty WG et al: Relative value of computed tomography and ultrasonography in the assessment of renal angiomyolipoma, *J CAT* 5:173-178, 1981.

Weg N et al: Liver lesions: improved detection with dual-detector-array CT and routine 2.5-mm thin collimation, *Radiology* 209:417-426, 1998.

Zerhouni EA et al: CT of the pulmonary nodule: a cooperative study, *Radiology* 160:319-327, 1986.

The authors would like to thank Marilyn Stuart and Mary Jane Li for their help in typing and preparing the manuscript. They also would like to thank the CT technologists who helped acquire the CT scans and Dean Malpass and Rhonda Lancaster for manuscript assistance.

Pediatric Computed Tomography

Son Nguyen* and Scott Lipson

Chapter Outline

*This chapter was originally written by Victoria Bigland, RTR; Gordon Culham, MD, FRCPC; and Kenneth Poskitt, MDCM, of the British Columbia Children's Hospital, Department of Radiology. It was revised for the second edition by Jeremy Lysne, RT(R)(CT), Department of Radiology, Denver Children's Hospital, and for the third edition by Dr. Scott Lipson, MD, Department of Radiology, Long Beach Memorial Medical Center, and Dr. Son Nguyen, MD, Department of Radiology, Miller Children's Hospital, Long Beach Memorial Medical Center.

The objective of the pediatric computed tomography (CT) examination is to acquire optimum diagnostic images with the minimum discomfort and radiation exposure to the patient. To this end, two basic tenets apply: (1) the technologist should be knowledgeable and well prepared and (2) the technologist should be honest and upfront with the patient and family. A well-prepared technologist plays an important role in avoiding delays and helps reduce the time the patient must be on the table of the CT scanner.

The CT technologist taking care of children should be honest in terms of the exact details of the CT examination. This helps ensure the cooperation of young patients and their parents during the procedure. The results can be successful, especially when the patient and parents are well informed. In most institutions, parents are encouraged to remain in the CT room during the examination.

In addition, a relaxed, nonthreatening environment helps gain the confidence and cooperation of the pediatric patient. Toys, books, and puzzles are a welcome diversion for the child who is waiting for a CT examination. In the CT room, interesting posters (Fig. 19-1) or pictures hung on the walls or ceiling help provide a friendly atmosphere. Young children are encouraged to bring a favorite blanket or cuddly toy with them for reassurance.

Fortunately, the current generation of multidetector CT (MDCT) scanners has made the CT examination much shorter and better tolerated by children. A trained CT technologist enlisting the cooperation of the parents is now able to scan the majority of children quickly, painlessly, and without sedating them.

MULTIDETECTOR CT

Differences Versus Single-Detector CT

MDCT is fundamentally different from single-slice spiral CT (SSCT). With SSCT a single detector

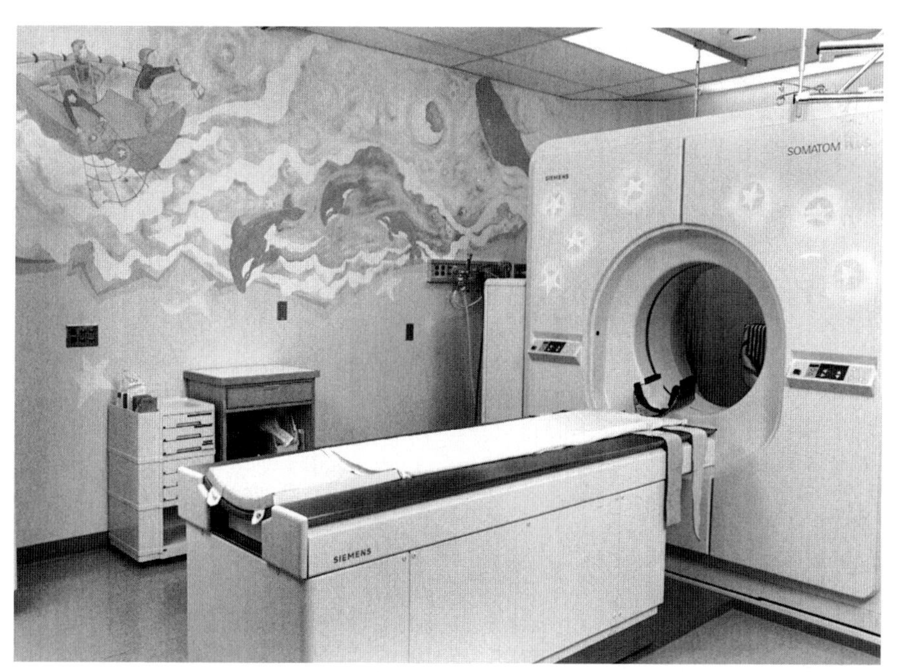

FIGURE 19-1 An interesting wall mural helps provide a friendly environment.

is present. The x-ray tube rotates around the patient, and a single image is produced for every rotation. The slice thickness of the image is determined by beam collimation. An MDCT scanner, however, contains multiple detector elements and can therefore generate multiple images from each rotation of the x-ray tube. Current CT scanners can yield up to 64 images per rotation. Image slice thickness is determined not by beam collimation but by the size of the detector elements that are used during the scan acquisition.

The size, number, and arrangement of detector elements are different for each scanner. Some scanners have detector elements that are of uniform size throughout the entire detector, whereas other scanners may contain central elements that are smaller and more peripheral elements that are larger. Detector elements may be combined to produce thicker slices and more coverage or used individually for higher-resolution images. The number of data channels present in the scanner determines the maximum number of images that can be produced per rotation. Each channel can use information from a single row or multiple detector rows. The scanner is named by the number of data channels present (e.g., a 16-slice scanner has 16 data channels capable of producing up to 16 images per gantry rotation). This scanner will have more than 16 rows of detector elements, however, because more than one row may be combined into a single channel.

Advantages of Multidetector CT in Pediatric Imaging

Advantages of MDCT are substantial for pediatric imaging. Faster scanners allow for substantially more rapid acquisition of data, producing better patient tolerance, reduced motion artifacts, and better use of contrast media. This is particularly important in pediatric imaging, where motion is a constant issue and scan time is of the essence. In addition, there is substantial improvement in spatial resolution. These qualities make MDCT especially useful in multiplanar and volume reconstructions and have opened up a plethora of new applications. Volumetric data acquisitions with very thin slices produce data sets that can be reconstructed in any plane with virtually no loss in image quality. This makes patient positioning for examinations easier and eliminates the need to obtain direct coronal images for examinations such as sinuses, temporal bone, and extremities. This helps keep radiation dose lower in children.

One inherent disadvantage with MDCT scanning is that the radiation dose may be increased when submillimeter slices are acquired. These thin slices will increase the effects of dose buildup of the radiation penumbra (the radiation penumbra is that portion of the radiation from a point source that falls outside the detector opening and therefore contributes to patient radiation dose but does not contribute to image formation). The thinner the slices, the more the penumbra effect can increase dose. This effect is dependent on the number of slices acquired per rotation and can be significant with four-slice scanners but is small with 16-slice scanners and negligible in 32- and 64-slice scanners.

New Pediatric Applications Possible with Multidetector CT

Many new applications and techniques for pediatric imaging are now possible with MDCT because of the ability to acquire thinner images in a shorter duration. These include three-dimensional (3D) volume- and surface-rendering techniques, allowing the radiologist to look at 3D relationships of anatomical structures, airway reconstructions, virtual bronchoscopy, and colonoscopy. CT angiography (CTA) by use of MDCT has blossomed, with detail never before possible. CTA has virtually replaced conventional angiography in many areas, including evaluation of the aorta and pulmonary arteries. CTA is useful in pediatric imaging, especially to delineate aortic arch anomalies, cardiac anomalies (before and after surgery), and aberrant vasculature, such as in cases of pulmonary sequestration or vascular malformations.

Cerebrovascular evaluation for aneurysms and vascular malformations is also helpful. Because of the speed of MDCT, it is frequently possible to obtain images with reduced contrast dose compared with older scanners. CTA offers many advantages compared with catheter angiography. It is noninvasive and safer and radiation dose is lower. CTA also allows evaluation of structures adjacent to and outside of the vasculature.

Another major growth area is orthopedic imaging. Characterization of fractures and congenital abnormalities of the skeletal system is greatly improved with advanced visualization techniques. MDCT allows for a single volumetric data set to be produced and reconstructed in any plane or projection. It is no longer necessary to scan patients in more than one plane. Current-generation scanners generate much less artifact in patients with metal hardware in place and are useful to evaluate patients who have undergone surgery with internal fixation devises.

BOX 19-1 *Procedure Preparation*

1. Have the patient's radiographic file available for consultation.
2. Review the order to make sure it is appropriate and that adequate clinical information is available. If there are any questions, contact the radiologist or ordering physician.
3. Obtain a protocol for the examination from the radiologist.
4. Register pertinent patient data into the CT system and select the appropriate parameters under which the CT examination is to be conducted.
5. Prepare the scanning room and have all necessary accessory equipment (e.g., immobilization devices, monitoring equipment) available for the procedure.
6. Prepare the necessary intravenous contrast media, if required.

ROLE OF THE CT TECHNOLOGIST

Patient Management

Pediatric patients need constant attention and monitoring. The technologist should work to ensure that the scanner is ready when the patient arrives and needed information such as clinical history and scan protocol has been determined. This will minimize delays and distractions that can interfere with the technologist's duty to care for the patient (Box 19-1).

The parents are usually an important ally of the technologist and should be included in the process whenever possible. One parent can be given a lead apron and remain in the room with the child during the entire procedure. This frequently helps reduce anxiety of both the child and the parent. If no parent is available, other ancillary staff such as nurses or assistants may be able to fill this role and comfort the child. The principal duty of the technologist, however, is to ensure that the scan is done safely, quickly, and accurately.

Neonatal Patients

To minimize the risk of infection to the neonatal patient, CT personnel who handle the infant should remove rings and watches, wash hands thoroughly with antibacterial soap, and always wear a cover gown. During the scanning procedure, it is important to maintain the infant's body temperature. This can be achieved by increasing the temperature in the CT scanning room before the arrival of the patient, wrapping the infant in a warm blanket, and covering the infant's head with a cap or small towel to prevent rapid heat loss. Equally important is placing a heating blanket under the infant positioned on the scanning table or focusing a heat lamp on the patient with special attention to the correct distance of the lamp from the patient. Finally, a nurse who accompanies the patient to the radiology department should monitor the patient's vital signs and body temperature throughout the CT examination.

Sedation

The use of sedation is inevitable in pediatric CT scanning. Image degradation from patient motion remains a problem. The introduction of MDCT has been a tremendous advance in pediatric imaging. Most scans can be completed in less than 30 seconds, and with current 16- to 64-slice scanners, scan times as short as 5 to 10 seconds can be routinely achieved while the highest image quality is maintained. This substantially decreases the need for sedation.

With MDCT sedation is rarely required for routine head and sinus studies, where some motion is tolerable. Sedation may still be required for studies requiring advanced multiplanar and volume reconstructions because motion artifact can significantly reduce the quality of these types of studies. Common examples would include studies of the temporal bone and CTA.

Sedation protocols and standards should be cooperatively established by the departments of radiology and anesthesiology to ensure high-quality care for the sedated patient. Any syndrome or condition with a respiratory risk that contraindicates sedation is recorded and brought to the attention of the radiologist. The decision to sedate a child should be a cooperative effort of the radiologist, the nurse, and the child's parent. Factors affecting the decision to sedate are summarized in Box 19-2.

Preparation for sedation requires patients to ingest nothing by mouth 4 to 6 hours for solid foods, 2 to 4 hours for formula or breast milk, and 2 hours for clear liquids before the examination. CT department personnel should inform parents of the correct preparation and sedation instructions at the time the examination is scheduled to help minimize any misunderstanding on the day of the examination. Any child who potentially may need sedation should be given preparation instructions for this at the time of scheduling. When the patient arrives in the radiology department, the CT technologist or the radiology nurse performs a careful assessment of the child's ability to undergo the CT examination without sedation.

BOX 19-2 *Sedation Assessment*

1. Consider the complexity of the CT study planned. (Is intravenous contrast required? Will 3D or multiplanar imaging be needed)
2. Explain the examination to the parents and child.
3. Consider the parents' opinion of the child's ability to cooperate.
4. Evaluate whether babies seem ready to sleep on their own. With older children, a visit to the scan room to observe another child being scanned may be helpful.
5. Observe the child in the scan room. A dry run is often useful to gauge whether the child will be able to cooperate.

Children less than 6 months of age rarely require sedation. Wrapping them in a warm blanket and providing them with a pacifier and use of a table restraint system to immobilize them can be all that is needed for a successful scan. Sleep deprivation is another technique that can be used with infants. With faster scanners, good patient communication, and the proper use of restraints, the need for sedation can be minimized.

For older infants and toddlers requiring sedation, oral or rectal chloral hydrate is the most commonly used drug. The typical starting dose is 50 to 75 milligrams (mg) per kilogram (kg) to a maximum dose of 100 mg/kg. This is generally effective and can be routinely administered by a radiology nurse under the direction of a radiologist.

Children older than toddler age can usually be talked through a CT study with the help of a parent. When this does not work, oral or intravenous (IV) midazolam (Versed) with or without morphine may be used for conscious sedation. Some children and toddlers may not adequately respond to these drugs and will require deep sedation with drugs such as IV pentobarbital sodium (Nembutal). This group may also include children with delayed development, sleep apnea, or chronic respiratory problems. Pentobarbital is generally administered by specially trained personnel such as a dedicated pediatric sedation team or anesthesiologists.

All sedation patients require continuous monitoring by nursing staff including pulse oximetry, blood pressure, and respiratory rate. Paradoxical hyperactivity and agitation is a side effect of chloral hydrate and has been reported with pentobarbital sodium as well. When this does occur, it is necessary to keep the child safely under observation until the effect passes.

Resuscitative supplies are kept in the CT scan room at all times. When the study is completed, the sedated child is moved to the recovery room for monitoring. Patients are discharged when they are easily aroused, have enough muscle tone to hold up their heads, and can drink clear fluids. The parents are given an information sheet about care of the sedated child that includes a telephone number to call if they have any concerns after their return home.

Immobilization

Immobilization of the child is essential to ensure patient safety and to provide images free of motion artifacts. For patients less than 5 years old, the immobilizer (Fig. 19-2) is a comfortable device that secures the patient's arms beside the head during body examinations. This device is secured to the patient scanning table with adhesive straps after the patient has been positioned.

Larger children are generally immobilized by other methods, such as adhesive straps placed under the mattress and over the patient. After the patient has been immobilized, the CT technologist should still carefully monitor the child by closed-circuit television or direct visualization.

Some time of immobilization is important in nearly every case. Sedated children should be gently immobilized with soft straps or paper tape. Cooperative older children should also have immobilization to help remind them not to move.

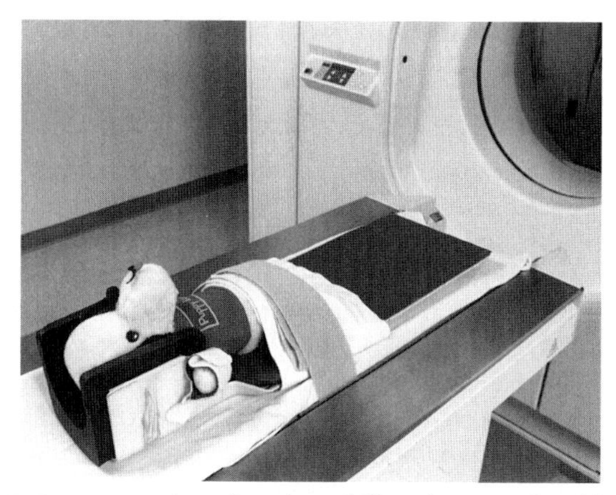

FIGURE 19-2 A patient immobilizer is a comfortable device to secure the pediatric patient.

Use of Intravenous Contrast Media

The routine use of nonionic contrast media almost eliminates minor reactions such as pain, nausea, vomiting, and urticaria. This is especially important in pediatric CT, and the use of nonionic contrast media is therefore recommended in those examinations requiring contrast media. The removal of these potential reactions and discomforts helps ensure the cooperation of the patient and provides a safer examination for the sedated child. Fortunately, severe allergic reactions to contrast media are rare in children. Informed consent should be obtained before IV contrast injection.

The dose of contrast material for children is 2 to 3 milliliters (ml)/kg to a maximum of 150 ml. Power injectors are now commonly used because they provide a constant rate of injection that allows more accurate timing of the bolus and better organ enhancement. The deciding factor for use of a power injector depends on the IV site and size. Only peripheral IV sites can be obtained on most children. The injection rate is determined by the size of the IV catheter; injection rates of 2-3 ml per second can be used with 22-gauge catheters, whereas a 24-gauge catheter can be injected at 1 to 2 ml per second. Butterfly-type needles and percutaneous indwelling central venous catheter lines are almost always hand injected rather than by use of power injectors.

Scan timing is very important for contrast enhanced imaging, particularly of the neck, chest, and body. Unlike in adult patients where routine scan delays are effective in most people, scan delay in children must be individualized depending on the size of the child, the site of the IV, the injection rate, and the duration of the scan. If a power injector is used, standard delays can be used in most patients. For neck and chest examinations, delays of 35 to 45 seconds are effective. For studies of the abdomen and pelvis, longer delays of 50 to 70 seconds are used. Infants generally require shorter delays because the volume of contrast injected is so small. When hand injection is used, the scan should start when the injection is almost complete. Timing for contrast-enhanced studies of the brain is less critical. These scans are usually begun after all of the contrast has been given.

Another option to determine scan delay to produce optimal vascular enhancement is available on most MDCT scanners (e.g., Toshiba's SureStart, General Electric's SmartPrep, Phillips Dose-Right). This software uses bolus-tracking to trigger the start of the scan. The operator places a region of interest (ROI) on a vessel or organ at the start of the study. Contrast injection is begun and serial low dose scans are performed in the same location. The enhancement curve is tracked in real time. The scan can be triggered automatically when the Hounsfield units (HU) reach a predetermined threshold or manually by the technologist on the basis of the visual appearance of the vessel. In children manual triggering is usually preferred because the small size of the vessels may make automatic triggering unreliable if the child moves at all. Bolus tracking is the preferred method to initiate the scan for CT angiography, but it can also be useful for scans of the neck, chest, and abdomen. One disadvantage of this technique is increased radiation dose to the region where the monitoring scan is performed.

Regardless of the injection type, it is important to monitor the IV site during injection. If manual injection is used, filling the contrast medium into smaller syringes facilitates injection compared with the use of a large syringe.

Radiation Protection

Growing cells are the most sensitive to radiation. For any particular milliamperage (mA), pediatric organ doses are higher compared with those of an adult. Because of these factors, and the cumulative effect over a lifetime of exposure, radiation exposure has a potentially higher risk for the pediatric patient than for the adult patient. It has been shown that even small radiation doses carry the same relative risk of cancer mortality as low-dose exposure for atomic bomb survivors. These radiation doses are in the range typically seen with CT scans with adult scan parameters not adjusted for children. Therefore, radiation protection is an integral part of the pediatric CT examination. The ALARA principle should be followed, in that radiation dose should be kept *as low as can be reasonably achieved.*

This issue has generated substantial interest in both the popular press and the radiology literature. It is the responsibility of every person involved with imaging pediatric patients to make sure that diagnostic scans are obtained with the minimum radiation dose. This goal requires a comprehensive approach that addresses all aspects of the CT examination from ordering procedures to examination planning to specific examination parameters chosen by the technologist at the CT console.

Scan Planning and Preparation

Radiation exposure control begins with a careful review of all orders to ensure that the study is indicated and appropriate. Some requests may need to be redirected to ultrasonography or magnetic resonance imaging (MRI), depending on the indication. Additional clinical information from the ordering physician may be needed to ensure that the proper study is performed the first time.

Once it is determined the examination is necessary, the proper protocol must be chosen. Coverage should be limited to the area of interest. Multiphase scans should be minimized in children. Scans both with and without contrast should not be performed routinely. Pediatric specific examination protocols should be created and used. Lead shielding should be routinely used to cover body parts that are outside the ROI. Particular attention should be made to avoid scanning sensitive areas such as the breasts, genitalia, and lens whenever possible.

Scan Parameters

Particular attention must be paid to many different scan parameters in order to minimize dose. Factors such as tube current (mA) and peak kilovoltage (kVp) have an obvious effect on radiation dose, but many other variables used in spiral/MDCT such as pitch, slice thickness, and rotation time can also significantly affect dose.

Increasing pitch is an effective way to decrease dose. A pitch of 1.5 can lower the dose by about 25% compared with a pitch of 1, whereas a pitch of 2 can reduce the exposure by about 50%. Shorter rotation times will also decrease dose. A rotation time of 0.5 seconds gives half the dose of a 1-second rotation time if all other parameters are constant. With MDCT scanners, very thin slice thickness (less than 1 millimeter [mm]) can result in increased dose secondary to overlapping of the radiation penumbra. This effect can be significant with four-slice scanners but is minor in scanners with 16 or more slices. Care should be used when acquiring submillimeter scans on a four-slice machine.

Slice thickness may be a consideration in pediatric patients. One inherent disadvantage with MDCT scanning is that the radiation dose may be increased when submillimeter slices are acquired. These thin slices will increase the effects of dose buildup of the radiation penumbra. The thinner the slices, the more the penumbra effect can increase dose. This effect is dependent on the number of slices acquired per rotation and can be significant with four-slice scanners but is small with 16-slice scanners and negligible in 32- and 64-slice scanners. In fact, 64-slice scanners can produce images of superior quality compared with scanners with fewer detectors with the same radiation dose (same scan parameters). Facilities using four-slice scanners should use submillimeter slices with caution in children.

Modification of dose parameters is the most straightforward and important method to reduce dose. There are two primary methods to optimize CT dose parameters. The first way is for the CT technologist to individually tailor the dose parameters for each patient on the basis of the patient's weight and the body part being imaged (Table 19-1). Alternatively, multiple different protocols can be created in the scanner for each type of examination on the basis of the patient's size/weight with appropriate kVp/mA parameters built into each protocol. Although this approach can be effective if the protocols are built and followed correctly, it is somewhat cumbersome and is easily subject to error if the technologist chooses the wrong protocol.

Recognizing the limitations of the previous methods, CT manufacturers have focused much attention on methods to control, monitor, and reduce the radiation dose from CT examinations. As a result, most MDCT scanners now have some form of automatic exposure control available. There are different techniques used by the CT manufacturers, but the basic principles are similar. The most common approach relies on attenuation measurements derived from the actual patient obtained during scout image acquisition to create a radiation dose profile for the examination that is individually tailored to that patient. The dose will actually vary during the examination depending on the attenuation of the body. For example, in a chest study the radiation dose will be much higher through the shoulders and much lower through the lungs. The most sophisticated systems now allow the operator to select appropriate image quality on the basis of noise levels and the scanner and then apply the appropriate tube current regardless of patient size. This relieves the operator of the need

TABLE 19-1 Recommended Dose Parameters for Pediatric Multidetector Computed Tomography

	DOSE PARAMETERS			
Weight (kg)	kV	mAs Chest	mAs Abdomen	mAs Head (120 kV)
<15	80	20	30	100
15-24	80-100	30	40	120
25-34	80-100	40	60	140
35-44	100	50	80	160
45-54	100-120	60	100	180
>55	120	60+	100+	200+

kV, Kilovolts.

to vary conditions on the basis of patient size or weight.

Finally, it is important to have a quality assurance program to consistently monitor the entire process to ensure that protocols are up to date, scan techniques are optimized, technologists understand and follow the protocols, and the CT scanner is properly maintained and tested with phantoms. Steps used to minimize radiation dose in children are summarized in Box 19-3.

CT OF THE HEAD, NECK, AND SPINE

Imaging of the head and spine in children depends on a number of factors, including the age of the child, medical condition, ability to cooperate, and above all the indication for the examination. These factors will determine which modality is best suited to the overall assessment of the patient's medical problem. The majority of neuroimaging examinations in children are performed with CT or MRI. The main exception to this is the neonate, in whom ultrasonography is the dominant imaging technique. Plain films have a small role, usually for the spine. Indications for diagnostic pediatric neuroangiography are limited and have been replaced by magnetic resonance angiography (MRA) and CTA. Catheter angiography is primarily a therapeutic tool used to treat children with aneurysms and vascular malformations.

Indications

With some exceptions, most indications for examination of the central nervous system (CNS) are best studied by MRI. MRI retains several advantages over CT for neuroimaging. MRI uses no

BOX 19-3 *Steps to Minimize Radiation Exposure*

1. Review all orders for appropriateness and clinical need.
2. Obtain a pediatric-specific protocol from the radiologist.
   a. Multiphase scanning should be minimized.
   b. Judicious use of very thin slices when a four-row MDCT is used
3. Shield sensitive areas whenever possible.
4. Select appropriate scan parameters on the basis of patient size and weight or use automatic exposure control methods when available.
   a. Refer to pediatric dose charts for mA and kilovolt values.
   b. Adjust pitch and scan time to minimize dose when appropriate.
5. Maintain a QC program to ensure that the scanner is functioning properly and that the protocols that have been set up are being followed correctly.

ionizing radiation and has inherently better soft tissue contrast that can be used to characterize normal anatomy and pathology of the CNS. CT has several advantages over MRI, primarily speed of acquisition and accessibility. CT is also superior to identify acute hemorrhage and calcifications and to characterize abnormalities of the bone.

CT of the Brain

Primary indications for CT over MRI include assessment of trauma in the acute phase (Fig. 19-3), detection of acute hemorrhage, and the detection of calcification such as in cases of prenatal TORCH (toxoplasmosis, other [congenital syphilis and viruses], rubella, cytomegalovirus, and herpes simplex virus) infections or postnatal infection such as cysticercosis. CT is also recommended for skull lesions and fractures (Fig. 19-3).

Either CT or MRI can adequately evaluate many other indications for brain imaging. In these instances CT is often preferred because it is quicker and easier to obtain and often can be done without sedation. Common indications include evaluation of hydrocephalus and shunt malfunction, screening evaluation for children with headaches or abnormal head size, and evaluation and follow-up of children with congenital abnormalities such as Chiari malformations or Dandy-Walker syndrome.

MRI is the preferred modality for evaluation of many other indications such as seizures, known or suspected brain tumors, acute and chronic ischemia, most CNS infections and inflammatory diseases, vascular malformations, congenital syndromes such as neurofibromatosis and tuberous sclerosis, diseases of white matter and demyelination such as acute disseminated encephalomyelitis (ADEM), and evaluation of the pituitary gland. Although MRI may be the study of choice in most instances, CT is frequently performed in these patients either in the acute setting when the child is in the emergency department or for follow-up after the initial evaluation and treatment. CT can also serve as the primary evaluation modality when MRI is not available.

CT of the Face and Neck

Primary indications for CT include assessment of facial and orbital trauma, evaluation of osseous abnormalities of the maxilla or mandible, assessment of the temporal bone and middle ear in

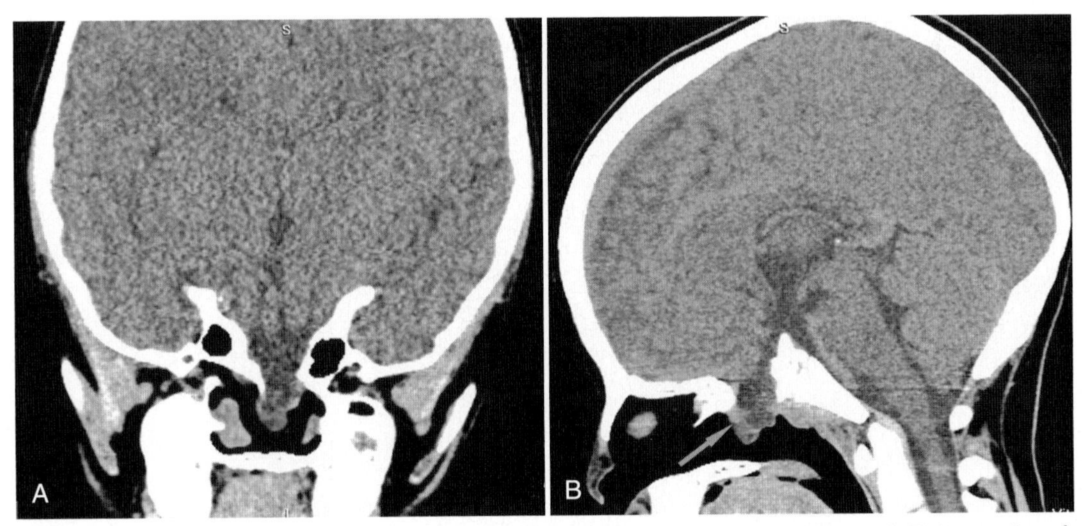

FIGURE 19-3 Sphenoidal encephalocele. High-resolution 0.5-mm coronal **(A)** and sagittal **(B)** images in soft tissue window. There is a left parasagittal defect in the sphenoid bone with herniation of meninges and cerebrospinal fluid into the sphenoid sinus. The pituitary tissue is shown at the bottom of the encephalocele *(arrow)*.

children with infection or hearing loss, evaluation of the sinuses for sinusitis, and evaluation of the airway. Either CT or MRI may be performed to evaluate the face and neck to characterize masses, enlarged lymph nodes, salivary gland evaluation, and infectious processes.

CT of the Spine

CT is primarily used to evaluate suspected spinal trauma. CT is also useful to characterize congenital bony abnormalities such as scoliosis, lesions of the vertebral bodies, and osteomyelitis (Fig. 19-4). MRI is the primary modality for evaluation of the spinal cord and tumors of the cord and canal. Evaluation for disk conditions is uncommon in pediatric patients but is preferable with MRI.

Patient Positioning

When positioning the patient for CT of the brain and face, it is essential to have the patient's head geometrically centered in the gantry to ensure artifact-free images. In this respect, the patient's head must be centered accurately from right to left in the head holder and from front to back in the gantry. Multiple small positioning sponges can be used to secure the patient's head in the head holder. For the accurate assessment of midline structures, care must be taken to position the head so that the right and left sides are symmetrical and not tilted.

Direct coronal images are important for evaluation of structures such as the orbits, sinuses, and temporal bone. When older-generation scanners are used, it is still important to obtain direct coronal images for these examinations. Newer MDCT scanners, particularly 16-slice and 64-slice scanners, have obviated the need to obtain direct coronal images. A single high-resolution data set can be reconstructed into any plane.

The coronal position is usually comfortable for the pediatric patient and is easily achieved with even sedated children. Patients are placed prone with the chin extended forward. The CT gantry is tilted to obtain images in the coronal plane. Occasionally, a patient cannot tolerate the coronal position. An alternate position is a Water's view, in which the patient's head is extended to maximum tolerance. With the aid of a scout view, the scans are prescribed as close to 90 degrees to the clivus as possible.

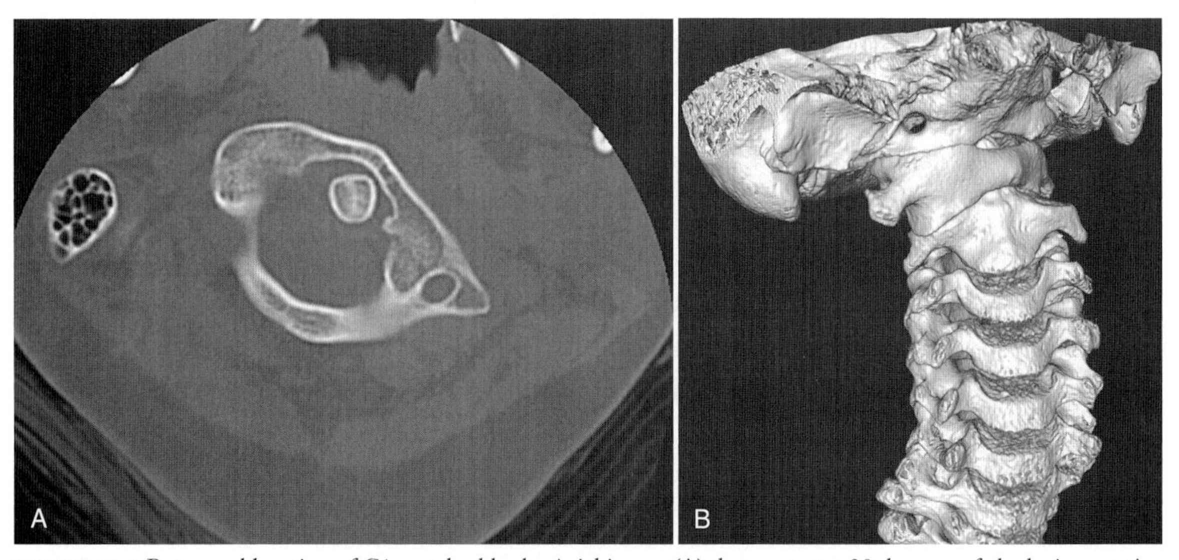

FIGURE 19-4 Rotary subluxation of C1 vertebral body. Axial image **(A)** demonstrates 30 degrees of clockwise rotation of C1 with respect to C2. The rotation is better demonstrated on the 3D surface-shaded display **(B)**.

Technical Considerations

Scans of the brain can be obtained with either conventional sequential axial images or with the helical technique. Some radiologists have traditionally felt that sequential technique produces images that are sharper with better contrast. This technique requires a very cooperative or sedated child and is particularly susceptible to motion artifacts. Helical scanning offers many benefits. The scans are quicker, less sensitive to motion, and generate fewer partial volume and streak artifacts, and, above all, high-resolution data sets can be obtained that can be reconstructed into different planes. With current-generation MDCT scanners it is generally possible to obtain image quality from helical scans that is equal or nearly equal to that of sequential scans. For these reasons, we prefer to use helical scanning in the brain for pediatric patients.

Scans of the face, sinuses, temporal bone, neck and spine should all be obtained helically for obvious reasons. Multiplanar images should routinely be generated and reviewed in these cases.

Most pediatric neurological scans can be performed without contrast. The most common indications such as trauma, headaches, and hydrocephalus do not require contrast. Certain indications such as known or suspected infection or neoplasm do benefit from contrast administration. When the brain is imaged, scans before and after contrast are generally obtained in these patients. However, for evaluation of the face and neck precontrast scans are usually not needed and will needlessly increase the radiation dose to the child.

Timing for contrast studies of the head and face is usually less critical than for body studies and CTA. Contrast can be administered by either hand injection or power injector and the scans begun once all the contrast is injected. If a rapid injection is performed, an additional 10- to 20-second delay should be applied before the scan is started.

As in all pediatric CT examinations, the technologist must be careful to ensure that scan parameters chosen for the study are appropriate to the size and age of the child.

Scanning Protocols

Scanning protocols are usually established to include information that covers data acquisition and reconstruction and image transfer. These protocols are intended to assist the technologist performing the CT examination and generally help increase the overall efficiency of the examination. Comprehensive examination protocols help ensure that the proper study is performed and minimize wasted time for both the technologist and the radiologist.

Acquisition parameters include patient position, prescan localization (scout view), scan range, acquisition slice thickness, pitch, gantry rotation speed, and specific dose parameters. Dose parameters can be determined by the technologist on the basis of the patient's age or weight or automatically chosen by the scanner by use of one of the automated exposure control programs. Reconstruction parameters include reconstruction algorithm (e.g., soft tissue, and bone), reconstructed slice thickness, and multiplanar or 3D reconstructions. The protocol should also describe which information is to be archived on PACS (picture archiving and communication system) or film and whether data should be sent to a 3D workstation for additional postprocessing.

Tables 19-2 through 19-4 are examples of generalized protocols of the head, orbit/sinus, temporal bone/IAC (internal auditory canal), and spine used for four-,16-, and 64-slice scanners. These protocols are generalizations and must be modified for each scanner. On 64-slice scanners, the mAs can be decreased slightly compared with 16-slice scanners for a comparable result. All manufacturers have some differences in detector configuration, scan features, and reconstruction options.

CT OF THE CHEST AND ABDOMEN

Body CT in children (unlike adults) is generally more of an ancillary imaging modality. Ultrasonography remains the primary screening modality for

TABLE 19-2 Pediatric Neurological Protocols: Techniques for Four-Slice Multidetector Computed Tomography

Scan Parameter	Brain	Orbit/Sinus	IAC	Neck	Spine
Scan mode	Helical	Helical	Helical	Helical	Helical
Coverage	Skull base to vertex	Top of orbits through area of interest	Temporal bone	Skull base to lung apex	Spine ROI
Gantry rotation speed	1 second	0.5 second	1 second	0.5 second	0.5 second
Detector slice thickness	2.5 mm	2.5 mm	1.25 mm	2.5 mm	2.5 mm
Pitch	1.0	1.25	1.0	1.25	1.0
Kilovolts	120	100-120	120	100-120	100-120
mA	60-100	50-100	50-100	50-100	50-100
Reconstruction slice thickness	3-5 mm	3 mm	1-2 mm	3 mm	3 mm
Reconstruction interval	3-5 mm	2 mm	1 mm	3 mm	2 mm
Algorithm	Soft tissue	Soft tissue, bone	Bone	Soft tissue	Soft tissue, bone
Multiplanar reconstructions	Optional	Coronal	Coronal	Sagittal, coronal	Sagittal, coronal
Contrast volume if needed	2 ml/kg	2 ml/kg		2 ml/kg	2 ml/kg

the abdomen and pelvis, but CT is a very important modality for many indications.

Indications

Trauma

CT is the modality of choice for examination of the abdomen after blunt injury or high-speed trauma to evaluate possible laceration of liver, spleen, pancreas, or kidney (Fig. 19-5). IV and oral contrast (through a nasogastric [NG] tube) should be used in trauma cases. It is usually not possible to give a substantial amount of oral contrast through an NG tube in an unconscious patient because of the risk of aspiration, but a small amount can be given to at least outline the duodenum.

Infections

The most common infections where CT is used in children are pneumonia, pyelonephritis, and appendicitis. IV contrast is needed when there is a pleural effusion or empyema. Oral or rectal contrast, with IV contrast, is needed to evaluate appendicitis and possible abscesses (Fig. 19-6). CT is often used in postoperative patients to look for abscess.

Tumors

CT is an integral part of the diagnostic workup and posttreatment assessment of pediatric solid tumors, including lymphoma (e.g., Burkitt's or Hodgkins) and abdominal tumors (e.g., Wilms' tumor of the kidney, neuroblastoma, rhabdomyosarcoma, and hepatoblastoma) (Fig. 19-7). The investigation of

TABLE 19-3 Pediatric Neurological Protocols: Techniques for 16-Slice Multidetector Computed Tomography

Scan Parameter	Brain	OrbitT/Sinus	IAC	Neck	Spine
Scan mode	Helical	Helical	Helical	Helical	Helical
Coverage	Skull base to vertex	Top of orbits through area of interest	Temporal bone	Skull base to lung apex	Spine ROI
Gantry rotation speed	0.5 second	0.5 second	0.5 second	0.5 second	0.5 second
Detector slice thickness	0.5-1.25 mm	0.5-1.25 mm	0.5 mm	0.5-1.25 mm	0.5-1.25 mm
Pitch	1.0	1.25	1.0	1.25	1.0
Kilovolts	120	100-120	120	100-120	100-120
mA	200+	100-200	100-200	100-200	100-200+
Reconstruction slice thickness	3-5 mm	2 mm	1 mm	3 mm	2 mm
Reconstruction interval	3-5 mm	2 mm	0.5-1 mm	3 mm	2 mm
Algorithm	Soft tissue	Soft tissue, bone	Bone	Soft tissue	Soft tissue, bone
Multiplanar reconstructions	Optional	Sagittal, coronal	Coronal	Sagittal, coronal	Sagittal, coronal
Contrast volume if needed	2 ml/kg	2 ml/kg		2 ml/kg	2 ml/kg

TABLE 19-4 Pediatric Neurological Protocols: Techniques for 64-Slice Multidetector Computed Tomography

Scan Parameter	Brain	Orbit/Sinus	IAC	Neck	Spine
Scan mode	Helical	Helical	Helical	Helical	Helical
Coverage	Skull base to vertex	Top of orbits through area of interest	Temporal bone	Skull base to lung apex	Spine ROI
Gantry rotation speed	0.4-0.5 second	0.4-0.5 second	0.4-0.5 second	0.4-0.5 second	0.4-0.5 second
Detector slice thickness	0.3-1.25 mm	0.3-1.25 mm	0.3-0.5 mm	0.3-1.25 mm	0.3-1.25 mm
Pitch	1.0	1.25	1.0	1.25	1.0
Kilovolts	120	100-120	120	100-120	100-120
mA	200+	100-200	100-200	100-200	100-200+
Reconstruction slice thickness	3-5 mm	2 mm	1 mm	3 mm	2 mm
Reconstruction interval	3-5 mm	2 mm	0.5-1 mm	3 mm	2 mm
Algorithm	Soft tissue	Soft tissue, bone	Bone	Soft tissue	Soft tissue, bone
Multiplanar reconstructions	Optional	Sagittal, coronal	Coronal	Sagittal, coronal	Sagittal, coronal
Contrast volume if needed	2 ml/kg	2 ml/kg		2 ml/kg	2 ml/kg

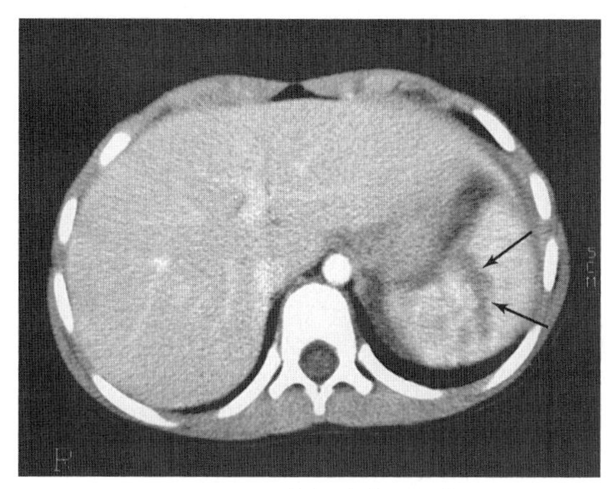

FIGURE 19-5 Splenic laceration.

these oncological diseases generally includes a noncontrast chest CT to look for lung metastases. Chest CT for mediastinal disease requires a contrast examination because unenhanced mediastinal vessels may mimic masses or adenopathy on a noncontrast scan.

CT of the Chest

CT of the chest is used to evaluate central and peripheral airways, pulmonary nodules, vascular anatomy, lung parenchyma, and congenital masses (lung cysts, cystic adenomatoid malformations) (Fig. 19-8). CT is an excellent modality to assess foreign body aspirations, when the material is of low density and does not show up well on chest x-ray. MDCT is also used to evaluate the trachea for stenosis, malacia, and atresia with virtual endoscopy (Fig. 19-9). Because these evaluations are limited by the ability of patients to hold the breath for the scan, the use of this technology may be limited in pediatrics. CT for infections, pleural effusions, and malignancy should be with IV contrast.

High-Resolution CT

High-resolution CT is sometimes performed on the pediatric patient for the assessment of parenchymal lung disease such as cystic fibrosis or bronchiectasis (Fig. 19-10). However, in most cases bronchiectasis can be well seen by using conventional CT, so high-resolution CT is not necessary. This consideration is important because an increased radiation dose is required to acquire the thinner images in high-resolution CT.

Patient Positioning

The patient can be placed head or feet first into the scanner. Placing the patient feet first may be less intimidating for young children. This position also allows the parent or technologist a clear view of the child for monitoring and comforting.

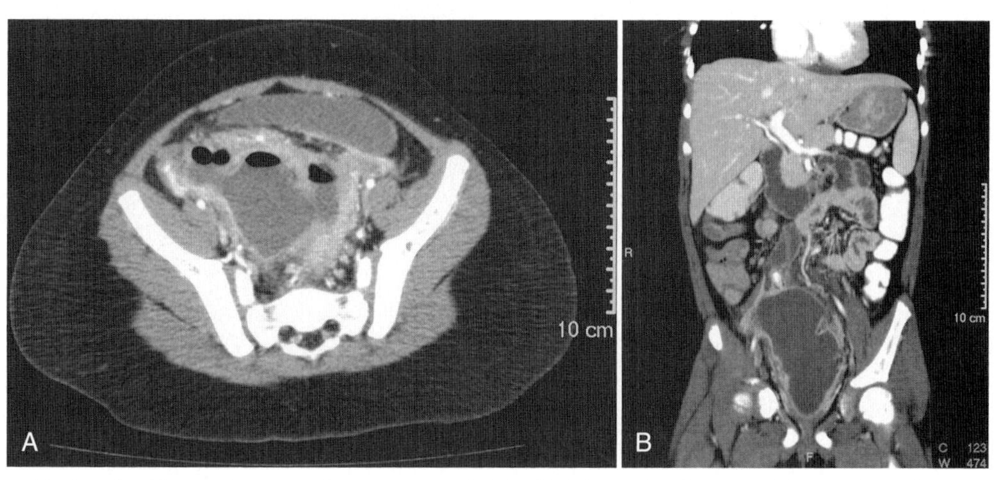

FIGURE 19-6 A, Abscess from perforated appendicitis. **B,** Coronal reformatted image from 3-mm axial images. Complex fluid collections with enhancing walls are present.

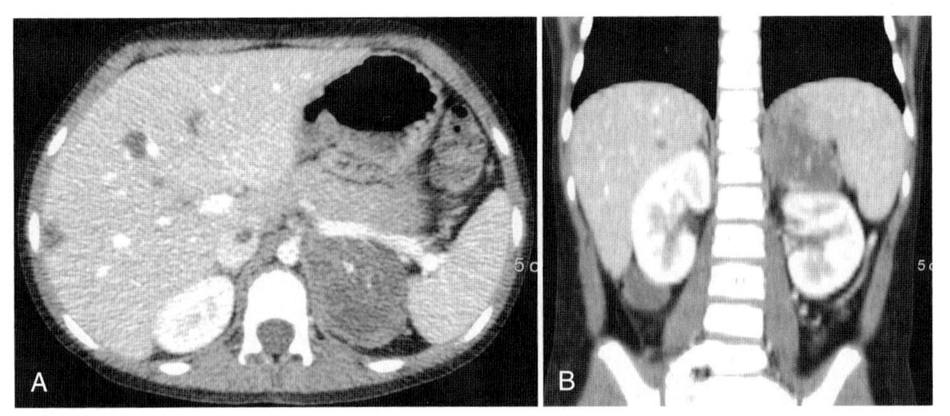

FIGURE 19-7 **A,** Neuroblastoma of the left adrenal gland. **B,** Coronal reformatted image clearly demonstrates suprarenal location of the calcified mass.

The patient must be centered correctly in the gantry, which may involve the use of immobilization sponges or blankets and tape.

Technical Considerations

For chest CT, shallow breathing in the young child will be adequate. Instructions for breath-hold may not work, and misregistration or motion artifacts are risked if the child takes another deep breath. Older children can be instructed to withhold their breaths, especially in high-resolution CT. Children on ventilators may be briefly taken off ventilation during image acquisition, provided they are monitored and can tolerate this action.

Scanning of the chest can be initiated by bolus tracking or can be started just before the end of contrast injection. Scans about 30 to 50 seconds after beginning injection will demonstrate adequate

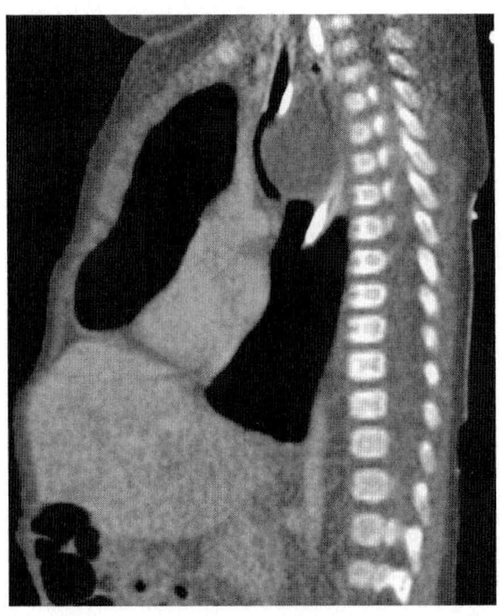

FIGURE 19-8 Esophageal duplication cyst. Location of cyst posterior to trachea is nicely demonstrated on sagittal image.

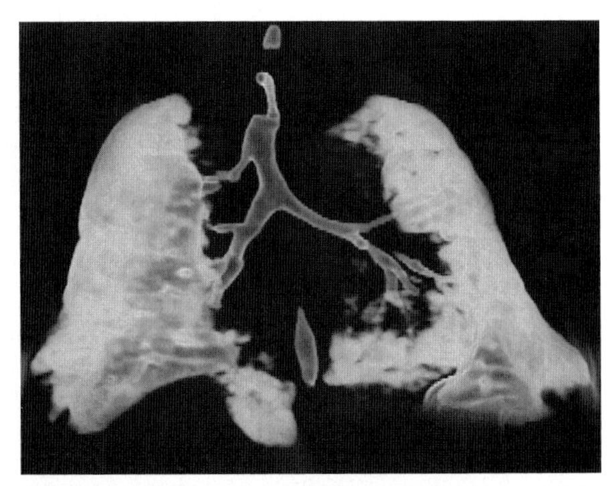

FIGURE 19-9 Aberrant bronchus (bronchus suis/pig bronchus). Airways reconstruction. Aberrant bronchus to right upper lobe directly from trachea is noted.

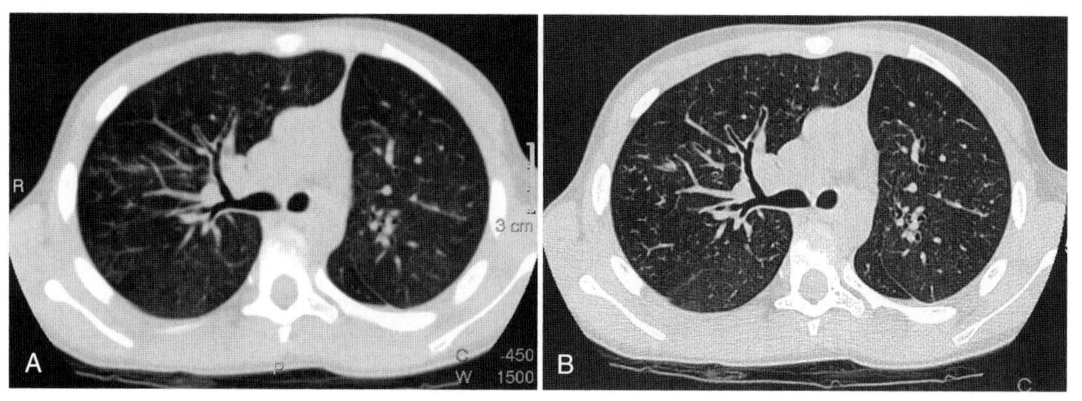

FIGURE 19-10 **A** and **B,** Normal lung, routine CT (3-mm axial slice) versus high-resolution CT (1-mm axial slice). Bronchial walls and diameters can be seen fairly well even with routine imaging.

vascular enhancement in older children. In infants, this time frame will be shorter, with maximal enhancement probably around 10 to 20 seconds after the beginning of injection. In infants, abdominal scans should begin sooner than the usual 70- to 90-second delay of adult scans, probably right at the end of the contrast bolus.

For abdominal and pelvic CT scans, oral contrast should always be used if the patient can tolerate it. This is especially important in the evaluation of intra-abdominal abscess or bowel obstruction. A long (at least 2-hour) preparation should be performed for studies where there may be conditions of the colon. For trauma patients, a small amount of oral contrast can be injected through the NG tube to delineate the duodenum. Rectal contrast may be used in cases of appendicitis. About 250 ml of contrast is usually adequate to opacify the colon in this patient population (5-15 years old), or contrast can be instilled by gravity drip until the patient feels full.

Noncontrast CT scans can be used to evaluate renal stones. Delayed scans (5-10 minutes) are needed to evaluate hemangiomas/hemangioendotheliomas. Renal excretion of contrast peaks at around 3 to 5 minutes after injection. Delayed scans to evaluate urinary tract obstruction should therefore be longer than this period (around 10 minutes after injection), with the patient placed prone because the kidneys drain anteriorly.

Scanning Protocols

Protocols for pediatric CT of the chest, abdomen, and pelvis are summarized in Tables 19-5 through 19-7.

MUSCULOSKELETAL CT

MDCT has had a significant impact on pediatric orthopedic imaging. Isotropic data acquisition with 3D reconstruction techniques has proved valuable for many different indications.

Indications

Complex Fractures

MDCT is the study of choice to evaluate complex fractures, particularly of the acetabulum/pelvis and the upper and lower extremities. Surface-rendered and multiplanar reconstructions can give the orthopedic surgeon a clear 3D picture of the fracture planes and are valuable in planning operative repair (Fig. 19-11). Segmentation of the images is very helpful to show the joint surfaces.

Tumors

Osseous tumors (e.g., Ewing's sarcoma and osteogenic sarcoma) are best imaged with MRI, which

TABLE 19-5 Pediatric Chest and Abdomen Protocols: Technique for Four-Slice Multidetector Computed Tomography

Scan Parameter	Chest	Abdomen/Pelvis
Scan mode	Helical	Helical
Coverage	Lower neck through lung base	Diaphragm to pubic symphysis
Gantry rotation speed	0.5 second	0.5 second
Detector slice thickness	2.5 mm	2.5 mm
Pitch	Variable	Variable
Kilovolts	80 (100-120 for >45 kg)	80 (100-120 for >45 kg)
mA		
<15 kg	40	50-70
15-24 kg	60	80
25-34 kg	80	100
35-44 kg	100	120-140
>45 kg	120-140	160-200
Reconstruction slice thickness	3 mm	3-5 mm
Reconstruction interval	3 mm	3-5 mm
Algorithm	Soft tissue and lung	Soft tissue and lung
Multiplanar reconstructions	Coronal	Coronal
Contrast volume (if needed)	2 ml/kg	2 ml/kg

TABLE 19-6 Pediatric Chest and Abdomen Protocols: Techniques for 16-Slice Multidetector Computed Tomography

Scan Parameter	Chest	Abdomen
Scan mode	Helical	Helical
Coverage	Lower neck through lung base	Diaphragm to pubic symphysis
Gantry rotation speed	0.5 second	0.5 second
Detector slice thickness	0.5-1.25 mm	0.5-1.25 mm
Pitch	Variable	Variable
Kilovolts	80 (100-120 for >45 kg)	80 (100-120 for >45 kg)
mA		
<15 kg	40	50-70
15-24 kg	60	80
25-34 kg	80	100
35-44 kg	100	120-140
>45 kg	120-140	160-200
Reconstruction slice thickness	3 mm	3 mm
Reconstruction interval	3 mm	3 mm
Algorithm	Soft tissue and lung	Soft tissue and lung
Multiplanar reconstructions	Coronal	Coronal
Contrast volume (if needed)	2 ml/kg	2 ml/kg

TABLE 19-7 Pediatric Chest and Abdomen Protocols: Techniques for 64-Slice Multidetector Computed Tomography

Scan Parameter	Chest	Abdomen
Scan mode	Helical	Helical
Coverage	Lower neck through lung base	Diaphragm to pubic symphysis
Gantry rotation speed	0.4-0.5 second	0.4-0.5 second
Detector slice thickness	0.5-1.25 mm	0.5-1.25 mm
Pitch	Variable	Variable
Kilovolts	80 (100-120 for >45 kg)	80 (100-120 for >45 kg)
mA		
<15 kg	40	50-70
15-24 kg	60	80
25-34 kg	80	100
35-44 kg	100	120-140
>45 kg	120-140	160-200
Reconstruction slice thickness	3 mm	3 mm
Reconstruction interval	3 mm	3 mm
Algorithm	Soft tissue and lung	Soft tissue and lung
Multiplanar reconstructions	Coronal	Coronal
Contrast volume (if needed)	2 ml/kg	2 ml/kg

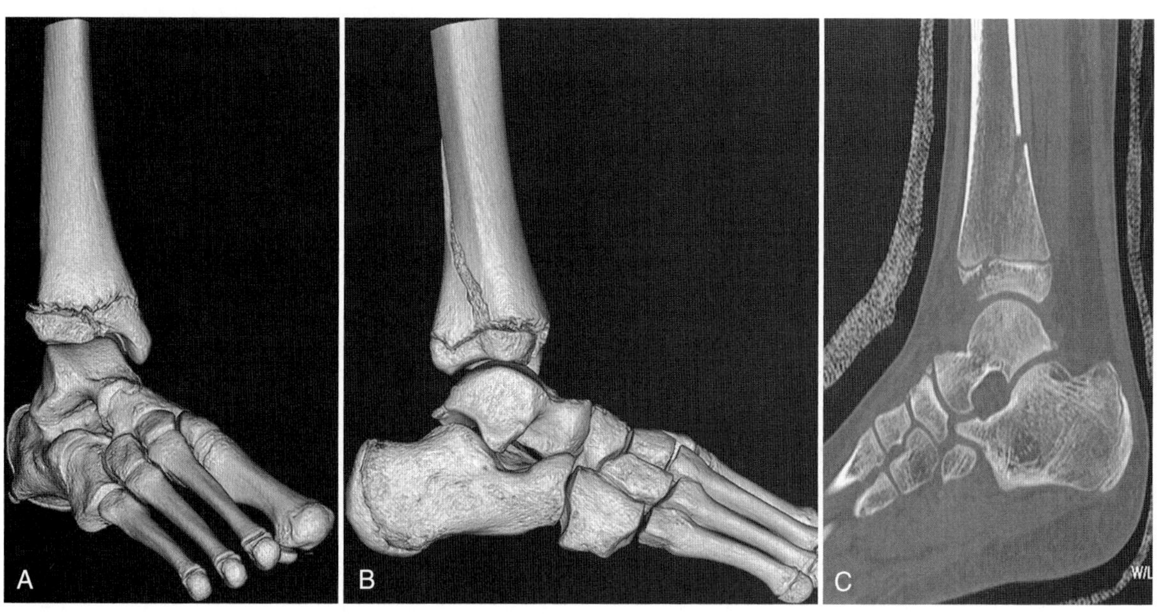

FIGURE 19-11 Salter 4 fracture of distal tibia. Surface (**A** and **B**) and sagittal reconstructions **(C)** demonstrate fracture line through metaphysis and epiphysis.

can delineate soft tissue and marrow involvement much better than CT. CT is used to visualize the cortex itself, or calcifications (Fig. 19-12). It is not good at defining soft tissue involvement.

Infections

Osseous infections are best evaluated using bone scan or MRI. The infection must be fairly aggressive and advanced to produce bony changes. CT findings may therefore be absent in early stages of an infection. Soft tissue infections are also better evaluated by MRI. CT may be used to delineate soft tissue abscesses. IV contrast must be used.

Deformities

CT can be used to evaluate femoral anteversion or tibial torsion and is also valuable in assessing congenital hip and shoulder dysplasias (Fig. 19-13). CT is also an excellent way to evaluate leg-length discrepancy. Imaging for this purpose can be done by using a low radiation dose method, which imparts lower radiation than the corresponding plain film study.

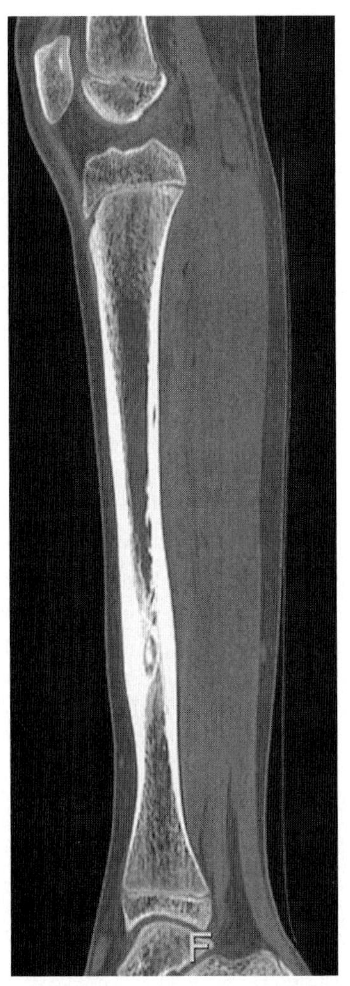

FIGURE 19-12 Osteoid osteoma. Sagittal reconstruction from 2-mm axial images shows cortical reaction and calcified nidus of lesion.

Patient Positioning

The area being imaged must be placed as close to the center of the gantry as possible and away from the body (if possible) to minimize scatter artifacts. For studies of deformities or leg-length studies, the ankles should be taped in the neutral (usually upright) position to eliminate movement and artifacts. Both legs should be as parallel to each other as possible. Always scan both extremities at the same time for leg length, tibial torsion, and femoral anteversion studies.

Technical Considerations

Because most cases of osseous tumors and infections are better evaluated by MRI, it should always be considered whether MRI is the more appropriate examination for the patient. IV contrast should be used whenever there is a question of soft tissue mass or infection. Contrast generally does not help for evaluation of the bone.

MDCT has eliminated the need to scan patients in multiple planes. A single isotropic acquisition can be performed and reconstructed to the desired planes on the scanner or workstation. It is therefore very important to use thin slice images whenever possible. Scans should be reconstructed with both a soft tissue and a bone filter. Bone algorithm produces higher quality multiplanar reconstructions,

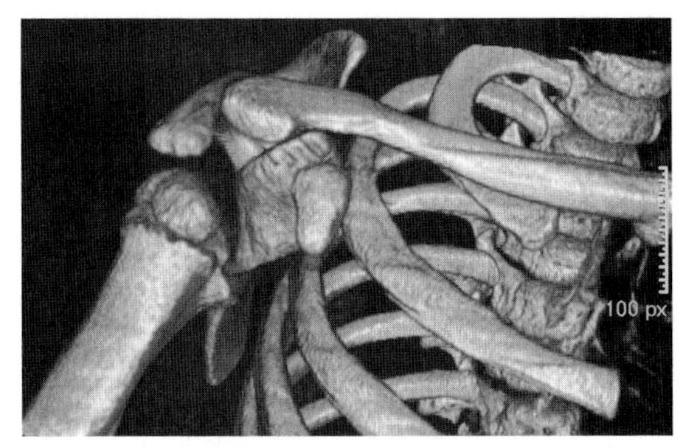

FIGURE 19-13 Chronic shoulder dislocation. Bone surface reconstruction clearly shows dysplastic glenoid and posterior dislocation of the flattened humeral head.

but the soft tissue algorithm produces smoother, better-looking 3D images.

Scans for alignment (e.g., tibial torsion) and leg-length studies can be done with a minimal radiation dose because high bone detail is not needed in these types of studies. All patients should have aggressive shielding of the body adjacent to the area being scanned.

Scanning Protocols

Generalized protocols for musculoskeletal CT are presented in Tables 19-8 through 19-10.

CT ANGIOGRAPHY

CTA and MRA have replaced diagnostic catheter angiography in children for almost all indications. Advantages of MRA include no ionizing radiation and no need for iodinated contrast. CTA, however, is much faster (better patient tolerance, less motion artifact) and has higher spatial resolution,

TABLE 19-8 Pediatric Bone Protocol: Technique for Four-Channel Multidetector Computed Tomography

Scan Parameter	Infant (<15 kg)	Toddler (15-25 kg)	Child (25-40 kg)	Teenager
Scan mode	Helical	Helical	Helical	Helical
Coverage	ROI	Same	Same	Same
Gantry rotation speed	0.5 second	0.5 second	0.5 second	0.5 second
Detector slice thickness	0.5-2.5 mm	0.5-2.5 mm	0.5-2.5 mm	0.5-2.5 mm
Pitch	Variable	Variable	Variable	Variable
Kilovolts	80	80-100	100	120
mA	40	50-70	70-90	120+
Reconstruction slice thickness	2 mm	2 mm	2 mm	2 mm
Reconstruction interval	2 mm	2 mm	2 mm	2 mm
Algorithm	Soft tissue, bone	Soft tissue, bone	Soft tissue, bone	Soft tissue, bone
Multiplanar reconstructions (as needed)	Coronal, sagittal, 3D	Coronal, sagittal, 3D	Coronal, sagittal, 3D	Coronal, sagittal, 3D
Contrast volume (if needed)	2 ml/kg	2 ml/kg	2 ml/kg	2 ml/kg

TABLE 19-9 Pediatric Bone Protocol: Technique for 16- and 64-Channel Multidetector Computed Tomography

Scan Parameter	Infant (<15 kg)	Toddler (15-25 kg)	Child (25-40 kg)	Teenager
Scan mode	Helical	Helical	Helical	Helical
Coverage	ROI	Same	Same	Same
Gantry rotation speed	0.4-0.5 second	0.4-0.5 second	0.4-0.5 second	0.4-0.5 second
Detector slice thickness	0.5-2.5 mm	0.5-2.5 mm	0.5-2.5 mm	0.5-2.5 mm
Pitch	Variable	Variable	Variable	Variable
Kilovolts	80	80-100	100	120
mA	40	50-70	70-90	120+
Reconstruction slice thickness	2 mm	2 mm	2 mm	2 mm
Reconstruction interval	2 mm	2 mm	2 mm	2 mm
Algorithm	Soft tissue, bone	Soft tissue, bone	Soft tissue, bone	Soft tissue, bone
Multiplanar reconstructions (as needed)	Coronal, sagittal, 3D	Coronal, sagittal, 3D	Coronal, sagittal, 3D	Coronal, sagittal, 3D
Contrast volume (if needed)	2 ml/kg	2 ml/kg	2 ml/kg	2 ml/kg

TABLE 19-10 Special Cases for Musculoskeletal Computed Tomography

	Scan Region (Scan Both Extremities at the Same Time)	Kilovolts/mA	Detector/Slice Reconstruction Interval
Leg-length discrepancy	Entire leg (above hip through ankle joint)	80-120 kV 40 mA	2.5-mm detector at 10-mm intervals
Femoral anteversion	(1)Femoral head and neck (Skip diaphysis) (2) Femoral condyles	Same	Same
Tibial torsion	(1)Tibial plateau (Skip diaphysis) (2) Tibial-talar joint (include fibula in field of view)	Same	Same

kV, Kilovolts.

which is important to evaluate small vessels in infants and children.

Indications

CTA is useful throughout the head and body primarily to evaluate vascular anomalies such as aberrant vessels, aneurysms and vascular malformations, and manifestations of congenital or acquired diseases such as sickle cell anemia, vasculitis, and thrombotic states (Figs. 19-14 and 19-15). CTA is also the test of choice for traumatic vascular injury.

Patient Positioning and Preparation

High-quality CTA requires motion-free images for 3D reconstructions. To this end, proper immobilization of the patient is essential. Infants can usually be immobilized without the need for sedation.

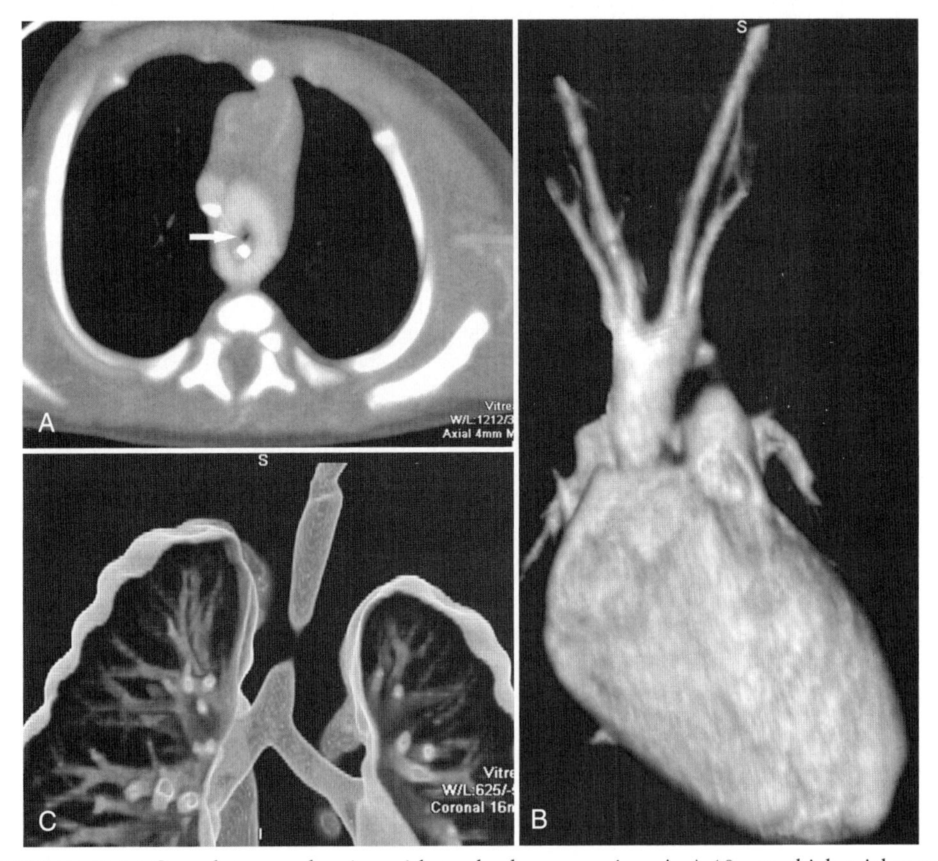

FIGURE 19-14 Complete vascular ring with tracheal compression. **A,** A 10-mm thick axial maximum intensity projection image demonstrates a complete vascular ring. The trachea *(white arrow)* is seen as a tiny dot of air. The esophagus has a high-density NG tube within it. The volume-rendered image **(B)** demonstrates a double aortic arch. The two arches are nearly symmetrical and both give rise to a subclavian and a carotid artery. Thin slab (11 mm) volume-rendered image with high transparency **(C)** shows a very high-grade tracheal compression resulting from the vascular ring.

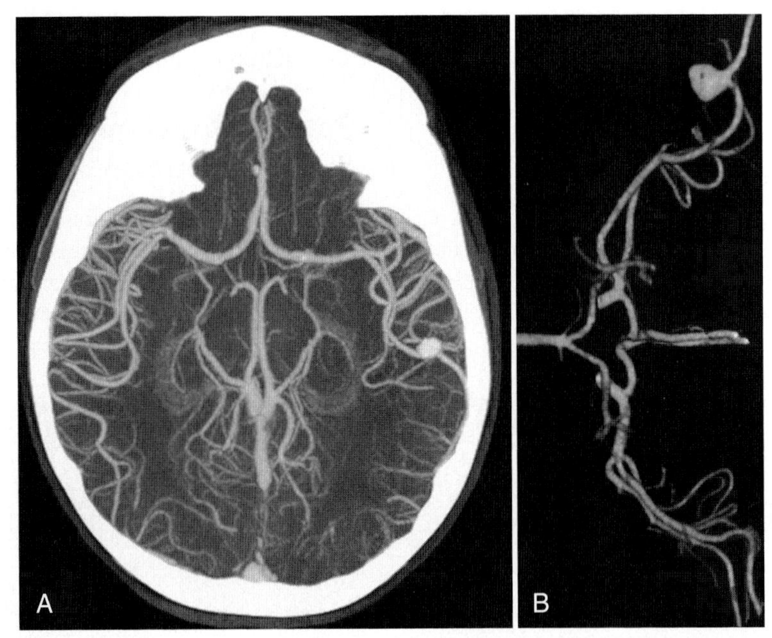

FIGURE 19-15 Mycotic middle cerebral artery aneurysm. Axial maximum intensity projection image **(A)** shows an aneurysm arising from a left peripheral middle cerebral artery branch artery. The relationship of the aneurysm to the vessel is better demonstrated on the volume-rendered image **(B)**.

Toddlers and young children may require sedation to obtain a good-quality study. CTA in older children can often be performed without sedation if proper coaching and parental support is provided. Older children should also be coached in breath holding, which is particularly important in chest studies.

For studies of the abdomen, it is important that patients do not receive any oral contrast because this will interfere with 3D reconstructions.

Technical Considerations

Successful CTA requires optimization of scan technique and contrast administration. Speed is important for image acquisition to minimize motion artifacts and maximize coverage and contrast density. The shortest rotation time available on the scanner should be used. Pitch values of 1.25 to 1.5 will also reduce scan time. Slice thickness is a trade-off between resolution and scan time (coverage). This can require a difficult decision with a four-slice scanner but is usually not a factor with 16-slice scanners. In general, the thinnest slice thickness that will allow adequate coverage within an appropriate scan time should be used.

Proper delivery of contrast media is essential for CTA. Power injection with a rate of at least 2 ml per second (3 ml/second is preferred) is strongly recommended. This can be easily achieved with a 22-gauge peripheral IV and occasionally achieved with a 24-gauge IV if the catheter is in an adequate vein. Hand injection and butterfly needles are not recommended for CTA. High-density contrast such as 350 to 380 mg of iodine per ml is also recommended because this will improve vascular enhancement.

The timing of the scan should be initiated with bolus-tracking software whenever possible because this will minimize the chance of error caused by mistiming the bolus. Scans can be triggered either manually on the basis of the visual

TABLE 19-11 Pediatric Computed Tomography Angiography Protocols: Techniques for Four-Slice Multidetector Computed Tomography

Parameters	Cerebral	Cardiothoracic	Abdominal
Detector slice thickness	1-2.5 mm	1-2.5 mm	1-2.5 mm
Pitch	1.2	1.2-1.5	1.2-1.5
Reconstructed slice thickness	1-2.5 mm	1-2.5 mm	1-2.5 mm
Reconstructed slice interval	1-1.5 mm	1-1.5 mm	1-1.5 mm
Gantry rotation time	0.5 second	0.5 second	0.5 second
Voltage	120 kV	120 kV	120 kV
Tube current	50-120 mA	50-120 mA	50-120 mA
Injection rate	2-3 ml/second	2-3 ml/second	2-3 ml/second
Scan timing	Bolus tracking	Bolus tracking	Bolus tracking
Reconstruction algorithm	Soft tissue	Soft tissue	Soft tissue
Contrast volume	2-3 ml/kg	2-3 ml/kg	2-3 ml/kg

appearance of the vessel or automatically when a certain threshold for HU is achieved. Empirical delays can also be used but will need to be varied depending on the size of the patient, the body part scanned, the IV site, the injection rate, and the presence of certain medical conditions such as heart disease.

After the scan, the thinnest slice thickness available should be reconstructed on the scanner and sent to PACS or the 3D workstation to allow for postprocessing of the images. Overlapping reconstructions are also helpful to improve reconstruction quality if the slice thickness of the data acquisition is greater than 1 mm.

Scanning Protocols

Generalized CTA protocols for four-, 16-, and 64-slice scanners are presented in Tables 19-11 and 19-12.

TABLE 19-12 Pediatric Computed Tomography Angiography Protocols: Techniques for 16- and 64-Slice Multidetector Computed Tomography

Parameters	Cerebral	Cardiothoracic	Abdominal
Detector slice thickness	0.5-0.75 mm	0.5 - 1.25 mm	0.5 - 1.25 mm
Pitch	1.2	1.2-1.5	1.2-1.5
Reconstructed slice thickness	0.5-0.75 mm	0.5 - 1.25 mm	0.5 - 1.25 mm
Reconstructed slice interval	0.5 mm	0.5-1 mm	0.5-1 mm
Gantry rotation time	0.5 second	0.5 second	0.5 second
Voltage	120 kV	120 kV	120 kV
Tube current	50-120 mA	50-120 mA	50-120 mA
Injection rate	2-3 ml/second	2-3 ml/second	2-3 ml/second
Scan timing	Bolus tracking	Bolus tracking	Bolus tracking
Reconstruction Algorithm	Soft tissue	Soft tissue	Soft tissue
Contrast volume	2-3 ml/kg	2-3 ml/kg	2-3 ml/kg

ADDITIONAL READINGS

Aitken GF et al: Leg length determination by CT digital radiograph, *AJR Am J Roentgenol* 144: 613-615, 1985.

Brenner DJ et al: Estimated risks of radiation-induced fatal cancer from pediatric CT, *AJR Am J Roentgenol* 176:289-296, 2001.

Chan FP et al: MDCT angiography of pediatric vascular diseases of the abdomen, pelvis, and extremities, *Pediatr Radiol* 35:40-53, 2005.

Daneman A: *Pediatric body CT*, New York, 1987, Springer-Verlag.

Donelly LF et al: Minimizing radiation dose for pediatric body applications of single-detector helical CT, *AJR Am J Roentgenol* 176:303-306, 2001.

Flodmark O et al: Periventricular leukomalacia radiologic diagnosis, *Radiology* 162:119-124, 1987.

Frush D, Donnelly LF: Helical CT in children: technical considerations and body applications, *Radiology* 209:37-48, 1998.

Frush D et al: Challenges of pediatric spiral CT, *Radiographics* 17:939-959, 1997.

Huda W et al: An approach for the estimation of effective radiation dose at CT in pediatric patients, *Radiology* 203:417-422, 1997.

Jacob RP et al: Tibial torsion calculated by computerized tomography, *J Bone Joint Surg* 62B:238-242, 1980.

Jacquenier M et al: Acetabular anteversion in children, *J Pediatr Orthop* 12:373-375, 1992.

Keeter S et al: Sedation in pediatric CT: national survey of current practice, *Radiology* 175:745-752, 1990.

Patterson A et al: Helical CT scan of the body: are settings adjusted for pediatric patients? *AJR Am J Roentgenol* 176:297-301, 2001.

Siegel MJ: Multiplanar and three-dimensional multidetector row CT of thoracic vessels and airways in the pediatric population, *Radiology* 229:641-650, 2003.

Ozonoff MB: *Pediatric orthopedic radiology*, ed 2, Philadelphia, 1992, WB Saunders.

Chapter 20

Quality Control for Computed Tomography Scanners

Mahadevappa Mahesh

Chapter Outline

WHAT IS QUALITY CONTROL?

What is quality control (QC), and how does it relate to computed tomography (CT) scanners? For CT scanners, *QC* may be defined as a program that periodically tests the performance of a CT scanner and compares its performance with some standard. If the scanner is performing suboptimally, then steps must be initiated to correct the problem. The goal of a QC program is to ensure that every image created by the CT scanner is a quality image. High-quality images provide the radiologist maximum information, improve the chances for correct diagnosis, and ultimately contribute to quality patient care.

The definition of QC consists of two parts. Quality assurance requires a measurement of the CT scanner's performance to ensure that the scanner is operating at some acceptable level. Unfortunately, quality assurance does not prescribe what to do if the standards are not met. Quality control carries the concept of quality assurance one step further—if the quality is inadequate, then steps are taken to correct the problem.

This simple definition does not attempt to describe how such a program might work or how to apply QC to a CT scanner. However, the remainder of this chapter describes aspects of a QC program for CT scanners and includes descriptions of some tests that have proven useful in QC testing. Descriptions of the testing instruments, an outline of necessary measurements, and hints on interpretation of the results are presented.

This chapter describes a generic QC program that can be adapted to almost any CT scanner system. As part of the purchase package, CT manufacturers often prescribe a daily QC program for use on their CT systems. Sometimes their QC program includes a specially furnished phantom or test object to be imaged with selected techniques. In some cases, internal software is used to interpret the measurements and to notify the operator of unsatisfactory results.

Unfortunately, manufacturers' tests are often restricted to images from one or two scans. The amount of information that can be gained from the images is limited. The tests described later in this chapter can be used to augment or to replace the manufacturers' tests. The information gained from these augmentation tests may prove useful in the assessment of additional aspects of the scanner's performance.

Many tests are based on QC tests published in the literature (Cacak, 1985; Burkhart et al, 1987; Cacak and Hendee, 1979; McCollough et al, 2004) and described in Report 99 of the National Council on Radiation Protection and Measurement (1988). More complex physics tests are outlined in Report 39 of the American Association of Physics in Medicine (1993). Although the tests are similar to those described in these references, the types and frequency of the QC tests may vary somewhat to reflect advances in CT scanner technology. One recent and significant advance of CT scanner technology has been the introduction of spiral/helical CT scanners. The "wind-up" cables that connect the moving and stationary parts of the CT scanner are eliminated through a series of sliding electrical contacts, or slip rings. Because no cables follow the moving part of the scanner, it is no longer necessary to stop and unwind the twisting cables after every scan. Consequently, the heavy motors, brakes, and clutches can be made lighter and the moving sections can be rotated faster, which allows for shorter scan times. These scanners can make a complete revolution of an x-ray tube (and sometimes detectors) in 0.5 second or less. Some CT scanners have multiple rows of detectors, which allow them to acquire data for several scan planes simultaneously. With this multiple-row detector computed tomography system, many images can be acquired very quickly. For example, if a CT scanner has 16 sets of detectors and can complete one revolution in 0.5 second, then 32 images can be acquired in 1 second. This is incredibly fast compared with the CT scanners from only a few years ago.

Because of their sliding electrical contacts, continuously rotating x-ray tube and detectors do not need to stop at the end of each scan. If necessary, the x-ray tube can merely stop the production of x rays while the bed advances to the next scan location. In fact, most CT scanners do not stop x-ray production to move the bed but instead allow the bed and patient to move continuously as the x-ray tube continues to rotate and data are collected. The pattern of the x-ray beam as it winds around the patient in a screw-like fashion is sometimes called *spiral/helical scanning*. Most of the QC tests described here are applicable to both spiral/helical CT scanners and more conventional scan-and-stop scanners. However, when tests involve a phantom, the alignment of the phantom to the x-ray beam is much easier if these QC tests are performed in the stationary-bed, single-scan mode. For most tests, the measurements performed in the stationary-bed mode closely resemble measurements performed in the spiral/helical mode.

Generally, some absolute standard of imaging performance exists that should be exceeded by the CT scanner. For example, the CT scanner may be required to always resolve a certain size (presumably small) object in a clinical image. Therefore, the QC program sets up an internal standard for high-contrast resolution capabilities of the scanner (e.g., the CT scanner must be able to image high-contrast objects at least as small as 0.75 millimeter [mm]). If the performance is below this standard (i.e., it cannot resolve small objects), then the scanner must be adjusted or repaired.

Some tests are too complex and require too much time for routine use. When a new CT scanner is installed, detailed acceptance test should be performed with the help of a medical physicist before patient scanning. The measurements performed at the time of acceptance test forms the baseline for future comparison of the scanner's performance. Depending on the skill, comfort level, and available time, the QC technician can select the tests to be performed and their frequency. A majority of the tests described in this chapter are designed to be performed by radiation technologists. For more complex tests, help can be sought from a medical physicist.

Experience has shown that if a QC program is to be effective, the tests must be objective, quantitative, easy, and quick. If the test results determine that the scanner is working at an acceptable level, then the results are merely recorded. If the results demonstrate that the scanner is not functioning well, alternative corrective procedures should be followed. The tests in this chapter suggest some alternative procedures to follow when acceptable limits are exceeded.

WHY QUALITY CONTROL?

The answer to the question, "Is a QC program needed for the CT scanner?" is usually "yes." Progressive hospitals and clinics that operate CT scanners and other complex instruments have long recognized the value of QC programs to maintain high performance standards for their patients. In addition, regulatory agencies increasingly demand that some standard of quality be maintained on x-ray units and other equipment that can potentially harm patients if the units are not performing optimally. These agencies frequently require that institutions using CT scanners verify the scanner's performance periodically (e.g., daily, monthly, annually) and often prescribe alternative measures if the performance standards are not met. To meet these regulatory requirements, a QC program must be operational.

In the case of CT scanners, the engineering is exceedingly complex. With so many mechanical and electronic parts involved in the creation of the images, there are many opportunities for the quality of the images to subtly and unnoticeably degrade. The mechanical parts of these complex, heavy instruments can wear slowly. Electronic parts can change characteristics and drift out of optimal adjustment. When this occurs, the CT scanner may no longer yield the same quality images as it did when it was in proper adjustment. Often, this wear and drift can be repaired or compensated, but the suboptimal imaging problems must first be recognized. Comparing modern

QC data with past data can demonstrate that the scanner is not performing as well as in the past.

A quality control program can be an important ally in many aspects of CT scanner service. For example, if the QC data are used to define the problem and its extent, the service person will be better able to correct a subtle image quality problem. If a measurable change can be quantitatively demonstrated to the service person, the necessity of repair will be more apparent, and the degree to which it should be repaired can be specified (i.e., "we want it to perform like new" or "as good as last August").

Often a QC program can result in reduced downtime. A good QC program may recognize weakened or marginally performing parts before complete failure, and unscheduled service may be avoided.

PRINCIPLES OF QUALITY CONTROL

Three basic tenets of quality control are as follows:

1. The QC must be performed on a regular periodic basis. Ideally, these tests might be performed between each patient examination. At this testing frequency, there would be maximal insurance that the CT scanner was always operating correctly. However, in reality, this very frequent QC attention is too costly in terms of the time taken from patient examinations. Some compromises must be made for the sake of time and effort.

It does seem prudent to perform certain quick tests on a daily basis. Less-important or more time-consuming tests might be performed less frequently (e.g., monthly), and the most complex tests might be performed semiannually or yearly. The institution's philosophy and its willingness to devote time to periodic QC tests often dictate which tests are performed and how often. To an administrator watching the revenues generated by a CT scanner, QC has a double affliction of requiring labor, which must be paid, and reducing the availability of the CT scanner for patients, which reduces revenue. A compromise must be reached that balances the effort and expense of a QC program with the expected benefits, such as better images, consistent images, reduced downtime, and legal and regulatory requirements.

2. The second tenet is prompt interpretation of the measurements. Data usually show that the CT scanner is operating within specified guidelines. But on those occasions when it is not, this fact must be recognized and some remedial action must be taken. This action may be as simple as notifying the physicist, service person, or radiologist, or it may be as aggressive as taking the unit out of service until it is repaired. But to institute this facet of the QC program, the person making the test must be able to recognize that the results are outside acceptable limits. Some mechanism should be in place that alerts the QC technician to errant behavior of the scanner. For example, on the data form for a particular test, acceptable limits of the data may be stated. From an inspection of the measured results, the QC technician can recognize immediately that the results are out of tolerance. Another method is to enter data into a computer, then instruct the computer to issue an appropriate alert when limits are exceeded. In the latter case, the temptation to sit on data for a few days or weeks before they are entered into the computer must be avoided. If a computer is to be relied on to make the necessary comparisons and if the program is to be effective, the data must be entered promptly.
3. The third tenet of good QC is faithful bookkeeping. If time and effort are to be expended to perform the tests, then the results should be recorded. These results should be maintained in a logbook, data form, or computer for a reasonable period, usually as long as the CT scanner is active (i.e., for its lifetime). Keeping good records is not just a tedious

exercise. These results will prove invaluable if the unit appears to be malfunctioning some time in the future. A comparison of past measurements with current results can easily demonstrate a change in performance (usually degradation). These data can also prove important to defend a lawsuit that might arise because of a reading of a CT image. For example, if litigation arises that is dependent on an interpretation (or misinterpretation) of a CT image and data can be produced from the QC logbook to demonstrate that the CT scanner was functioning satisfactorily at the time of interpretation, then the CT scanner is removed as a source of blame for the interpretation.

QUALITY CONTROL TESTS FOR CT SCANNERS

The methods described in the remainder of this chapter provide some details of the testing procedure, the equipment required, interpretation of the results, some suggestions for acceptable limits, and how often the test should be performed. The tests are listed in approximate order of importance, with some weighting of the tests according to the ability to perform the test quickly and easily.

Choosing a Technique for Quality Control Measurements

The selection of technique for the QC tests depends on the type of CT scanner and the test being performed. Many variables can be selected for each test, including peak kilovoltage (kVp), milliamperage (mA), scan time, slice width, type of algorithm, x-ray filter type, and focal spot size. The number of possible combinations of techniques is usually overwhelming, and the best that can be done is to select one or two representative techniques. In general, the technique should remain the same for a specific test from day to day. However, the technique for one test does not have to be the same as the technique for other tests. A good rule of thumb is to use a technique that matches a frequently used clinical technique. One method to select a QC technique is to choose the most frequently used head or body technique and use it for the tests. As many tests as possible should be performed with this technique, with the understanding that deviations may be required for some tests.

Test Frequency

It is usually necessary to limit the more complex tests to annual surveys, those occasions when the CT scanner is being initially tested for acceptance, and subsequent occasions when the deterioration of image quality is suspected. It is good practice to repeat appropriate tests after replacement of a major component such as an x-ray tube or after the performance of extensive service or adjustments. If data from CT scanner images are used quantitatively or if the precision of an image is used for accurately localizing tissue (e.g., to perform biopsies or plan radiation therapy treatment), the frequency of appropriate tests should be increased.

Limits of a "Passing" Test

What are acceptable limits? How big should the window of acceptable values be for each test described here before the CT scanner is considered "out of tolerance"? These complex questions depend on the technology of the unit being tested, the type of test instrument being used, and the imaging technique.

Perhaps more important than the actual value of the measured variable is a change in the variable between measurements. A CT scanner that is operating the same today as it did yesterday should produce nearly the same results when the test is repeated. After acceptable limits are established, a quick inspection of the measurements can identify deviant values. Past history can provide good insight into what the values have been. A range

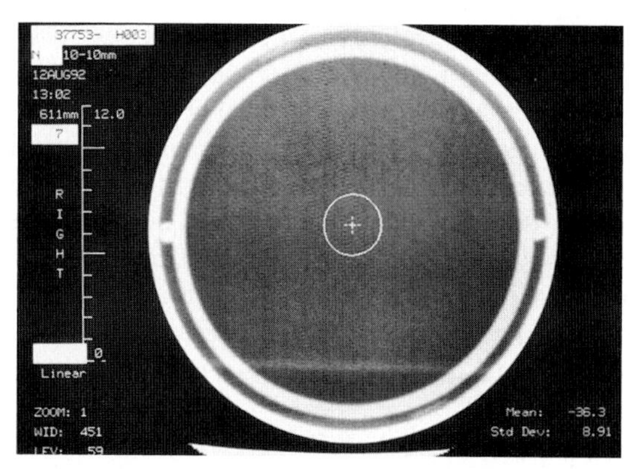

FIGURE 20-1 CT scanner image of a uniform water phantom. The ROI is placed in the center of the water-filled phantom to measure the average CT number and the standard deviation of the CT numbers inside the ROI. In this case, the average or "mean" CT number measures −36.3, which is not acceptable.

that includes most values when the unit was operating optimally can be easily determined from an inspection of past values. Of course, it is never absolutely certain that the CT scanner was operating optimally in the past when these supposedly "good" readings were taken. But if the readings were taken when the unit was new or believed to be functioning well, then they can be presumed to be "good" readings and used as a standard. Some generic limits are suggested in the following sections.

Quality Control Tests

QC tests are proposed in this section. Suggestions are given regarding the following: phantom or equipment, expected results, acceptance limits, possible causes of failure, and frequency of tests.

TEST 1 Average Computed Tomography Number of Water (Computed Tomography Number Calibration)

PHANTOM OR EQUIPMENT: A simple water-filled cylindrical plastic container about 20 centimeters (cm) in diameter. Commercial phantoms are available for this test and are often provided by the CT manufacturer, but some institutions have used 1-gallon plastic containers from liquid laundry bleach. The bleach, of course, is replaced with water.

MEASUREMENT: Take an axial scan through the water phantom at the usual technique. Reconstruct the image of the water phantom. Examine the region of interest (ROI) feature available on the imaging monitor of most scanners to verify that the scanner can measure the average of the CT numbers of the pixels inside the ROI. Enlarge the ROI area to include an area of about 2 to 3 cm^2 (or about 200 to 300 pixels). Position the ROI near the center of the phantom image and measure the average CT number (Fig. 20-1).

Two media that serve as calibration points for CT numbers are water and air. Occasionally (e.g., once a month), move the ROI outside the phantom into the region of the image that is known to contain air. Check the average CT number of air. It should be −1000 if the CT scanner is calibrated properly.

EXPECTED RESULTS: The average CT number of water should be very close to zero.

ACCEPTANCE LIMITS: If the average CT number of water is more than 3 CT numbers away from 0 (i.e., outside the range −3 to ++3), the CT scanner fails the test. The CT number of air should be −1000 ± 5.

POSSIBLE CAUSES OF FAILURE: Miscalibration of the algorithm that generates the CT number. If a recalibration does not help, notify the service person. Usually the manufacturer provides a procedure to recalibrate the CT number scale.

FREQUENCY: This should be performed at the time of installation as part of acceptance test and daily thereafter.

TEST 2 Standard Deviation of Computed Tomography Number in Water

PHANTOM OR EQUIPMENT: A simple water-filled cylindrical plastic container about

20 cm in diameter (the same phantom used in Test 1).

MEASUREMENT: Use the same image as in Test 1 (see Fig. 20-1). Position the ROI near the center of the phantom image and measure the standard deviation of the CT number.

EXPECTED RESULTS: Typical values are in the range of two to seven CT numbers. The actual value will depend on the dose at the location of the ROI, which depends on the kVp, mA, scan duration, slice width, and phantom size. The standard deviation of the CT number also depends on the type of reconstruction algorithm (can be higher with sharp algorithm compared with smooth algorithm) and the position of the ROI (slightly smaller at the edge of the phantom compared with the center). Ensure that the technique is the same each day and that the standard deviation is measured at the same place each time (e.g., the center of the phantom).

ACCEPTANCE LIMITS: Ideally, the standard deviation should be very small. The actual acceptance limits must be determined by examination of past measurements that were presumably performed when the performance of the CT scanner was good. The technique must stay the same for this measurement from day to day. If the standard deviation starts to increase, this indicates a "noisier" image with more variation in pixel-to-pixel CT numbers and poorer low-contrast resolution.

POSSIBLE CAUSES OF FAILURE: Something is causing a noisier image, such as decreased dose (x-ray tube output) or increased electronic noise of the x-ray detectors, amplifiers, or A/D (analog-to-digital) converters. Notify the service person.

FREQUENCY: This should be performed at the time of installation as part of acceptance test and daily thereafter.

TEST 3 High-Contrast Resolution

PHANTOM OR EQUIPMENT: High-contrast (contrast difference of 10% or greater) resolution pattern in an imaging phantom. Although a variety of patterns are available to perform high-contrast tests, including patterns for generating modulation transfer function measurements, a quick and easy test pattern is most suitable for QC tests. One such pattern consists of a series of rows of holes drilled in plastic (Fig. 20-2). Each row contains a set of holes (usually five) of constant diameter with the centers of the holes two diameters apart. The holes decrease in size from one row to the next. If the holes are drilled in acrylic and filled with water, the contrast is about 20%. If the holes are filled with air, the contrast is about 100%. Either filling is satisfactory. Another pattern consists of eight aluminum bar patterns (4-12 line pairs/cm) embedded in a tissue equivalent material.

MEASUREMENT: On the axial CT image (Fig. 20-3), determine the smallest row of holes in which all holes can be clearly seen. The smaller the holes that can be clearly seen,

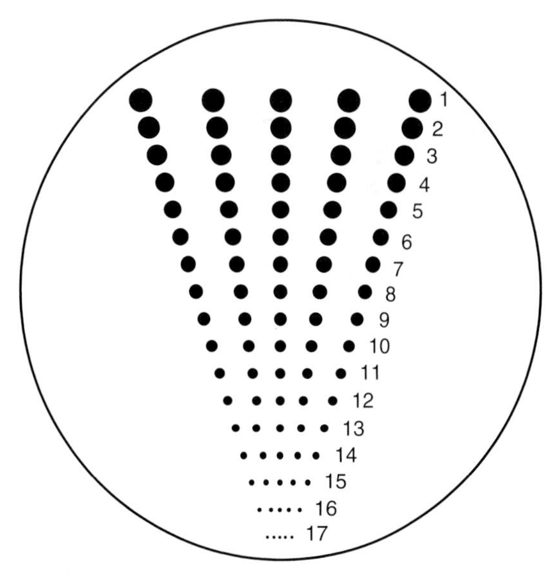

FIGURE 20-2 Hole pattern for a high-contrast phantom test object. The test pattern consists of rows of holes of various sizes drilled in plastic. Each row contains five holes of the same diameter. In a row of constant sizes, the holes are separated by two diameters from center to center.

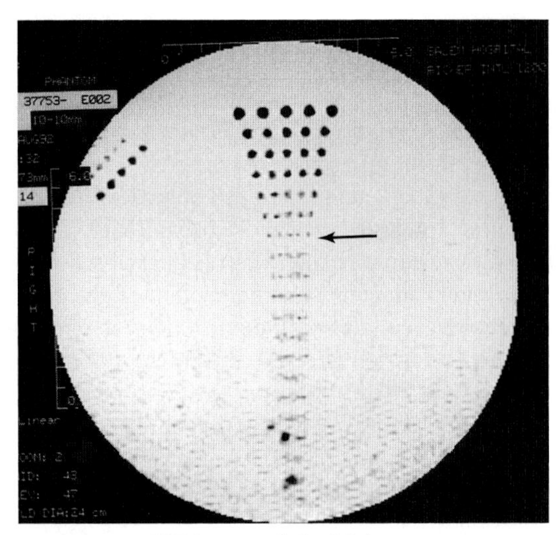

FIGURE 20-3 CT image of the high-contrast test pattern shown in Figure 20-2. The CT scanner is judged by the smallest row in which all five holes can be seen *(arrow)*.

the better the performance of the CT scanner. Be certain that all holes can be seen in the image. Sometimes it appears that one fewer hole is seen in the row than is actually in the phantom. This is usually a phase reversal phenomenon and should not be counted as a complete set of holes. On the other hand, the bar pattern where the bars and spaces are distinctly visualized indicates the level of high-contrast resolution.

EXPECTED RESULTS: Most modern CT scanners have a high-contrast resolving power slightly smaller than 1 mm by using a typical head image technique. Therefore, they will be able to visualize a complete set of holes in some of the rows in the range of 0.75 to 1.0 mm. With the highest resolution technique available to a particular scanner, some CT scanner manufacturers claim to be able to visualize holes as small as 0.25 mm.

ACCEPTANCE LIMITS: This baseline number should be established at the time of the acceptance test when the CT scanner is working well by scanning the phantom and noting the smallest set of holes that can be seen. This initial measurement becomes the baseline for future tests. Subsequent tests can be compared with this baseline. Alternatively, the manufacturer's specifications for this test can be used to verify that the performance of the CT scanner is at least as good as the specifications.

POSSIBLE CAUSES OF FAILURE: Enlarged focal spot in the x-ray tube, excessive mechanical wear in the motion of the gantry, mechanical misalignments or poor registration of electromechanical components, vibrations, or detector failures. If the resolution has degraded from the baseline, inform the service person.

FREQUENCY: This should be performed at the time of installation as part of acceptance test and biannually thereafter.

TEST 4 Low-Contrast Resolution

PHANTOM OR EQUIPMENT: Low-contrast resolution pattern in imaging phantom. A quick and easy test pattern of low-contrast test objects consists of a series of holes (2 to 8 mm diameter) drilled in polystyrene. The holes are filled with liquid (often water) to which has been added a small amount some other material (usually methanol or sucrose) to bring the liquid's CT number close (about 0.5% different) to that of the plastic itself. One such pattern (Fig. 20-4) consists of a series of rows of holes drilled in relatively thick plastic. Each row contains holes of a constant diameter. The holes decrease in size from one row to the next. In a CT image, the holes appear to have a density similar to their surround (i.e., the holes have low contrast).

Another technique is to use partial voluming by making the plastic very thin (e.g., a plastic membrane). Low contrast in the image is achieved by a different principle than the solid plastic type of low-contrast phantom. The membrane type of phantom consists of a thin membrane containing a pattern of holes (the same pattern shown in Fig. 20-4). The membrane is stretched across a plane of the phantom and is then immersed in water. The CT x-ray beam, as visualized from its edge (Fig. 20-5), strikes mostly water. But a small fraction of the beam is absorbed by the plastic, forming a faint (low-contrast) image of the hole pattern. By varying the thickness of the plastic relative to the width of the x-ray beam, the contrast can be varied.

In both techniques, the contrast of the object is difficult to calculate. In QC testing, it is sufficient that the contrast be constant between tests. The contrast should be selected so that the standard test image shows about 50% of the holes. At that level of hole imaging, a decrease in low-contrast imaging performance will result in the visualization of fewer rows of holes.

MEASUREMENT: On the CT image, determine the smallest row of holes in which all holes can be clearly seen. The smaller the holes that can be seen at a particular technique, the better the performance of the CT scanner. A sample of a "low-noise" (high-dose) image and a "high-noise" (low-dose) image are shown in Figure 20-6. In the low-noise image, more sets of smaller objects can be seen.

EXPECTED RESULTS: The smallest holes that can be imaged by modern CT scanners should be 4 to 5 mm in diameter or smaller for 0.5% contrast objects. Perhaps more important, the minimum size of holes visualized should not increase over the life of the scanner.

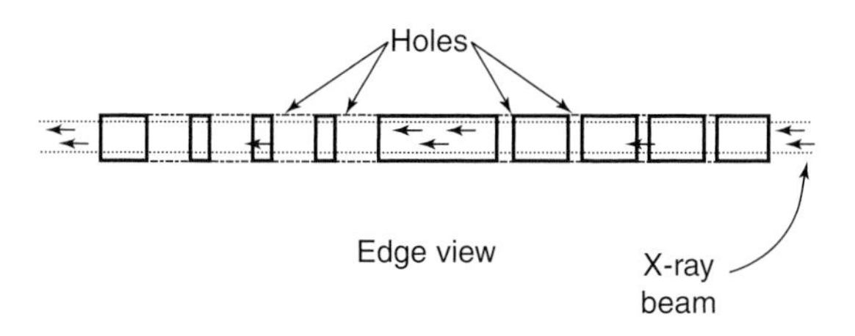

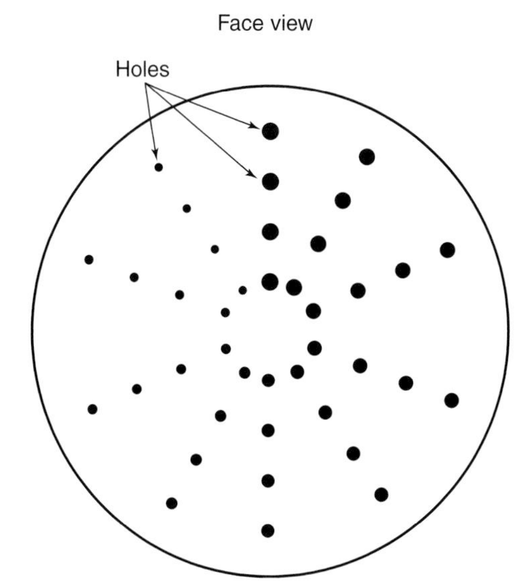

FIGURE 20-4 "Solid plastic" type of low-contrast phantom test object that consists of a pattern of holes (face view) drilled in a piece of plastic with the holes filled with liquid. The low-contrast aspect of this test object is achieved by adjusting the absorption characteristics of the water solution to nearly match (about 0.5% difference) the absorption of the plastic.

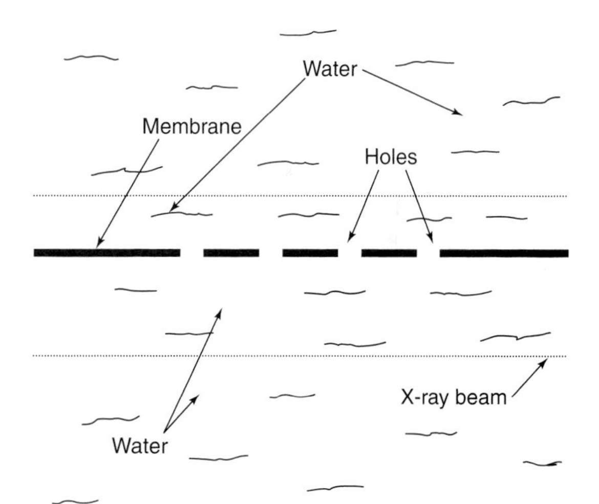

FIGURE 20-5 Edge view of a membrane of partial-volume type of low-contrast test object. The presence of the thin membrane alters the absorption characteristics very slightly wherever there is membrane. Where the membrane is not present (i.e., in the holes), the absorption is that of just water. The slight difference in absorption characteristics between the water and the water-plus-membrane combination produce a low-contrast test pattern that appears as the hole pattern in the membrane.

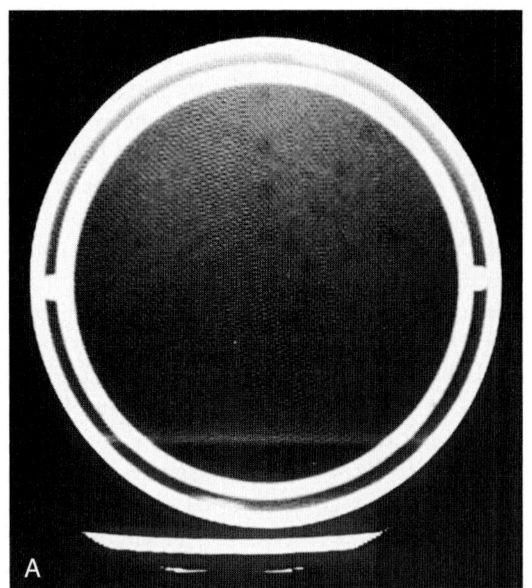

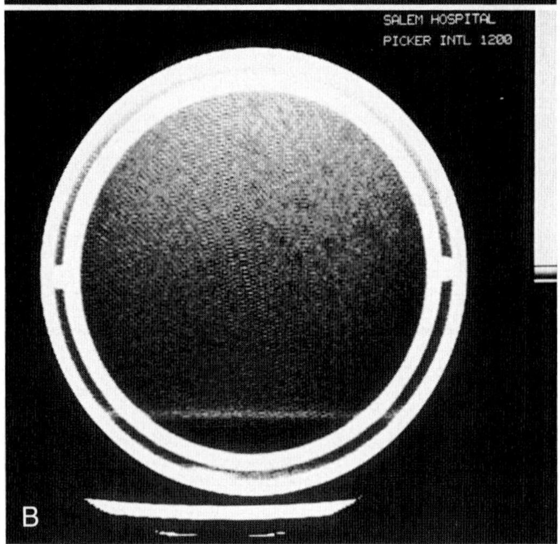

FIGURE 20-6 Low-noise **(A)** and high-nose **(B)** low-contrast images produced with a membrane-type low-contrast test object obtained from a high-dose (low noise) CT scan and a low-dose (high noise) type of scan.

ACCEPTANCE LIMITS: The number of holes that can be visualized varies widely between techniques. For example, if a partial volume phantom is used, the apparent contrast of the object depends on the thickness of the membrane and the slice width of the image. In addition, an increase in mA value of the scan technique will usually reduce the noise in the image and will permit smaller holes to be visualized. Therefore a baseline scan at a chosen technique (usually a commonly used head technique) performed when the scanner is functioning well can serve as baseline against which future images can be compared. This technique, once chosen, should not be changed from day to day.

A smoothing algorithm filter can also reduce the apparent statistical fluctuations between pixels. These algorithms produce images with smaller standard deviations and usually permit visualization of smaller low-contrast objects by sacrificing some high-contrast resolution. Therefore it is important to always use the same reconstruction algorithm to compare repeated results from this test.

POSSIBLE CAUSES OF FAILURE: A higher noise level in the image usually causes reduced low-contrast resolution. Some possible sources of increased noise are decreased dose, decreased mA values, or any other factor that will reduce the x-ray tube output, such as a tungsten coating build-up on the inside of older x-ray tubes. Increased electronic noise is also possible and may arise from noise in the x-ray detectors, amplifiers, or A/D converters. The service person should be informed of decreasing low-contrast resolution and asked to perform further diagnosis.

FREQUENCY: This should be performed at the time of installation as part of acceptance test and biannually thereafter.

TEST 5 Accuracy of Distance-Measuring Device

PHANTOM OR EQUIPMENT: An object with two or more small objects that have a precisely known spatial relationship (i.e., the distance between them is precisely known). One such object is a large "+" pattern of small holes in a plastic phantom (Fig. 20-7). The holes are precisely 1 cm apart, and the size of the "+" is large enough to fill most of the image.

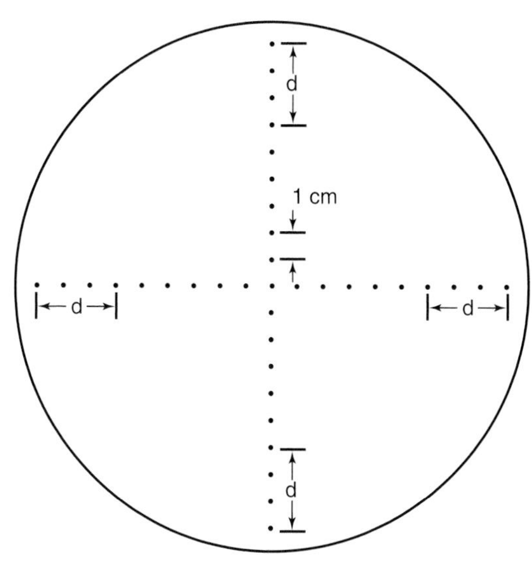

FIGURE 20-7 A pattern of holes to measure image distortion. The pattern consists of a series of holes arranged in a "++" pattern that spans the diameter of the phantom. The holes are exactly 1 cm apart.

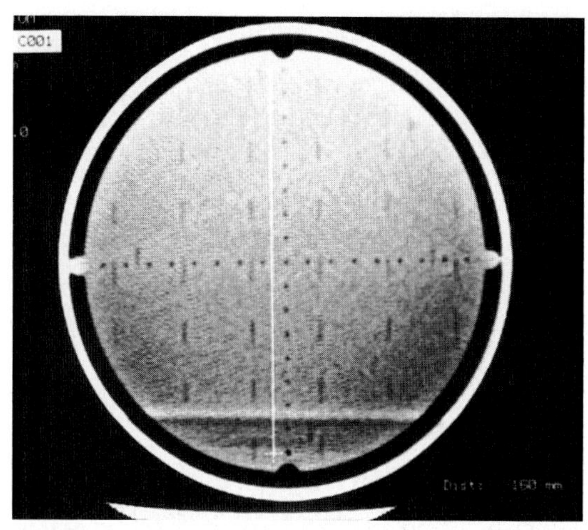

FIGURE 20-8 Testing the distance-measuring device by measuring the distance between two holes separated by a precisely known distance. In this case the measured distance *(Dist)* between two holes spaced 16 cm apart is 160 mm (perfect).

Some institutions have used an image of a regular square grid that covers most of the field of view. One source of square grids is a type of fluorescent light fixture that uses square grid light diffusers made of plastic with a square spacing of about 0.5 inch (12 mm). With a moderate amount of effort, the grids can be cut to fit inside a phantom or scanned in air (no phantom).

MEASUREMENT: With use of the distance-measuring feature available on the video monitors of most scanners, measure the distance between two well-visualized holes near the periphery of the phantom, one near the top and one near the bottom (Fig. 20-8). Repeat the measurement between two holes, moving right to left. If required, a diagonal measurement between two holes can be made and the true distance can be calculated by the Pythagorean theorem.

EXPECTED RESULTS: The distance indicated by the CT scanner should agree with the true distance as determined by counting the spaces between the two holes.

ACCEPTANCE LIMITS: Disagreement of 1 mm or less is good. Disagreement of greater than 2 mm should be corrected.

POSSIBLE CAUSES OF FAILURE: Reconstruction algorithm may be improperly calibrated. If the manufacturer has not provided the user with a means to recalibrate the algorithm, a service person should be notified.

FREQUENCY: This should be performed at the time of installation and annually thereafter.

TEST 6 Uniformity or Flatness of Computed Tomography Number

PHANTOM OR EQUIPMENT: A simple cylindrical plastic container about 20 cm in diameter (the same phantom used for Test 1).

MEASUREMENT: Using the ROI feature available on most CT scanners, measure the CT number of water near the top, bottom, right, and left of the phantom (Fig. 20-9). Use an ROI large enough to cover an area of 200 to 300 pixels. Compare with the measurement in Test 1.

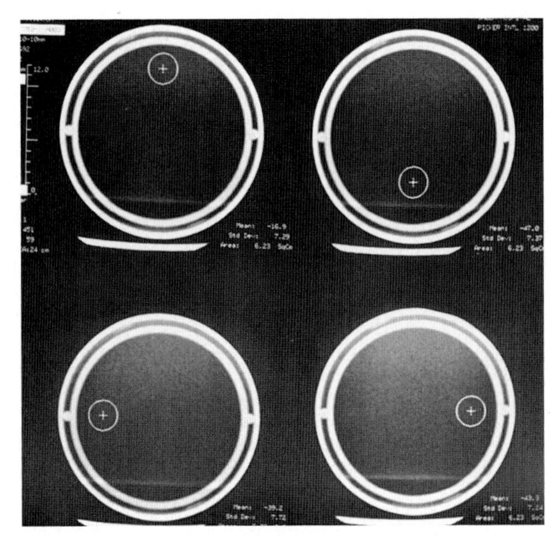

FIGURE 20-9 Use several ROIs to measure flatness. In a homogenous water phantom, the CT number should measure zero at any location in the phantom. In these images, the CT number at the top measures −16.9 and the rest of the image has values in the range of −37 to −47. This image is unacceptable because it is not "flat."

EXPECTED RESULTS: Ideally, the CT number of water will be zero at all points in the phantom.

ACCEPTANCE LIMITS: If the CT number anywhere in the phantom differs by more than five CT numbers from the average CT number collected from all measurements, then the CT image does not have a uniform or *flat* image. If the CT number is high in the center and low near the perimeter of the phantom, the image exhibits *capping*. A low value in the center relative to the edges exhibits *cupping*.

POSSIBLE CAUSES OF FAILURE: Often capping and cupping are the result of the hardening of the x-ray beam as it penetrates the phantom. Near the edges of the phantom, the x-ray beam does not penetrate as much phantom material, and the beam is softer (i.e., it has a lower average energy). To arrive at the center, the x rays must penetrate more phantom material and are harder near the center of the phantom. Because the effective energy of the x rays determines the absorption characteristics of the x rays, the absorption characteristics of water change slightly from center to edge in the phantom. Because the CT number is calculated from the number of x rays absorbed, slight differences in CT number may indicate differences of the average energy of the x-ray beam at various points in the phantom. Some CT scanners have software corrections built into the algorithm that compensate for these x-ray beam hardening effects, and these corrections sometimes overcompensate or undercompensate for the beam hardening. The service person may be able to adjust the algorithm to compensate for an unflat image.

FREQUENCY: This should be performed at the time of installation as part of acceptance test and monthly/biannually thereafter.

TEST 7 Hard Copy Output

PHANTOM OR EQUIPMENT: A stepped gray-scale image generated by the computer such as SMPTE (Society of Motion Picture and Television Engineers) pattern and a film densitometer.

MEASUREMENT: Display the SMPTE pattern on the display monitor. Adjust the display contrast so that both 95% and 100% patches are clearly separated. The 5% patch should just be visible inside of the 0% patch. The area of the 0% patch should be almost black. The 95% patch should be visible inside the 100% patch. Print the image and display on a viewbox to ensure the visibility of 5% and 95% patch (McCollough et al, 2004) (Fig. 20-10).

EXPECTED RESULTS: The same image should be reproduced with the hard copy device each time the image is recorded.

ACCEPTANCE LIMITS: If the hard copy image is unable to display both 5% and 95% patches, examine the display setting and also the printer setting. If the condition still exists, then investigate further with service person to reset the hard copy printer settings.

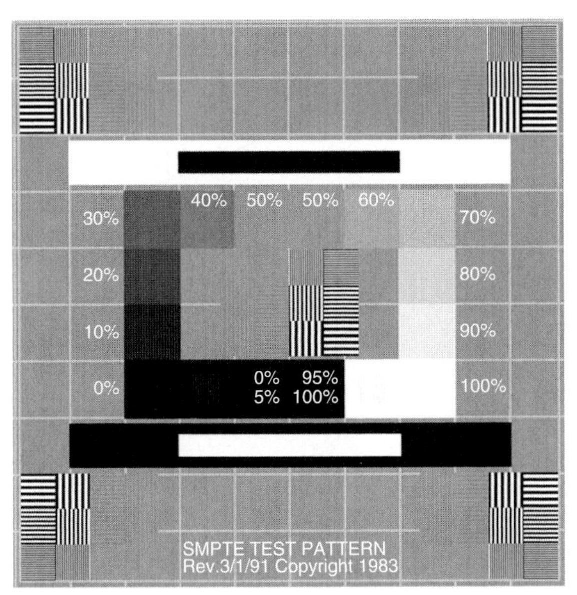

FIGURE 20-10 SMPTE image for checking hard copy output. A film image of this pattern is processed and visualized to examine the visibility of 5% and 95% squares. (From Carter CE, Veale BL: *Digital radiography and PACS*, St. Louis, 2008, Mosby/Elsevier.)

POSSIBLE CAUSES OF FAILURE: Most frequently, drifts in the optical density of films from the camera can be traced to problems in the film processing. However, if the processor has been eliminated as a source of the problem, then the camera must be assumed to be the errant instrument. Sometimes the video monitor, laser, or other light device used to expose the film has changed its output. In this case a service person should be called for repairs.

FREQUENCY: This should be performed at the time of installation as part of acceptance test and annually thereafter.

TEST 8 Accuracy of Localization Device

PHANTOM OR EQUIPMENT: A test object with a target that can be aimed for in the localization image and a gauge that indicates how far the resulting CT images fall from the target. One example of this phantom is a set of two small holes drilled in plastic that are perpendicular to each other but at 45 degrees to the plane of the image. A cross-sectional drawing of the device is shown in Figure 20-11. The two holes are offset slightly and do not intersect. The localization target is centered on the point where the two holes appear to intersect in the localization image, and a scan is performed. After the CT

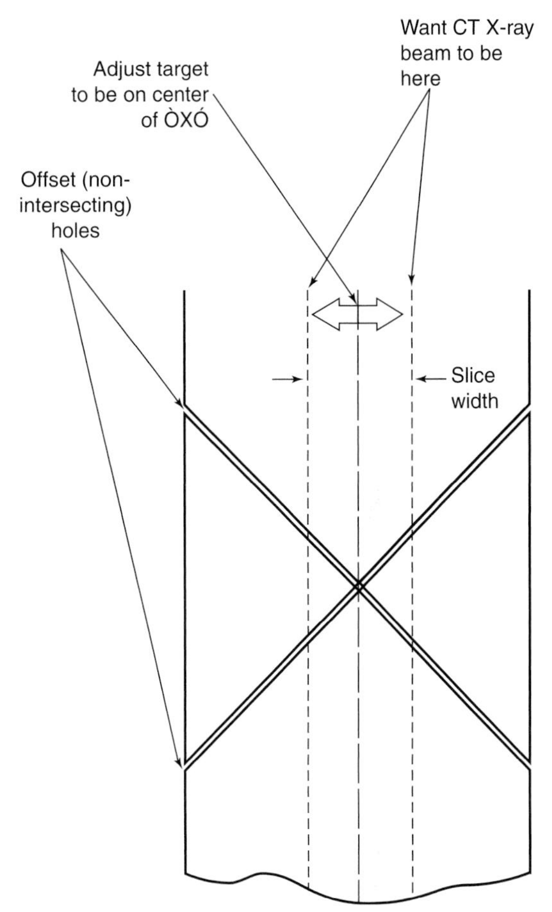

FIGURE 20-11 Target pattern to test localization device. After this section is imaged with the localization image, the CT image is targeted directly on the spot where the two holes tilted 45 degrees to the scan plane appear to cross. Then a scan is performed and an image at the targeted location is reconstructed. In the image, the relative location of the two slanted holes indicates the position of the scan relative to the target.

image is reconstructed, the holes should appear directly opposite each other with perfect alignment between the holes. If there is offset in the holes, the scan is not being performed where the localization image shows it to be.

MEASUREMENT: Image the phantom by using the localization device (sometimes called a *scout* or *targeting* image). With this localization image, set up the scanner to make a single scan at a certain thickness so that the center of the scan is directly on the intersection of the holes. Make a scan and reconstruct the image. At the very least, both holes should appear in the CT image. If they do not, then the localization device is so poorly adjusted that the width of the x-ray beam does not intersect the plastic section in which the holes are drilled. If the localization device is working properly, the image of the two holes should appear exactly side by side (Fig. 20-12). If the holes are not aligned, then the center of the slice is off target. The distance that the center of the CT image is located from its targeted position (the intersection of the holes) can be quantified by measuring the amount of offset of the two holes in the image. By using the distance measuring device on the video monitor (the measurement can be made with a ruler on the video monitor or on the hard copy image if there is no distortion in these devices and if appropriate compensation for the magnification of the image is made), measure the distance from the tip of one hole to the tip of the other hole (Fig. 20-13). The distance that the center of the CT slice is from the targeted location is equal to the length L.

Repeat the test at other slice widths.

Note that the lengths of the holes on the image, measured from end to end, are a direct measurement of the width of the CT slice. See Test 12 for a more thorough description of why this is so.

EXPECTED RESULTS: In the ideal case, the holes should be exactly aligned.

ACCEPTANCE LIMITS: If the measured value of L is 3 mm or greater, the localization device is out of adjustment and a service person should be called.

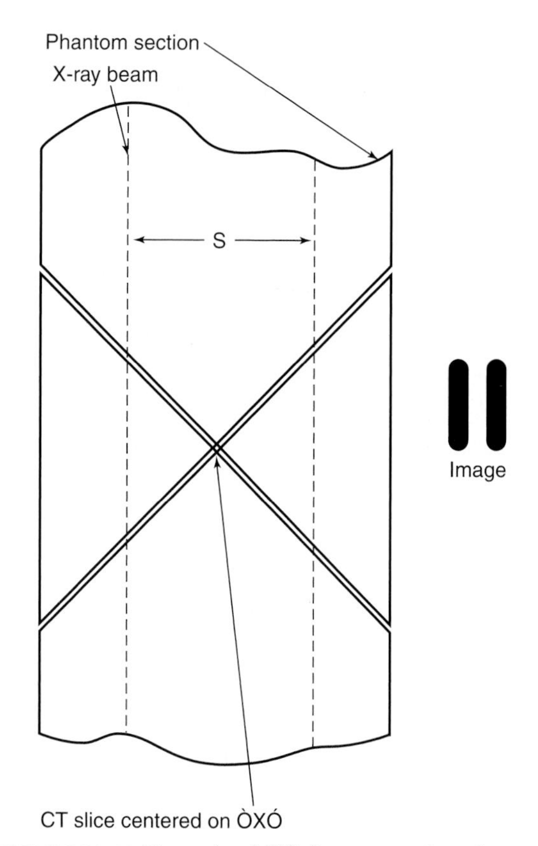

FIGURE 20-12 Example of CT slice centered on the spot where the holes appear to cross. If the two holes are aligned as shown, the localization feature is on target.

POSSIBLE CAUSES OF FAILURE: Miscalibration of the patient bed positioning mechanisms is usually the cause, although a software problem is also possible.

FREQUENCY: This should be performed at the time of installation as part of acceptance test and annually thereafter.

TEST 9 Bed Indexing

PHANTOM OR EQUIPMENT: A single piece of x-ray film. A 10 × 12-inch "Ready-pak" film (Kodak) works particularly well.

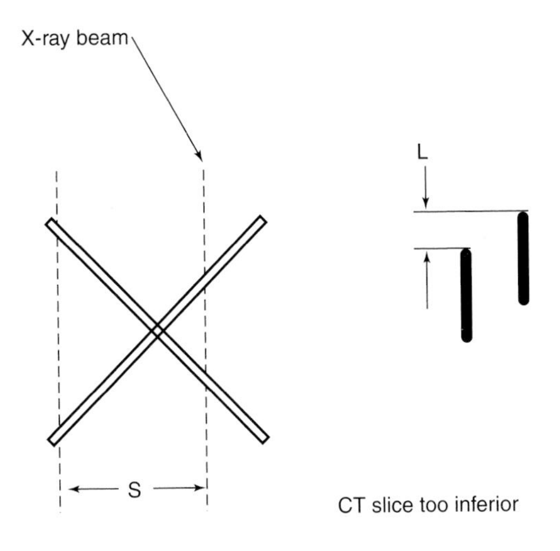

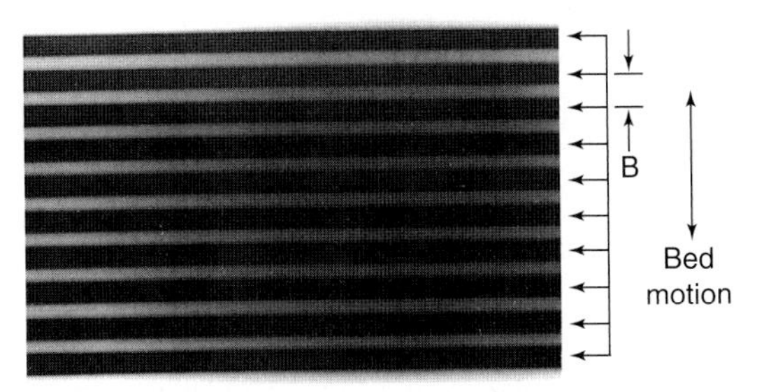

FIGURE 20-14 Measurement of bed indexing from an exposed x-ray film. The series of dark lines on the film are produced by several scans through a piece of x-ray film, moving the bed after each scan. The distance between the lines *(B)* is a measure of the distance that the patient bed has moved between scans.

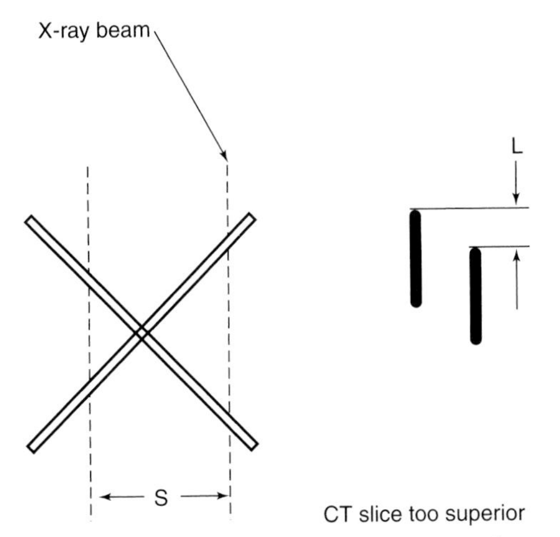

FIGURE 20-13 Measurement of *L* for slice localization accuracy. If the two holes appear offset in the image, the error in the localization feature can be determined by measuring the offset of the lines *L*.

MEASUREMENT: The x-ray film is taped to the patient table; the length of the film is parallel to the length of the table. The scanner is programmed to perform a series of 10 to 12 scans; each scan is 10 mm from the preceding scan with the slice width set to the smallest width available (less than 5 mm). The bed is loaded with at least 100 pounds (50 kilograms [kg]) of material to simulate the weight of a patient. When the scan is initiated, the x-ray beam exposes a series of narrow bands on the film (Fig. 20-14). With a ruler, measure the distance between the bands to determine how much the film (and bed) has moved between each scan.

EXPECTED RESULTS: The distance from center to center of the exposed bands on the film is expected to be 10 mm, or whatever the scan spacing was chosen to be.

ACCEPTANCE LIMITS: A series of 10 scans (nine interscan spacings) should create a series of exposed bands exactly 90 mm from the first to the last band. If the measured length of this band distance differs by more than 1 mm, the bed movement is not accurate and a service person should be notified.

POSSIBLE CAUSES OF FAILURE: Excessive slippage in the bed drive mechanism or miscalibration of the bed position indicators. Notify a service person.

FREQUENCY: This should be performed at the time of installation as part of acceptance test and annually thereafter.

TEST 10 Bed Backlash

PHANTOM OR EQUIPMENT: Two small lengths of masking tape, a pencil, and a ruler.

MEASUREMENT: The patient bed is loaded with at least 100 pounds (50 kg) of material to simulate the weight of a patient. The bed is moved to a convenient location to serve as a zero point. Two strips of masking tape are placed adjacent to each other, one on the edge of the movable part of the bed, the other on a part of the bed that does not move (Fig. 20-15). A pencil mark is placed on each piece of tape so that the two marks are exactly opposite each other. The CT scanner is programmed to move the bed automatically about 150 to 200 mm in 10- or 20-mm increments in one direction (for example, bed into scanner), and then return to its original (zero) starting location. After all the motions, the mark on the moving bed should return to its original position opposite the stationary mark. A measurement of the distance between the two marks indicates if there are mechanical discrepancies ("backlash") in the patient bed.

This measurement should be repeated driving the bed in the opposite direction as the first test.

If there is a position readout on the bed, the readout should be tested by driving the bed in and out about 200 to 300 mm and then returning the bed to its original position, as determined by the readout. Again, the marks on the tape should align if there is no backlash.

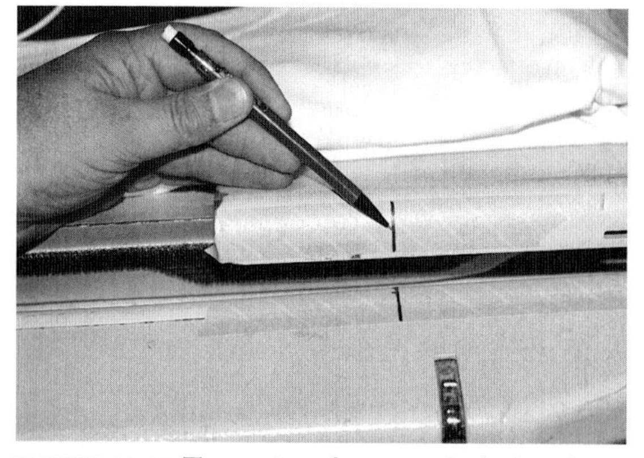

FIGURE 20-15 Two strips of tape on the bed to determine bed backlash for both the moveable and stationary parts of the bed. The two pencil marks opposite each other define the starting or zero location of the bed.

EXPECTED RESULTS: The marks on the two pieces of tape should always align when the bed is returned to its starting (zero) location.

ACCEPTANCE LIMITS: If the bed does not return to its starting position within 1 mm, then a service person should be notified.

POSSIBLE CAUSES OF FAILURE: Various types of mechanical backlash in the gears, belts, and pulleys driving the table, or slippage of the sensors that indicate the position of the bed. A service person can usually adjust the bed drive mechanism to eliminate this problem.

FREQUENCY: This should be performed at the time of installation as part of acceptance test and annually thereafter.

TEST 11 Light Field Accuracy

PHANTOM OR EQUIPMENT: A piece of x-ray film. The same piece of film used for Test 9 can be used for this test.

MEASUREMENT: Tape a sheet of "Ready-pak" film to the patient bed. Raise the patient bed so that the film is approximately centered (vertically) in the gantry opening. Turn on the external or internal light field (some CT scanners use a laser beam) that indicates the location of the first scan. With a needle or other sharp object (e.g., a penknife), poke two very small holes through the paper wrapper of the film and into the film (Fig. 20-16). The two holes should be exactly on top of the light field, with one hole near the left edge of the film and the other on the right edge. These holes, which will be visible after the film is processed, will indicate the location of the light field.

If an external light field was used, move the bed into position for the first scan. Make a medium-technique scan with the slice width set to the minimal width. The radiation should produce a narrow dark band on the film that indicates

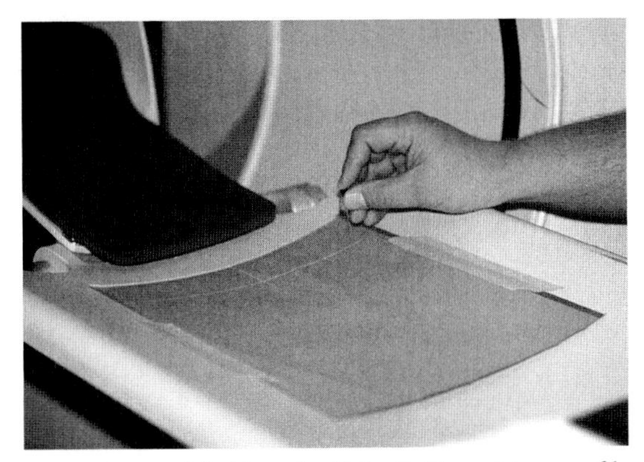

FIGURE 20-16 Marking the light field position on film with a needle. Two small holes are poked into the film at the center of the light field. The film is then scanned (exposed) with a narrow beam slice to produce a darkened stripe of the film where the radiation field hit the beam. The needle marks indicate the location of the light field. The position of the light field and the radiation field should coincide.

where the radiation struck the film. Process the film and examine the location of the dark band relative to the two pinholes.

EXPECTED RESULTS: If the light field is correctly centered on the radiation field, which is also the position of the image, the dark exposed band caused by the radiation should be centered on both pinholes.

ACCEPTANCE LIMITS: The light field should be coincident with (i.e., on top of) the radiation field to within 2 mm.

POSSIBLE CAUSES OF FAILURE: Often the optical field light system is out of alignment. Less frequently, the x-ray tube may have been installed off center. Notify your service person.

FREQUENCY: This should be performed at the time of installation as part of acceptance test and annually thereafter.

TEST 12 Slice Width (Nonspiral/Nonhelical Scanner)

PHANTOM OR EQUIPMENT: A phantom with a thin wire or a hole oriented at a 45-degree angle to the scan plane. The test object described in Test 8 will work.

Do not rely on the measurement of the width of the radiation bands on film to determine the slice width.

MEASUREMENT: A series of at least three scans are performed through the 45-degree hole. The scans should include a selection of possible beam widths available on the CT scanner. A selection of three slice thicknesses—narrow, medium, and wide—is usually sufficient. With use of the distance-measuring device on the reconstructed image, measure the length of the hole visible on the image. When the hole is oriented at 45 degrees to the incoming radiation beam, the projection of the hole onto the CT image is the same length as the width of the x-ray beam that strikes the detectors (Fig. 20-17).

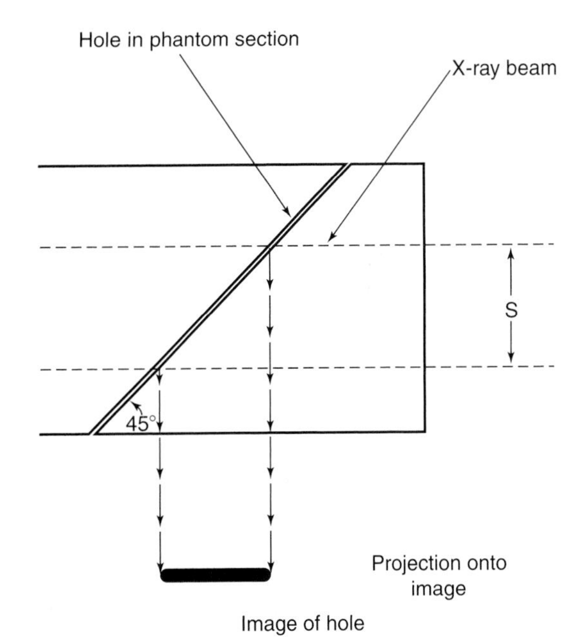

FIGURE 20-17 X-ray beam intersecting a hole angled at 45 degrees through a thick plastic plate. As a radiation beam with a certain actual width strikes a hole or wire oriented at 45 degrees to the radiation beam, the beam intersects a certain width of that hole. When that width of hole is projected onto an image, the length of the hole in the image is exactly the same as the width of the radiation beam.

EXPECTED RESULTS: The beam width measured from the image should agree with the set (i.e., nominal) beam width.

ACCEPTANCE LIMITS: For slice widths 7 mm and greater, the measured slice width should agree with the nominal slice width to within 2 mm or less. Unfortunately, at narrower slice widths, the discrepancy between nominal and measured slice widths often becomes greater. For example, at nominal slice widths of 2 to 3 mm, the measured beam width may be twice the nominal slice width.

POSSIBLE CAUSES OF FAILURE: Miscalibration of the mechanism (e.g., shutters or collimators) that collimates that portion of the x-ray beam that reaches the detectors. Notify a service person.

FREQUENCY: This should be performed at the time of installation as part of acceptance test and annually thereafter.

TEST 13 Pitch and Slice Width (Spiral/Helical Scanner)

NOTE: A single test may be used to determine both the slice width and pitch of spiral/helical CT scanners. For a CT scanner with a single array of detectors, the *pitch* is defined as the ratio of bed movement (mm) that occurs during one complete revolution to the slice width (mm). For CT scanners with a single array of detectors, the slice width is determined by collimator spacing.

In the case of CT scanners with several (e.g., four) arrays of detectors that enable several slices of data to be acquired simultaneously, the definition of pitch must be clarified. In these multiarray cases, the slice width is usually determined by the size of the detectors, not by the collimator. By a logical extension, the new definition of *pitch* is still the ratio of the distance the bed moves (mm) during one complete revolution to the slice width (mm). But it should be realized the detector size is determining the slice width, and it is not unusual to see pitch settings of 4 to 8 on these multiarray units.

PHANTOM OR EQUIPMENT: A phantom with a small diameter wire, several centimeters long, placed in the center of the scan plane at 45 degrees to the scan plane. This test involves several adjacent scans, which may be either single scans separated by bed indexing between scans, or if the scanner is capable of spiral/helical scanning, several revolutions of the x-ray tube while the bed moves several centimeters.

Do not rely on the measurement of the width of the radiation bands on film to determine the slice width.

MEASUREMENT: For an axial scanner, set up the scanner to perform a series of five or six single scans with a constant bed indexing between the scans. Analysis of this test is easier if the slice width is selected to be the same as the bed indexing (e.g., set the bed indexing = slice width = 10 mm). For spiral/helical scans from a single array CT scanner, set the bed index the same as the slice width (pitch = 1). For a multiarray CT scanner, set the bed indexing equal to the slice width multiplied by the number of detector arrays used. Perform the scans of the wire and reconstruct the images. For spiral/helical scans, make sure that the data from the same 360-degree arc is used to reconstruct each image. To measure the slice width, use the distance-measuring device on the reconstructed image. Measure the length of the wire visible on the image. When the wire is oriented at 45 degrees to the incoming radiation beam, the projection of the wire onto the CT image is the same length as the width of the x-ray beam that strikes the wire (Fig. 20-18, *A*).

From this same set of images, the slice overlap or gap may be determined. To do this, overlay any two adjacent images, electronically if possible. If the images cannot be added electronically (some scanners do not have this feature), then make a film copy of the two images. Cut the adjacent images from the hard copy film and manually overlay them on a viewbox.

EXPECTED RESULTS: First, the beam width measured from the image should agree with the

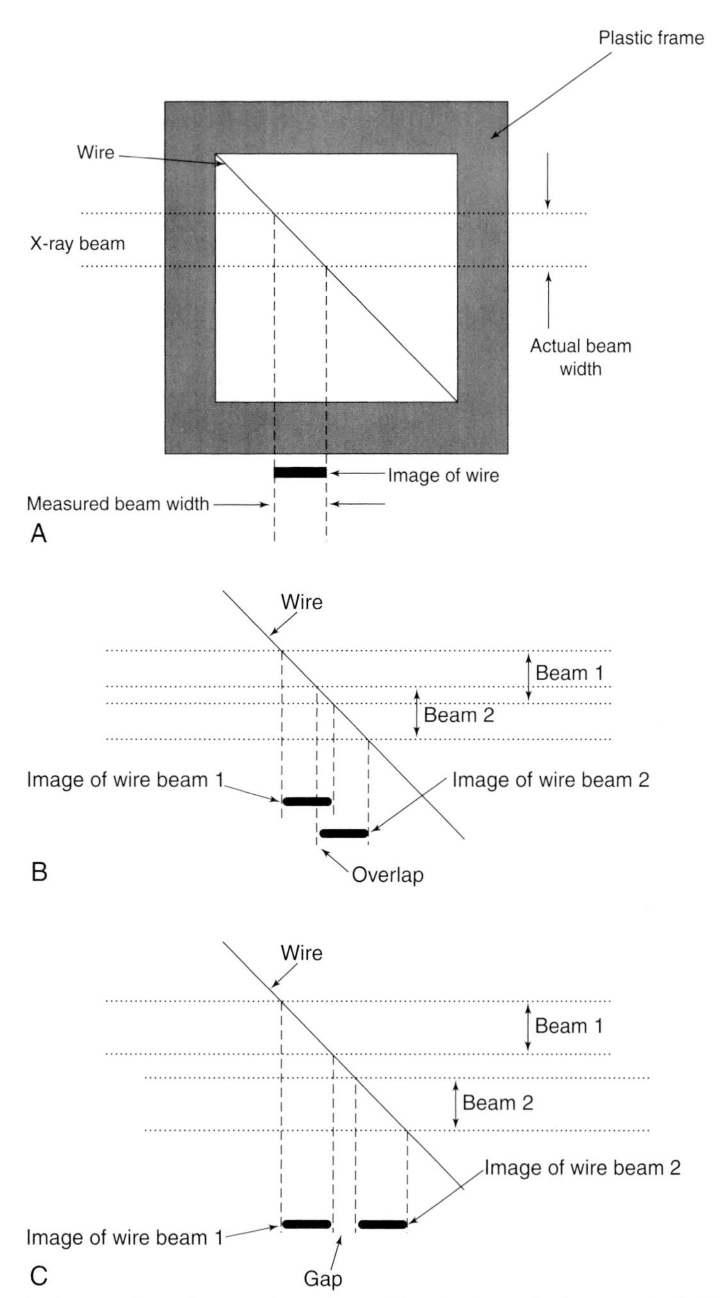

FIGURE 20-18 A, A several centimeters long (e.g., 10 cm) piece of wire stretched 45 degrees diagonally across a plastic frame serves as an object that projects the beam width directly to the CT scanner image. **B,** Overlaying the images from adjacent slices allows a comparison of the relative location of the adjacent slices. If adjacent slices overlap, the ends of the wire on the overlaid images will also overlap. **C,** If the adjacent slices are too far apart, a gap will appear in the overlaid images.

set or nominal beam width by use of a technique similar to that described in Test 12. Next, examine the images for correct pitch by looking at the overlaid images. The image of the wires (inclined at 45 degrees) should appear in different positions in the two images. If the bed indexing is exactly the same as the slice width, the images of the wire segments should just touch at the two ends of the wire that are closest to each other. If the ends of the wire seem to overlap as shown in Fig. 20-18, *B*, this indicates that the adjacent slices also overlap. If the two images of the wires do not touch at the ends as shown at the bottom of Fig. 20-18, *C*, the adjacent slices also have a gap between them. Ideally, the ends of the wires will just touch. Either overlap or a gap indicates that the bed indexing is not the same as the slice width. If the bed indexing test (Test 9) verifies the bed indexing accuracy, then the slice width is usually at fault.

ACCEPTANCE LIMITS: For slice widths 7 mm and greater, the measured slice width should agree with the nominal slice width to within 2 mm or less. The gap or overlap between adjacent slices should be less than 3 mm. Unfortunately, at narrower slice widths and bed index settings, the discrepancy between nominal and measured often becomes greater and these values may be relaxed somewhat.

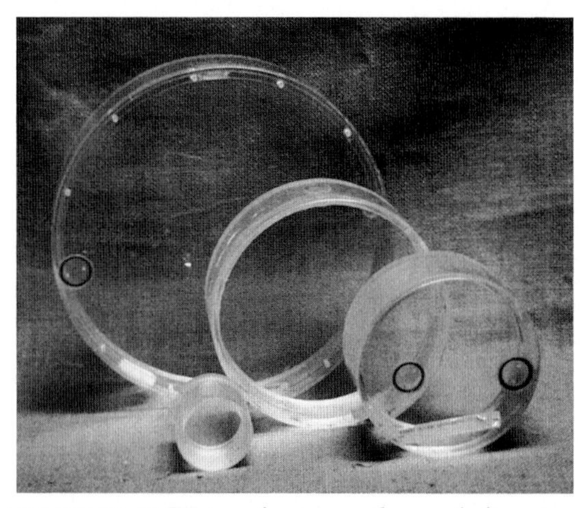

FIGURE 20-19 Water phantoms of several diameters. A selection of water phantom sizes is used to test whether the CT number of water changes as the phantom (patient) size changes.

POSSIBLE CAUSES OF FAILURE: Errors in beam width are usually caused by miscalibration of the mechanism (e.g., shutters or collimators) that collimates the portion of the x-ray beam reaching the detectors. Overlap or gaps in adjacent images or improper pitch settings may be caused by inaccuracies in the bed indexing (see Test 9) or more frequently, inaccuracy in the slice width setting. In either case, notify a service person.

FREQUENCY: This should be performed at the time of installation as part of acceptance test and annually thereafter.

TEST 14 Computed Tomography Number Versus Patient Position

PHANTOM OR EQUIPMENT: A simple cylindrical plastic container about 20 cm in diameter (the same phantom used for Test 1).

MEASUREMENT: At least five scans of the same phantom at the same technique are performed. However, the position of the phantom in the gantry should be changed for each scan. Place the phantom near the center of the gantry (use this image as the "standard"), top, bottom, and right and left sides. Set the ROI feature available on the video monitor to about 200 to 300 mm^2 (or 200 to 300 pixels) and measure the average CT number of water at the center of the phantom (not the center of the image) in each image.

EXPECTED RESULTS: The average CT number of water should always be zero, independent of the position of the phantom in the CT scanner.

ACCEPTANCE LIMITS: If the average CT number varies by more than five CT numbers from the CT number at the center of the CT scanner, there may be a problem with the symmetry of the CT scanner.

POSSIBLE CAUSES OF FAILURE: Various asymmetries in the CT scanner system. Consult a service person.

FREQUENCY: This should be performed at the time of installation as part of acceptance test and annually thereafter.

TEST 15 Computed Tomography Number Versus Patient Size

PHANTOM OR EQUIPMENT: Three or four water-filled phantoms, each of different diameters (Fig. 20-19). Typical diameters are 30 cm (body), 20 cm (adult head), and 15 cm (pediatric head). Figure 20-19 also shows a very small phantom (8 cm in diameter) that models extremities.

MEASUREMENT: A scan of each phantom size at the same technique is performed. The size of the phantoms should cover the sizes of the anatomy used clinically. For each CT scan, set the CT scanner field of view just large enough to view the entire phantom. Set the ROI feature available on the video monitor to about 200 to 300 mm^2 (or 200 to 300 pixels) and measure the average CT number of water at the center of each phantom image.

EXPECTED RESULTS: The average CT number of water should always be zero, independent of the size of the phantom.

ACCEPTANCE LIMITS: The average CT number of water should vary no more than 20 CT numbers from the smallest to the largest phantom.

POSSIBLE CAUSES OF FAILURE: Some CT scanners have electronic circuitry that compensates for the wide range of x-ray intensities that activate the detectors. The intensity of the x-ray signal depends on the amount of tissue that the x rays penetrate before they strike the detector. Improper compensation for the number of x rays that reach the detector may cause the calibration of CT for water and other materials to shift from the ideal value. A service person is usually required to trace the problem.

FREQUENCY: This should be performed at the time of installation as part of acceptance test and annually thereafter.

TEST 16 Computed Tomography Number Versus Algorithm

PHANTOM OR EQUIPMENT: A simple cylindrical plastic container about 20 cm in diameter (the same phantom used for Test 1).

MEASUREMENT: Perform a single scan of the phantom. If possible, use the same raw data to construct the image several times, each time using a different reconstruction algorithm or filter. If it is not possible to use the same data for several reconstructions, rescan the phantom using a different algorithm for each image.

EXPECTED RESULTS: The average CT number of water should always be zero, independent of the type of algorithm used to reconstruct the image.

ACCEPTANCE LIMITS: The average CT number should vary no more than three CT numbers from one algorithm to the next.

POSSIBLE CAUSES OF FAILURE: Miscalibration of the algorithm. If a recalibration of the CT scanner does not remedy the problem, a service person should be notified.

FREQUENCY: This should be performed at the time of installation as part of acceptance test and annually thereafter.

TEST 17 Computed Tomography Number Versus Slice Width

PHANTOM OR EQUIPMENT: A simple cylindrical plastic container about 20 cm in diameter (the same phantom used for Test 1).

MEASUREMENT: A few scans of the water phantom are performed at the same technique; however, the nominal slice width is changed between each scan. The slice widths used should cover the sizes of slice widths used clinically. Set the ROI feature available on the video monitor to about 200 to 300 mm^2 (or 200 to 300 pixels) and measure the average CT number of water at the center of each phantom image.

EXPECTED RESULTS: The average CT number of water should always be zero, independent of the slice width.

ACCEPTANCE LIMITS: The average CT number should vary no more than three CT numbers from one slice width to the next.

POSSIBLE CAUSES OF FAILURE: Miscalibration of the electronic detection circuitry or algorithm, especially the part that compensates for changes in x-ray intensity striking the detectors. Notify the service person.

FREQUENCY: This should be performed at the time of installation as part of acceptance test and annually thereafter.

TEST 18 Noise Characteristics

PHANTOM OR EQUIPMENT: A simple cylindrical plastic container about 20 cm in diameter (the same phantom used for Test 1).

MEASUREMENT: A few scans of the water phantom are performed at different mAs and different slice widths, with all other parameters constant. The settings should start at the smallest mA value available and fast scans (low mAs) and increase to the highest mA value and slow scans (high mAs). Set the ROI feature available on the video monitor to about 200 to 300 mm^2 (or 200 to 300 pixels) and measure the standard deviation (not the average) of the CT number of water at the center of each phantom image.

EXPECTED RESULTS: The noise in the image is proportional to the standard deviation of the CT number measured in a homogeneous medium (water). Generally, the standard deviation of the CT numbers in the ROI (σ) should decrease as the mA values and slice width are increased, keeping all other parameters constant (Brooks and Di Chiro, 1976). At lower mA values, the dependence is $\sigma \infty$ (mA • Slice width)– 1/2.

The low mA region is called the *photon noise region* and is statistical in nature. On a sheet of graph paper, plot the standard deviation versus *(mAs × Slice width)*– 1/2 (Fig. 20-20). As the mA value is increased, the standard deviation will decrease; eventually the image noise will not be limited by the number of photons. At that point, the noise will become more or less constant and characteristic of the inherent electronic noise of the CT scanner.

ACCEPTANCE LIMITS: The noise curve that was obtained when the CT scanner was new should not change appreciably with age. Be especially sensitive to increased standard deviation as the CT scanner ages in the high-mA portion of the curve, in which the noise is dominated by electronic components.

POSSIBLE CAUSES OF FAILURE: Anything that can cause the noise of the system to change, such as changed sensitivity of the detectors, increased noise in the detector amplification circuits, or reduced photon output per mA. Notify the service person.

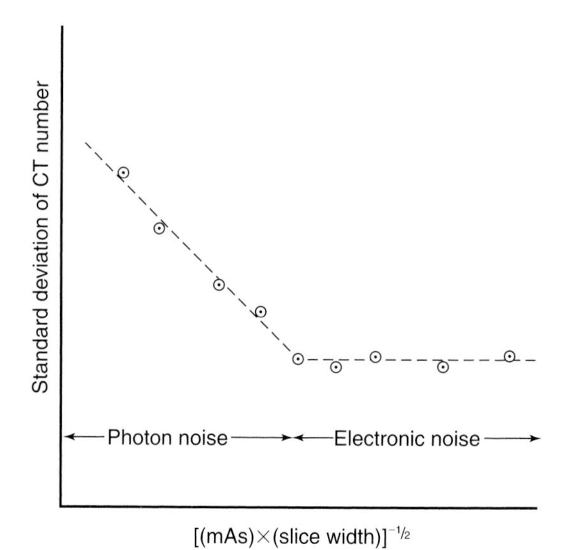

FIGURE 20-20 Standard deviation of CT number *(Noise versus mA × slice width)* – 1/2. The noise decreases gradually in the photon noise (low-dose) region and assumes an approximately constant value at high-dose levels. In the high-dose region, the noise is mostly inherent electronic noise that cannot be easily reduced.

FREQUENCY: This should be performed at the time of installation as part of acceptance test and annually thereafter.

TEST 19 Radiation Scatter and Leakage

PHANTOM OR EQUIPMENT: An integrating or total exposure/dose survey meter (Geiger counter) or large volume ion chamber and a head-size water phantom. An integrating exposure meter is essential for these measurements. A simple dose-rate meter is not very satisfactory because of the wide variation in dose received as the CT gantry rotates.

MEASUREMENT: Insert the head phantom into the scan plane to provide radiation scatter for the measurements. Put on a lead apron normally used for fluoroscopic procedures. Position the radiation detector at the location where the radiation measurement will be performed, and initiate a scan. It may be helpful to have a colleague initiate the scan during these measurements. Measure the total radiation emitted at that location per one complete scan. Repeat the measurements for several locations, paying particular attention to locations where attending personnel might stand during a scan. To determine an attendant's total radiation dose, simply multiply the number of attending scans by the dose per scan at the attendant's location during the scans.

EXPECTED RESULTS: The results will vary according to location and distance from the scanner. Usually, the highest exposure rate will be next to the patient and close to the scanner (Fig. 20-21).

ACCEPTANCE LIMITS: None.

POSSIBLE CAUSES OF FAILURE: If the exposure rate is exceedingly high (>25 milliroentgens/scan), there may be a problem with the collimation system or the x-ray tube shielding. In that case, notify the service person.

FREQUENCY: This should be performed at the time of installation as part of acceptance test and annually thereafter.

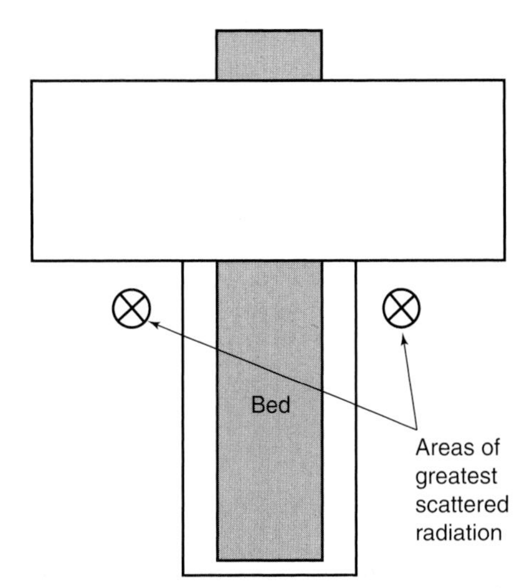

FIGURE 20-21 Top view of a CT scanner suite showing areas of highest radiation intensity near a CT scanner *(f)*.

REFERENCES

American Association of Physics in Medicine: *Specifications and acceptance testing of computed tomographic scanners*, Report 39, New York, 1993, American Association of Physics in Medicine.

Brooks RA, Di Chiro G: Statistical limitations in x-ray reconstructive tomography, *Med Phys* 3:237-240, 1976.

Burkhart RL et al: CT quality assurance in the mid-1980s, *Appl Radiol* 25-37, 1987.

Cacak RK: Design of a quality assurance program. *The selection and performance of radiographic equipment*, Baltimore, 1985, Williams & Wilkins.

Cacak RK, Hendee WR: Performance evaluation of a fourth-generation computed tomography (CT) scanner, *Proc Soc Photo-optic Instr Eng* 173:194-207, 1979.

McCollough CH et al: The phantom portion of the American College of Radiology (ACR) Computed Tomography (CT) accreditation program: practical tips, artifact examples, and pitfalls to avoid. *Med Phys* 31:2423-2441, 2004.

National Council on Radiation Protection and Measurements: *Quality assurance for diagnostic imaging*, Report 99, pp 120-124, Bethesda, Md, 1988, National Council on Radiation Protection and Measurements.

Spiral Versus Helical

Spiral or helical CT: right or wrong?

From: Willi A. Kalender, PhD
Siemens Medical Systems
Henkestrasse 127, D-91050 Erlangen, Germany

Editor:

The term spiral computed tomography (CT) was first made public at the 1989 RSNA scientific assembly (1). Peter Vock, MD, from Switzerland and myself, not native speakers of the English language, had had some trouble in deciding on the name for the technique. Both spiral and helical appeared to be acceptable to us—helical was possibly more precise (which is very important to the Swiss), and spiral was more readily understandable. Authoritative dictionaries of the English language told us that both terms were correct. Having walked up and down spiral staircases with spiral binders under our arms without any problems, we believed that the term spiral might be more readily understood and accepted intuitively. Indeed, the term was accepted. However, in several of our communications, we stressed that spiral and helical can be considered as synonyms (2).

Apparently, a controversy arose in the past 1-2 years, as documented by letters to editors of scientific journals (3,4). The authors made very intelligent and acceptable statements voting for either one of the terms. I think that the discussion is unnecessary. There is no right or wrong term; both terms should be kept as synonyms.

Last, but not least, for yet another reason I recommend that the scientific community and their journals stay away from deciding that one term is right and the other one is wrong. There are some commercial implications and interests connected to the terms, and any decision might be misinterpreted. For what I hope are understandable reasons, I will continue to use the original term spiral CT in my communications; however, it shall not imply a decision about which term is right and which term is wrong.

REFERENCES

1. Kalender WA, Seissler W, Vock P. Single-breathhold spiral volumetric CT by continuous patient translation and scanner rotation (abstr). Radiology 1989;173(P):414.
2. Kalender WA. Technical foundations of spiral CT. Semin Ultrasound CT MR 1994; 15: 81-89.
3. Towers MJ. Spiral or helical CT? (letter). AJR 1993; 161: 901.
4. Mintz RD. Spiral vs helical: a matter of precision (letter). AJR 1994; 162:1507.

Editor's note.—We concur; hereafter, *Radiology* will accept either term.

Stanley S. Siegelman, MD
Editor, *Radiology*

Letter to editor, *Radiology* 193:583, 1994.

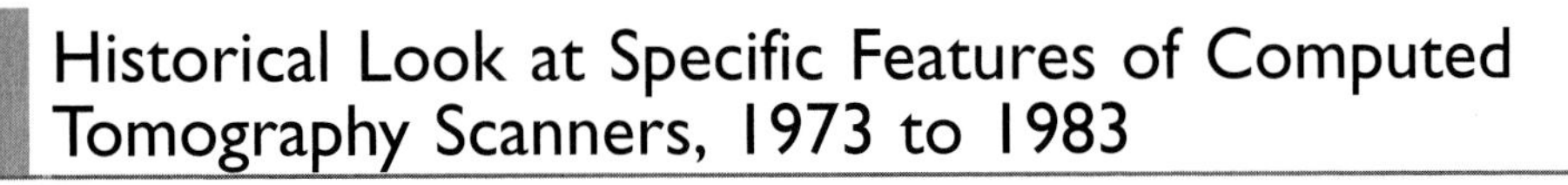

Appendix B

Historical Look at Specific Features of Computed Tomography Scanners, 1973 to 1983

YEAR	DEVELOPMENTS
1973	EMI is sole manufacturer and delivers 60-head computer tomographs with 6.5-minute scan time.
1974	Siemens brings similar unit, Siretom, to clinical use as first x-ray company; Ledley presents his whole-body ACTA scanner, which is built by Pfizer in the following year; Ohio Nuclear announces the whole-body Delta-Scan 50 with 2.5-minute scan time; Artronix announces a rotation system for a 9-second computer tomograph with water-compensating body.
1975	EMI presents the 60-second head unit CT 1010 and the 20-second whole-body computer tomograph 5005; GE presents a 10-second mamma unit CT/M with rotation system as pilot project, announces the 5-second whole-body unit CT/T and sells the 270-second head unit CT/N of the Neuroscan Company; Siemens takes the Delta-Scan 50 into the worldwide sales program (apart from United States and Canada) and afterward the following Delta-Scan types as well, up to 1977.
1976	Ohio Nuclear introduces the 18.8-second Delta-Scan 50 FS, Pfizer the 20-second computer tomograph 0200 FS, and Philips the 20-second Tomoscan, and thus follow the EMI unit CT 5005; Syntex shows a 12-second whole-body computer tomograph with translation-rotation system that is, however, dropped in the following year; Elscint introduces the 10-second whole-body computer tomograph Scanex (also with translation-rotation); AS & E presents the ring detector system for 5-second scan time; Siemens introduces the Somatom with crystal semiconductor detector and instant image.
1977	Ohio Nuclear comes in the spring with the Delta-Scan 2000 series and thus "shoots down" the Delta-Scan 50 FS prematurely; three manufacturers announce at the RSNA meeting at the end of the year ring detector systems without showing image results: EMI, Picker, and Artronix; Philips announces the 5-second whole-body Tomoscan 300 and thus makes the just-available Tomoscan 200 into a special offer unit; Syntex 60 is added to the Philips sales program as neurocomputer tomograph Tomoscan 100; Syntex drops out of the computed tomography field in the following year; CGR takes over the sale of the Pfizer units and afterward those of the Varian scanner and brings the 20-sec head unit ND 8000 onto the market.
1978	Syntex, AS & E, Searle "bail out"; Pfizer takes over technology and production of the AS & E scanner; EMI distributes Searle computer tomographs because their own CT 7070 is not yet ready; Elscint exploits the translation-rotation system up to a minimum scan time of 5.8 seconds.

YEAR	DEVELOPMENTS
1979	CGR announces its own whole-body unit CE 10,000 with 1024 xenon detectors, of which the first head scans were shown only 2 years later; Siemens is successful in breaking through to the American market with the Somatom 2; all x-ray firms except for Picker prefer the rotation system with the traveling detector.
1980	EMI drops out of the computer tomography field; GE takes over the service, apart from in the United States and Canada, where Omnimedical takes over servicing and finally continues in the following year with the CT 7070 modified as Quad 1; Elscint brings a hybrid computer tomograph onto the market with the Exel 1002 with translation-rotation for high resolution and 1.9-second rotation with only 280 detectors; Pfizer shows CT images from its new ring detector with 2400 elements and a resolution of 0.4 mm.
1981	Pfizer "bails out"; Picker is taken over by the British GEC; GE and Siemens present at the RSNA meeting the CT 9800 and the Somatom DR, with minimum scan times of 1.3 and 1.4 seconds, respectively.
1981 to 1983	Eight manufacturers still represented with worldwide activities; among these, GE has the peak position in the United States, Siemens in Europe, and Toshiba in Japan.

From Dümmling K: 10 years' computed tomography: a retrospective view, *Electromedica* 52:13-28, 1984.

Appendix C

Physics of Cardiac Imaging with Multiple-Row Detector Computed Tomography*

Mahadevappa Mahesh, MS, PhD
Dianna D. Cody, PhD

Coronary heart disease (CHD) represents the major cause of morbidity and death in Western populations (American Heart Association, 2003). In 2003 alone, more than 450,000 deaths were associated with CHD in the United States; that translates to nearly one of every five deaths (American Heart Association, 2003). The economic burden on health care as a result of CHD is also enormous. Advances in multiple-row detector computed tomography (CT) technology have made it feasible for imaging the heart and to evaluate CHD noninvasively. Calcium scoring, CT angiography, and assessment of ventricular function can be performed with multiple-row detector CT (Mahnken et al, 2005). Coronary artery calcium scoring (Budoff et al, 2003; Ulzheimer and Kalender, 2003) allows patients at intermediate risk for cardiovascular events to be risk stratified. Coronary arterial anatomy and both noncalcified and calcified plaques are visible at coronary CT angiography (Dewey et al, 2004; Pannu et al, 2006b). Vessel wall disease and luminal diameter are depicted, and secondary myocardial changes may also be seen (Dewey et al, 2004; Pannu et al, 2006b; Schoenhagen et al, 2004).

Although the prime diagnostic tool to evaluate and treat CHD is coronary angiography (an x-ray fluoroscopy-guided procedure) and the fluoroscopically guided images are considered the standard of reference for comparing coronary artery image quality, the procedure is invasive and requires longer examination times than CT angiography, including patient preparation and recouping times. Images obtained with 16-row and 16+-row detector CT scanners are increasingly becoming comparable to those of the standard of reference (Hoffman et al, 2004).

The prospect of imaging the heart and coronary arteries with CT has been anticipated since the development of CT more than 3 decades ago. The lack of speed and poor spatial and temporal resolution of previous generations of CT scanners prevented meaningful evaluation of the coronary arteries and cardiac function. Most early assessments of the coronary arteries with CT were performed with electron beam CT, developed in the early 1980s (McCollough and Morin, 1994). Electron-beam CT has been used mostly for noninvasive evaluation of coronary artery calcium (Detrano, 1996), but other applications including assessment of coronary artery stenosis have been reported in limited cases. However, electron-beam CT is expensive and is not widely available.

Recent advances in CT technologies, especially multiple-row detector CT, have dramatically changed the approach to noninvasive imaging of cardiac disease. With submillimeter spatial resolution (<0.75 millimeters [mm]), improved temporal resolution (80-200 milliseconds [ms]) (Mahesh, 2006), and electrocardiographically (ECG) gated or triggered mode of acquisition, the current generation of CT scanners (16- to 64-row detectors) makes cardiac imaging possible (Flohr et al, 2005; Gerber et al, 2004; Klingenbeck-Regn, 1999, 2002; Nikolaou et al, 2004, Pannu et al, 2003) and has the potential to accurately characterize the coronary tree.

The purpose of this article is to describe the physics of cardiac imaging with multiple-row detector CT.

From the Russell H. Morgan Department of Radiology and Radiological Science, Johns Hopkins University School of Medicine, Baltimore, Md (M. M.), and the Department of Imaging Physics, University of Texas M.D. Anderson Cancer Center, Houston, Tex (D. D. C)

*From *Radiographics* 27:1495-1509, 2007. Reprinted by permission of the Radiological Society of North America and the authors.

The factors affecting temporal and spatial resolution are discussed along with scan acquisition and reconstruction methods, reconstruction algorithms, reconstruction interval, pitch, radiation dose, and geometric efficiency.

KEY ISSUES IN CARDIAC IMAGING WITH MULTIPLE-ROW DETECTOR CT

The primary challenge required to image a rapidly beating heart is that the imaging modality should provide high temporal resolution. It is necessary to freeze the heart motion to image coronary arteries located close to heart muscles because these muscles show rapid movement during the cardiac cycle. Because the most quiescent part of the heart cycle is the diastolic phase, imaging is best if performed during this phase. Hence, it is required to monitor the heart cycle during data acquisition. The subject's ECG is recorded during scanning because the image acquisition and reconstruction are synchronized with the heart motion. Also, the imaging modality should provide high spatial resolution to resolve very fine structures such as proximal coronary segments (right coronary ascending and left anterior descending arteries) that run in all directions around the heart. These requirements impose greater demands on multiple-row detector CT technology. One of the primary goals of the rapid development of CT technology has been to achieve these demands to make cardiac CT imaging a clinical reality.

UNDERSTANDING THE PHYSICS OF CARDIAC IMAGING

To better demonstrate and understand the necessity for high temporal resolution in cardiac imaging, Figure C-1 shows how the length (in time) of the diastolic phase changes with heart rates. The least amount of cardiac motion is observed during the diastolic phase; however, the diastolic phase narrows with increasing heart rate. With rapid heart rates, the diastolic phase narrows to such an extent that the temporal resolution needed to image such subjects is less than 100 ms. The desired temporal resolution for motion-free cardiac imaging is 250 ms for heart rates up to 70 beats per minute and up to 150 ms for heart rates greater than 100 beats per minute. Ideally, motion-free imaging for all phases requires temporal resolution to be around 50 ms. The standard of reference for comparing the temporal resolution obtained with multiple-row detector CT is fluoroscopy, wherein the heart motion is frozen during dynamic imaging to a few milliseconds (1-10 ms). Therefore, the demand for high temporal resolution implies decreased scan time required to obtain data needed for image reconstruction; the scan time is usually expressed in milliseconds.

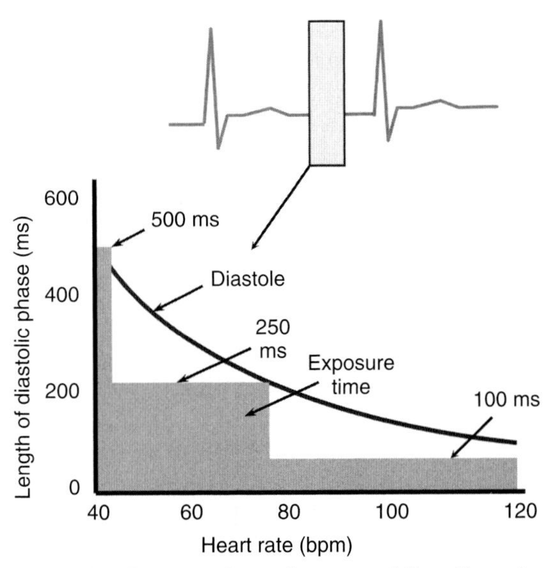

FIGURE C-1 Diagram shows the range of diastolic regions for varying heart rates. The desired temporal resolution for cardiac CT is approximately 250 milliseconds *(ms)* for average heart rates of less than 70 beats per minute *(bpm)*; for higher heart rates, the desired temporal resolution is approximately 100 ms.

The demand for high spatial resolution that enables the visualization of various coronary segments (such as the right coronary artery, left anterior descending artery, and circumflex artery) that run in all directions around the heart with decreasing diameter is high. These coronary segments range from a few millimeters in diameter (at the apex of the aorta) and decrease to a few submillimeters in diameter as they traverse away from the aorta in all directions. The need to image such small coronary segments requires small voxels, and this is key to cardiac imaging with multiple-row detector CT. Spatial resolution is generally expressed in line pairs per centimeter or line pairs per millimeter. Like temporal resolution, the standard of reference for comparing spatial resolution is the resolution obtained during fluoroscopy. However, one of the major goals of multiple-row detector CT technology development has been to obtain similar spatial resolution in all directions, also expressed as *isotropic spatial resolution* (Mahesh, 2002).

In addition, a sufficient contrast-to-noise ratio is required to resolve small and low-contrast structures such as plaques. In CT, low-contrast resolution is typically excellent. However, it can degrade with the increasing number of CT detectors in the z direction as a result of increased scattered radiation that can reach detectors in the z direction. It is important to achieve adequate low-contrast resolution with minimum radiation exposure. The need to keep the radiation dose as low as reasonably possible is essential for any imaging modality that uses ionizing radiation.

Overall, cardiac imaging is a very demanding application for multiple-row detector CT. Temporal, spatial, and contrast resolution must all be optimized with an emphasis on minimizing radiation exposure during cardiac CT imaging.

Temporal Resolution

There are a number of factors that influence the temporal resolution achieved with multiple-row detector CT scanners. Among them, the key factors are the gantry rotation time, acquisition mode, type of image reconstruction, and pitch.

Gantry Rotation Time

Gantry rotation time is defined as the amount of time required to complete one full rotation (360 degrees) of the x-ray tube and detector around the subject. The advances in technology have considerably decreased the gantry rotation time to as low as 330 to 370 ms. The optimal temporal resolution during cardiac imaging is limited by the gantry rotation time. The faster the gantry rotation, the greater the temporal resolution achieved. However, with increasing gantry rotation speed, there is also an increase in the stresses on the gantry structure because rapid movement of heavy mechanical components inside the CT gantry results in higher gravitational forces, making it harder to achieve a further reduction in gantry rotation time. In fact, even a small incremental gain in the gantry rotation time requires great effort in the engineering design.

In the past, the minimum rotation time was as high as 2 seconds; in the past few years, gantry rotation time has decreased steadily to less than 400 ms. As discussed in the previous section and in Figure C-1, because the currently available gantry rotation time is not in the desired range for obtaining reasonable temporal resolution, various methods have been developed to compensate, such as different types of scan acquisitions or image reconstructions to further improve temporal resolution.

Acquisition Mode

For imaging the rapidly moving heart, projection data must be acquired as fast as possible to freeze the heart motion. This is achieved in multiple-row detector CT either by prospective ECG triggering or by retrospective ECG gating (Desjardins and Kazerooni, 2004).

Prospective Electrocardiographic Triggering

Prospective ECG triggering is similar to the conventional CT "step-and-shoot" method. The patient's cardiac functions are monitored through ECG signals continuously during the scan. The CT technologist sets up the subject with ECG monitors and starts the scan. Instructions are built into the protocol to start the x rays at a desired distance from the R-R peak, for example, at 60% or 70% of the R-R interval. The scanner, in congruence with the patient's ECG pulse, starts the scan at the preset point in the R-R internal period (Fig. C-2). The projection data are acquired for only part of the complete gantry rotation (i.e., a partial scan).

The minimum amount of projection data required to construct a complete CT image is 180 degrees plus the fan angle of the CT detectors in the axial plane. Hence, the scan acquisition time depends on the gantry rotation time. The best temporal resolution that can be achieved in the partial scan mode of acquisition is slightly greater than half the gantry rotation time. Once the desired data are acquired, the table is translated to the next bed position and, after a suitable and steady heart rate is achieved, the scanner acquires more projections. This cycle repeats until the entire scan length is covered, typically 12 to 15 centimeters (cm) (depending on the size of the heart).

With multiple-row detector CT, the increasing number of detectors in the z direction allows a larger volume of the heart to be covered per gantry rotation. For example, by use of a multiple-row detector CT scanner capable of obtaining 16 axial sections (16 rows of detectors with 16 data acquisition system channels in the z direction) and with each detector width of 0.625 mm, the technologist can scan a 10-mm (16 × 0.625 mm) length per gantry rotation. Similarly, with a 64-section multiple-row detector CT scanner (64 rows of detectors with 64 data acquisition system channels) and each

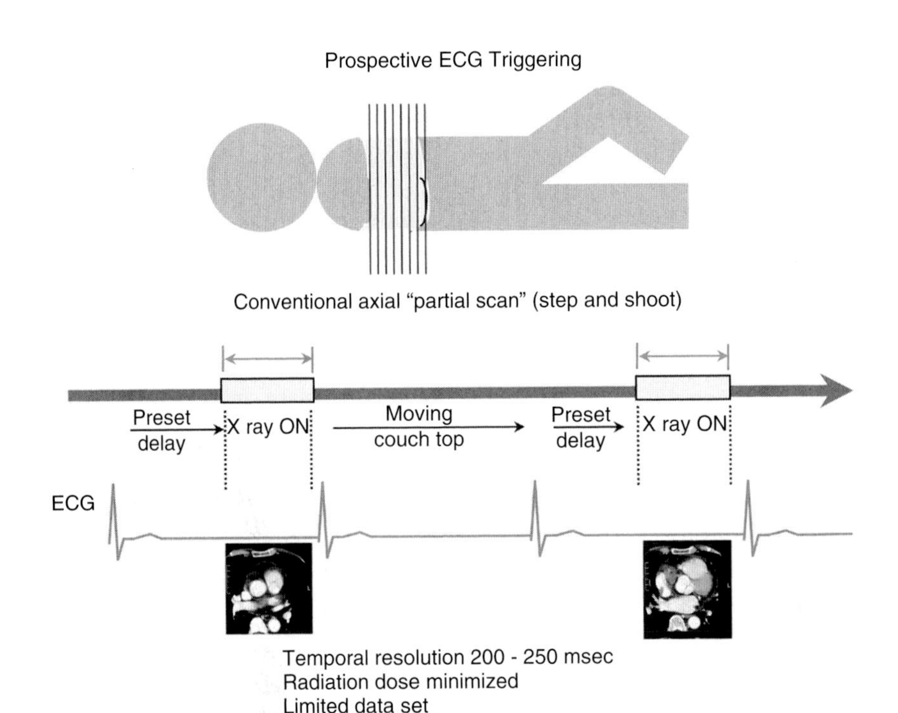

FIGURE C-2 During the prospective ECG-triggered scan mode, the patient's ECG is continuously monitored, but the x rays are turned on at predetermined R-R intervals to acquire sufficient scan data for image reconstruction. The table is then moved to the next location for further data acquisition. These types of scans are always sequential and not helical and result in a lower patient dose because the x rays are on for a limited period. Calcium scoring scans are typically performed in this scan mode.

detector 0.625 mm wide, about 40 mm per gantry rotation can be scanned. Typically, the cardiac region ranges from 120 to 150 mm, which can be covered in three to four gantry rotations with a 64-row detector CT scanner. This has a major advantage in terms of the decreased time required for breath holding to minimize motion artifacts (critical when sick patients are scanned).

One of the advantages of the prospective triggering approach is reduced radiation exposure because the projection data are acquired for short periods and not throughout the heart cycle. Temporal resolution with this type of acquisition can range from 200 to 250 ms. Prospective triggering is the mode of data acquisition used for calcium scoring studies because calcium scoring analysis is typically performed in axial scan mode. The scan technique such as tube current (milliamperes) for a calcium scoring protocol can be quite low, yielding low radiation dose because calcium has a high CT number and is easily visible even with a noisier background. Also, each data set is obtained during the most optimal ECG signal to reduce motion artifacts.

Retrospective Electrocardiographic Gating

Retrospective gating is the main choice of data acquisition in cardiac coronary artery imaging with multiple-row detector CT. In this mode, the subject's ECG signals are monitored continuously, and the CT scan is acquired continuously (simultaneously) in helical mode (Fig. C-3). Both the scan projection data and the ECG signals are recorded. The information about the subject's heart cycle is then used during image reconstruction, which is performed retrospectively, hence the name *retrospective gating*. The image reconstruction is performed either with data corresponding to partial scan data or with segmented reconstruction.

In segmented reconstruction, data from different parts of the heart cycle are chosen so that the sum of the segments equates to the minimal partial scan data required for image reconstruction. This results in further improvements in temporal resolution. Temporal resolution with this type of acquisition can range from 80 to 250 ms.

The disadvantage of the retrospective gating mode of acquisition is the increased radiation dose because the data are acquired throughout the heart cycle, although partial data are actually used in the final image reconstruction. Also, because this scan is performed helically, the tissue overlap specified by the pitch factor is quite low, indicating excessive tissue overlap during scanning, which also increases radiation dose to the patients. The need for low pitch values or excessive overlap is determined by the need to have minimal data gaps in the scan projection data required for image reconstruction. The need for low pitch values is discussed in detail in the section on pitch.

Reconstruction Method

Cardiac data acquired with either prospective ECG triggering or retrospective ECG gating are used in reconstructing images. High temporal resolution images are obtained by reconstructing the data either with partial scan reconstruction or with multiple-segment reconstruction.

Partial Scan Reconstruction

Among the methods of image reconstruction in cardiac CT, the most practical solution is the partial scan reconstruction. Partial scan reconstruction can be used for both prospective triggering and retrospective gating acquisitions. The minimum amount of data required to reconstruct a CT image is at least 180 degrees plus the fan angle of data in any axial plane. This determines the scan time to acquire projection data needed for partial scan reconstruction and also limits the temporal resolution that can be achieved from an acquisition. The CT detectors in the axial plane of acquisition extend in an arc that covers at least a 30- to 60-degree fan angle. Therefore, during partial scan reconstruction, the scan data needed for reconstruction are obtained by rotating the x-ray tube by 180 degrees plus the fan angle of the CT detector assembly (Fig. C-4).

If the gantry rotation time is 500 ms, the time required to obtain the minimum scan data is slightly greater than half the gantry rotation time.

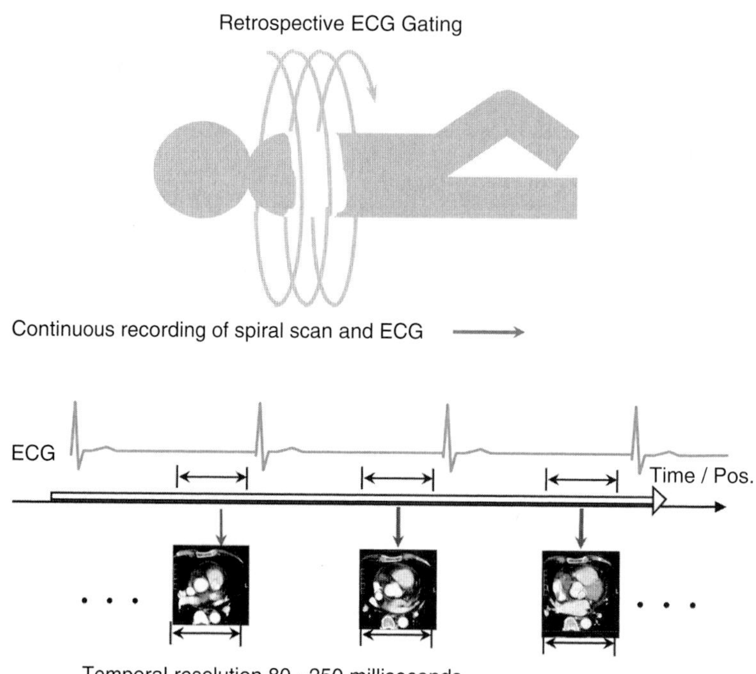

FIGURE C-3 During the retrospective ECG-gated scan mode, the patient's ECG is continuously monitored and the patient table moves through the gantry. The x rays are on continuously, and the scan data are collected throughout the heart cycle. Retrospectively, projection data from select points within the R-R interval are selected for image reconstruction. Radiation dose is higher in this type of scan mode compared with that in the prospective triggering mode. *Pos*, Position.

This means that, for a gantry rotation of 500 ms, the scan time for acquiring data for partial scan reconstruction is around 260 to 280 jms. This value represents the limit of temporal resolution that can be achieved through partial scan reconstruction. To achieve further improvements in temporal resolution, the CT manufacturers are driving scanner gantry rotation time faster and faster. To date, the fastest commercially available gantry rotation time is 330 ms. In such scanners, the partial scan reconstruction temporal resolution can be as high as 170 to 180 ms. At the same time, the gravitational force generated from rapid gantry motion is growing exponentially and is reaching a limit for the existing technology. The demand for even higher temporal resolution has led to the development of dual-source CT, and some are even considering developing multiple x-ray source CT scanners.

Multiple-Segment Reconstruction

The primary limitation to achieving high temporal resolution with the partial scan approach is the gantry rotation time. To achieve even higher temporal resolution, multiple-segment reconstruction was developed (Flohr et al, 2005). The principle behind multiple-segment reconstruction is that the scan projection data required to perform a partial scan reconstruction are selected from various sequential heart cycles instead of from a single heart cycle (Fig. C-4). This is possible only with a

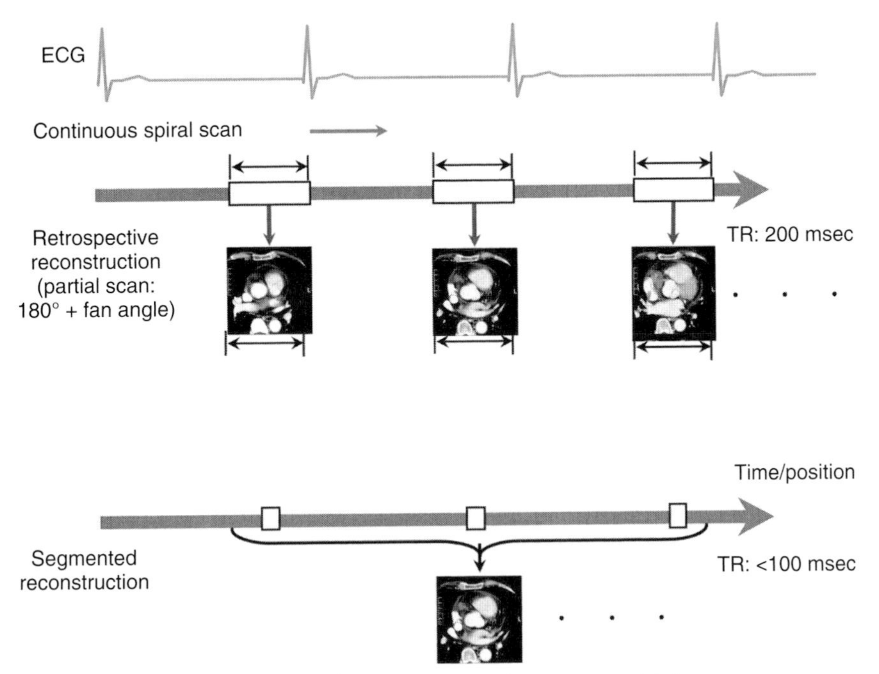

FIGURE C-4 Differences between partial scan reconstruction versus multiple-segment reconstruction. *Top*, During partial scan reconstruction, sufficient data from a prescribed time range within the R-R interval of one cardiac cycle are selected for reconstruction. *Bottom*, In multiple-segment reconstruction, sufficient data segments of the same phase from multiple cardiac cycles are selected for image reconstruction. Higher temporal resolution *(TR)* can be achieved with this type of reconstruction. *msec*, Milliseconds.

retrospective gating technique and a regular heart rhythm. The CT projection data are acquired continuously throughout many sequential heart cycles.

The multiple-segment reconstruction method selects small portions of projection data from various heart cycles so that, when all the projections are combined, they constitute sufficient data to perform partial scan reconstructions. For example, if the technologist chooses to select half of the data set required for partial scan reconstruction from one heart cycle and the rest from another heart cycle, this results in temporal resolution that is about one fourth of the gantry rotation time. This is done by using projection data from two separate segments of the heartbeat cycle for image reconstruction. Further improvement in temporal resolution can be achieved by cleverly selecting projection data from three or four different heart cycles, resulting in temporal resolution as low as 80 ms.

In general, with multiple-segment reconstruction, the temporal resolution can range from a maximum of $T_R/2$ to a minimum of $T_R/2M$, where T_R is the gantry rotation time (seconds) and M is the number of segments in adjacent heartbeats from which projection data are used for image reconstruction. Usually, M ranges from 1 to 4.

$$TR_{max} = \frac{T_R}{2M}$$

If T_R = 400 ms and M = 1, then TR_{max} is as follows:

$$TR_{max} \geq \frac{T_R}{2} \geq 200\,\text{ms}$$

If T_R = 400 ms and M = 2, then TR_{max} is as follows:

$$TR_{max} \geq \frac{T_R}{4} \geq 100\,\text{ms}$$

If T_R = 400 ms and M = 3, then TR_{max} is as follows:

$$TR_{max} \geq \frac{T_R}{6} \geq 67\,\text{ms}$$

The advantage of multiple-segment reconstruction is the possibility to achieve high temporal resolution. The disadvantage is that, because projection data sets are obtained from different heartbeat cycles, a misregistration caused by rapid motion can result in the degradation of image spatial resolution. This method also allows selection of different packets of data for reconstructing an image for patients with irregular heart rates.

Overall, the temporal resolution of cardiac CT depends on the gantry rotation time. A gantry rotation time of 330 to 500 ms is possible with 16- to 64-channel multiple-row detector CT scanners. With such rapid gantry rotation time, one can achieve a temporal resolution of 80 to 250 ms through multiple- and partial-segment reconstruction, respectively. Temporal resolution improves with multiple-segment reconstruction (Fig. C-5); however, the spatial resolution can degrade as a result of misregistration of motion artifacts because projection data sets are selected from different heartbeats.

With both types of reconstruction, there is a demand for a significant amount of projection overlap during data acquisition, which is indicated by the pitch. Usually, the pitch ranges from 0.2 to 0.4 for cardiac CT protocols. This is quite different from routine body CT protocols, which are typically performed with pitch values of 0.75 to 1.50.

Spatial Resolution

There are a number of factors that influence the spatial resolution achieved with multiple-row detector CT scanners. Among them are the detector size in the longitudinal direction, reconstruction algorithms, and patient motion.

Effect of Detector Size

The effect of detector size in the z direction or out-of-plane spatial resolution is very significant

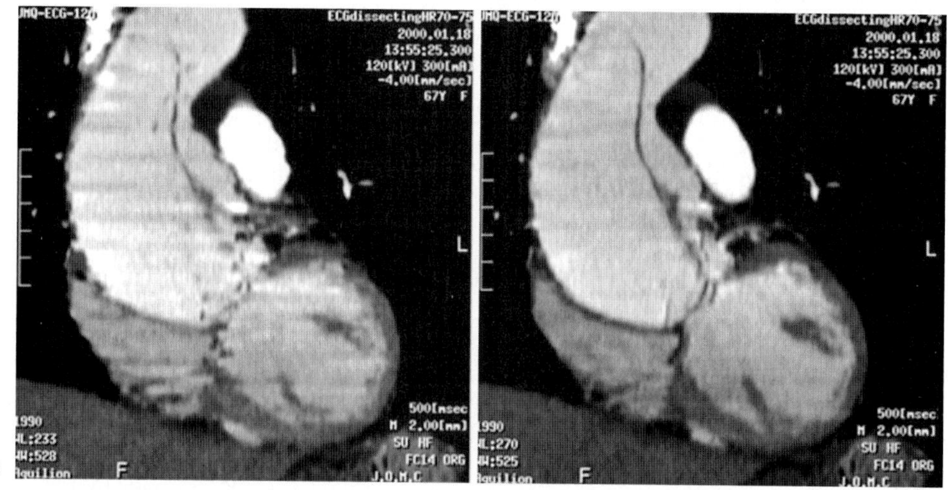

FIGURE C-5 Effect of temporal resolution on reconstructed images from the same patient. **A,** Partial scan reconstruction with temporal resolution of approximately 250 milliseconds. **B,** Multiple-segment reconstruction (two segments) yields a temporal resolution of approximately 105 milliseconds. The stairstep artifacts are less visible and the structures in the sagittal plane have a smooth edge compared with the appearance of partial scan reconstruction.

and has become one of the driving forces in the advancement of multiple-row detector CT technology. Also, larger volume coverage in combination with a larger number of thin images requires more detectors in the z direction, which is the hallmark of technological advance in multiple-row detector CT. On the other hand, scan plane or axial spatial resolution has been very high from the beginning and is dependent on the scan field of view (SFOV) and image reconstruction matrix. Axial pixel size is the ratio of SFOV to image matrix; for example, for a conventional 512 × 512 matrix, the transverse pixel size for a 25-cm SFOV is 0.49 mm. On the other hand, the longitudinal or z-axis resolution mainly depends on the image thickness. The z-axis spatial resolution (image thickness) ranges from 1 to 10 mm in conventional (nonhelical) and in helical single-row detector CT. With multiple-row detector CT, the z-axis detector size is further reduced to submillimeter size.

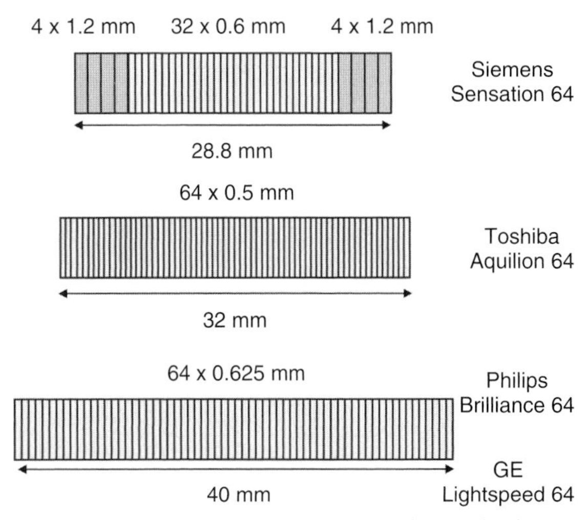

FIGURE C-6 Detector array designs for multiple-row detector CT scanners that can yield 64 sections per gantry rotation.

Initially, with the introduction of multiple-row detector CT technology, the thinnest detector size was 0.5 mm and there were only two such detectors. However, within a few years, the technology improved to provide 16 of these thin detectors, ranging from 0.625 to 0.5 mm. With 64-section multiple-row detector CT scanners, the detector array designs are as shown in Fig. C-6; 64 thin detectors (0.625 mm) are currently available, resulting in z-axis coverage of up to 40 mm per gantry rotation (Mahesh, 2006). The increased spatial resolution with multiple-row detector CT scanners is demonstrated in Figure C-7. Cardiac CT images can be comparable in delineating details of the coronary vessels to the cardiac images obtained with fluoroscopy (Hoffman et al, 2004).

Reconstruction Interval

The reconstruction interval defines the degree of overlap between reconstructed axial images. It is independent of x-ray beam collimation or image thickness and has no effect on scan time or patient exposure. The reason for decreased reconstruction interval (or increased overlap) is to improve z-axis resolution, especially for three-dimensional (3D) and multiplanar reformation (MPR) images. If a diagnosis is made on the basis of only axial images, the reconstruction interval is not an issue. But frequently, physicians are also reading MPR and 3D images; this is especially true for cardiac CT.

For example, in a single examination the same cardiac data set (acquired at 0.5-mm detector configuration) was reconstructed with three different values of reconstruction interval (Fig. C-8). Overlapping axial images results in a relatively large number of images but can also result in improved lesion visibility in MPR and 3D images without increasing the patient dose. For routine MPR and 3D applications, a 30% image overlap is generally sufficient (1-mm section thickness with 0.7-mm reconstruction interval). For cardiac images, at least 50% overlap is desirable (0.5-mm section thickness with 0.25-mm reconstruction interval).

It should be recognized that too much overlap results in a large number of images, increases reconstruction time, can result in longer interpretation periods, and can put undue strain on image handling overhead costs (image transfer, image display, image archiving, and so forth) with no significant gain in image quality.

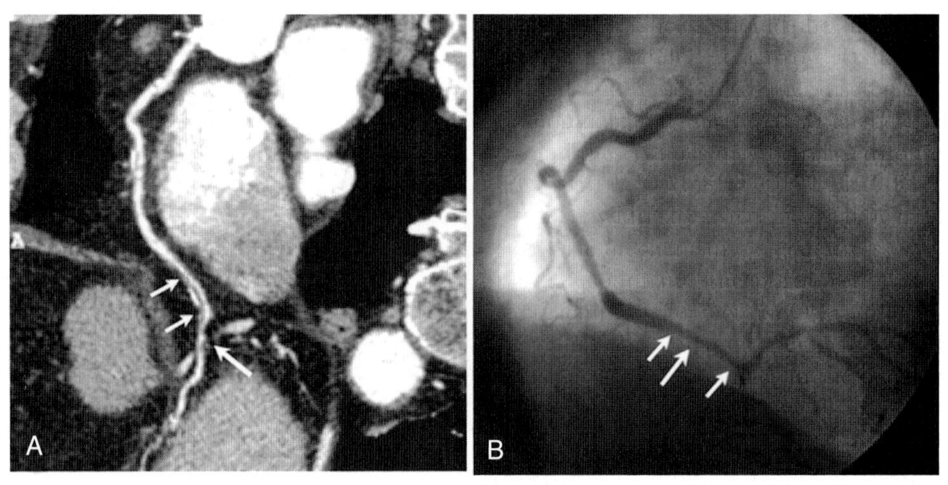

FIGURE C-7 Images from cardiac CT angiography **(A)** and fluoroscopically guided coronary angiography **(B)** show a right coronary artery *(long arrow)* with calcification *(short arrows)*. The spatial resolution and delineation of details of CT angiography are comparable with those of coronary angiography. (Reprinted with permission from Hoffmann MH et al: Noninvasive coronary imaging with MDCT in comparison to invasive conventional coronary angiography: a fast-developing technology, *AJR Am J Roentgenol* 182:601-608, 2004.)

Overall, spatial resolution in the axial or x-y plane has always been quite high and is on the order of 10 to 20 line pairs per centimeter. The z-axis spatial resolution is influenced by the detector size, reconstruction thickness, and other factors such as pitch and is around 7 to 15 line pairs per centimeter. The efforts toward obtaining isotropic resolution are leading further developments in multiple-row detector CT technology.

Pitch

The concept of pitch was introduced with the advent of spiral CT; it is defined as the ratio of table increment per gantry rotation to the total x-ray beam width (International Electrotechnical Commission, 2002; Mahesh et al, 2002) (Fig. C-9). Pitch values less than 1 imply overlapping of the x-ray beam and higher patient dose; pitch values greater than 1 imply a gapped x-ray beam and reduced patient dose (Mahesh, 2002). Cardiac imaging demands low pitch values because higher pitch values result in data gaps (Fig. C-10), which are detrimental to image reconstruction. Also, low pitch values help minimize motion artifacts, and certain reconstruction algorithms work best at certain pitch values, which are lower than 0.5 in cardiac imaging. Typical multiple-row detector CT pitch factors used for cardiac imaging range from 0.2 to 0.4.

The pitch required for a particular scanner is affected by several parameters, as shown in the following equation. For single-segment reconstruction (partial scan acquisition), the pitch factor is influenced heavily by the subject's heart rate (Ohnesorge et al, 2002).

$$P \leq \left(\frac{N-1}{N}\right)\frac{T_R}{T_{RR}+TQ}$$

where N = number of active data acquisition channels, T_R = gantry rotation time (milliseconds), T_{RR} = time for a single heartbeat (milliseconds), and T_Q = partial scan rotation time (milliseconds). For heart rates of 45 to 100 beats per minute (T_{RR} of 1333-600 ms), T_R of 500 ms, and T_Q of 250 to 360 ms, the

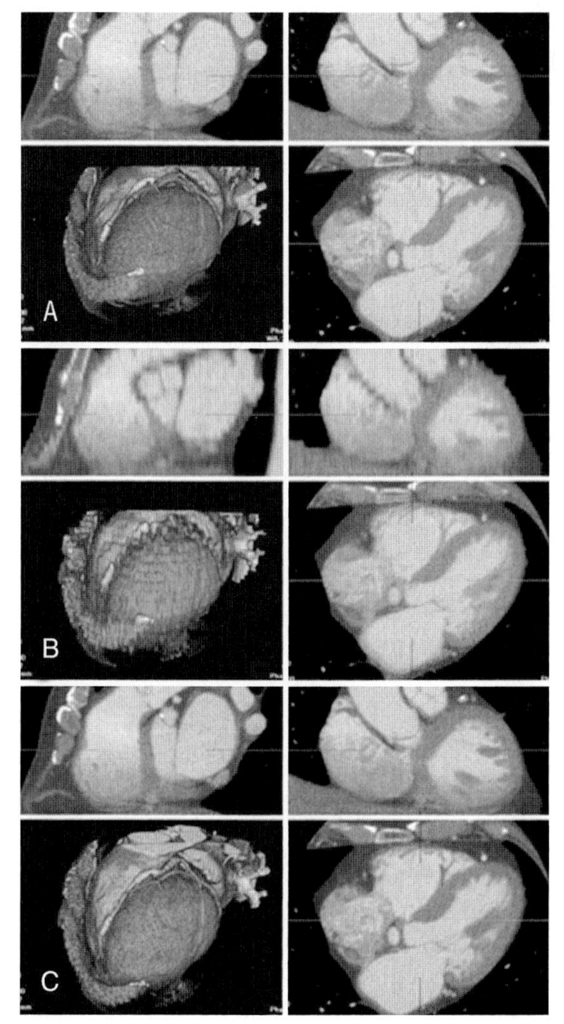

FIGURE C-8 Effect of reconstruction interval on image quality. All three sets of images are from the same data set reconstructed with 0.5-mm section thickness. However, the reconstruction intervals are different, which affects the number of reconstructed images and 3D image quality. **A,** A reconstruction interval of 0.3 mm yields 301 images and implies a 60% overlap. **B,** A reconstruction interval of 5 mm yields only 19 images and results in a staggered appearance of 3D images. **C,** A reconstruction interval of 0.5 mm yields 184 images and results in image quality similar to that of a. Normally, a 50% overlap is sufficient for optimum image quality for MPR and 3D images.

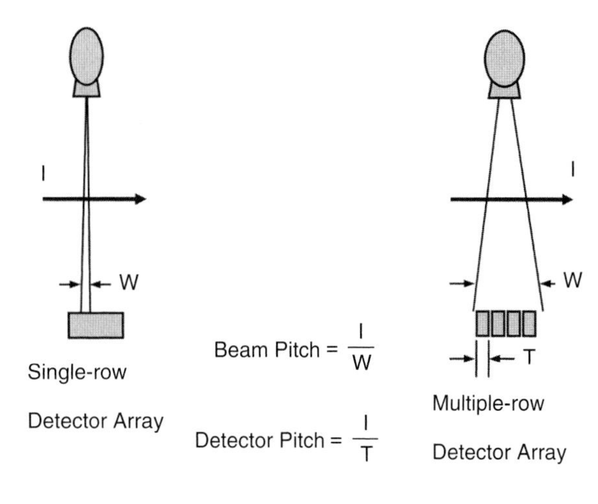

FIGURE C-9 Pitch is defined as the ratio of table feed per gantry rotation to the total x-ray beam width. This definition is applicable to both single-row detector CT and multiple-row detector CT (International Electrotechnical Commission, 2002). *I*, Table travel (mm) per rotation; *N*, number of active data acquisition channels; *T*, single data acquisition channel width (mm); *W*, beam width (mm).

required pitch factor ranges from 0.375 to 0.875. At higher pitch, there are substantial data gaps. As a result, most cardiac CT protocols require injecting β-blockers (Pannu et al, 2006a) to lower the subject's heartbeat within the desirable range of less than 70 beats per minute.

When the subject's heart rates are rapid and difficult to control, the diastolic ranges are smaller, so images are reconstructed by multiple-segment reconstruction to improve temporal resolution. With multiple-segment reconstruction, the number of segments used in the reconstruction further restricts the pitch factors.

$$P \leq \left(\frac{N + M - 1}{NM}\right)\frac{T_R}{T_{RR}}$$

where N = number of active data acquisition channels, M = number of segments or subsequent heart cycles sampled, T_R = gantry rotation time

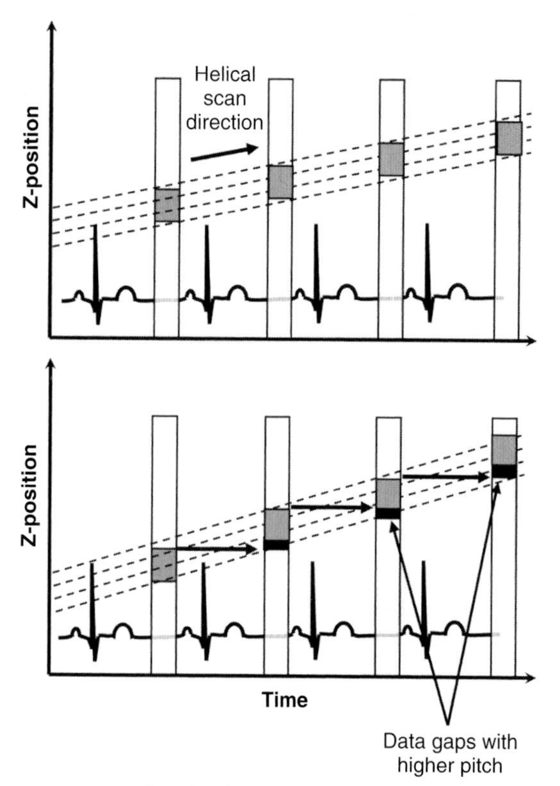

FIGURE C-10 Graphs demonstrate the necessity for scanning at low pitch values during helical cardiac CT data acquisition. If the table feed becomes greater than the beam width, it results in a data gap, which is detrimental for image reconstruction.

(milliseconds), and T_{RR} = time for a single heartbeat (milliseconds). For a heart rate of 60 beats per minute with a T_R of 400 ms, $N = 16$, and $M = 2$, the required pitch is ≈ 0.21; similarly, for $M = 3$, the required pitch is ≈ 0.15.

The pitch factor plays a significant role in improving both the temporal and spatial resolution but at the same time has a dramatic effect on the overall radiation dose delivered during a cardiac CT examination. Because radiation dose is inversely proportional to the pitch, the low pitch values characteristic of cardiac CT protocols substantially increase radiation dose to patients undergoing cardiac imaging with multiple-row detector CT.

In cardiac CT imaging, the need for high spatial and temporal resolution in turn requires the pitch values to be as low as 0.2 to 0.4. This results in a radiation beam overlap of nearly 80% to 60%, respectively, and an increase in radiation dose of up to a factor of five times compared with a pitch of 1. Hence, proper choice and optimization of pitch factor is critical in cardiac imaging. In fact, the demand for reducing radiation dose and faster scans is driving the technology to introduce either an even higher number of thin detectors in the z direction (256 rows) or flat-panel technology so that the entire cardiac area can be covered in a single gantry rotation without the necessity for tissue overlap (low pitch values).

Radiation Risk

One of the disadvantages of cardiac imaging with multiple-row detector CT is its use of ionizing radiation. The radiation dose delivered is highly dependent on the protocol used in cardiac CT (Gerber et al, 2005). Among the most widely known protocols such as calcium scoring studies, the effective dose is relatively small, 1-3 millisieverts (mSv) (Hunold et al, 2003). However, for retrospective gating, used for coronary vessel stenosis assessment and CT angiography, effective doses of 8 to 22 mSv and higher have been reported. By comparison, the radiation dose of an uncomplicated diagnostic coronary angiography study performed under fluoroscopic guidance ranges from 3 to 6 mSv (Hunold et al, 2003; Mahesh, 2006) and for typical body CT protocols ranges from 2 to 10 mSv (Morin et al, 2003) (Table C-1). Across the board, radiation doses are higher with multiple-row detector CT compared with the doses delivered with electron beam CT and fluoroscopically guided diagnostic coronary angiography and similar procedures (Hunold et al, 2003). One approach to reduce the high dose associated with retrospective gating, called ECG dose modulation (Jakobs et al, 2002), is directed at reducing the tube current during specific parts of the cardiac cycle, particularly during systole, where image quality is already degraded by

TABLE C-1 Typical Effective Doses for Various Cardiac Imaging and Routine Computed Tomography Procedures

Imaging Procedures	Modality	Effective Dose (mSv)*
Cardiac procedures		
Calcium scoring	Electron-beam CT	1.0-1.3
	Multiple-row detector CT	1.5-6.2†
Cardiac CT angiography	Electron-beam CT	1.5-2.0
	Multiple-row detector CT	6†-25
Cardiac SPECT with ^{99m}Tc or ^{201}Tl	Nuclear medicine	6.0-15.0
Coronary angiography (diagnostic)	Fluoroscopy	2.1†-6.0
Chest radiography	Radiography	0.1-0.2
Routine CT procedures		
Head CT	Multiple-row detector CT	1-2
Chest CT	Multiple-row detector CT	5-7
Abdominal and pelvic CT	Multiple-row detector CT	8-11

CT, Computed tomography; *SPECT*, single-photon emission CT; ^{99m}*Tc*, technetium 99m; ^{201}*T1*, thallium 201.
*10 mSv = 1 rem.
†Indicated data are from Hunold P et al: Radiation exposure during cardiac CT: effective doses at multi-detector row CT and electron-beam CT, *Radiology* 226:145-152, 2093.

motion artifacts and these portions of the cardiac cycle are not used in the image reconstruction. When dose modulation is implemented, a 10% to 40% dose reduction (Jakobs et al, 2002) can be achieved; however, the savings must be evaluated for each specific CT protocol. It is important that any steps taken to reduce radiation exposure should not jeopardize the image quality because poor image quality may result in repeat scans, which would result in additional radiation doses to patients.

Geometrical Efficiency

Dose efficiency (also called geometric efficiency) is of particular concern with the earlier four-channel multiple-row detector CT scanners, for which the x-ray photon beam has to be quite uniform as it strikes the detector array. This requirement means that the natural shadowing of the beam (penumbra) attributable to the finite-sized focal spot is intentionally positioned to strike the neighboring nonactive detector elements. Thus, some amount of radiation transmitted through the patient does not contribute to image generation. The width of the penumbra is fairly constant with each scanner, generally in the range of 1 to 3 mm.

The proportion of radiation wasted relative to the overall width of the x-ray beam varies with the protocol used. If very thin images are required and the overall x-ray beam width is small—5 mm, for example—then the proportion of wasted x rays could be 20% to 60% (resulting in a dose efficiency of 40%-80%). If thin images are not required and a wider x-ray beam can be used—20 mm, for example—then the proportion of wasted x-rays would be 5% to 15% (resulting in a dose efficiency of 85%-95%). Dose efficiency may be displayed on the scanner console. More recent multiple-row detector CT scanners have been engineered so that this problem is very much diminished.

Artifacts

In cardiac imaging, owing to the inherent nature of imaging a rapidly moving organ, there arise many unique artifacts (Choi et al, 2004; Nakanishi et al, 2005); among them, the most common artifacts are

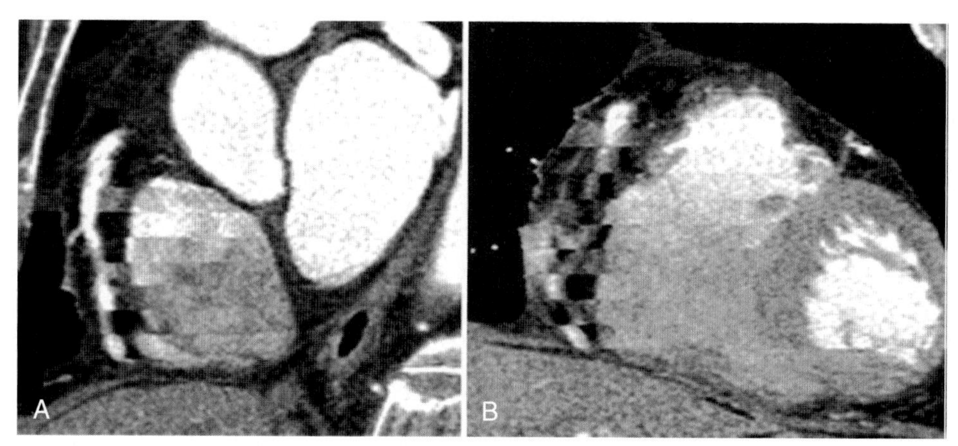

FIGURE C-11 Left anterior oblique **(A)** and anterior **(B)** MPR images show cardiac pulsation artifacts resulting from a rapid heartbeat. (Reprinted with permission from Nakanishi T et al:. Pitfalls in 16-detector row CT of the coronary arteries, *Radiographics* 25:425-440, 2005.)

due to cardiac pulsation (Nakanishi et al, 2005). Figure C-11 shows disconnect in the lateral reconstructed image as a result of pulsation. These types of artifacts are minimized by multiple-segment reconstruction or by scanning at even higher temporal resolution on the order of 50 milliseconds. The second types of artifacts are the banding artifacts resulting from increased heart rate during the scan. In the example shown in Figure C-12, the heart rate varied from 51 to 69 beats per minute during the scan and resulted in banding artifacts (Nakanishi et al, 2005). The other types of cardiac artifacts commonly observed are due to incomplete breath holding. These types of artifacts are not observed on axial images but are visible on coronal or sagittal views (Fig. C-13).

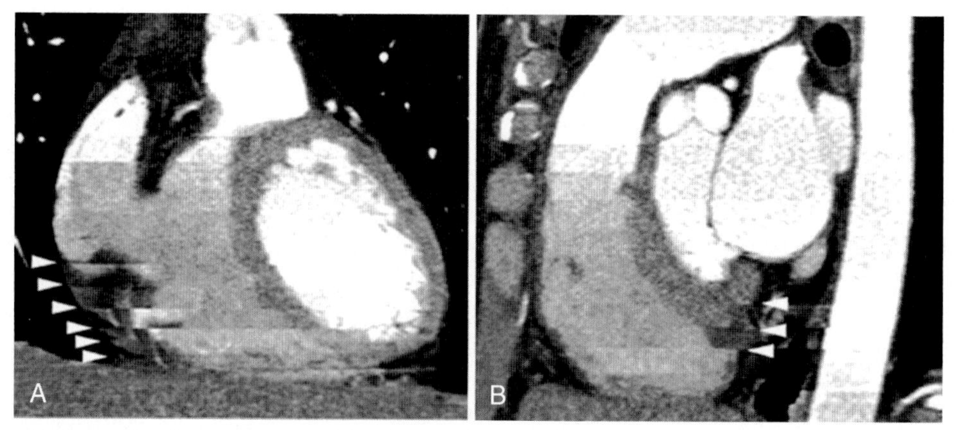

FIGURE C-12 Banding artifacts resulting from an increased heart rate from 51 to 69 beats per minute. Coronal **(A)** and sagittal **(B)** reformatted images of the heart obtained from CT data show banding artifacts *(arrowheads)*. (Reprinted with permission from Nakanishi T et al:. Pitfalls in 16-detector row CT of the coronary arteries, *Radiographics* 25:425-440, 2005.)

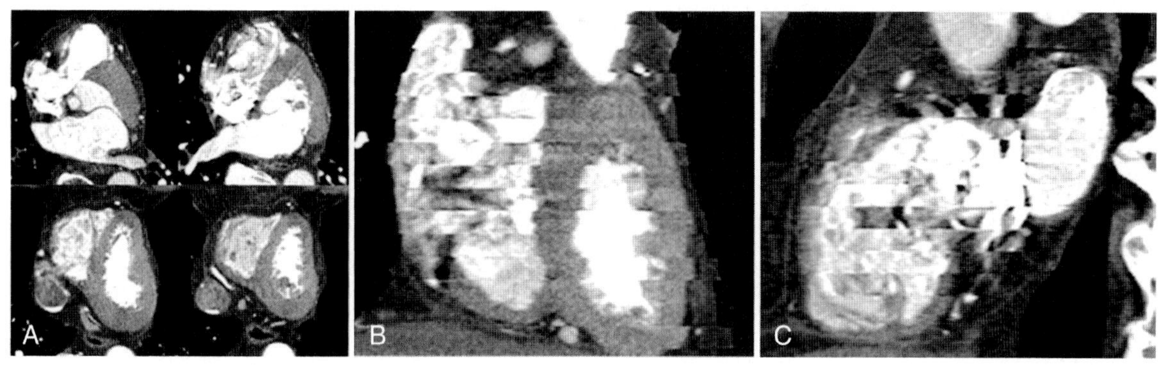

FIGURE C-13 Artifacts resulting from incomplete breath holding. **A,** Axial images show no motion artifacts. Coronal **(B)** and sagittal **(C)** reformatted images show banding artifacts. (Reprinted with permission from Nakanishi T et al: Pitfalls in 16-detector row CT of the coronary arteries, *Radiographics* 25:425-440, 2005.)

When subjects with previous stents or coils in the coronary artery undergo CT imaging, we observe streak artifacts around these highly attenuating objects. Often these artifacts can dominate the artery region and obscure other structures. As shown in Figure C-14, the metallic structures appear on axial images with no streak artifact but are very distinct and disturbing in coronal or sagittal planes (Nakanishi et al, 2005). These types of artifacts are to some extent handled by special artifact reduction software developed by manufacturers. The blooming artifacts are caused primarily by the combination of very highly attenuating objects and the inherent limiting resolution of the scanner.

FUTURE DIRECTIONS IN CARDIAC IMAGING

The demand for higher temporal and spatial resolution has already led to the development of a dual-source CT scanner (Flohr et al, 2006) and a 256-row detector CT scanner (Mori et al, 2005). In dual-source CT, there are two x-ray tubes positioned 90 degrees apart providing 64 axial sections for a complete gantry rotation, which yields further improvement in temporal resolution. As mentioned earlier, the minimum amount of data needed to reconstruct an image is 180 degrees plus the fan

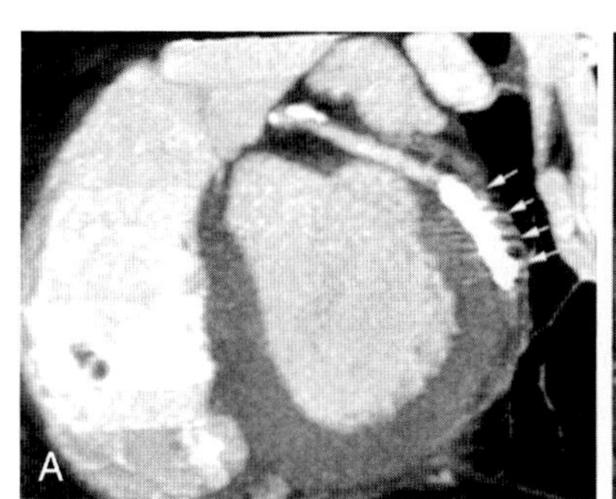

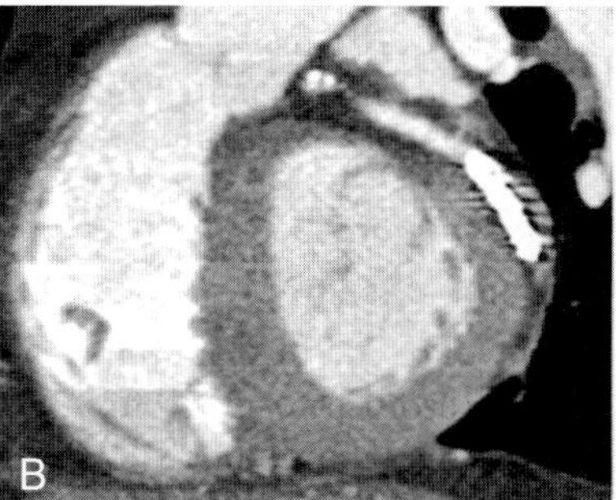

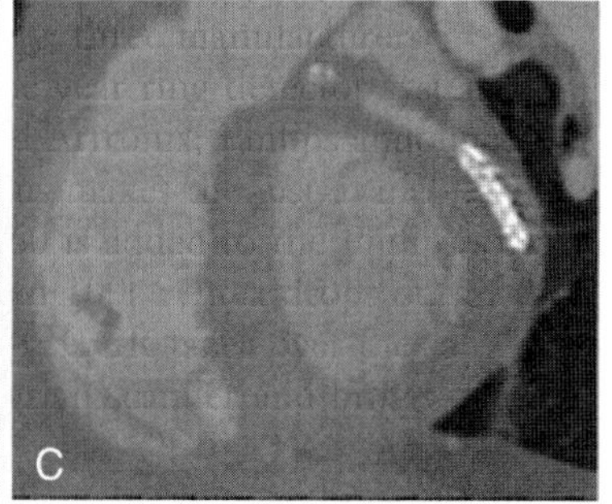

FIGURE C-14 Streak artifacts visible in the presence of a stent. Thin-slab maximum intensity projection image **(A),** MPR image **(B),** and thin-slab maximum intensity projection image obtained with a wide window **(C)** show streak artifacts *(arrows in a)*. (Reprinted with permission from Nakanishi T et al:. Pitfalls in 16-detector row CT of the coronary arteries, *Radiographics* 25:425-440, 2005.)

angle; therefore, with two tubes positioned at 90 degrees, it is sufficient to acquire data for one fourth of a gantry rotation and then coordinate the data from two sets of detectors to reconstruct the image. This can yield temporal resolution as low as one fourth the gantry rotation speed. With scanner gantry rotation speeds at below 330 ms, the temporal resolution can be as low as 80 ms. With this scanner, the pitch factor may be increased for higher heart rates with a potential to reduce radiation dose.

Similarly, the demand for higher spatial resolution has led to the development of a 256-row detector CT scanner, which can cover the entire heart in one gantry rotation (12.8-cm beam width at isocenter). In the 256-row detector CT scanner, the 256 detectors in the longitudinal direction can cover an area of 12.8 mm per gantry rotation and therefore can eliminate the need for overlapping pitch. In this type of scanner, it is possible to obtain complete data from one heart cycle, further diminishing the need for excessive tissue overlaps (low pitch values) and therefore reducing radiation dose and also reducing motion artifacts. Ideally, the combination of a 256-row detector assembly in the dual-source CT scanner would be phenomenal because that would not only give high temporal resolution but also high spatial resolution with minimal motion artifacts.

CONCLUSIONS

Cardiac imaging is a highly demanding application of multiple-row detector CT and is possible only because of recent technological advances. Understanding the tradeoffs between various scan parameters that affect image quality is key in optimizing protocols that can reduce patient dose. Benefits from an optimized cardiac CT protocol can minimize the radiation risks associated with these cardiac scans. Cardiac CT has the potential to become a reliable tool for noninvasive diagnosis and prevention of cardiac and coronary artery disease.

REFERENCES

American Heart Association: *International cardiovascular disease statistics*, Dallas, Tex, 2003, American Heart Association.

Budoff MJ et al: Clinical utility of computed tomography and magnetic resonance techniques for noninvasive coronary angiography, *J Am Coll Cardiol* 42:1867-1878, 2003.

Choi HS et al: Pitfalls, artifacts, and remedies in multidetector row CT coronary angiography, *Radiographics* 24:787-800, 2004.

Desjardins B, Kazerooni EA: ECG-gated cardiac CT, *AJR Am J Roentgenol* 182:993-1010, 2004.

Detrano RC: Coronary artery scanning using electron beam computed tomography, *Am J Card Imaging* 10:97-100, 1996.

Dewey M et al: Coronary artery disease: new insights and their implications for radiology, *Eur Radiol* 14:1048-1054, 2004.

Flohr TG et al: Multi-detector row CT systems and image-reconstruction techniques, *Radiology* 235:756-773, 2005.

Flohr TG et al: First performance evaluation of a dual-source CT (DSCT) system, *Eur Radiol* 16:256-268, 2006.

Gerber B et al: Physical principles of cardiovascular imaging, In St John Sutton M, Rutherford J, editors: *Clinical cardiovascular imaging: a companion to Braunwald's heart disease*, Philadelphia, 2004, Elsevier-Saunders.

Gerber TC et al: Techniques and parameters for estimating radiation exposure and dose in cardiac computed tomography, *Int J Cardiovasc Imaging* 21:165-176, 2005.

Hoffmann MH et al: Noninvasive coronary imaging with MDCT in comparison to invasive conventional coronary angiography: a fast-developing technology, *AJR Am J Roentgenol* 182:601-608, 2004.

Hunold P et al: Radiation exposure during cardiac CT: effective doses at multi-detector row CT and electron-beam CT, *Radiology* 226:145-152, 2003.

International Electrotechnical Commission: *Medical electrical equipment, part 2-44: particular requirements for the safety of x-ray equipment for computed tomography*, IEC Publication No. 60601-2-44, Geneva, Switzerland, 2002, International Electrotechnical Commission.

Jakobs TF et al: Multi-slice helical CT of the heart with retrospective ECG gating: reduction of radiation exposure by ECG-controlled tube current modulation, *Eur Radiol* 12:1081-1086, 2002.

Klingenbeck-Regn K et al: Subsecond multi-slice computed tomography: basics and applications, *Eur J Radiol* 31:110-124, 1999.

Klingenbeck-Regn K et al: Strategies for cardiac CT imaging, *Int J Cardiovasc Imaging* 18:143-151, 2002.

Mahesh M: Search for isotropic resolution in CT from conventional through multiple-row detector, *Radiographics* 22:949-962, 2002.

Mahesh M: Cardiac imaging: technical advances in MDCT compared with conventional x-ray angiography. In Boulton E, editor: *US cardiology 2006: the authoritative review of the clinical and scientific issues relating to cardiology with perspectives on the future*, pp 115-117, London, UK, 2006, Touch Briefings, (http://www.touchcardiology.com).

Mahesh M et al: Dose and pitch relationship for a particular multi-slice CT scanner, *AJR Am J Roentgenol* 177:1273-1275, 2001.

Mahnken AH et al: Multislice spiral computed tomography of the heart: technique, current applications, and perspective, *Cardiovasc Intervent Radiol* 28: 388-399, 2005.

McCollough CH, Morin RL: The technical design and performance of ultrafast computed tomography, *Radiol Clin North Am* 32:521-536, 1994.

Mori S et al: Clinical potentials of the prototype 256-detector row CT-scanner, *Acad Radiol* 12:148-154, 2005.

Morin RL et al: Radiation dose in computed tomography of the heart, *Circulation* 107:917-922, 2003.

Nakanishi T et al: Pitfalls in 16-detector row CT of the coronary arteries, *Radiographics* 25:425-440, 2005.

Nikolaou K et al: Advances in cardiac CT imaging: 64-slice scanner, *Int J Cardiovasc Imaging* 20:535-540, 2004.

Ohnesorge B et al: *Multi-slice CT in cardiac imaging*, Heidelberg, Germany, 2002, Springer.

Pannu HK et al: Current concepts in multi-detector row CT evaluation of the coronary arteries: principles, techniques, and anatomy, *Radiographics* 23:S111-S125, 2003.

Pannu HK et al: Beta-blockers for cardiac CT: a primer for the radiologist, *AJR Am J Roentgenol* 186 (6 Suppl 2):S341-S345, 2006a.

Pannu HK et al: Coronary CT angiography with 64-MDCT: assessment of vessel visibility, *AJR Am J Roentgenol* 187:119-126, 2006b.

Schoenhagen P et al: Noninvasive imaging of coronary arteries: current and future role of multi-detector row CT, *Radiology* 232:7-17, 2004.

Ulzheimer S, Kalender WA: Assessment of calcium scoring performance in cardiac computed tomography, *Eur Radiol* 13:484-497, 2003.

A

Page numbers followed by f indicate figures; t, tables, b, boxes.

D

E

N

S

T

Z